Beckmann and Ling's
Obstetrics and Gynecology
EIGHTH EDITION

Beckmann and Ling's Obstetrics and Gynecology

EIGHTH EDITION

American College of Obstetricians and Gynecologists

with

LEAD AUTHORS

Robert Casanova, MD, MHPE, FACOG
Adjunct Professor, Department of Medical Education, Assistant Dean for Clinical Sciences Curriculum, Assistant Vice Dean Medical Education Covenant Branch Campus, Texas Tech University Health Sciences Center, Lubbock, Texas

Alice Chuang, MD, MEd, FACOG
Professor, Department of Obstetrics and Gynecology, Clerkship Director, University of North Carolina School of Medicine, Chapel Hill, North Carolina

Alice R. Goepfert, MD, FACOG
Professor, Department of Obstetrics and Gynecology, Associate Dean for Graduate Medical Education and Designated Institutional Official, University of Alabama School of Medicine, University of Alabama at Birmingham, Birmingham, Alabama

Nancy A. Hueppchen, MD, MSc, FACOG
Associate Professor, Department of Gynecology and Obstetrics, Associate Dean for Undergraduate Medical Education, Johns Hopkins University School of Medicine, Baltimore, Maryland

Patrice M. Weiss, MD, FACOG
Professor, Department of Obstetrics and Gynecology, Virginia Tech Carilion School of Medicine, Executive Vice President and Chief Medical Officer, Carilion Clinic, Roanoke, Virginia

ORIGINAL AUTHORS

Charles R. B. Beckmann, MD, MHPE, FACOG
Former Professor of Obstetrics and Gynecology, Thomas Jefferson University College of Medicine, Former Director, Offices of Ambulatory Care and of OB-GYN Academic Affairs, Department of Obstetrics and Gynecology, Albert Einstein Medical Center, Philadelphia, Pennsylvania

Frank W. Ling, MD, FACOG
Clinical Professor, Department of Obstetrics and Gynecology, Vanderbilt University School of Medicine and Meharry Medical College, Nashville, Tennessee; Partner, Women's Health Specialists, PLLC, Germantown, Tennessee

William N.P. Herbert, MD, FACOG
Former William Norman Thornton Professor and Chair, Professor Emeritus, Department of Obstetrics and Gynecology, University of Virginia, Charlottesville, Virginia

Douglas W. Laube, MD, MEd, FACOG
Professor and former Chair, Department of Obstetrics and Gynecology, University of Wisconsin School of Medicine and Public Health, Madison, Wisconsin; Past President (2006–2007), American College of Obstetricians and Gynecologists

Roger P. Smith, MD, FACOG
The Robert A. Munsick Professor of Clinical Obstetrics and Gynecology, Director, Medical Student Education, Director, Division of General Obstetrics and Gynecology, Department of Obstetrics and Gynecology, Indiana University School of Medicine, Indianapolis, Indiana

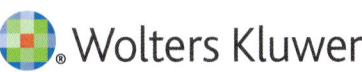

Philadelphia • Baltimore • New York • London
Buenos Aires • Hong Kong • Sydney • Tokyo

Not authorised for sale in United States, Canada, Australia, New Zealand, Puerto Rico, and U.S. Virgin Islands.

Acquisitions Editor: Matt Hauber
Development Editor: Laura Horowitz/Andrea Vosburgh
Editorial Coordinator: Laura Horowitz/Annette Ferran
Editorial Assistant: Brooks Phelps
Marketing Manager: Mike McMahon
Production Project Manager: Bridgett Dougherty
Design Coordinator: Steve Druding
Manufacturing Coordinator: Margie Orzech
Prepress Vendor: Newgen Knowledge Works Pvt. Ltd., Chennai, India

8th edition
Copyright © 2019 Wolters Kluwer.

Copyright © 2014, 2010, 2006, 2002, 1998, 1995, 1992 by Lippincott Williams & Wilkins, a Wolters Kluwer business.

All rights reserved. This book is protected by copyright. No part of this book may be reproduced or transmitted in any form or by any means, including as photocopies or scanned-in or other electronic copies, or utilized by any information storage and retrieval system without written permission from the copyright owner, except for brief quotations embodied in critical articles and reviews. Materials appearing in this book prepared by individuals as part of their official duties as U.S. government employees are not covered by the above-mentioned copyright. To request permission, please contact Wolters Kluwer at Two Commerce Square, 2001 Market Street, Philadelphia, PA 19103, via email at permissions@lww.com, or via our website at lww.com (products and services).

9 8 7 6 5 4 3 2 1

Printed in China

9781496353092
Library of Congress Cataloging-in-Publication Data
available upon request

This work is provided "as is," and the publisher disclaims any and all warranties, express or implied, including any warranties as to accuracy, comprehensiveness, or currency of the content of this work.

This work is no substitute for individual patient assessment based upon healthcare professionals' examination of each patient and consideration of, among other things, age, weight, gender, current or prior medical conditions, medication history, laboratory data and other factors unique to the patient. The publisher does not provide medical advice or guidance and this work is merely a reference tool. Healthcare professionals, and not the publisher, are solely responsible for the use of this work including all medical judgments and for any resulting diagnosis and treatments.

Given continuous, rapid advances in medical science and health information, independent professional verification of medical diagnoses, indications, appropriate pharmaceutical selections and dosages, and treatment options should be made and healthcare professionals should consult a variety of sources. When prescribing medication, healthcare professionals are advised to consult the product information sheet (the manufacturer's package insert) accompanying each drug to verify, among other things, conditions of use, warnings and side effects and identify any changes in dosage schedule or contraindications, particularly if the medication to be administered is new, infrequently used or has a narrow therapeutic range. To the maximum extent permitted under applicable law, no responsibility is assumed by the publisher for any injury and/or damage to persons or property, as a matter of products liability, negligence law or otherwise, or from any reference to or use by any person of this work.

LWW.com

The new lead authors would like to dedicate the eighth edition to the original authors who paved the way with the first six editions and invited us to collaborate on the seventh. We hope to continue the long tradition with this edition. In addition, we would like to dedicate this edition to the medical students who have inspired us and to the women who, as patients, have entrusted us with their care. Finally, we want to thank our families who supported us through the edits and rewrites.

About the Authors

Drs. Beckmann and Ling embarked on the project that would become this textbook as a response to the conventional wisdom of the day that medical students should "know all of Williams." They decided that this was unreasonable and opted to write a "core" textbook based on the APGO Learning Objectives instead. The rules were simple: fully address the objectives but only with essential information, not all that the author knows (i.e., the task was to decide what NOT to include, a much more difficult task than writing all you know). They also noted a lot of "here at ... we do…" kind of text, also useless, and agreed not to do that. In addition, they noted that many of the figures and some tables really added nothing, hence the rule that a figure or table must be able to "stand alone" and teach. If it could not pass that test, it was not worthy of the book.

The first two editions were well received, but it was only when they added information they knew students were being asked on rounds (despite the first two rules) that the book gained its present popularity.

Thus, from the earliest planning meetings for the first edition of *Obstetrics and Gynecology*, the authors have remained focused on the needs of the primary audience, medical students rotating through their clerkship in this specialty. Having medical education as a primary focus of their respective academic careers has made this team of authors uniquely positioned to create an effective learning tool. In this eighth edition, the "second generation" of leading ob/gyn clinician–educators took over as lead authors for each chapter. They, too, have dedicated their careers to enhancing the quality of women's health through medical education. As evidence of their collective involvement and success in ob/gyn education, the author team features the following current and past achievements:

University Educational and Administrative Appointments

Department Chair	4
Department Vice-Chairs	5
Fellowship Directors	1
Residency Directors	8
Student Clerkship Directors	11
Assistant/Associate Deans	7
Department Director of Undergraduate Medical Education	2
President Academy of Educators	1
Designated Institution Official	1
Chief Medical Officer	1

National Organizations
American College of Obstetricians and Gynecologists (College)

President	1
Committee Chair	3
District Chair	1
SASGOG Board	1

Association of Professors of Gynecology and Obstetrics (APGO)

President	3
Council Member	7
Undergraduate Medical Education Committee Chair	2
Undergraduate Medical Education Committee Member	7
Academic Scholars and Leaders, Scholar	4
Academic Scholars and Leaders, Faculty	2
Academic Scholars and Leaders, Advisors	6

American Board of Obstetrics and Gynecology (ABOG)

President	1
Vice President	1
Board Examiner	8
Chairman of the Board	1

Council on Resident Education in Obstetrics and Gynecology (CREOG)

Chairman	1
Vice Chair	1
Education Committee Chair	3
Council Member	4
Program Chair	3
InTraining Exam	2

Other National Educational Activities and Honor

National Test Committee Member	5
National Test Committee Reviewer	4
Peer-Reviewed Educational Research Publications	214
Medical Student Teaching Award	57
Resident Teaching Award	12
Resident Review Committee Member	5
District IV Mentor Award	2

The authors remain committed to not only including the most up-to-date evidence-based information but also presenting it in a fashion that meets the needs of the ever-evolving adult learner. This eighth edition of *Beckmann and Ling's Obstetrics and Gynecology* is the latest step in our collective journey in the field of women's health education.

Foreword

Welcome to one of the most innovative and useful textbooks in obstetrics and gynecology. The chapters in this book are organized around the Association of Professors of Gynecology and Obstetrics (APGO) Medical Student Education Objectives, tenth edition. In fact, each chapter of *Beckmann and Ling's Obstetrics and Gynecology*, eighth edition, begins with the relevant APGO Educational Topics, learning objectives, and a clinical case to set context. The body of the text will give you the information needed to achieve the learning objectives. The APGO educational objectives were created by the APGO Undergraduate Medical Education Committee. This committee consists of renowned medical educators, clerkship directors, and program directors from across the United States and Canada. The objectives are revised on a regular basis to assure currency and relevance in developing a curriculum for the obstetrics and gynecology clerkship. Students on their first, or even elective, obstetrics and gynecology clerkship experience will find that these objectives guide learning and mastery of the concepts needed to succeed in their ob-gyn clerkship. Through this organization, the text is easy to read, yet is very complete in giving all the information necessary to master the learning objectives.

APGO is an organization dedicated to providing optimal resources and support to educators who inspire, instruct, develop, and empower the women's healthcare providers of tomorrow. APGO has proudly provided 55 years of service to students and faculty. APGO's resources are designed to assist faculty and students in meeting their educational goals. Through its Web site, www.apgo.org, medical students will find a host of useful modules and resources to aid in their learning of obstetrics and gynecology. The APGO Undergraduate Web-Based Interactive Self-Evaluation (uWISE) is an interactive self-exam designed to help medical students acquire the necessary basic knowledge in obstetrics and gynecology, regardless of future medical specialty choice. This self-learning resource is a widely used tool in gaining an understanding of the fundamental concepts in obstetrics and gynecology. The APGO Web site has many other useful tools for students and educators to use in their development. Most medical school programs are members and can provide students and faculty members with free access to the rich and robust resources on this Web site.

We at APGO wish you an enjoyable and successful journey through your learning experience in obstetrics and gynecology.

Maya M. Hammoud, M.D., M.B.A.
Association of Professors of Gynecology and Obstetrics President-Elect
Donna Wachter
Association of Professors of Gynecology and Obstetrics Executive Director

Preface

The primary goal of this book, which has evolved since its inception more than 20 years ago, is to provide foundational knowledge about obstetrics and gynecology that all medical students need to successfully complete an obstetrics and gynecology clerkship, to pass national standardized examinations in this content area and to competently care for women in their future practice regardless of specialty. The field of medicine continues to change, and we have strived to ensure our text has as well. We hope that practitioners of all backgrounds and training who care for women will find this book helpful in their practice and their educational endeavors. This edition promises to fulfill these goals better than ever before.

In publication since 1992, *Obstetrics and Gynecology* features chapters extensively revised and reviewed in a team-style fashion among the authors, rather than written by individual authors. This collaborative effort serves the dual purpose of cross-checking content accuracy as well as preserving continuity throughout the text while maintaining the focus on the needs of the reader.

In addition, *Obstetrics and Gynecology* is proud to continue its fruitful collaboration with the American College of Obstetricians and Gynecologists (College)—the leading group of professionals providing health care to women. With over 52,000 members, the College maintains the highest clinical standards for women's health care by publishing practice guidelines, technology assessments, and opinions emanating from its various committees on a variety of clinical, ethical, and technologic issues. These guidelines and opinions were rigorously applied as evidence-based resources in the writing of each chapter.

This eighth edition has incorporated many suggestions offered by users of past editions to make it even more user-friendly. Key features of this edition include the following:

- The book has been restructured and helpfully divided into six units: I. General Obstetrics and Gynecology, II. Obstetrics, III. Medical and Surgical Problems in Pregnancy, IV. Gynecology, V. Reproductive Endocrinology and Infertility, and VI. Gynecologic Oncology and Uterine Leiomyoma.
- Also designed to enhance organization and readability, additional subheadings demarcate topics and break up long passages. An ancillary benefit is that anyone seeking to merely review a chapter can more quickly scan through headings to locate relevant spots.
- Chapter opening and closing cases frame the chapter material in a clinical context to aid learning and recall.
- The interior is color-coded by section to facilitate navigation. The design is understated and elegant to provide an appropriate background for the text.
- The Common Medical Problems in Pregnancy chapter has been separated into several smaller chapters specific to each topic for increased depth as well as easier assimilation.
- The Ethics chapter includes a paramount consideration in women's health care—Patient Safety.
- The Gynecologic Procedures chapter has been updated to reflect the latest techniques, including minimally invasive as well as robotic surgery.
- Several new ultrasounds of common disorders and anomalies such as bicornuate uterus and Müllerian anomaly have been added to the art program.

Continuing the innovations unveiled in the sixth edition, other popular features that will assist the medical student in reading, studying, and retaining key information include the following:

- Correlation of chapters with the tenth edition of *Medical Student Educational Objectives* published by the Association of Professors of Gynecology and Obstetrics (APGO). The Educational Topic Area numbers and titles employed in this text are used with permission of APGO. The use of these objectives has been invaluable to educators and students alike. The complete version of the APGO *Medical Student Educational Objectives* is available through their Web site at www.apgo.org.
- The artwork in the book has been rendered in full color and in an anatomical style familiar to today's medical students. Great care has been taken to construct illustrations that teach crucial concepts. Photos have been chosen to illustrate key clinical features, such as those associated with sexually transmitted diseases. Other photos provide examples of the newest imaging techniques used in obstetrics and gynecology.
- Integration of the latest information and guidelines regarding several key topics.
- Appendices include the latest versions of the Well-Woman Care: Assessments and Recommendations by Age Group, the American College of Obstetricians and Gynecologists Antepartum Record and Postpartum Form and the Edinburgh Postpartum Depression Scale.
- An extensive package of study questions is available in an online format at the Lippincott Williams & Wilkins student Web site.
- Chapters are concise, yet eminently readable, and focused on key clinical aspects.
- Shaded, italicized text provides critical clinical "pearls" focusing on specific issues encountered in gynecologic and obstetric practice.
- An abundance of lists, boxes, and tables provides rapid access to crucial points.

- We are justifiably enthusiastic about the significant changes that have been made to this edition, and we believe that they will be of tremendous benefit to medical students and other readers who need core information for the primary and obstetric–gynecologic care of women. As a new generation enters the health care professions and the dynamics of providing health care continue to change, women's health care remains central to the promotion of our society's health and well-being. This eighth edition of *Beckmann and Ling's Obstetrics and Gynecology* intends to be at the forefront of medical education for this new generation of health care providers and will continue its authors' commitment to providing the most reliable evidence-based medical information to students and practitioners.

Acknowledgments

We extend our appreciation to Matt Hauber at Wolters Kluwer for his seemingly tireless help and encouragement during the arduous preparation of the eighth edition of *Obstetrics and Gynecology*. We continue to be grateful for the innovative art provided by Rob Duckwall and Dragonfly Media Group for this edition and Joyce Lavery for previous editions and for the thoughtful indexing of Barbara Hodgson, which adds to the usefulness of the book for new learners. A special "shout out" goes to our development editor Laura Horowitz, whose wisdom and insight into the educational process as well as the needs of the reader can be seen throughout the final product. We would especially like to thank the original authors, RB, Frank, Bill, Doug, and Roger for the opportunity to collaborate with them on this time-honored text.

Contents

SECTION I GENERAL OBSTETRICS AND GYNECOLOGY

1. Women's Health Examination and Women's Health Care Management   1
2. The Obstetrician–Gynecologist's Role in Screening and Preventive Care   14
3. Ethics, Liability, and Patient Safety in Obstetrics and Gynecology   22
4. Embryology and Anatomy   29

SECTION II OBSTETRICS

5. Maternal–Fetal Physiology   43
6. Preconception and Antepartum Care   56
7. Genetics and Genetic Disorders in Obstetrics and Gynecology   72
8. Intrapartum Care   86
9. Abnormal Labor and Intrapartum Fetal Surveillance   98
10. Immediate Care of the Newborn   112
11. Postpartum Care   120
12. Postpartum Hemorrhage   127
13. Multifetal Gestation   134
14. Fetal Growth Abnormalities: Intrauterine Growth Restriction and Macrosomia   140
15. Preterm Labor   147
16. Third-Trimester Bleeding   152
17. Premature Rupture of Membranes   158
18. Post-term Pregnancy   163
19. Ectopic Pregnancy and Abortion   167

SECTION III MEDICAL AND SURGICAL DISORDERS IN PREGNANCY

20. Endocrine Disorders   177
21. Gastrointestinal, Renal, and Surgical Complications   184
22. Cardiovascular and Respiratory Disorders   191
23. Hematologic and Immunologic Complications   201
24. Infectious Diseases   209
25. Neurologic and Psychiatric Disorders   219

SECTION IV GYNECOLOGY

26. Contraception   225
27. Sterilization   239
28. Vulvovaginitis   245
29. Sexually Transmitted Infections   250
30. Pelvic Support Defects, Urinary Incontinence, and Urinary Tract Infection   262
31. Endometriosis   271
32. Dysmenorrhea and Chronic Pelvic Pain   279
33. Disorders of the Breast   285
34. Gynecologic Procedures   295
35. Human Sexuality   304
36. Sexual Assault and Domestic Violence   312

SECTION V REPRODUCTIVE ENDOCRINOLOGY AND INFERTILITY

37 Reproductive Cycles   321
38 Puberty   327
39 Amenorrhea and Abnormal Uterine Bleeding   332
40 Hirsutism and Virilization   337
41 Menopause   345
42 Infertility   353
43 Premenstrual Syndrome and Premenstrual Dysphoric Disorder   363

SECTION VI GYNECOLOGIC ONCOLOGY AND UTERINE LEIOMYOMA

44 Cell Biology and Principles of Cancer Therapy   369
45 Gestational Trophoblastic Neoplasia   374
46 Vulvar and Vaginal Disease and Neoplasia   379
47 Cervical Neoplasia and Carcinoma   389
48 Uterine Leiomyoma and Neoplasia   402
49 Cancer of the Uterine Corpus   406
50 Ovarian and Adnexal Disease   415

Appendices

A The American College of Obstetricians and Gynecologists Well-Woman Recommendations by Age Group   427
B The American College of Obstetricians and Gynecologists Antepartum Record and Postpartum Form   433
C Edinburgh Postnatal Depression Scale (EPDS)   449

Index   451

General Obstetrics and Gynecology

CHAPTER 1
Women's Health Examination and Women's Health Care Management

This chapter deals primarily with APGO Educational Topic Areas:

TOPIC 1 HISTORY
TOPIC 2 EXAMINATION
TOPIC 3 PAP TEST AND DNA PROBES/CULTURES
TOPIC 4 DIAGNOSIS AND MANAGEMENT PLAN
TOPIC 5 PERSONAL INTERACTION AND COMMUNICATION SKILLS

Students should be able to refine their communication and clinical care skills in taking a pertinent comprehensive medical history and assessing risk and patient adherence to health care recommendations. They should be able to perform a comprehensive breast and pelvic exam, including a Pap test and appropriate screening. They should be able to use this information to formulate a diagnosis and management plan while communicating important findings and recommendations to the patient, incorporating her socioeconomic and cultural context, as well as her gender identity (heterosexual, lesbian, gay, bisexual, or transgender).

CLINICAL CASE

On a pleasant, rather warm summer's day, a 72-year-old woman comes to your office with her daughter for her "annual examination." She is pleasant, happy, and alert, dressed in a brightly colored dress matched with a heavy sweater. Your notes indicate that she uses your office for her general as well as gynecologic health care and that it has been over 7 years since her last visit. Review of her records shows a pattern of general good health with two successful term pregnancies and a postpartum tubal ligation during her twenties followed at age 38 years by a diagnostic laparoscopy for pelvic pain and heavy menstrual bleeding that revealed multiple uterine fibroids and very mild endometriosis. She subsequently had a total abdominal hysterectomy without oophorectomy, and her mild endometriosis was successfully treated with nonsteroidal anti-inflammatory medications until an unremarkable menopause at age 49 years. All previous Paps, and laboratory and imaging studies were normal. She is 5 ft. 4 in. tall and weighs 142 lb. Her blood pressure is 112/65 mm Hg with normal pulse, temperature, and respirations. Her interval history and review of systems is unremarkable with the exception of often feeling cold and complaining that her skin has of late felt dryer than previously. Her physical examination is unremarkable. She asks for her sweater while waiting for her examination, complaining that she is cold and tells you she is worried about being overweight since she has gained a few pounds over the past few years. Her daughter remarks that her mother complains constantly that the temperature of her room is set too low.

INTRODUCTION

Obstetrics was originally a separate branch of medicine, and **gynecology** was a division of surgery. Over time, an increasing knowledge of the pathophysiology of the female reproductive tract led to a natural integration of these two areas, and obstetrics and gynecology merged into a single specialty. After completing an approved residency, the obstetrics and gynecology specialist may practice *general obstetrics* (care of the woman during pregnancy, labor, and the postpartum period) and *gynecology* (traditionally care of the female reproductive organs and breasts, but now encompassing comprehensive women's health care from before puberty to beyond the menopause). They may also choose subspecialty practice by completing fellowships in any of the four subspecialty areas recognized by the American Board of Obstetrics and Gynecology (ABOG). *Maternal–fetal medicine* deals with high-risk pregnancies and prenatal diagnosis. *Gynecologic oncology* focuses on the treatment of malignancy of the reproductive tract and associated organ systems. *Reproductive endocrinology–infertility* addresses problems in conception and gynecologic endocrine disease. *Female pelvic medicine and reconstructive surgery* (often referred to as *urogynecology*) deals with advanced pelvic surgery and urologic problems involving the female urogenital system. Fellowships not recognized by the ABOG include *minimally invasive surgery*, *family planning*, and *adolescent gynecology*.

Currently, many obstetrician–gynecologists also provide routine general medical care for women throughout their lives. Thus, obstetrician–gynecologists must have additional knowledge and skills in the primary and preventive health care needs of women and must be able to identify situations where they may provide care and those in which referral to other specialists is appropriate. The demographics of women in the United States are undergoing profound change. A woman born today will live 81 or more years, experiencing menopause at the age of 51 to 52 years. Unlike previous generations, women will spend more than one third of their lives in menopause. The absolute number and the proportion of all women over age 65 years are projected to increase steadily through 2040 (Fig. 1.1). These women will expect to remain healthy (physically, sexually, and mentally) throughout their lives including their "menopause years." Physicians must keep the needs of this changing population in mind in their practice of medicine, especially in the provision of primary and preventive gynecologic care.

The care of women in their menopausal years will become an increasingly large part of the practice of gynecology in the 21st century.

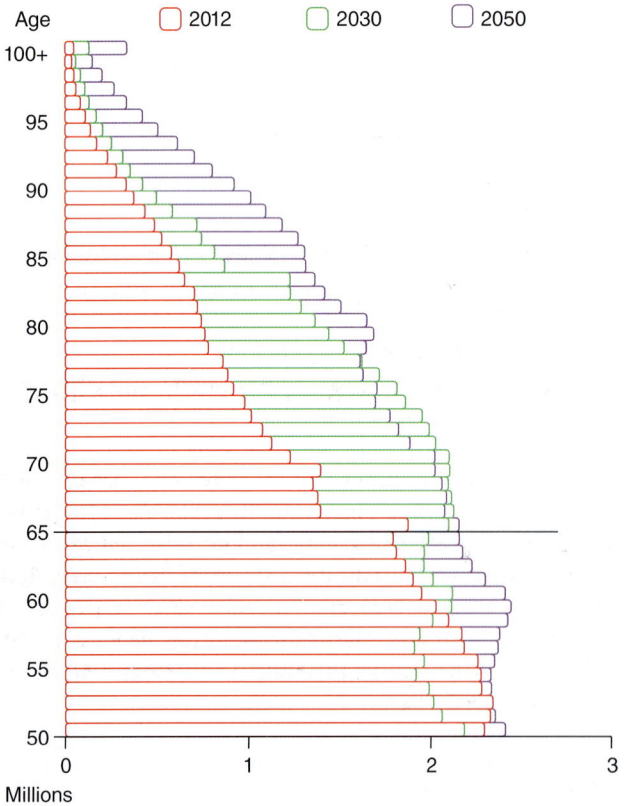

FIGURE 1.1. The U.S. population demographics. (Adapted from the U.S. Census Bureau.)

Obstetrician–gynecologists must be able to establish an empathic, trusting professional relationship with patients and be able to perform a general and women's health history and physical examination, using this information to formulate a comprehensive management plan. Finally, obstetrician–gynecologists must fully understand the concepts of evidence-based medicine and incorporate them into their scholarship and practice in the context of a well-established pattern of lifelong learning and self-evaluation.

This chapter directly addresses the initial or "new patient visit" for gynecology and primary/preventive care as well as a first visit for obstetric care (a "new OB" visit). Subsequent return visits are generally shorter and more focused. Obtaining complete information is an essential basis of good health care. Age-appropriate health care screening and preventive and primary health care are discussed in Chapter 2. An up-to-date comprehensive medical record should include information from history taking, physical examination, and laboratory and radiology testing. Information from referrals and other medical services outside the purview of the obstetrician–gynecologist should be integrated into the medical record.

● ESTABLISHING AN EFFECTIVE PATIENT–PHYSICIAN PARTNERSHIP

The patient encounter begins with an appropriate greeting that deserves special attention because of the importance of initial impressions at the start of the patient–physician partnership. After verifying the patient's identity, the patient should be asked how she prefers to be addressed—by first name, surname, or nickname. Transgender patients should be asked what pronouns they prefer. For example: "Good morning, I am Dr. Jones. Are you Janet Moore? How would you like to be addressed? … What brings you in today?" A handshake is commonly used.

A friendly but neutral greeting allows the patient to frame her response in a comfortable environment, be it a problem, a concern, or another issue.

High-quality health care outcomes are facilitated by the use of a patient–physician partnership. Communication in which the physician demonstrates empathy and sympathy is characteristic of such a partnership. Using *empathic communication skills*, a physician strives to "project" himself or herself into the patient's life and imagine the situation from the patient's point of view. Thus, empathy goes beyond sympathy wherein the physician knows the patient's emotions from his or her side of the partnership but does not view or feel them from the unique perspective of the patient. Empathic communication promotes the physician's fullest understanding of the patient's situation, which improves trust, the quality of information (and, thus, diagnostic accuracy), patient compliance with the decisions the patient and physician make, and the satisfaction of both the patient and physician. Seemingly counterintuitively, the use of empathic communication throughout the patient encounter actually shortens the time of the visit because when a patient's emotional concerns are not acknowledged by the

TABLE 1.1 STEPS OF A PATIENT-CENTERED PARTNERSHIP WOMEN'S HEALTH CARE VISIT

Steps[a]	Description	Useful Empathic Communications and Visit Supporting Actions
1	Opening the visit (patient focused)	Welcome patient and introduce yourself. Ask patients how they wish to be addressed. Ensure patient's readiness and privacy. Remove communication barriers by silencing cell phone. Ensure patient comfort and put patient at ease using empathic communication skills.
2	Identifying the CC or reason for visit and other problems or issues (patient-focused part of visit)	Indicate the time available for visit. Obtain the list of all the problems and issues the patient wishes to discuss and identify health care issues needing attention based on medical record. Summarize and finalize the agenda; negotiate specifics if there are too many items and plan another visit to address remaining items.
3	HPI or CC (active listening by physician used with equal focus on patient and physician)[b]	Ask open-ended questions; use silence and nonverbal communication. Pay more attention to patient than to your documentation. Obtain detailed information on HPI or CC, including patient's emotional status.
4	Detailed HPI or CC, physical examination, past medical history, and ROS (physician-focused part of visit) An unexpected finding on physical examination may add another item to the agenda, either for the present visit or for a future visit	Use focused as well as open-ended communications. Careful attention to chronology of problem or of symptoms is especially valuable because it may play a crucial role in diagnosis or progression of illness. Explain and ask permission to document visit by writing or using electronic medical record. Perform physical examination, asking the patient's permission before starting. If pelvic examination is required, again ask permission and have an attendant present during examination to assist the physician and as a chaperone regardless of the physician's sex. A good rule is "talk before you touch."
5	Partnership identification of problems or issues and agreement on management plans (shared patient and physician focus)	Summarize conversation and confirm accuracy of information. Agree on management plan, including follow-up visits.

[a] Overlapping with time for each based on the nature of the patient's visit.
[b] Consistent use of empathic communication skills.
Adapted with permission from ACOG Committee Opinion 423, Washington, DC: American College of Obstetricians and Gynecologists; January 2009, Motivational Interviewing: A Tool for Behavior Change.

physician, the patient will continue to make multiple attempts to express these concerns until they are addressed, often lengthening the visit in the process. Empathic communication is a learned skill that facilitates a good patient–physician partnership and the most efficient use of the time available for patient encounters.

Another characteristic of a good patient–physician partnership is that the physician spends about the same amount of time listening as talking during the first two thirds of a patient visit. This kind of communication, called motivational interviewing, replaces the traditional approach of "advice giving" and gives way to "reflective listening." The patient is encouraged to talk, and the physician actively listens, periodically confirming what has been heard. Because the information gained is of better quality and the patient's needs are met during the encounter, time-consuming "late-arising concerns" (significant issues brought up after a degree of closure has been reached on the primary problems) are less likely to occur. Building a strong and trusting patient–physician partnership is central to good women's health care.

The steps of this kind of patient–physician partnership and visits follow a productive pattern outlined in Table 1.1.

THE WOMEN'S HEALTH EVALUATION: HISTORY AND PHYSICAL EXAMINATION

When organized effectively, data gathered in a woman's health evaluation are critical in facilitating patient management. Record keeping is now turning to electronic medical records, whose advantages include elimination of both transcription errors and illegible information, automated follow-up with reminders of tests and consultations, simultaneous creation of billing information, and organization and rapid availability of an entire patient's chart.

Medical History

The medical history includes the chief complaint (CC), problem, or concern; history of present illness (HPI); a past history that includes a gynecologic history, obstetric history, family health history, and social history; and a review of system (ROS).

Chief Complaint

The CC is a concise statement describing the symptom, problem, condition, diagnosis, physician-recommended return, or other reasons for the patient visit. A CC may not be present if the patient is seeing the obstetrician–gynecologist for preventive care.

History of Present Illness

HPI is a chronologic description of the development of the patient's CC, or if the office visit is for primary care, chronology applies to the other components of the history. Establishing *chronology* can be important because chronological organization often suggests a specific disease or narrows consideration of illness to an organ system. Sometimes, the onset of symptoms is easily identified because of its abruptness. In other cases, the onset is insidious, making it difficult for a patient to identify a specific time. When the onset of symptoms is slow, patients are often unable to accurately identify when the symptom began. Asking in the context of a recognizable date prior to the visit (e.g., a holiday) will often allow the patient to provide better chronological information. This technique may be useful in any history taking, not just for the CC.

Past History

Past history includes information about sexual health history as well as medical, surgical, or psychiatric illnesses and/or treatments the patient has had, including the diagnosis, the medical and/or surgical treatment, and the results. Questions about previous surgery of any kind should include the name of the procedure; indication; when, where, and by whom the surgery was performed; and the results. Operative notes may contain useful information. A previous surgeon's notes describing findings consistent with the effects of a pelvic infection should prompt the physician to ask specifically about a history of sexually transmitted infections (STIs) such as gonorrhea or *Chlamydia* that can cause these findings but the interview should also query into previous herpes, genital warts, hepatitis, AIDS, and syphilis as well as about vaginitis and vaginal discomfort. Vaginitis and STIs are often confused. Careful history taking is needed to differentiate vaginitis or cervicitis from pelvic inflammatory disease. This can avoid delay in appropriate evaluation and treatment, which can have long-term impact on a woman's reproductive health.

Explaining the differences while obtaining this history is an excellent opportunity to use empathic and motivational communication skills to build and enhance the patient–physician partnership. The patient's immunization history should be obtained to update adult immunization schedules and discuss new vaccines like the human papillomavirus (HPV) vaccine.

Gynecologic History

The gynecologic history includes the menstrual history, which begins with **menarche**, the age at which menses began. The basic **menstrual history** includes the following:

- Last menstrual period
- Length of periods (number of days of bleeding)
- Number of days between periods
- Any recent changes in periods

Episodes of bleeding that are "light but on time" should be noted as such, because they may have diagnostic significance. Sometimes women disregard such an episode when asked when they last had a menstrual period, so it is often useful to specifically ask if there had been any "light" bleeding, which may represent an actual ovulatory cycle. Determining a last menstrual period may be made difficult by an episode of "light vaginal bleeding." Specific questioning is often helpful in understanding whether a woman's last menstrual cycle was normal or abnormal. Estimation of the amount of menstrual flow can be made by asking whether the patient uses pads or tampons, how many are used during the heavy days of her flow, and whether they are soaked or just soiled when they are changed. It is normal for women to pass clots during menstruation, but normally they should not be larger than the size of a dime. Specific inquiry should be made about **irregular bleeding** (bleeding with no set pattern or duration), **intermenstrual bleeding** (bleeding between menses), and **postcoital bleeding** (bleeding immediately after coitus).

The menstrual history may include **premenstrual symptoms**, such as anxiety, fluid retention, nervousness, mood fluctuations, food cravings, variations in sexual feelings, and difficulty sleeping. Cramps and discomfort during menses are common but abnormal when they interfere with daily activities of living or when they require more analgesia than provided by non-narcotic analgesia. Menstrual pain is mediated through prostaglandins and should be responsive to nonsteroidal anti-inflammatory drugs. Inquiry about duration (both how long the patient has noted this pain and how long each episode of pain lasts), quality, radiation of the pain to areas outside the pelvis, and association with body position or daily activities completes the pain history.

The term **menopause** refers to the cessation of menses for greater than 1 year. **Perimenopause** is the time of transition from menstrual to nonmenstrual life when ovarian function begins to wane, often lasting 1 to 2 years. Significant and disruptive perimenopausal symptoms are often very disturbing and require focused attention when they are identified. Timely specific treatment is often indicated. The perimenopausal period often begins with increasing menstrual irregularity and varying or decreased flow and is associated with hot flushes, nervousness, mood changes, and decreased vaginal lubrication with sexual activity as well as altered libido (see Chapter 41).

The gynecologic history includes known gynecologic illnesses and how they were treated. The history also lists surgeries the woman has had, including what was done, why it was done, when it was done, and by whom. These details are often available by obtaining copies of the surgical dictations (operative reports), which often provide crucial diagnostic information.

The gynecologic history also includes a **sexual history**. Taking a sexual history is facilitated by behaviors, attitudes, and direct statements by the physician that project a nonjudgmental manner of acceptance and respect for the patient's gender identity and lifestyle. Nonjudgmental methods of inquiring about the sexual history without hindering an open discussion about sexual orientation include the following questions:

Have you ever been sexually active?
Tell me about your partners.
Who are you sexually attracted to? Males, females, or both?

A good opening question is, "Please tell me about your sexual partner or partners." These questions are gender neutral and also give the patient considerable latitude for response. However, these questions must be individualized to each patient. As our society is steadily showing more understanding of patients who are lesbian, gay, bisexual, or transsexual (LGBT), the suggested opening questions may quickly be followed by exploration of gender identity. It is well documented that these patients often receive substandard care. Barriers include concerns about confidentiality, lack of health insurance as these patients may be barred from participating in their partners' employment benefits, caregiver attitudes, and limited understanding of their own health risks.

Effective care, including screening for STIs, requires that physicians and their female patients engage in a comprehensive and open discussion not only about sexual identity but also about sexual and behavioral risks. The latter is followed by a discussion of means to lessen the risk of STI acquisition. All women should be screened for STIs based on the same risk factors regardless of orientation. Data that should be elicited in the sexual history include whether the patient is currently or ever has been sexually active, the lifetime number of sexual partners, the partners' gender/s, and the patient's current and past methods of contraception. A patient's **contraceptive history** should include the method currently used, when it was begun, any problems or complications, the patient's satisfaction with the method, and desire for pregnancy. Previous contraceptive methods and the reasons they were discontinued may prove relevant. If no contraceptive actions are being taken, inquiry should be made as to why, which may include the desire for conception or concerns about contraceptive options as understood by the patient. A serious error is to assume that patients with same-sex partners do not need contraception. Open discussion of this possibility is an important part of the contraceptive care of these patients. Additionally, these patients may not be aware of their need for Pap tests but may be at risk too due to previous or current heterosexual contact as well as HPV transmission through shared sex toys. Finally, patients should be asked about behaviors that put them at high risk for the acquisition of HIV, hepatitis, or other STIs including noncoital sexual activity such as oral and anal intercourse.

Obstetric History

The basic obstetric history includes the patient's **gravidity**, or number of pregnancies (Box 1.1). A pregnancy can end in a live birth, miscarriage, premature birth (less than 37 weeks of gestation), or an abortion. Details about each live birth are noted, including birthweight of the infant, sex, number of weeks at delivery, and type of delivery. The patient should be asked about any pregnancy complications, such as diabetes, hypertension, and preeclampsia, and whether she has a history of depression or anxiety, before, during, or after a pregnancy. A breastfeeding history is also useful information.

Preconception Counseling and Care

Preconception care can improve the outcome of pregnancy by planning conception itself as well as by identifying and managing illness before conception. This reduces the potential ill effects of preexisting illness on the mother and fetus.

Preconception counseling includes a discussion of the following with the patient:

- Family planning and pregnancy spacing
- Immunization status
- Genetic history (both maternal and paternal)
- Teratogens; environmental and occupational exposures
- Assessment of socioeconomic, educational, and cultural context

If a patient has a history of **infertility** (generally defined as *failure to conceive for 1 year with sufficiently frequent sexual encounters*), questions concerning both partners should cover previous diseases or surgery that may affect fertility, pregnancy histories (previous children with the same or other partners), duration that conception has been attempted, and the frequency and timing of sexual intercourse. Evaluation is recommended after 6 months of failed attempts in women over 35 years old in the face of waning fertility.

Family History

The **family history** should list illnesses occurring in first-degree relatives, such as diabetes, cancer, osteoporosis, and heart diseases. Information gained from the family history may indicate a genetic predisposition for a hereditary disease. This information may guide selection of specific tests or other interventions for the surveillance of the patient and perhaps other family members.

BOX 1.1 Common Terms Used to Describe Parity

Gravida	A woman who is or has been pregnant
Primigravida	A woman who is in or who has experienced her first pregnancy
Multigravida	A woman who has been pregnant more than once
Nulligravida	A woman who has never been pregnant and is not currently pregnant
Primipara	A woman who is pregnant for the first time or who has given birth to only one child
Multipara	A woman who has given birth two or more times
Nullipara	A woman who has never given birth or who has never had a pregnancy progress beyond the gestational age of an abortion

Review of Systems

The ROS is an inventory of body systems, obtained through a series of questions, which seeks to identify symptoms that the patient has experienced or is experiencing. Equally important are **pertinent negatives**, information derived from focused leading questions seeking the presence or absence of symptoms of illness. Pertinent negatives are often as important as positive responses in the ROS. For example, the ROS for urinary tract infection (UTI) and bladder function might include these questions, "Are you urinating more frequently than usual? How often? Does it burn when you urinate?" Increasingly frequent urination and pain with urination are often symptoms of UTI. "Do you feel you have completely emptied your bladder after you urinate? Do you lose urine accidentally when you laugh, sneeze, or cough?" These screening questions can identify problems with bladder function and pelvic support (see Chapter 30).

Physical Examination

The general physical examination serves to detect abnormalities suggested by the medical, surgical, or gynecologic history as well as unsuspected asymptomatic problems. Specific information the patient gives during the history should guide the physician to areas of physical examination that may not be surveyed in a routine screening. The extent of the examination is generally determined by the patient's complaints, what is being medically managed by other clinicians, and what is medically indicated from history. Three of these are of special importance to obstetric and gynecologic care: the breast examination, the abdominal examination, and the pelvic examination. Any examination warrants thorough handwashing before touching the patient.

Any request for a chaperone to also attend the physical examination should be met, regardless of the physician's sex or whether the request is made by the patient or the physician. In general, a chaperone is a wise preventive precaution. When chaperones are present during the physical examination, the physician should provide a separate opportunity for private conversation between him or herself and the patient.

Vital Signs

Every physical examination begins with vital signs: temperature; pulse; blood pressure; height; weight; and a derived value, the body mass index (see Chapter 2). The physician should comment on the vital signs and explain the health implications of any abnormal findings. The American Heart Association and American College of Cardiology issued new, more stringent, guidelines for hypertension in 2017 (Table 1.2) eliminating prehypertension, and defining high blood pressure as readings of 130 mm Hg and higher systolic or 80 and higher diastolic. The new guidelines may double the number of women under 45 years of age classified as hypertensive who will require extra vigilance during and after pregnancy.

Breast Examination

The breast examination by a physician remains the best means of early detection of breast cancer when combined with appropriately scheduled mammography. The results of the breast examination

TABLE 1.2 BLOOD PRESSURE CATEGORIES

Blood Pressure Category[a]	Systolic Blood Pressure (mm Hg)[b]	Diastolic Blood Pressure (mm Hg)[b]
Normal	<120	and <80
Elevated	120–129	and <80
Stage 1 hypertension	130–139	or 80–89
Stage 2 hypertension	140 or higher	90 or higher
Hypertensive crisis	>180	>120

[a] Based on Whelton, P.K., et al., 2017, doi.org/10.1161/HYP.0000000000000065.
[b] Systolic blood pressure at or after first two heart sounds; diastolic blood pressure just before disappearance of heart sounds. Blood pressure taken seated after 5 minutes of quiet with appropriately sized blood pressure cuff; diagnostic value is the average of two or more measurements taken at two or more office visits.

may be expressed by description or diagram, or both, usually with reference to the quadrants and tail region of the breast or by allusion to the breast as a clock face with the nipple at the center (Fig. 1.2).

The breasts are first examined by **inspection**, with the patient's arms at her sides, and then with her hands pressed against her hips, and/or with her arms raised over her head (Fig. 1.3). If the patient's breasts are especially large and pendulous, she may be asked to lean forward so that the breasts hang free of the chest, facilitating inspection. Tumors often distort the relations of these tissues, causing disruption of the shape, contour, and symmetry of the breast or position of the nipple. Some asymmetry of the breasts is common, but marked differences or recent changes deserve further evaluation.

Discolorations or ulcerations of the skin of the breast, areola, or nipple, or edema of the lymphatics that causes a leathery puckered appearance of the skin (referred to as *peau d'orange* or "like the skin of an orange") are abnormal. A clear or milky breast discharge is usually bilateral and associated with stimulation or elevated prolactin levels (**galactorrhea**). Bloody discharge from the breast is abnormal and usually unilateral; it usually does not represent carcinoma, but rather inflammation of a breast structure with intraductal papilloma is often found. Evaluation is necessary to exclude malignancy. Pus usually indicates infection, although an underlying tumor may be encountered.

Very large breasts may pull forward and downward, causing upper back pain and stooped shoulders. Disabling pain and posture are usually considered appropriate indications for insurance to cover breast reduction surgery (reduction mammoplasty).

Palpation follows inspection, first with the patient's arms at her sides and then with the arms raised over her head. This part of the examination is usually done with the patient in the supine position. The patient may also be seated, with her arm resting on the examiner's shoulder or over her head, for examination of the most lateral aspects of the axilla. Palpation should be done with slow, careful maneuvers, using the flat part of the fingers rather than the tips. The fingers are moved up and down in a wavelike motion, moving the tissues under them back and forth, so that any breast masses that are present can be more easily felt. The examiner should decide upon a specific pattern of examination (e.g., in spiral, radial, and longitudinal strips)

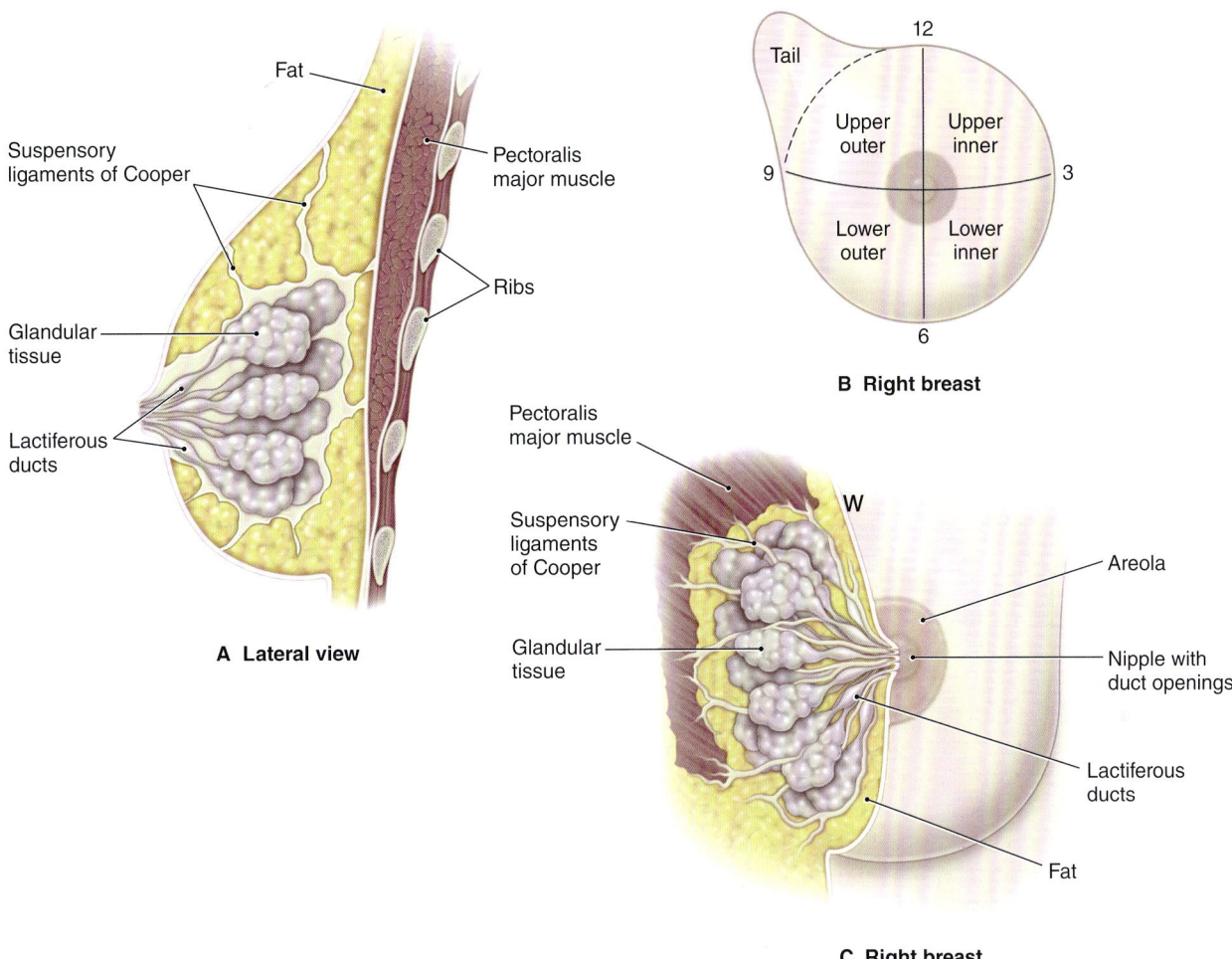

FIGURE 1.2. Clinical anatomy and associated examination schema of the breast.

and become facile with it so as to routinely include the entire breast, including the axillary tail. If masses are found, their size, shape, consistency (i.e., soft, hard, firm, and cystic), and mobility as well as their position should be determined. Women with large breasts may have a firm ridge of tissue located transversely along the lower edge of the breast. This is the inframammary ridge and is a normal finding.

The examination is concluded with gentle pressure inward and then upward at the sides of the areola to express fluid. If fluid is noted on inspection or is expressed, it should be sent for culture and sensitivity and cytopathology.

Counseling Breast Self-Awareness

Current recommendations emphasize that physicians encourage women to develop greater **breast self-awareness**, which may, for some women, include **breast self-examination (BSE)**. Breast self-awareness is generally defined as a woman's awareness of the normal appearance and feel of her breasts. The awareness of something being wrong has been shown to correlate with 50% to 70% of women subsequently being found to have breast cancer. Thus, enhanced breast self-awareness is associated with an increased likelihood of earlier detection of breast cancer.

This may be especially important for women who have had a recent "normal physician breast examination" or negative mammogram and yet actually have breast cancer. Encouraging breast self-awareness may include BSE if desired and may be of value in women at higher risk for breast cancer (e.g., first-degree relatives with breast cancer). Routine teaching of BSE is no longer generally recommended because it is associated with a high incidence of false-positive findings, leading to unnecessary testing including breast biopsy. For a woman who does request instruction in BSE, emphasis should be placed on observing her breasts in a mirror with her arms raised, looking for changes in the shape or contour of her breasts or discolorations. This is followed by gentle systematic palpation of the breasts with the flat of her fingers, including up into the armpits, wherein lies the axillary tail of the breast. Abnormal findings may include lumps, bumps, changes in breast texture, and unusual discomfort. When gentle squeezing of the nipples expresses blood or pus, this abnormal finding should be reported to the physician.

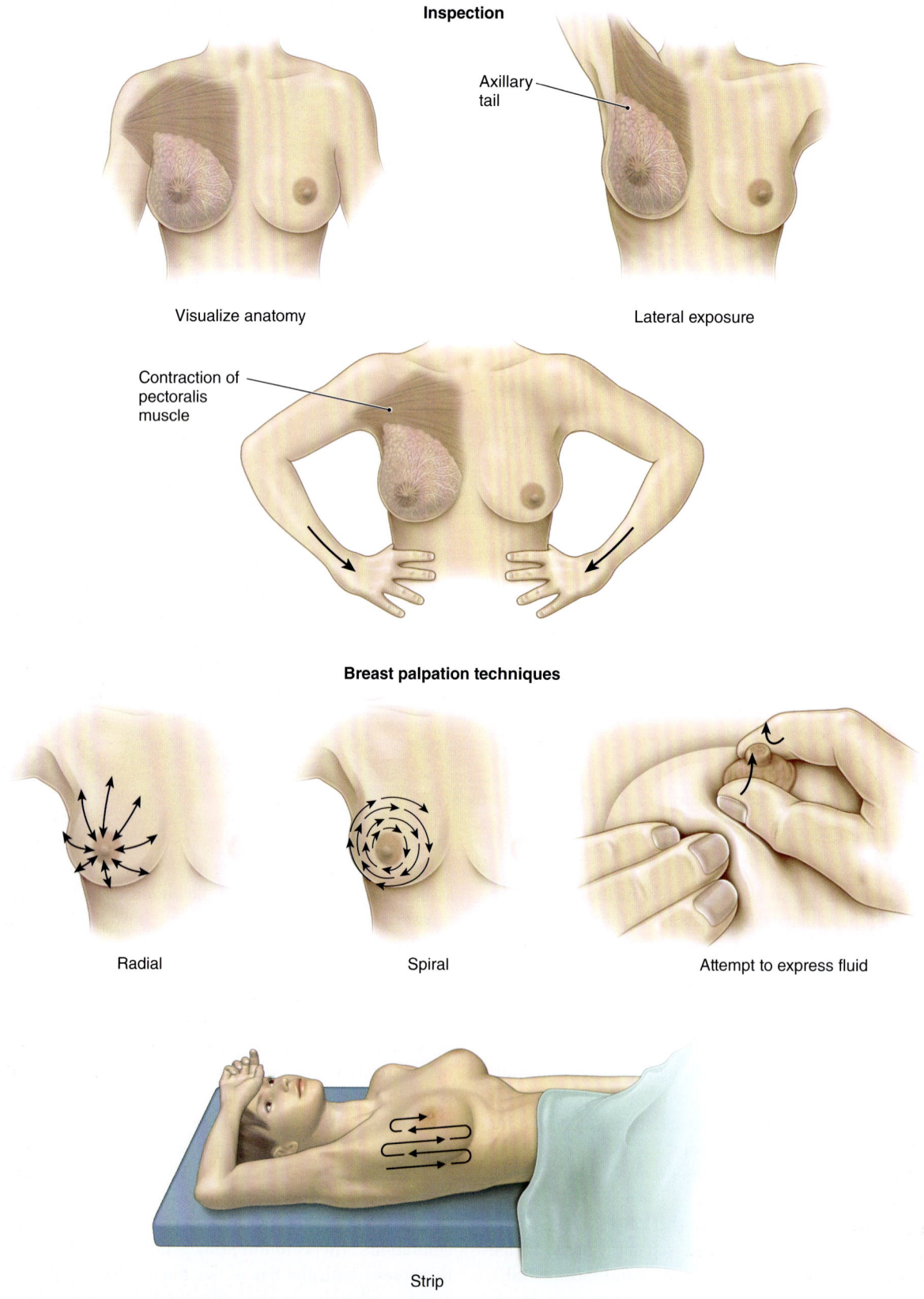

FIGURE 1.3. Breast examination. Regardless of your preferred method, accuracy is attained by systematic practice and by ensuring full coverage of the breast tissue, including the axillary tail.

Pelvic Examination

There has been much debate about the need for a pelvic examination on an annual basis for asymptomatic women not needing a Pap. In 2014, the American College of Physicians recommended that clinicians stop performing routine annual pelvic examinations due to lack of evidence that there was any benefit to the asymptomatic patient. But many clinicians claim they can detect many gynecologic conditions during a pelvic examination in otherwise asymptomatic women, including cancers of the vulva and vagina; cervical infections and lesions; uterine fibroids; and ovarian cysts and tumors. The American College of Obstetricians and Gynecologists (ACOG) continues to recommend an annual pelvic examination for women 21 years and older.

To assure comfort during the pelvic examination, an empty bladder is necessary. If needed, a "clean-catch" urine specimen is obtained from the mid-portion of her urinary stream after the patient has wiped her external genitals with the supplies provided. This kind of urine specimen may be used for urine culture with sensitivity testing as well as chemical testing. Abdominal and pelvic examinations require relaxation of the muscles. Techniques that help the patient to relax include encouraging the patient to breathe in through her nose and out through her mouth, gently and regularly, rather than holding her breath, and helping the patient to identify specific muscle groups (such as the abdominal wall or the pelvic floor) that need to be looser.

Communication with the patient during the examination is important. Everything that is going to happen during the pelvic examination should be explained before it occurs. Following the precept "talk before you touch" avoids anything unexpected.

An abrupt or stern command such as "Relax now; I'm not going to hurt you" may raise the patient's fears, whereas a statement such as "Try to relax as much as you can, although I know that is a lot easier for me to say than for you to do" sends two messages: 1) that the patient needs to relax, and 2) that you recognize that it is difficult, both of which demonstrate patience and understanding. Saying something such as "Let me know if anything is uncomfortable, and I will stop and we will try to do it differently" tells the patient that there might be discomfort but that she has control and can stop the examination if discomfort occurs. Likewise, stating "I am going to touch you now" is helpful in alleviating surprises. Using these statements demonstrates that the examination is a cooperative effort, further empowering the patient in facilitating care.

Position of the Patient and Examiner

The patient is asked to sit at the edge of the examination table, and an opened draping sheet may be placed over the patient's lap and knees. If a patient requests that a drape not be used, the request should be honored.

Positioning the patient for examination begins with the elevation of the head of the examining table to approximately 30° from horizontal. This serves three purposes: 1) it allows eye contact between the patient and physician and facilitates communication between the patient and physician during the entire examination; 2) it relaxes the abdominal wall muscle groups, making abdominal and pelvic examinations easier; and 3) it allows the physician to observe the patient for responses to the examination, which may provide valuable information (e.g., the nonverbal communication of wincing as evidence of discomfort during the abdominal and bimanual examinations). The physician or an assistant should help the patient lie back, slide down to the end of the examination table until her buttocks are at the edge of the table, place her feet in the footrests, bend her knee, and open her legs (**lithotomy position**) as shown in Figure 1.4. After the patient is in position, a drape may be placed over the patient's legs and adjusted so that it does not obscure the clinician's view of the perineum or obscure eye contact between patient and physician.

The physician should sit at the foot of the examining table, with the examination lamp adjusted to shine on the perineum. The lamp is optimally positioned in front of the physician's chest a few inches below the level of the chin, at approximately an arm's length distance from the perineum. The physician should glove both hands. After contact with the patient, there should be minimal contact with equipment such as the lamp.

Inspection and Examination of the External Genitalia

The pelvic examination begins with the inspection and examination of the external genitalia. Inspection should include the mons pubis, labia majora, labia minora, perineum, and perianal area. Inspection continues as palpation is performed in an orderly sequence, starting with the clitoral hood, which may be pulled back to inspect the glans proper. The labia are spread laterally to allow inspection of the introitus and outer vagina. The urethral meatus and the areas of the urethra and Skene glands should be inspected. The sequence of inspection and then palpation should be included in the thorough examination of the external genitalia. The forefinger is placed an inch or so into the vagina to gently milk the urethra. A culture should be taken of any discharge from the urethral opening. The forefinger is then rotated posteriorly to palpate the area of the Bartholin glands between that finger and the thumb (Fig. 1.5).

Speculum Examination

The next step is the **speculum examination.** The parts of the speculum are shown in Figure 1.6. There are two types of specula in common use for the examination of adults. The **Pederson**

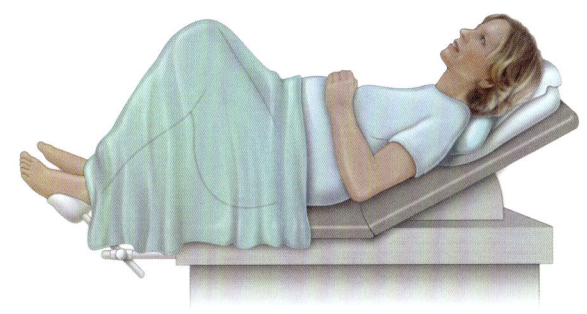

FIGURE 1.4. Lithotomy position during a pelvic examination.

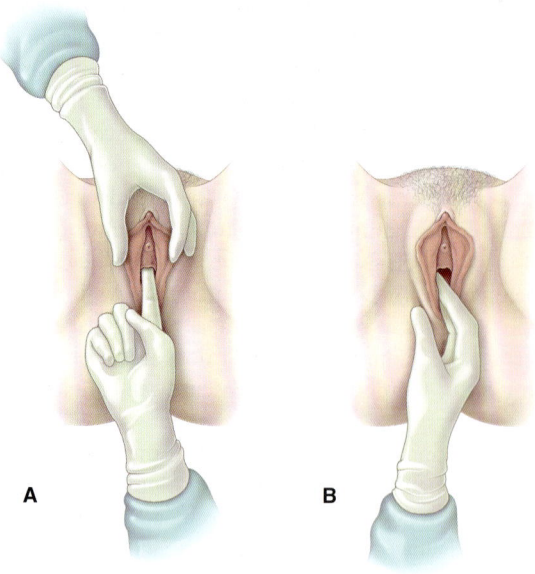

FIGURE 1.5. Palpation of the Bartholin, urethral, and Skene glands. (A) Palpation of urethral and Skene glands and "milking" of urethra. (B) Palpation of Bartholin glands.

speculum has flat and narrow blades that barely curve on the sides. The Pederson speculum works well for most nulliparous women and for postmenopausal women with atrophic, narrowed vaginas. The **Graves speculum** has blades that are wider, higher, and curved on the sides; it is more appropriate for most parous women. Its wider, curved blades keep the looser vaginal walls of multiparous women separated for visualization. A Pederson speculum with extra narrow blades may be used for visualizing the cervix in pubertal girls. Selection of the correct type of speculum is a key aspect of the comfortable and complete speculum examination. The speculum should be warmed either with warm water or by holding it in the examiner's hand. In some settings, the speculum is already stored on a heating pad. Warming the speculum is done for the comfort of the patient and to aid with insertion.

Speculum insertion should take into account the normal anatomic relations. As illustrated in Figure 1.7, by inserting the speculum along the axis of the vagina, minimal force is needed, and comfort is maximized. Until recently, the use of lubricants was avoided because of interference with cytologic interpretation, although this is less of a concern with liquid-based Pap test techniques. Situations that may require lubricant use are encountered infrequently and include examination of some prepubertal girls, some postmenopausal women, and patients with irritation or lesions of the vagina.

Most physicians find that control of pressure and movement of the speculum are facilitated by holding the speculum with the dominant hand. The speculum is held by the handle with the blades completely closed. The first two fingers of the opposite hand are placed on the perineum laterally and just below the introitus; pressure is applied downward and slightly inward until the introitus is opened slightly. If the patient is sufficiently relaxed, this downward pressure on the perineum causes the

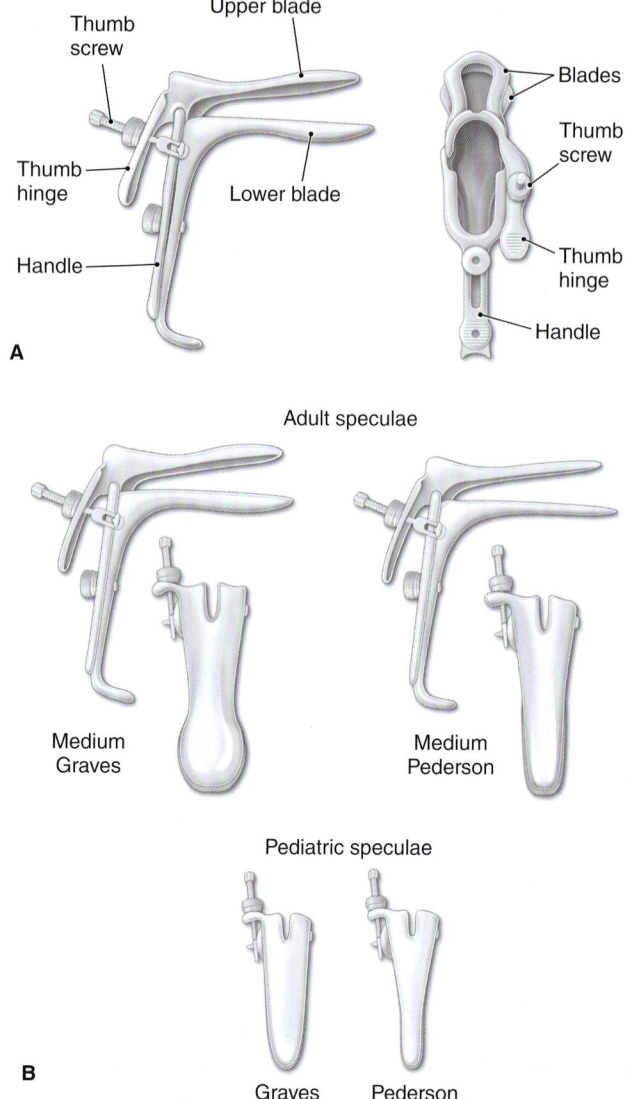

FIGURE 1.6. The vaginal speculum. (A) Parts of the vaginal speculum. (B) Types of vaginal specula.

introitus to open, allowing for easier insertion of the speculum. The speculum is initially inserted in a horizontal plane with the width of the blades oblique to the vertical axis of the introitus. The speculum is then directed posteriorly at an approximately 45° angle from horizontal; the angle is adjusted as the speculum is inserted, so that the speculum slides into the vagina with minimal resistance. If the patient is not relaxed, posterior pressure from a finger inserted in the vagina sometimes relaxes the perineal musculature.

As the speculum is inserted, a slight continuous downward pressure is exerted so that distension of the perineum is used to create space into which the speculum may advance. Taking advantage of the distensibility of the perineum and vagina posterior to the introitus is a crucial concept for the efficient and comfortable manipulation of the speculum examination (and later for the bimanual and rectovaginal examination). Pressure superiorly causes pain in the sensitive area of the urethra and

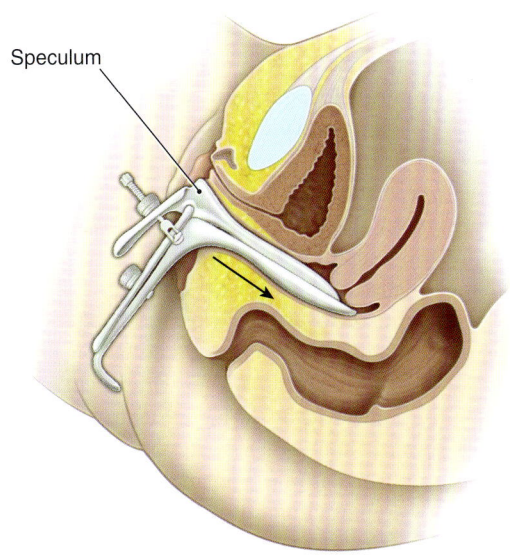

FIGURE 1.7. Speculum insertion.

clitoris and should be intentionally avoided. The speculum is inserted as far as it will go, which, in most women, means insertion of the entire speculum length. The speculum is then opened in a smooth and deliberate fashion. With slight tilting of the speculum, the cervix slides into view between the blades of the speculum. The speculum is then locked into the open position using the thumbscrew. Failure to find the cervix most commonly results from not having the speculum inserted far enough, often due to fear of causing patient discomfort. Keeping the speculum fully inserted while opening the speculum does not result in discomfort.

When the speculum is locked into position, it usually stays in place without being held. For most patients, the speculum is opened sufficiently by use of the upper thumbscrew. In some cases, however, more space is required. This may be obtained by gently expanding the vertical distance between the speculum blades by the use of the screw on the handle of the speculum. With the speculum in place, the cervix and the deep lateral vaginal vault may be inspected and specimens obtained of any discharge or lesion. Before obtaining samples for the Pap test, the patient should be told that she may feel a slight "scraping" sensation but no pain. Specimens are collected to fully evaluate the transformation zone, where cervical intraepithelial neoplasia is more likely to be encountered. Specimens are obtained from the exocervix and endocervix and either plated on slides, which are immediately fixed with a preservative spray, or placed in a liquid collection medium (Fig. 1.8).

Speculum withdrawal also allows for inspection of the vaginal walls. After telling the patient that the speculum is to be removed, the blades of the speculum are opened slightly by putting pressure on the thumb hinge, and the thumbscrew is completely loosened. Opening the speculum blades slightly before starting to withdraw the speculum avoids pinching the cervix between the blades. The speculum is withdrawn approximately 1 in. before pressure on the thumb hinge is slowly released. The speculum is withdrawn slowly enough to allow inspection of the vaginal walls. The blades of the speculum are naturally brought together by vaginal wall pressure. As the end of the speculum blades approaches the introitus, there should be no pressure on the thumb hinge, as otherwise the anterior blade can flip up, hitting the sensitive vaginal, urethral, and clitoral tissues.

Bimanual Examination

The **bimanual examination** uses both a "vaginal" hand and an "abdominal" hand to entrap and palpate the pelvic organs. The bimanual examination begins by exerting gentle pressure on the abdomen approximately halfway between the umbilicus and the pubic hair line with the abdominal hand, while inserting the index and middle fingers of the vaginal hand into the vagina to approximately 2 in. and gently pushing downward, distending the vaginal canal. The patient is asked to feel the muscles being pushed on and to relax them as much as possible. Then both the index and middle fingers are advanced into the vagina until

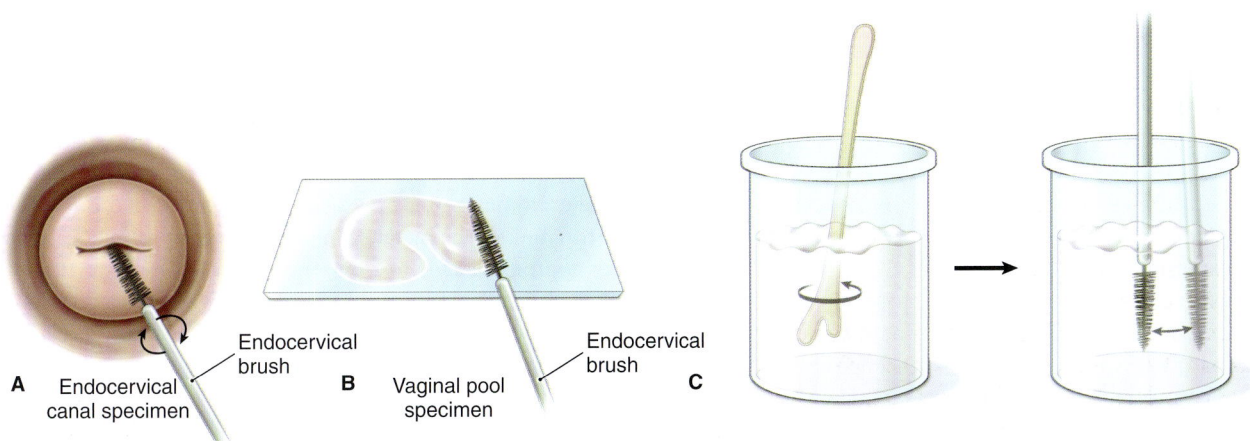

FIGURE 1.8. Pap test collection. (A) Obtaining endocervical portion of Pap test. (B) Spread specimen before fixation within 10 seconds. (C) Placement of specimens in liquid collection medium.

they rest at the limit of the vaginal vault in the posterior fornix behind and below the cervix. A great deal of space may be created by posterior distension of the perineum. Occasionally, only the index finger of the vaginal hand can be comfortably inserted.

During the bimanual examination, the pelvic structures are "caught" and palpated between the abdominal and vaginal hands. Whether to use the dominant hand as the abdominal or vaginal hand is a question of personal preference. A common error in this part of the pelvic examination is failure to make effective use of the abdominal hand. Pressure should be applied with the flat part of the fingers, not the fingertips, starting midway between the umbilicus and the hairline, moving downward in conjunction with upward movements of the vaginal hand. The bimanual examination continues with the circumferential examination of the cervix for its size, shape, position, mobility, and the presence or absence of tenderness or mass lesions (Fig. 1.9).

Bimanual examination of the uterus is accomplished by lifting the uterus up toward the abdominal fingers so that it may be palpated between the vaginal and abdominal hands. The uterus is evaluated for its size, shape, consistency, configuration, and mobility; for masses or tenderness; and for position. The uterus may tilt on its long axis (from cervix to fundus, **version**) yielding three positions (**anteverted**, **midposition**, and **retroverted**). It may also tilt on a shorter axis (from just above or at the area of the lower uterine segment, **flexion**) yielding two positions (**anteflexed** and **retroflexed**) (see Fig. 4.12). The retroverted, retroflexed uterus has three particular clinical associations: 1) it is especially difficult to estimate gestational age by bimanual examination during the first trimester of pregnancy, 2) it is associated with dyspareunia and dysmenorrhea, and 3) its position behind and below the sacral promontory may lead to the obstetric complication of uterine inculcation. **Cervical position** is often related to uterine position. A posterior cervix is often associated with an anteverted or midposition uterus, whereas an anterior cervix is often associated with a retroverted uterus. Sharp flexion of the uterus, however, may alter these relations.

The bimanual examination technique varies somewhat with the position of the uterus. Examination of the anterior and midposition uterus is facilitated with the vaginal fingers lateral and deep to the cervix in the posterior fornix. The uterus is gently lifted upward to the abdominal fingers and a gentle side-to-side "searching" motion of the vaginal fingers is combined with steady pressure and palpation by the abdominal hand to determine the characteristics of the uterus.

Examination of the retroverted uterus may be more difficult. In some cases, the vaginal fingers may be slowly pushed below or at the level of the uterine fundus, after which gentle pressure exerted inward and upward causes the uterus to antevert, or at least to move "upward," somewhat facilitating palpation. Then, palpation is accomplished as in the normally anteverted uterus. If this cannot be done, a waving motion with the vaginal fingers in the posterior fornix must be combined with an extensive rectovaginal examination to assess the retroverted uterus.

Bimanual examination of the adnexa to assess the ovaries, fallopian tubes, and support structures begins by placing the vaginal fingers to the side of the cervix, deep in the lateral fornix. The abdominal hand is moved to the same side, just inside the flare of the sacral arch and above the pubic hairline. Pressure is then applied downward and toward the symphysis with the abdominal hand, at the same time lifting upward with the vaginal fingers. The same movements of the fingers of both hands used to assess the uterus are used to assess the adnexal structures, which are brought between the fingers by these maneuvers to evaluate their size, shape, consistency, configuration, mobility, and tenderness as well as to palpate for masses. Special care must be taken when examining the ovaries, which are sensitive even in the absence of pathology. The ovaries are palpable in normal menstrual women approximately half of the time, whereas palpation of ovaries in postmenopausal women is less common.

Rectovaginal Examination

When indicated, a **rectovaginal examination** forms part of the complete pelvic examination on initial and annual examination as well as at interval examinations whenever clinically indicated (e.g., when there is suspicion of a posterior pelvic mass or in the evaluation of chronic pelvic pain).

The rectovaginal examination is begun by changing the glove on the vaginal hand and using a liberal supply of lubricant. The examination may be comfortably performed if the natural inclination of the rectal canal is followed: upward at a 45° angle for approximately 1 to 2 cm, then downward (Fig. 1.10). This is accomplished by positioning the fingers of the vaginal hand as for the bimanual examination, except that the index finger is also flexed. The middle finger is then gently inserted through the rectal opening and inserted to the "bend" where the angle turns downward. The index (vaginal) finger is inserted into the vagina, and both fingers are inserted until the vaginal finger rests in the posterior fornix below the cervix, and the rectal finger rests as far as it can go into the rectal canal. Asking the

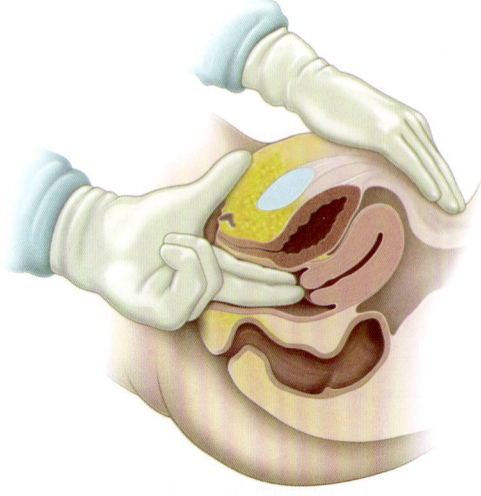

FIGURE 1.9. Bimanual examination of the uterus and adnexa.

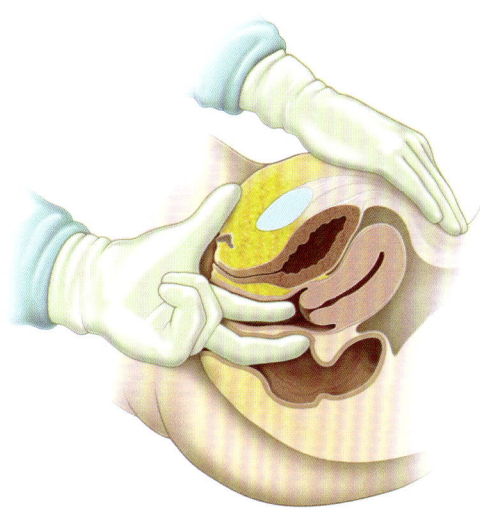

FIGURE 1.10. Rectovaginal examination.

patient to bear down as the rectal finger is inserted is not necessary and may add to the tension of the patient. Palpation of the pelvic structures is then accomplished, as in their vaginal palpation. The uterosacral ligaments are also palpated to determine if they are symmetrical, smooth, and nontender (as normally) or if they are nodular, slack, or thickened. The rectal canal is evaluated, as are the integrity and function of the rectal sphincter. After palpation is complete, the fingers are rapidly but steadily removed in a reversal of the sequence of movements used on insertion. Care should be taken to avoid contamination of the vagina with fecal matter.

At the conclusion of the pelvic examination, the patient is asked to move back up on the table and, thereafter, to sit up.

DIAGNOSIS, MANAGEMENT, AND CONTINUITY OF CARE

Depending on the reason for the patient's visit—either for a specific medical problem or for a preventive examination, further assessments and management plans are established. If a problem exists, the history and physical findings help establish a differential diagnosis (i.e., a list of possible underlying causes of the problem). Tests are ordered to try to further identify the most likely diagnosis. A presumptive diagnosis is made, and a management plan agreed upon between the patient and physician. Amelioration of symptoms and other evidence of treatment success confirm the diagnosis. If unsuccessful, the physician is led to further evaluation and consideration of new management plans.

If the patient has had a preventive health care examination, issues that arise during the history and physical examination and a long-term plan for addressing these issues should be discussed. The patient and physician agree on a plan of action, which may include behavior modification, lifestyle modification, referral to another physician or health care or social services professional, or referral to community resources. Screening tests and immunizations that are appropriate for the patient should also be administered (see Chapter 2).

CLINICAL FOLLOW-UP

You assure her of her good general health and recommend age-appropriate screening examinations. Discussion of her weight using height and weight tables does not initially reassure her, but she is more reassured after an explanation of her normal calculated body mass index and how it is more accurate in evaluating her weight. You perform the standard screening examinations she should have had by her age, including complete blood count, metabolic panel with lipids, and thyroid-stimulating hormone (TSH) as well as mammogram and bone density studies, and express the hope that you may be able to help with her constantly feeling cold. Subsequently, her overdue TSH is found to be significantly elevated. With thyroid hormone replacement, much of her sensation of feeling cold resolves over the next few months with a commensurate improvement in the quality of her life and a modest decrease in weight.

thePoint® Visit http://thePoint.lww.com/activate for an interactive USMLE-style question bank and more!

CHAPTER 2

The Obstetrician–Gynecologist's Role in Screening and Preventive Care

This chapter deals primarily with APGO Educational Topic Areas:

TOPIC 3   PAP TEST AND DNA PROBES/CULTURES
TOPIC 7   PREVENTIVE CARE AND HEALTH MAINTENANCE

Students should be able to counsel patients on important preventive medicine and health maintenance topics in women's health care, including topics such as immunization, diet, and exercise. They should be able to describe appropriate screening protocols for cancer, cardiovascular disease, and osteoporosis.

CLINICAL CASE

A pleasant 57-year-old moderately obese, insulin-dependent diabetic, menopausal woman is seen for routine gynecologic care. She feels well generally but complains that she has constant perineal itching. Another physician has treated her for recurrent vulvovaginal candidiasis over the past 5 years, using topical antifungal and steroidal cream preparations. She is a 1-pack-per-day smoker who has unsuccessfully tried to quit multiple times in the past. On physical examination, you find hyphae on a potassium hydroxide preparation from her vagina and also notice three areas of slight discoloration on both labia majora. You explain your concern about the relationship of continued vulvar pruritus and vulvar carcinoma and recommend a punch biopsy of one of the discolored areas of her labia. She consents, and two specimens are obtained. You also treat her with systemic and topical antifungal medications and suggest she see her internist to review her diabetic management. Again you discuss smoking cessation.

INTRODUCTION

As the population ages, the health care needs of women will change, and thus the provision of primary and preventive care in the obstetric and gynecologic setting must evolve to meet these needs. The obstetrician–gynecologist is in a unique position to provide screening, preventive care, and counseling to women, which can have a positive impact on quality of life as well as morbidity and mortality.

PREVENTIVE CARE

Preventive care encompasses both primary and secondary prevention and is both beneficial and cost-effective over time. In **primary prevention** an attempt is made to eliminate or ameliorate risk factors for disease and, thus, prevent its occurrence or modify its severity. Primary prevention may include health education and behavioral interventions to promote a healthier lifestyle including immunizations, fitness and nutrition, hygiene, smoking cessation, personal safety, and safe sex. **Secondary prevention** focuses on **screening tests** for diseases that are performed when the patient is usually asymptomatic, allowing prompt intervention that reduces morbidity and mortality. Screening tests are performed as part of periodic health assessments (often called "annual examinations") that afford an opportunity to evaluate and counsel patients based on their age and risk factors.

Primary preventive care concerning sexually transmitted diseases (STDs) is found in Chapters 28 and 29. Similar care to increase the quality of life of newborn and mother before, during, and after pregnancy is found in Chapter 6.

IMMUNIZATIONS

In the United States, vaccination programs that focus on infants and children have reduced the occurrence of many childhood diseases. However, many adolescents and adults are still affected by vaccine-preventable diseases such as influenza, varicella, hepatitis A, hepatitis B, measles, rubella, and pneumococcal pneumonia. Obstetrician–gynecologists and other clinicians who provide primary care to women have opportunities to counsel women on the need for immunizations and may administer them or refer the patient to a facility that does provide them.

The clinician should attempt to gather a complete immunization history from each patient including risk factors indicating the need for immunization. Previous vaccination records are particularly valuable if the patient is in doubt about her immunization history. In lieu of a clear history, the physician should assume that a patient has not been immunized and proceed accordingly. The recommended vaccinations for women are listed in Box 2.1. Because immunization recommendations do change, it is useful to know that the most current recommendations can be accessed at the Centers for Disease Control and Prevention's (CDC) National Immunization Program Web page (www.cdc.gov/vaccines).

BOX 2.1 Recommended Vaccinations for Women (Also See Appendix A)

Recommended immunization schedule for adults 19 years or older by age group, United States, 2017

Vaccine	19–21 years	22–26 years	27–59 years	60–64 years	≥65 years
Influenza[1]	1 dose annually				
Td/Tdap[2]	Substitute Tdap for Td once, then Td booster every 10 yrs				
MMR[3]	1 or 2 doses depending on indication				
VAR[4]	2 doses				
HZV[5]				1 dose	
HPV—Female[6]	3 doses				
HPV—Male[6]		3 doses			
PCV13[7]					1 dose
PPSV23[7]	1 or 2 doses depending on indication				1 dose
HepA[8]	2 or 3 doses depending on vaccine				
HepB[9]	3 doses				
MenACWY or MPSV4[10]	1 or more doses depending on indication				
MenB[10]	2 or 3 doses depending on vaccine				
Hib[11]	1 or 3 doses depending on indication				

- ▨ Recommended for adults who meet the age requirement, lack documentation of vaccination, or lack evidence of past infection
- ▨ Recommended for adults with additional medical conditions or other indications
- ☐ No recommendation

Prevention of cervical neoplasia and cancer with the use of the human papillomavirus (HPV) vaccine is discussed in detail in Chapter 47. The American College of Obstetricians and Gynecologists (College) recommends initial vaccination for girls ages 11 to 12 years. Although obstetrician–gynecologists do not routinely care for girls in this age group, they are in a unique position to advocate for the use of the vaccine for females ages 13 to 26 years (the catch-up vaccination period). During a health care visit with a girl or a woman in the age range for vaccination, an assessment of the patient's HPV vaccine status should be conducted and documented in the patient record. The HPV vaccine is most effective when given before any exposure to HPV infection, but sexually active women who were exposed to HPV prior to vaccination can receive and benefit from the vaccine. Women should be informed that HPV immunization reduce the incidence of anogenital cancer and genital warts. This may include cervical intraepithelial neoplasia (CIN) and condylomatous vulvar disease. HPV vaccination should not be given during pregnancy but may be given to breastfeeding mothers.

SECONDARY PREVENTION: PERIODIC ASSESSMENT AND SCREENING

Periodic assessments conducted at regular intervals (i.e., annually) are an integral part of preventive health care and include screening, evaluation, and counseling. Recommendations for periodic health assessments and screening vary by age group and are based on risk factors as well as epidemiologic information (see Appendix A). This care starts with a thorough medical history, physical examination, and appropriate laboratory testing. The history, physical examination, and results of laboratory tests help guide interventions and counseling and may reveal additional risks that require targeted screening or evaluation.

The recommendations presented in Appendix A have been selected from a variety of sources taking into account factors such as the leading causes of morbidity and mortality in each age group as well as chronic health conditions that limit activity of adults (e.g., arthritis or other musculoskeletal disorders and circulatory disorders) that become more prevalent as women age.

Characteristics of Screening Tests

The principle behind routine screening is to detect the presence of disease in asymptomatic individuals without specific risk factors. Disease detection in this **sojourn time interval** allows maximum decrease in morbidity and mortality. The diseases screened for should be prevalent in the population and amenable to early intervention. Screening tests are currently available for a variety of cancers, metabolic disorders, and STDs. Examples of screening tests are Pap test and mammography.

Not every disease can be detected by screening, and screening is not cost-effective or feasible for every disease. The concepts of **sensitivity** and **specificity** are used to describe the efficacy of screening tests in detecting a disorder. The *sensitivity* of a test is the proportion of affected individuals that test positive on the screening test. The *specificity* is the proportion of unaffected individuals that test negative on the screening test. An effective screening test should be both sensitive (it has a high detection rate) and specific (it has a low false-positive rate). Other criteria for effective screening tests pertain to the population being tested and the disease itself (Box 2.2).

Cancer Screening

The Pap smear (cervical cancer) and mammography (breast cancer) are the only recognized effective screening tests for gynecologic cancers. There is no screening test with the requisite sensitivity and specificity to detect ovarian cancer. Women should be educated about the unique early signs and symptoms of ovarian cancer that may aid in earlier diagnosis (see Chapter 50). Likewise, screening tests are not available for endometrial, vaginal, or vulvar cancers. A history of postmenopausal bleeding (endometrial cancer) or chronic and persistent vulvar itching (vulvar cancer) may be useful, but for these neoplasms, as well as for cervical cancer, a tissue biopsy is needed to identify either frank invasion or a precursor lesion. Endometrial, vulvar, and vaginal biopsies are not screening tests.

Despite adequate primary and secondary screening, women remain at risk for the development of various kinds of carcinoma. This information may be of use in helping to explain the importance of such testing to the patient and her family (Table 2.1).

Breast Cancer

Breast cancer is the most commonly diagnosed cancer among women in the United States with a lifetime risk of 1 in 8 (about 12%), and it is the second leading cause of cancer-related death in women, second only to lung cancer. It is important that clinicians assess each patient's breast cancer risk by taking a thorough history because the recommendations for screening differ based on risk factors. The Gail model, a validated tool, is available online (http://www.cancer.gov/bcrisktool/) and may be used to estimate a patient's risk of developing breast cancer (also see Chapter 33).

For women at average risk, there are three major screening examinations for breast cancer: **clinical breast examination**, **screening mammography**, and **patient self-screening**. The American College of Obstetricians and Gynecologists recommends the following:

Clinical breast examination:

- Women aged 25 to 39 years—may be offered every 1 to 3 years
- Women aged 40 years and older—may be offered annually
- These recommendations may be adjusted based on risk

Mammography:

- Offer starting at 40 years and initiated at ages 40 to 49 if patient desires
- Recommend no later than 50 years if not initiated earlier
- Annually or biennially
- Continue until age 75
- Continue beyond 75 years based on shared decision-making process

---

BOX 2.2 Criteria for Screening Tests

Criteria for the Disease
- Asymptomatic period long enough to allow detection
- Prevalent enough to justify screening
- Treatable; treatment in an asymptomatic stage (preferably a superior treatment)
- Sufficient effect on quality and/or length of life

Criteria for the Test
- Sensitive
- Specific
- Safe
- Affordable
- Acceptable to patients

Criteria for the Population to Be Tested
- High disease prevalence
- Accessible
- Compliant with testing and treatment

TABLE 2.1 FEMALE RISK OF DEVELOPING GYNECOLOGIC CANCERS

Site of Cancer	Lifetime Risk of Developing
Breast	12.32 (1 in 8)
Uterine corpus	2.78 (1 in 36)
Ovary	1.31 (1 in 76)
Cervix	0.64 (1 in 156)

Data from American Cancer Society. *Lifetime Risk of Developing or Dying from Cancer.* 2016. https://www.cancer.org/cancer/cancer-basics/lifetime-probability-of-developing-or-dying-from-cancer.html

Breast self-examination:

- Not universally recommended
- Breast self-awareness is to be encouraged and supported by physicians

Ultrasound and magnetic resonance imaging (MRI) have no current role in screening women at average risk but are used as adjunctive tests. Ultrasound may be of value in evaluating inconclusive mammographic findings, differentiating solid from cystic masses, evaluating women with dense breasts, and guiding needle biopsies. It may also be used for MRI candidates with gadolinium contrast allergy, claustrophobia, or other barriers. In addition to yearly mammography, MRI is also recommended for women at very high risk of developing breast cancer (greater than 20% lifetime risk according to family history of risk assessment or who have BRCA gene mutations or a first-degree relative with BRCA gene mutation).

Breast cancer is covered in detail in Chapter 33.

Cervical Cancer

CIN is the precursor lesion to cervical cancer. CIN may regress spontaneously, but in some cases CIN 2 and CIN 3 may progress to cancer over time. **Exfoliative cytology**, specifically the **Pap test** (either slide or liquid based) with or without high-risk HPV identification, allows early diagnosis in most cases. The reduction in mortality from cervical cancer since the Pap test was introduced in the 1940s is testimony to the success of this screening program. It is estimated that 50% of women diagnosed with cervical cancer never had a Pap smear and an additional 10% did not have a Pap smear within 5 years of diagnosis.

New technologies and recommendations continue to evolve for cervical cancer screening.

The following are recommendations for cervical cancer screening for average-risk women based on the U.S. Preventive Services Task Force as well as the American Cancer Society, the American Society for Colposcopy and Cervical Pathology, and the American Society for Clinical Pathology:

- Younger than 21 years: should not be screened regardless of age of sexual initiation or other behavior-related risk factors, with the exception of women who are infected with HIV or who are otherwise immunocompromised.
- Ages 21 to 29 years: recommend screening every 3 years with cytology alone. Cotesting should not be performed on women younger than 30 years. Annual screening should not be performed.
- Ages 30 to 65 years: cotesting with cytology and HPV testing every 5 years is preferred. Screening every 3 years with cytology is acceptable. Annual screening should not be performed.
- Liquid-based and conventional methods of cervical cytology collection are acceptable for screening.
- Older than 65 years: screening by any method should be discontinued after age 65 with evidence of adequate negative prior test results and no history of CIN 2 or higher.
  - Adequate negative prior screening
    ◊ 3 consecutive negative cytology reports within the previous 10 years
    ◊ 2 consecutive negative cotesting reports within the past 10 years, the most recent within the past 5 years
- Routine cytology and HPV testing should be discontinued in women who have had a total hysterectomy (removal of cervix) and no history of CIN 2 or greater in the past 20 years.
- Women with a history of CIN 2, CIN 3, or adenocarcinoma in situ should continue screening for a total of 20 years after spontaneous regression or after appropriate management of CIN 2, CIN 3, or adenocarcinoma in situ, even if it extends the screening past age 65 years.
- Exceptions: The following risk factors may require more frequent cervical cancer screening than recommended in the routine screening guidelines:
  - Women who are infected with HIV
  - Women who are immunocompromised
  - Women who were exposed to diethylstilbestrol in utero
  - Women previously treated for CIN 2, CIN 3, or cancer

Cervical cancer is covered in detail in Chapter 47.

Colorectal Carcinoma

With nearly 65,000 new cases of **colorectal cancer** annually in women and over 24,000 deaths, colorectal cancer is the third leading cause of cancer death in women after lung cancer and breast cancer. Screening is appropriate and recommended because it is usually preceded by adenomatous polyps; early detection (preinvasive or early invasive stage) thus allows effective management for most patients.

Screening for colorectal cancer is recommended for all women at average risk, starting at age 50 years for average risk women and 45 years for African-American women. The College recommends stopping routine screening at age 75 years. The preferred method is **colonoscopy** performed every 10 years.

Other acceptable screening tests include the following:

- Annual high-sensitivity **fecal occult blood testing** or **fecal immunochemical testing**. Note that these tests require 2 or 3 stool samples, therefore a single sample collected by digital exam is not adequate.
- Flexible sigmoidoscopy every 5 years.
- Computed tomography colonography (virtual colonoscopy) every 5 years.
- Fecal DNA, interval not established.

Abnormalities found through any screening method other than colonoscopy require referral for diagnostic colonoscopy. Different recommendations apply to women at increased risk.

SEXUALLY TRANSMITTED DISEASES

Appropriate STD screening in nonpregnant women depends on the age of the patient and the assessment of risk factors (Box 2.3). Because of the risk that STDs pose in pregnancy, pregnant women are routinely screened for syphilis, HIV, chlamydia, and gonorrhea. STDs are covered in detail in Chapter 29.

Human Immunodeficiency Virus

The demographics of the HIV epidemic have changed over the last two decades. Prevalence has increased among adolescents, women, persons who reside outside metropolitan areas, and heterosexual men and women. Many are not aware that they are infected.

HIV testing is recommended for all women, and targeted testing is recommended for women with risk factors. The College and the CDC recommend that all females aged 13 to 64 years should be screened for HIV at least once and then annually based on risk factors; therefore, obstetrician–gynecologists should review their patients' risk factors annually and assess the need for retesting. Repeat HIV testing should be offered at least annually to women who

- Are injection drug users.
- Have sex partners who are injection drug users.
- Have sex partners who are HIV-infected.
- Exchange sex for drugs or money.
- Have had more than one sex partner since their most recent HIV test.

Obstetrician–gynecologists should also encourage women and their prospective sex partners to be tested prior to initiating a new sexual relationship. Periodic retesting could be considered even in the absence of risk factors, depending on clinical judgment and the patient's wishes.

The most common screening test is the **enzyme-linked immunosorbent assay** (**ELISA**), which is performed on a blood sample. There are also ELISA tests that use saliva or urine. A positive (reactive) ELISA must be confirmed by a supplemental test, such as the Western blot, to make a positive diagnosis.

Chlamydia Infection

Infection caused by **Chlamydia trachomatis** *is the most commonly reported bacterial STD in the United States and is often asymptomatic.* Over 1.5 million cases of chlamydia were reported to the CDC in 2015, a rate of 479 per 100,000, an increase of 6% since 2014. If untreated, chlamydia can cause significant long-term complications including infertility, ectopic pregnancy, and chronic pelvic pain. Diagnosing chlamydia promptly is necessary to prevent these complications.

The College and the CDC recommend annual screening for chlamydia in sexually active women younger than 25 years and asymptomatic women aged 25 years and older who are at high risk for infection. Nucleic acid amplification tests (NAATs) of endocervical swab specimens can identify infection in asymptomatic women with high specificity and sensitivity. NAATs of vaginal swabs and urine samples have comparable sensitivity and specificity.

Gonorrhea Infection

Over 395,000 cases of gonorrhea were reported in 2015, a rate of 124 per 100,000, an increase of 13% since 2014. Infection can be symptomatic with cervicitis and vaginal discharge, or it may be asymptomatic. Gonorrhea may lead to pelvic inflammatory disease, which is associated with long-term morbidity due to chronic pelvic pain, ectopic pregnancy, and infertility. The College and the CDC recommend annual screening for gonorrhea in sexually active women younger than 25 years and for asymptomatic women aged 25 years and older who are at high risk for infection. Screening can be done by cervical cultures or by newer techniques, such as NAATs and nucleic acid hybridization tests, that have better sensitivity with comparable specificity (see Chapter 29).

Syphilis

Syphilis is not a common disease in the United States, but the rate has increased over the last few years. About 23,900 cases of primary and secondary syphilis were diagnosed in 2015, which translates to a rate of 8 cases per 100,000, an increase of 19% since 2014.

Syphilis is a systemic disease caused by the bacterium *Treponema pallidum*. If untreated, syphilis may progress from a primary infection characterized by a painless ulcer (chancre) to secondary and tertiary infections. Signs and symptoms of secondary infection include skin manifestations and lymphadenopathy; tertiary infection may cause cardiac or ophthalmic manifestations, auditory abnormalities, and gummatous lesions. Serologic tests may be negative in the early stages of infection. The College and the CDC recommend annual syphilis screening for women at increased risk (see Box 2.3).

All pregnant women should be serologically screened as early as possible in pregnancy and again at delivery. Due to the possibility of a false-negative result in the early stages of infection, patients who are considered at high risk or who are from areas of high prevalence should be retested at the beginning of the third trimester.

BOX 2.3 — **Risk Factors for Sexually Transmitted Diseases**

- History of multiple sex partners
- Sexual partner with multiple sexual contacts
- Sexual contact with individuals with culture-proved STD
- History of repeated STDs
- Attendance at clinics for STDs

Used with permission from American College of Obstetricians and Gynecologists. Annual Women's Health Care. http://www.acog.org/About_ACOG/ACOG_Departments/Annual_Womens_Health_Care.

Screening is done with nontreponemal tests such as the Venereal Disease Research Laboratory test or rapid plasma reagin. These tests are followed by a confirmatory fluorescent treponemal antibody absorbed or *T. pallidum* particle agglutination. The specificity of the nontreponemal tests may be reduced in the presence of other conditions such as pregnancy, collagen vascular disease, advanced cancer, tuberculosis, malaria, and rickettsial diseases.

Metabolic and Cardiovascular Disorders

Routine screening can also be applied to noninfectious and noncancerous diseases, such as metabolic disorders and cardiovascular disease. Women should be evaluated for lifestyle issues and risks based on a history and physical examination. In many cases, early identification of risk factors and appropriate interventions are key components of disease prevention.

Osteoporosis

Osteoporosis affects approximately 9% of American women ages 50 years and older, and another 49% have **osteopenia**, or low bone mineral density (BMD). Osteoporosis-associated fracture, especially of the hip and spine, are leading causes of morbidity and mortality, increasing in proportion to age. Osteoporosis is a complication of menopause that is largely preventable with screening strategies, lifestyle modifications, and pharmacologic interventions.

BMD is an indirect measure of bone fragility. BMD is measured using dual-energy x-ray absorptiometry of the hip or the lumbar spine. The results are expressed in standard deviations compared with a reference population stratified by age, sex, and race. The **T-score** is expressed as the standard deviation from the mean peak BMD of a normal, young adult population; and the **Z-score** is expressed as the standard deviation from the mean BMD of a reference population of the same sex, race, and age as the patient. Z- and T-scores are used for hip and spine measurements. The World Health Organization (WHO) defines a normal BMD T-score as ≥−1.

Osteopenia (low bone mass) is defined as a T-score between −1 and −2.5. Osteoporosis is defined as a T-score ≤−2.5. Because of variance in the measurements obtained by the different commercial devices and at different sites, T- and Z-scores cannot be used as true screening tests, but they are good predictors of the risk of fracture. When these scores indicate low bone mass, the **fracture risk assessment tool (FRAX)** can be used in women older than age 40 years to predict their risk of fracture in the next 10 years. Developed in collaboration with the WHO, FRAX can be used to guide decisions about interventions including lifestyle changes and medical therapy to prevent or slow bone loss.

The College recommends BMD testing for all women starting at age 65 years. BMD testing should also be performed in younger postmenopausal women who have at least one risk factor for osteoporosis or fracture (Box 2.4). In addition, postmenopausal women who experience a fracture should have BMD testing to ascertain if they are osteoporotic; if so, treatment for osteoporosis is added to the therapy for fracture. Certain diseases or medical conditions (e.g., Cushing disease, hyperparathyroidism, hypophosphatasia, inflammatory bowel disease, lymphoma, and leukemia) and certain drugs (e.g., phenobarbital, phenytoin, corticosteroids, lithium, and tamoxifen) are associated with bone loss. Women with these conditions or taking these drugs may need to be tested more frequently.

Women should be counseled on the risks of osteoporosis and related fractures. Additional preventive measures include the following:

- Adequate calcium consumption (1,000 to 1,300 mg/day, depending on age) using dietary supplements if dietary sources are not adequate
- Adequate vitamin D consumption (600 to 800 international units daily, depending on age) and exposure to the natural sources of this nutrient
- Weight-bearing and muscle-strengthening exercises to reduce falls and prevent fractures
- Smoking cessation
- Moderation of alcohol intake
- Fall prevention strategies

Osteoporosis is covered in detail in Chapter 41.

Diabetes Mellitus

Diabetes mellitus is a group of disorders that share hyperglycemia as a common feature. Even when symptoms are not present, the disease can cause long-term complications. Ideally, it should be detected and treated in its early stages. A screening fasting blood glucose test is recommended for women beginning at age 45 years and every 3 years thereafter.

Screening should be considered in all adults who are overweight (BMI ≥25 kg/m^2) and have additional risk factors such as the following:

BOX 2.4   When to Screen for Bone Density before Age 65 Years

Bone density should be screened in postmenopausal women younger than 65 years if any of the following risk factors are noted:

- Medical history of a fragility fracture
- Body weight less than 127 lb
- Medical causes of bone loss (medications or diseases)
- Parental medical history of hip fracture
- Current smoker
- Alcohol abuse
- Rheumatoid arthritis

Used with permission from American College of Obstetricians and Gynecologists. Osteoporosis, Practice Bulletin No. 129. Washington, DC: American College of Obstetricians and Gynecologists; September 2012.

TABLE 2.2 SCREENING AND DIAGNOSTIC CRITERIA FOR DIABETES MELLITUS

Test	Prediabetes Screening[a]	Diabetes Diagnosis[b]
Fasting plasma glucose	100–125 mg/dL (impaired fasting glucose)	Greater than or equal to 126 mg/dL
2-h, 75-g oral glucose tolerance test	140–199 mg/dL (impaired glucose tolerance)	Greater than or equal to 200 mg/dL
Hemoglobin A1C	5.7–6.4%	Greater than or equal to 6.5%
Random plasma glucose	N/A	Greater than or equal to 200 mg/dL in patients with classic symptoms of hyperglycemia or hyperglycemic crisis

[a] If screening results are negative, screen again in 3 years; if screening results are positive, repeat screening using the same method, if possible.
[b] If the results of two different tests are both above diagnostic thresholds, the diagnosis of diabetes is confirmed.
Data from Standards of medical care in diabetes—2014. American Diabetes Association. *Diabetic Care* 2014;37 (Suppl 1):514–580.
Reprinted with permission from *Guidelines for Women's Health Care,* 4th ed. The American Congress of Obstetricians and Gynecologists.

- Physical inactivity
- First-degree relative with diabetes
- High-risk race/ethnicity (e.g., African-American, Latino, Native American, Asian American, Pacific Islander)
- Women who were diagnosed with gestational diabetes or gave birth to a newborn weighing more than 9 lb
- Hypertension (BP ≥140/90 mm Hg) or on therapy for hypertension
- HDL cholesterol <35 mg/dL and/or triglyceride level >250 mg/dL
- Women with polycystic ovarian syndrome
- Hemoglobin A1C ≥5.7%
- Other clinical conditions associated with insulin resistance such as severe obesity and acanthosis nigricans
- History of cardiovascular disease

Screening methods and criteria are noted in Table 2.2.

Thyroid Disease
Thyroid disease is often asymptomatic and, if untreated, can lead to serious medical conditions including the appearance of dementia in older adults. Because hypothyroidism in older women can present as dementia, thyroid-stimulating hormone levels should be tested every 5 years starting at age 50 years in women without risk factors.

Earlier or more frequent screening may be appropriate in women with a strong family history of thyroid disease or with an autoimmune disease (evidence of subclinical hypothyroidism may be related to unfavorable lipid profiles).

Hypertension
It is estimated that approximately 30% of adults ages 20 years and older have **hypertension**, which is defined as a systolic blood pressure ≥140 mm Hg or a diastolic blood pressure ≥90 mm Hg. Hypertension is one of the most important risk factors for heart disease and cerebrovascular accidents, two of the three leading causes for mortality among women. Hypertension is also a leading cause of mortality. About a third of those with hypertension do not know they have it. Because hypertension is often asymptomatic, the College recommends screening for hypertension annually for women and girls ages 13 years and older. **Prehypertension** (120–139/80–89) should prompt a review for comorbid conditions and more frequent evaluation of blood pressure.

Lipid Disorders
Coronary heart disease (CHD) is a leading cause of death for both men and women in the United States and accounts for approximately 500,000 deaths each year. Abnormal cholesterol levels have been linked to atherosclerosis as well as cardiovascular and cerebrovascular disease. Physicians and patients alike should be reminded that a 1% reduction in serum cholesterol levels results in a 2% reduction in CHD rates. Lipid levels are monitored by measuring **low-density lipoprotein, high-density lipoprotein,** and **triglycerides.** Approximately one in five adult Americans have a high total cholesterol level (≥240 mg/dL).

Current guidelines recommend that women without risk factors have a lipid profile assessment every 5 years, beginning at age 45 years. Earlier screening may be appropriate in women with risk factors such as family history of familial hyperlipidemia or premature cardiovascular disease (<50 years for men and <60 years for women). Other risk factors include previous personal history of CHD or noncoronary atherosclerosis (e.g., abdominal aortic aneurysm, peripheral artery disease, carotid artery stenosis) as well as personal or family history of peripheral vascular disease, obesity, diabetes mellitus, and multiple CHD risk factors (e.g., tobacco use and hypertension).

Obesity
Obesity is associated with increased risk for heart disease, type 2 diabetes, hypertension, and certain types of cancer (e.g., endometrial, colon, and breast), sleep apnea, osteoarthritis,

BOX 2.5 Body Mass Index

- BMI <18.5 = underweight
- BMI 18.5–24.9 = normal weight
- BMI 25–29.9 = overweight
- BMI 30–34.9 = obesity (Class I)
- BMI 35–39.9 = obesity (Class II)
- BMI ≥40 = extreme obesity (Class III)

National Heart, Lung, and Blood Institute and North American Association for the Study of Obesity. The Practical Guide: Identification, Evaluation, and Treatment of Overweight and Obesity in Adults. Bethesda, MD: National Institutes of Health; 2000.

gallbladder disease, and depression. Measurement of height and weight and the calculation of BMI are recommended as part of the periodic assessment (Box 2.5). Obese people with a BMI of 30 or more have up to two-fold increased risk of death. Behavioral therapy is the most common treatment, although bariatric surgery is an option to be considered for those who are morbidly obese and have proven refractory to treatment. Because of the consistent and often severe side effects of bariatric surgery, it should be considered a treatment of last resort and every effort made to use behavioral treatment and perhaps medications prior to such surgery.

Other Conditions

Finally, the annual exam is an ideal setting to screen for abuse, depression, and psychosocial issues such as stress, feeding and eating disorders, and nonsuicidal self-injury behavior.

CLINICAL FOLLOW-UP

The patient returns in 3 weeks and reports that her itching is somewhat improved and that her general physician had made a slight adjustment in her insulin regimen. She is concerned about the continued vulvar itching, however, given your previous discussion. You inform her that both vulvar biopsies revealed early vulvar malignancy. Because she is disheartened by this news, you reassure her that you are optimistic about a good outcome for this problem and have arranged an immediate consultation with a gynecologic oncologist. Subsequently, your consultant informs you that her very early noninvasive vulvar malignancy has been successfully treated, returning her to routine care in your practice and thanking you for the referral.

---

thePoint® Visit **http://thePoint.lww.com/activate** for an interactive USMLE-style question bank and more!

CHAPTER 3

Ethics, Liability, and Patient Safety in Obstetrics and Gynecology

This chapter deals primarily with APGO Educational Topic Area:

TOPIC 6 LEGAL AND ETHICAL ISSUES IN OBSTETRICS AND GYNECOLOGY

Students should gain an appreciation for the legal importance of confidentiality and informed consent. They should define basic principles of ethics and apply them to clinical dilemmas in obstetrics and gynecology. They should understand the role of obstetrician–gynecologists as advocates in women's health.

CLINICAL CASE

A 27-year-old attorney is referred from her general physician who has provided her general gynecologic care including contraception since puberty. Until recently, her care had been unremarkable, but in the past 18 months she was seen five times, complaining of a foul-smelling vaginal discharge. On the first visit, *Trichomonas vaginalis* was diagnosed and treated, with negative results for other investigations for sexually transmitted diseases. Your consulting physician notes that his discussion with her about her sexual history and safe sexual practices was met with a very reserved attitude that he found somehow disconcerting. She had also indicated that she wished no further discussion of the topic. On her subsequent four visits to her general physician with the complaint of an increasingly foul-smelling vaginal discharge, he could make no clinical diagnosis. She had become more and more unhappy and requested a consultation with a specialist who could find the infection causing her discharge. Visiting you, the specialist, she is insistent that there is a significant problem that she expects you to resolve. Unlike the quite specific and detailed discussion of her discharges, she is disconcertingly vague and elusive about her social history except that she had taken a leave of absence from her new legal practice for unspecified reasons. She tells you that you should spend your time dealing with vaginal discharge rather than unrelated and unimportant other issues.

INTRODUCTION

Patients and their physicians sometimes find themselves facing a dilemma choosing or implementing a clinical management decision, even when there is sufficient medical information to provide one or more logical management plans. Such dilemmas may involve ethical, moral, economic, or religious issues for the patient, patient's family, or the physician. They may also come from conflicts between the law and choice of management decision. Unfortunately, pressures felt by physicians and health care systems engendered by medical liability concerns often add to the dilemma. In some instances, these dilemmas may involve issues of omission or commission with respect to patient safety. In this chapter, we explore these three areas (ethics, medical liability, and patient safety) with the goal of helping the patient, physician, and others involved in such dilemmas to arrive at the best management options.

ETHICS

Physicians often encounter ethical dilemmas in the process of clinical decision making (clinical management). The use of an organized ethical framework in such situations is valuable in ensuring that evaluating situations and making decisions can be done in a systematic manner, rather than based on the physician's emotions, personal bias, or social pressures. There are several perspectives and frameworks that may be used, including principle-based ethics, care ethics, feminist ethics, communitarian ethics, case-based ethics, and virtue-based ethics, as seen in Table 3.1. One of these systems, **principle-based ethics**, is widely used because of its simple, user-friendly structure. Table 3.2 shows how the four principles of principle-based ethics might be used. It is important to note that no single perspective or framework can be applied to every clinical situation. One must also remember that they are not mutually exclusive and in fact may complement each other as they focus on different aspects of the ethical questions.

Principle-Based Ethics

Principle-based clinical management is based on systematic review of the case using four ethical principles:

1. Respect for **patient autonomy** acknowledges an individual's primary right to hold views, make choices, and take actions based on her beliefs or values independent of those of the physician, medical care system, or society as well as free of extrinsic controlling influences and limited understanding.

TABLE 3.1	CONTEMPORARY APPROACHES TO ETHICAL DECISION MAKING
Approach	Description
Principle-based ethics	Systematic approach based on four principles: autonomy, beneficence, nonmaleficence, and justice
Care ethics	Good decisions result from character traits such as sympathy, compassion, fidelity, love, and friendship inherent in interpersonal relationships
Feminist ethics	Care based in equality of care for men and women and the right of women to equal consideration and treatment
Communitarian ethics	Care based upon shared values, goals, and ideals of community rather than of the individual
Case-based ethics	Care based on previous cases and the accumulated scientific knowledge of them, understanding that this may change with new information
Virtue-based ethics	Care based on the character of the physician facilitated by qualities of character such as trustworthiness, prudence, fairness, fortitude, temperance, integrity, self-effacement, and compassion

TABLE 3.2	A PRINCIPLE-BASED ETHICAL APPROACH TO CLINICAL DECISION MAKING
Ethical Principle	Ethical Concerns
AUTONOMY Respect for the patient's right to self-determination	Knowing what the patient wants
BENEFICENCE The duty to promote the good of the patient	Evidence-based diagnosis and management
NONMALEFICENCE The duty not to inflict harm or injury	Impact of management on the patient's life
JUSTICE Assuring the patient is given what is "due"	The preferences of the patient, the needs of society, and the boundaries upon management placed by law

Respect for autonomy provides a strong moral foundation for the informed consent process in which a patient, adequately informed about her medical condition and available therapies, freely chooses specific treatments or no treatment. Attempting to override patient autonomy to promote what the clinician perceives as in a patient's best interests is termed *paternalism* and violates the principle of autonomy. Autonomy does not preclude the physician from providing a management recommendation based on evidence-based medicine and the physician's experience and judgment, as long as it is clearly understood that the physician does not expect or require the patient to follow the recommendation. Instead, it may be factored in as part of the patient's decision making.

2. **Beneficence** is the obligation to promote well-being by helping the patient make the best possible medical or surgical management decision, literally doing "good." It is the responsibility of the physician to always act for the benefit of the patient. In balancing beneficence with respect for autonomy, the clinician should define the patient's best interests as objectively as possible.

3. **Nonmaleficence** follows from beneficence, obliging the physician to not harm or cause or allow injury to the patient. The well-known maxim *primum non nocere* ("first, do no harm") comes from this ethical principle. This also includes the physician's obligation to maintain medical competence through study, application, and enhancement of medical knowledge and skills as well as to address and rehabilitate any behavior that diminishes the physician's capability to practice, such as substance abuse. Moreover, the physician should avoid any discrimination on the basis of race, color, religion, national origin, political viewpoints, financial status, or any other factor as well as to eschew any conflicts of interest. The application of these principles consists of balancing benefits and harms, both intentional harms and those that can be anticipated to arise despite the best intentions (e.g., unwanted adverse effects of medication or complications of surgical treatment).

4. **Justice** is the physician's obligation to render to the patient what is due or owed. It is the most complex of the ethical principles, in part because of the physician's role in the allocation of limited medical resources. Justice is the obligation to treat equally those who are alike or similar according to whatever criteria are selected. Individuals should receive equal treatment, unless scientific and clinical evidence establishes that they differ in ways that are relevant to the treatments in question.

Steps for Ethical Clinical Management

Using a stepwise, systematic approach to a difficult clinical situation based on an ethical foundation has been consistently found to benefit patients, their families, physicians, the health care system (including the hospital), and society. An example of such an application is found in Box 3.1.

There are seven steps in the decision-making process.

1. *Identify the decision makers.* The first step in clinical management is to answer the question: "Whose decision is it?" The patient is presumed to have the **capacity** to choose among evidence-based, medically acceptable management alternatives or to refuse treatment. Capacity depends on the patient's ability to understand information and appreciate the implications of the information presented and may vary among individuals. Capacity must not be confused with **competence** (authority to make decisions). Competence is a narrow legal determination made by health care professionals with

> **BOX 3.1** One Case Study: Five Approaches
>
> Although several approaches to ethical decision making may all produce the same answer in a situation that requires a decision, they focus on different, though related, aspects of the situation and decision.
>
> Consider, for instance, how they might address interventions for fetal well-being if a pregnant woman rejects medical recommendations or engages in actions that put the fetus at risk.
>
> 1. A **principle-based approach** would seek to identify the principles and rules pertinent to the case. These might include beneficence–nonmaleficence to both the pregnant woman and her fetus, justice to both parties, and respect for the pregnant woman's autonomous choices. These principles cannot be applied mechanically. After all, it may be unclear whether the pregnant woman is making an autonomous decision, and there may be debates about the balance of probable benefits and risks of interventions to all the stakeholders as well as about which principle should take priority in this conflict. Professional codes and commentaries may offer some guidance about how to resolve such conflicts.
> 2. A **virtue-based approach** would focus on the courses of action to which different virtues would and should dispose the obstetrician–gynecologist. For instance, which course of action would follow from compassion? From respectfulness? And so forth. In addition, the obstetrician–gynecologist may find it helpful to ask more broadly: Which course of action would best express the character of a good physician?
> 3. An **ethic of care** would concentrate on the implications of the virtue of caring in the obstetrician–gynecologist's special relationship with the pregnant women and with the fetus. In the process of deliberation, individuals using this approach generally would resist viewing the relationship between the pregnant woman and her fetus as adversarial, acknowledging that most of the time women are paradigmatically invested in their fetus' well-being and that maternal and fetal interests usually are aligned. If, however, a real conflict does exist, the obstetrician–gynecologist should resist feeling the need to take one side or the other. Instead, he or she should seek a solution in identifying and balancing his or her duties in these special relationships, situating these duties in the context of a pregnant woman's values and concerns, instead of specifying and balancing abstract principles or rights.
>
> Using another example, consider a case of a pregnant woman in preterm labor who refuses admission to the hospital for bed rest or tocolytics. Harris combines a care or relational perspective with a feminist perspective to provide a "much wider gaze" than a principle-based approach might:
>
>> The clinician would focus attention on important social and family relationships, contexts or constraints that might come to bear on [a] pregnant [woman's] decision making, such as her need to care for other children at home or to continue working to support other family members, or whatever life project occupied her, and attempt to provide relief in those areas....[Often] fetal well-being is achieved when maternal well-being is achieved.*
>
> 4. As this example suggests, a **feminist ethics approach** would attend to the social structures and factors that limit and control the pregnant woman's options and decisions in this situation and would seek to alter any that can be changed. It also would consider the implications any intervention might have for further control of women's choices and actions—for instance, by reducing a pregnant woman, in extreme cases, to the status of "fetal container" or "incubator."
> 5. Finally, a **case-based approach** would consider whether there are any relevant similar cases that constitute precedents for the current one. For instance, an obstetrician–gynecologist may wonder whether to seek a court order for a cesarean delivery that he or she believes would increase the chances of survival for the child-to-be but that the pregnant woman continues to reject. In considering what to do, the physician may ask, as some courts have asked, whether there is a helpful precedent in the settled consensus of not subjecting a nonconsenting person to a surgical procedure to benefit a third party, for instance, by removing an organ for transplantation.†
>
> *Harris LH. Rethinking maternal-fetal conflict: gender and equality in perinatal ethics. Obstet Gynecol 2000;96:786–791. In American College of Obstetricians and Gynecologists. Ethical Decision Making in Obstetrics and Gynecology. ACOG Committee Opinion 390. Washington DC: American College of Obstetricians and Gynecologists, 2007. Used with permission.
> †In re A.C., 572 A.2d 1235 (D.C. Ct. App. 1990).

expertise in this determination (psychologists, psychiatrists, or others), by attorneys, or by a judge. Understanding the difference between patient capacity and patient competency is crucial in emotion-filled, difficult clinical decision-making situations. If a patient is determined to be legally incompetent, or if the physician believes the patient does not have the capacity for decision making, a **surrogate decision maker** must be identified. In the absence of a durable power of attorney, family members may be called on to render proxy decisions. In some situations, the court may be called upon to appoint a guardian.

A surrogate decision maker should strive to make the decision that the patient would have wanted or, if the patient's wishes are not known, that will promote the best interests of the patient. In emergency situations, physicians may have to assume this role for a limited time while an appropriate decision maker is identified. In the obstetric setting, a pregnant woman is considered the appropriate decision maker for the fetus that she is carrying.

2. *Collect data* in as objective a manner as possible. Consultation is often useful to facilitate this task.
3. *Identify and evaluate all medically appropriate management options*.
4. *Systematically evaluate these options.* After elimination of any unethical options, the remaining choices are reviewed, and the "best management" is chosen. The values of the patient generally will be the most important consideration as decision making proceeds.
5. *Identify ethical conflicts and set priorities.*
6. *Select the option that can best be justified.*
7. *Reevaluate the decision after it is acted on based on the clinical outcomes.* If the management did not adequately resolve the problem, a reevaluation of all the information and another management plan may be used. Valuable questions at this time include, "Was the best possible decision made?" and "What lessons can be learned from the discussion and resolution of the problem?"

It is important for the individual physician to find or develop guidelines for decision making that can be applied consistently in facing ethical dilemmas. The American College of Obstetricians and Gynecologists (College) and many other such professional organizations provide guidelines that often facilitate this important task for physicians.

Sometimes, however, a medical or surgical management results in an adverse and/or unexpected outcome. Offering the physician's best, honest understanding of what happened and why to the patient (and her family and other stakeholders) is a clear ethical responsibility of physicians, as is the clear documentation of this discussion in the medical record. When the patient or patient's family questions this explanation, the specter of medical liability (sometimes misidentified as medical malpractice) looms.

MEDICAL LIABILITY

When an outcome is perceived to be less than optimal, a medical liability action (i.e., lawsuit) could ensue. Such situations are best prevented by the practice of evidence-based medicine as well as clear, honest, and complete communication between patient and physician. Appropriately detailed documentation in the medical record is very important.

Informed Consent

Providing "informed consent" is actually a process that is a component of the care that should be provided by all physicians every day with every patient. Simply stated, it involves the physician apprising a woman of the various options available for both her preventive care and specific problems. The process of informed consent is the responsibility of the physician and cannot be delegated to others. Discussion should also cover the findings and information that is presently known as well as any further investigations that may be recommended, including their indications, risks, benefits, and alternatives. The patient should also be made aware that she has the option of no treatment. If another physician's assistance is desired, a consultation or referral may be of benefit. Throughout these discussions, the patient is given the opportunity to ask questions which the physician answers fully. This process spans each action of every physician from giving an aspirin for a headache to major surgery. In actual practice, **informed consent** is of particular importance as part of major management decisions and procedures, such as childbirth and surgery. Appropriate documentation of the process includes the signing of an **informed consent form** that states that the above process has been followed and that the patient agrees to the suggested management plan (or to no treatment at that time). The patient, a witness, and, usually, the physician sign the document that is placed in the medical record. Often a copy is given to the patient.

Sometimes, however, the patient or family still questions the decisions and outcomes. In this circumstance, medical liability litigation may ensue.

Confidentiality

Respect for autonomy includes the patient's right to decide how and to whom their personal information will be shared. Breaches of confidentiality undermine trust in the patient–clinician relationship and ultimately patient care. In rare cases, breaches may be justified to protect the patient from serious harm.

Conflicts of Interest

Potential conflicts of interest should be resolved with the best interest of the patient in mind. The prescription of drugs, devices, or treatments should be based on medical indications and should not be affected by direct or indirect interests or commercial promotions from pharmaceutical firms or other third parties. The health care provider should disclose any actual or potential conflict of interest that may be viewed as significantly affecting the patient's care. Consultation with other practitioners or an ethics committee may be warranted.

Medical Liability Action

Medical liability action can be a significant source of fear and anxiety for the physician. Understanding the components of such an action is helpful, as is the recognition that in the current system of jurisprudence, a lawsuit can be brought by the patient or family irrespective of the actual quality of medical care rendered. Obtaining assistance from resources such as the "risk manager" of the health care system or practice as well as legal counsel is vital.

The components of a legal action vary from state to state, but some are common in most situations:

- A **certificate of merit**, a short written statement, usually by a physician knowledgeable in the issues of the action, saying that there is sufficient information to support a medical liability action, must be approved by a court in order for litigation to proceed.
- The **plaintiff(s)** (the patient or sometimes the family of the patient) and the **defendant(s)** (the physician[s], hospital[s], and/or health care system involved in the case) are identified.
- The plaintiff files a **complaint** specifying what the plaintiff believes to be wrong and why.
- Counsel for each party requests the **medical records** and any other relevant information (laboratory records, billing and financial records, and some communications). Some information is considered **exempt** (**privileged**, i.e., it cannot be used) such as communications with counsel.

Expert witnesses are retained by each party. They are expected to be knowledgeable about the medicine involved in the case. They should not be influenced by who retains them or how much they are paid for their services. In practice, experts often serve as advocates for the client represented by the attorney who hired the expert. Many professional organizations now provide guidelines for these individuals. The College does publish such guidelines. The opinions of these individuals are to be based solely on the medical information and their knowledge of the issues.

Differentiating between Maloccurrence and Malpractice
Medical maloccurrence is defined as undesirable outcome irrespective of the quality of care provided. For an outcome to be considered **medical malpractice**, it must be demonstrated to have resulted from negligence (i.e., the care provided fell below the expected standard of care).

Medical malpractice differs from medical maloccurrence by the demonstration of negligence.

After review of all available information and the opinions of the expert witnesses, counsel for the plaintiff and defendant have three primary options: 1) agree upon a **settlement**, with a specific financial compensation being given to the plaintiff, usually not involving public disclosure; 2) agree that the case for malpractice is inadequate with the result that the complaint is withdrawn ("dropped") usually without public disclosure; and 3) disagree about whether or not malpractice has occurred, resulting in the matter being taken to **court** where a trial ensues.

● PATIENT SAFETY

In the Institute of Medicine report, "To Err Is Human: Building a Safer Health System in 2000," patient safety and medical errors were noted to play a significant role in patient injury and death. As a result, patient safety and error reduction have become paramount for health care professionals and health care systems.

Patient safety refers to a systems analysis of medical errors that maintains individual accountability while minimizing individual blame. The first set of National Patient Safety Goals was established by the Joint Commission in 2003 and is modified annually. The goals are designed to be explicit, evidence based, and measurable.

The American College of Obstetricians and Gynecologists promotes the following six principles to promote patient safety.

1. ***Develop a culture of patient safety*** focusing on systems of care instead of individuals. According to the Agency for Healthcare Research and Quality, effective safety cultures include the following:
   - Acknowledgment of the high-risk nature of an organization's activities and the determination to achieve consistently safe operations.
   - A blame-free environment (also known as a *just culture*) where individuals are able to report errors or near misses without fear of reprimand or punishment.
   - Encouragement of collaboration across ranks and disciplines to seek solutions to patient safety problems.
   - Organizational commitment of resources to address safety concerns.

2. ***Implement recommended safe medication practices*** to improve legibility of written notes, ensure completeness of medical orders, avoid nonstandard abbreviations, "Always lead, never follow" (use a leading 0 for doses less than 1 unit [e.g., 0.1, not .1] and never use a trailing 0 after a decimal point [e.g., 1 mg, not 1.0 mg]), provide reasons for giving medication as well as parameters for prn drugs, and limit verbal orders to urgent situations, making sure they are written by the receiving individual.

3. ***Reduce the likelihood of surgical errors*** by using preprocedure verification processes, marking the operative site, and performing "time outs" before surgery (see Figure 3.1).

4. ***Improve handwashing*** to try to reduce the 90,000 patient deaths related to hospital-associated infections.

5. ***Improve communications with health care providers*** ensuring complete and accurate information, especially during transitions of care. The most common cause of preventable adverse outcome is communication error. A **hand-off**, or *sign-out*, is the transfer of patient information from one responsible provider or team to another. Hand-offs should be interactive with the opportunity for the receiving provider/s to ask questions and clarify points of care. Using standardized medical terminology avoids errors in communication. The setting for hand-offs must be free of distractions to enhance communication and decrease interruptions. Patient confidentiality must be maintained, and only those involved in the care of the patient should be privy to protected health care information. The hierarchy of personnel, particularly in teaching settings, may also interfere with the transfer of important information. Every

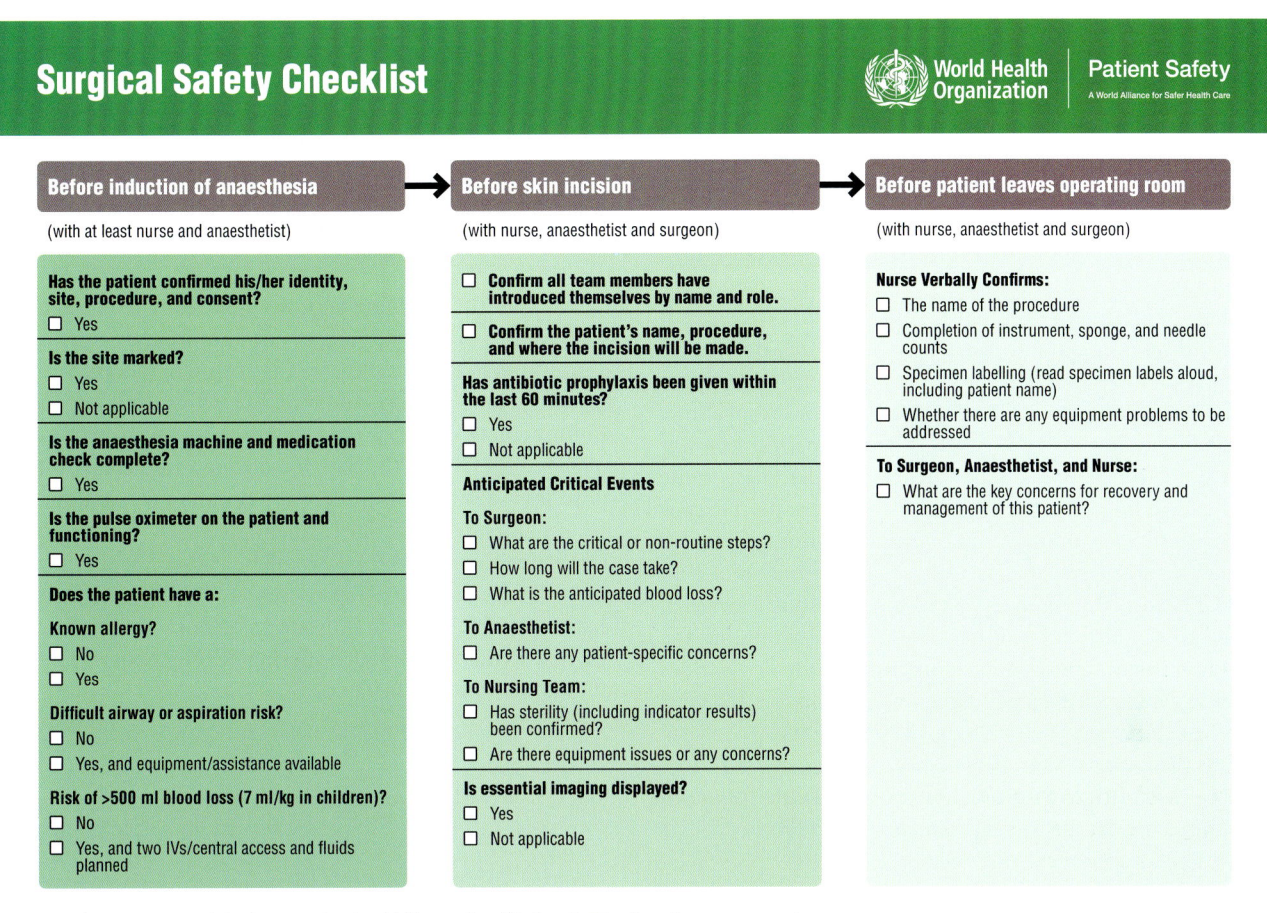

FIGURE 3.1. The WHO Surgical Safety Checklist.
From the WHO Surgical Safety Checklist. Retrieved from http://www.who.int/patientsafety/safesurgery/checklist/en/. Copyright World Health Organization 2009. All rights reserved.

member of the health care team that is present should be encouraged to participate. The method of communication may be a significant barrier to the effective transfer of vital information. Structured forms of communication such as the situation-background-assessment-recommendation technique should be considered so as to ensure that all members of the interprofessional team are speaking the same language. Critical attention to all aspects of patient hand-off is crucial to the development of a culture of safety.

6. **Improve communication with patients** by establishing a partnership and creating a meaningful dialogue, which is paramount to the physician–patient relationship. Improving communication with patients, listening to their concerns, and facilitating active partnerships should be central to any patient safety strategy. Providers should speak slowly, use nonmedical language, and not only allow but encourage questions.

Informed consent is a process of communication—not merely a form or sheet of paper that requires a signature. With informed consent, the patient should understand her diagnosis, recommended treatment, potential complications, and treatment options. She should always be made aware that she has the right to refuse treatment. In reality, clinical decision making is a continuum with the physician leading the discussion on one end and patients making the decision on the other end. Physicians need to inform patients how test results will be communicated, in both outpatient and inpatient locations. Lab results tracking strategies should be developed for the office and may include logbooks or computer prompts. The goal should be to communicate every test result to the patient on a timely basis. When the patient is hospitalized, the physician is obligated to use the hospital information system and inform the patient of results and their meaning when they become available. Improved communication with patients helps strengthen the physician–patient relationship that has been shown to increase patient satisfaction, increase diagnostic accuracy, increase compliance with therapeutic recommendations, and improve quality of care.

CLINICAL FOLLOW-UP

At the patient's first visit, you determine that she does not use female vaginal hygiene products, has not changed her bathing materials including soap, and has no allergies. Her medical history is negative, including, specifically, diabetes. Her pelvic examination is negative with no discharge, lesions, etc. You perform a series of screening and diagnostic tests. Upon her return visit, you note that all the tests were negative. She again complains that the discharge continues. Your repeat pelvic examination with wet preparations is again unrewarding. Because of the association of recurrent symptoms of foul-smelling vaginal discharge without diagnosis with the possibility of sexual abuse, or perhaps even assault, you use your best empathic communication skills to probe this issue further. Initially, she is quite resistant, reminding you of her legal rights and your peril in proceeding with further unimportant questions. Although you are aware that this strongly stated request is entirely consistent with her ethical right of autonomy, you are simultaneously aware of your ethical responsibilities of beneficence, understanding the growing harm with failure to recognize an episode or episodes of sexual violence. She begrudgingly gives permission for your office counselor to join the discussion and, finally, the young lady discloses a sexual assault by a coworker after an office happy hour 3 days before the first visit to her general physician when *T. vaginalis* was discovered. Tearfully, she said that she had told nobody of the assault because she was ashamed that she had not taken the obvious precautions to prevent such an attack. She continues that she is sure that you are failing to find the "dirty" infection she knows she still has. You and your staff immediately begin therapy for her now recognized rape trauma syndrome, assuring her she is not at fault and supporting her desire for health. You indicate that you will remain available to her and arrange a follow-up visit, but with support she agrees to an immediate visit to a rape treatment program that your staff arranged for later in the day. You also receive permission to disclose this information to the rape trauma program and also to her general physician. She further agrees that she needs to make a police report that you know will be part of the first evaluation she will receive at the trauma center. While remaining deeply distressed, she is able to indicate some hope for the future, noting that so many people are offering help without any indication of judgment of "her behavior."

thePoint® Visit http://thePoint.lww.com/activate for an interactive USMLE-style question bank and more!

CHAPTER 4
Embryology and Anatomy

Students should be able to describe basic development of the early human embryo, particularly as it relates to reproductive anatomy. They should be able to describe normal prepubertal, reproductive, and menopausal anatomy of the reproductive tract.

CLINICAL CASE

You are performing a total abdominal hysterectomy and bilateral salpingo-oophorectomy on a patient with a diagnosis of severe endometriosis and chronic disabling pelvic pain that inhibits a normal professional or personal lifestyle and is unresponsive to nonnarcotic analgesia. You have found dense pelvic adhesions, especially in the areas of the posterior cul-de-sac, disrupting normal anatomic relationships. Your dissection has proceeded through the utero-ovarian ligaments and is now approaching the level of the cervical os. You are concerned about inadvertent damage to the ureter because of the difficulty in dissection of the dense adhesions as well as the possibility of alteration of the normal anatomic relationships, especially that of the ureter. Supracervical hysterectomy is not an option because the patient has had severe cervical dysplasia and cervical conization. A preoperative discussion about the possible need for supracervical hysterectomy in the event of dense adhesions had also revealed the patient's firm desire for removal of the cervix due to the stress involved in her past workup for dysplasia, its treatment, and current follow-up.

INTRODUCTION

An understanding of reproductive anatomy and its developmental precursors is important for learners in their ability to apply basic diagnostic and therapeutic principles in patient care.

Knowledge of the embryology and anatomy of the female genital system is helpful in understanding both normal anatomy and the congenital anomalies that occur. Embryology may be useful in many areas of gynecologic and obstetric practice. For example, in gynecologic oncology, embryology can assist clinicians in predicting the growth and routes of spread of gynecologic cancers; in urogynecology and pelvic reconstructive surgery, it can enhance a surgeon's comprehension of the components of pelvic support and possible defects. It can also play a key role in understanding and diagnosing various aspects of sexual dysfunction.

Note: Throughout this chapter, "weeks of gestation" and "weeks of development" are used to describe embryologic events. *Weeks of gestation* is generally based on last menstrual period, whereas *weeks of development* connote post-fertilization age. Clarification and consistency here are important.

EMBRYOLOGY

The ovaries, fallopian tubes, uterus, and upper portion of the vagina are derived from the intermediate mesoderm, whereas the external genitalia develop from genital swellings in the pelvic region. Beginning in the fourth week (post-fertilization) of development, the intermediate mesoderm forms the **urogenital ridges** along the posterior body wall. As their name implies, these ridges contribute to the formation of the urinary and genital systems (Fig. 4.1). The gonads, genital ducts, and external genitalia all pass through an indifferent (undifferentiated) stage in which it is not possible to determine sex based on the appearance of these structures. The genetic sex of an embryo is determined by the sex chromosome (X or Y) carried by the sperm that fertilizes the oocyte. The Y chromosome contains a gene called *SRY* (**sex-determining region on Y**) that encodes a protein called **testis-determining factor**. When this protein is present, the embryo develops male sex characteristics. The ovary-determining gene is *WNT4*; when this gene is present and *SRY* is absent, the embryo develops female characteristics. Gonads become structurally male or female by the 7th week of development, and external genitalia become differentiated by the 12th week.

The influence of androgens is crucial in the normal development of the external genitalia. Any condition that increases the level of androgen production in a female embryo will cause developmental anomalies. For example, the genetic disease **congenital adrenal hyperplasia** (**CAH**) causes a decreased production of cortisol that results in a compensatory increase in androgens. The genitalia of female fetuses with CAH are ambiguous, that is, neither normal female nor normal male.

Development of the Ovary

Ovaries are homologous to the testes in the male. Both male and female gonads begin development as **gonadal** or **genital ridges** that form during the fifth week of gestation (not to be confused with weeks of development) from the **urogenital ridges**. Fingerlike bands of epithelial cells project from the surface of the gonad into each gonadal ridge, forming irregularly shaped **primary sex cords**. Growth of these cords into the gonadal ridge results in the creation of an outer cortex and an inner medulla in the indifferent gonad.

Primordial germ cells that give rise to gametes appear in the wall of the yolk sac (now called the *umbilical vesicle*) during the third week of development (see Fig. 4.1). From this location, primordial germ cells migrate along the allantois in the connecting stalk to the dorsal mesentery of the hindgut and then into the gonadal ridges, where they become associated with the primary sex cords by the sixth week. In the female, the primordial germ cells become **oogonia**, which divide by mitosis during fetal life; no oogonia are formed after birth. If the primordial germ cells fail to migrate to the genital ridges, the ovary does not develop.

By approximately the 10th week of development, the undifferentiated gonad has developed into an identifiable ovary. Primary sex cords degenerate, and secondary sex cords or **cortical cords** appear. These cords extend from the surface epithelium into the underlying mesenchyme (Fig. 4.2, right column of figure). By approximately 16 weeks of gestation, cortical cords in the ovary organize into **primordial follicles**. Each follicle eventually consists of an oogonium, derived from a primary germ cell, surrounded by a single layer of squamous follicular cells, derived from the cortical cords. Follicular maturation begins when the oogonia enter the first stage of meiotic division (at which point they are called **primary oocytes**). Oocyte development is then arrested until puberty, when one or more follicles are stimulated to continue development each month (see Chapter 38).

In male embryos, the primary sex cords do not degenerate; instead, they develop into **seminiferous** (or **testis**) **cords** that eventually give rise to the rete testis and seminiferous tubules (see Fig. 4.2, left column of figure). A layer of dense connective tissue (the **tunica albuginea**) separates the seminiferous cords from the surface epithelium, which eventually becomes the testis. Cortical cords do not form in the male embryo.

As they develop, gonads descend from their starting point high up in the primitive body cavity, where they are attached to a mesenchymal condensation called the **gubernaculum**. Ovaries move caudally to a location just below the rim of the true pelvis immediately adjacent to the fimbriated end of the fallopian tubes. The testis, on the other hand, continues to descend, eventually migrating through the anterior abdominal wall just superior to the inguinal ligament. The gubernaculum in the female fetus eventually forms the ovarian and round ligaments (see Figs. 4.2 and 4.3).

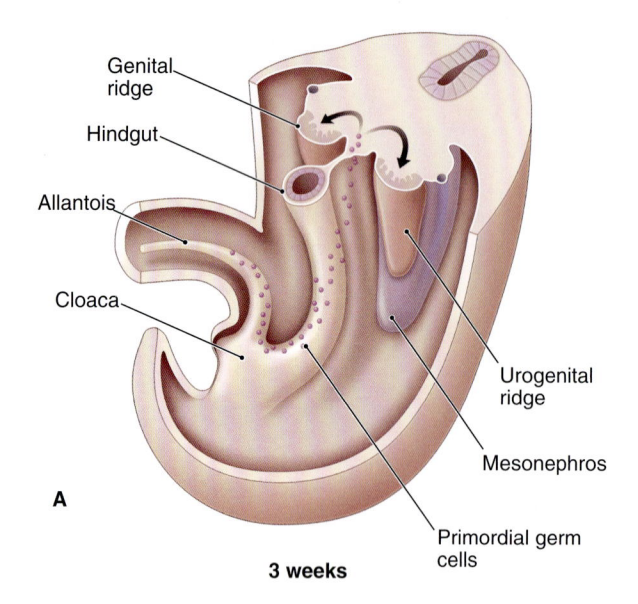

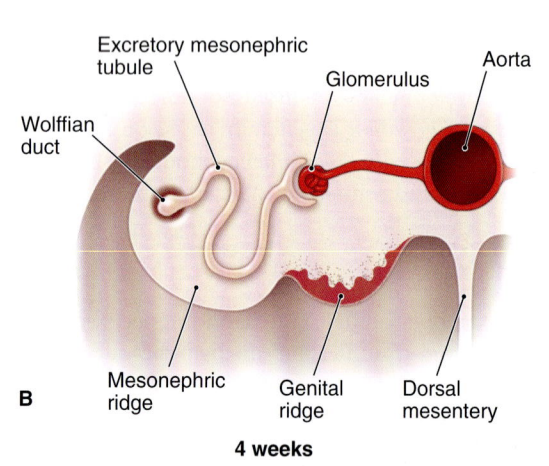

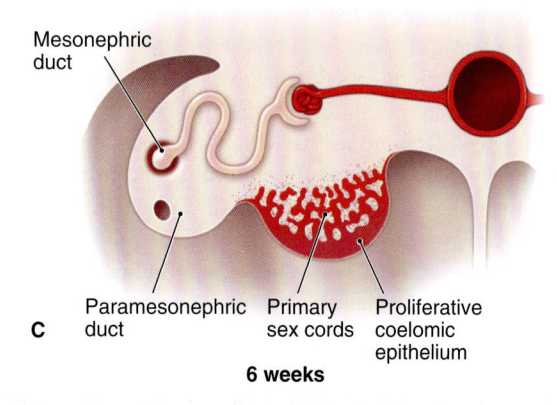

FIGURE 4.1. Early development of the urogenital system. **(A)** Beginning at approximately 3 weeks of gestation, urogenital ridges arise along the posterior wall of the coelomic cavity. Primordial germ cells migrate across the allantois into the genital ridges. **(B)** and **(C)** These transverse sections through the lumbar region of the human embryo show development of the indifferent gonad from the genital ridges at 4 and 6 weeks of gestation. (Modified from Sadler TW. *Langman's Medical Embryology*. 10th ed. Baltimore, MD: Lippincott Williams & Wilkins; 2006:240–241.)

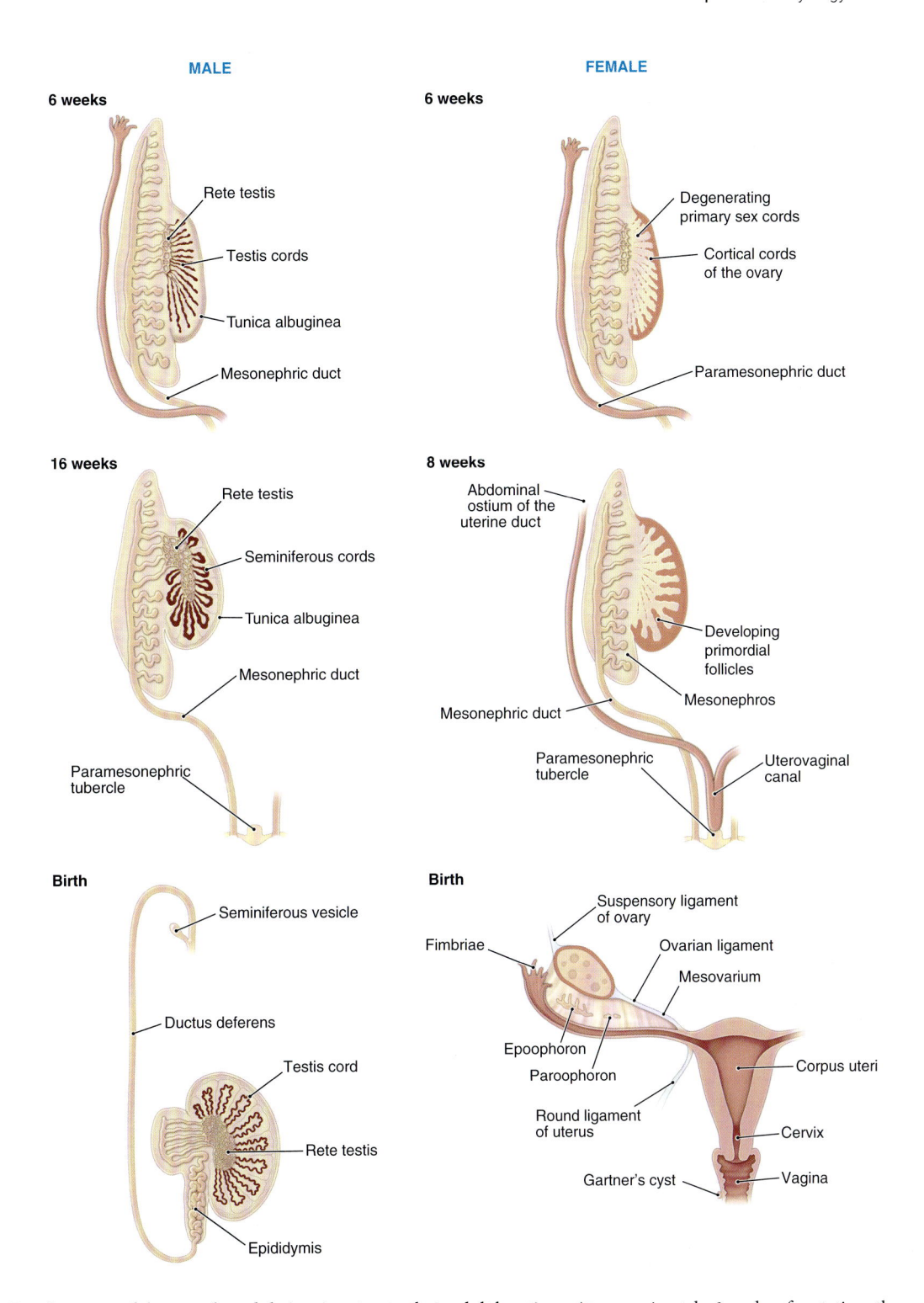

FIGURE 4.2. Development of the gonads and their migration to their adult locations. At approximately 6 weeks of gestation, the gonads have differentiated into either male or female. In male embryos, the mesonephric ducts develop into the main genital tracts (ductus deferens). In female embryos, the paramesonephric ducts develop into the uterus, uterine tubes, and parts of the vagina. (Modified from Sadler TW. *Langman's Medical Embryology.* 10th ed. Baltimore, MD: Lippincott Williams & Wilkins; 2006:243, 245.)

FIGURE 4.3. Route of the migrating gonads in a female fetus. (**A**) At 2 months, the early gonads are located high up in the coelomic cavity attached to the gubernaculum. (**B**) The gubernaculum migrates through the anterior abdominal wall just above the inguinal ligament; this process also takes place in the male embryo. (**C**) The ovaries arrest their descent in the ovarian fossa, immediately subjacent to the uterus on either side. (From Moore KL, Dalley AF. *Clinically Oriented Anatomy*. 5th ed. Baltimore, MD: Lippincott Williams & Wilkins; 2006:Fig. 2.14.)

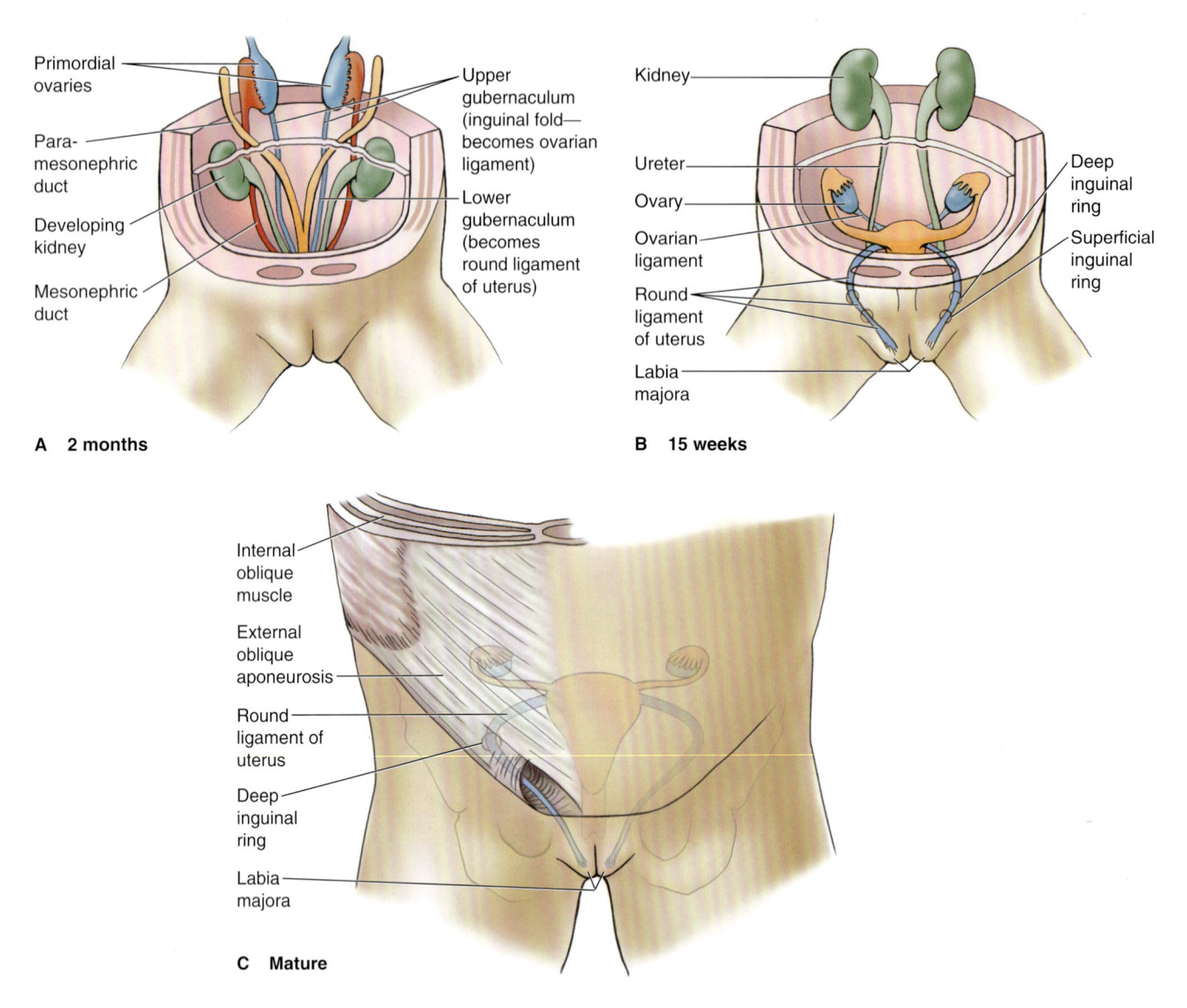

Development of the Genital Ducts

In both male and female embryos, two pairs of ducts develop—the **mesonephric (wolffian)** and **paramesonephric (Müllerian) ducts**. As with the gonad, these ducts pass through an indifferent stage in which both pairs of ducts are present in both the male and the female embryo. Differentiation of the female ductal system is not dependent on development of the ovaries (Fig. 4.4).

In the male embryo, the mesonephric ducts, which drain the embryonic mesonephric kidneys, eventually form the epididymis, ductus deferens, and ejaculatory ducts. In the female embryo, the mesonephric ducts disappear. The paramesonephric ducts persist to form major parts of the female reproductive tract (the fallopian tubes, uterus, and upper portion of the vagina). Paramesonephric ducts begin as invaginations of the epithelium covering the urogenital ridges, eventually forming longitudinally oriented tubes. The cranial end of each duct opens into the body (future peritoneal) cavity. The ducts grow caudally until the two caudal ends contact the posterior wall of the urogenital sinus. This contact induces the posterior wall to proliferate and form the **vaginal plate** that eventually gives rise to the lower portion of the vagina. Meanwhile, the lower ends of the paramesonephric ducts fuse to form the upper portion of the vagina, cervix, and uterus. The cranial portion of each duct remains separated and forms the fallopian tube on each side. As the ducts move toward fusion in the midline, they carry a fold of peritoneum with them that becomes the **broad ligament**.

Development of the External Genitalia

The **cloaca** is formed from a dilatation of the caudal end of the hindgut and is covered exteriorly by the cloacal membrane. Eventually, the cloaca is separated into the urogenital sinus anteriorly and the anorectal canal posteriorly by the **urorectal septum**. This septum forms from a collection of mesoderm in the pelvic floor that grows downward during the fifth to the eighth weeks of gestation to reach the **cloacal membrane**. At the same time, the **genital tubercle** develops at the cranial end of the cloacal membrane, while **labioscrotal swellings** and **urogenital folds** appear on each side (Fig. 4.5A). The genital tubercle enlarges in both the male and the female (Fig. 4.5B). In the presence of estrogens and the absence of androgens, external genitalia are feminized. The genital tubercle develops into the clitoris (Fig. 4.5C). The unfused urogenital folds form the labia minora, and the labioscrotal swellings become the labia majora (Fig. 4.5D). At approximately 15 weeks of gestation, transabdominal ultrasonography can often distinguish between the two sexes.

● ANATOMY

Bony Pelvis

The bony **pelvis** is composed of the paired innominate bones and the sacrum. The innominate bones are joined anteriorly to form the **symphysis pubis**, and each is articulated posteriorly with the sacrum through the sacroiliac joint (Fig. 4.6). The **sacrum** is composed of five or six sacral vertebrae, which are fused in adulthood. The sacrum articulates with the coccyx inferiorly and with the fifth lumbar vertebra superiorly.

The pelvis is divided into the **greater pelvis** (**false pelvis**) and the **lesser pelvis** (**true pelvis**), which are separated by the linea terminalis. The greater pelvis distributes the weight of the abdominal organs and supports the pregnant uterus at term. The greater pelvis is bounded by the lumbar vertebrae posteriorly, an iliac fossa bilaterally, and the abdominal wall anteriorly. The true pelvis contains the pelvic viscera, including the uterus, vagina, bladder, fallopian tubes, ovaries, and the distal rectum and anus. It is formed by the sacrum and coccyx posteriorly and by the ischium and pubis laterally and anteriorly.

In obstetrics, it is important to assess the size of the pelvis to determine whether it appears to be of adequate capacity for vaginal birth. This evaluation is based on the diameters of the pelvic outlet, pelvic inlet, and midpelvis. Measurement of these diameters is called **pelvimetry** and can be estimated during the bimanual portion of the pelvic examination or more accurately measured radiographically with x-ray or computed tomography. One of the most important measurements is that of the **obstetric conjugate** (Fig. 4.7), which is the narrowest

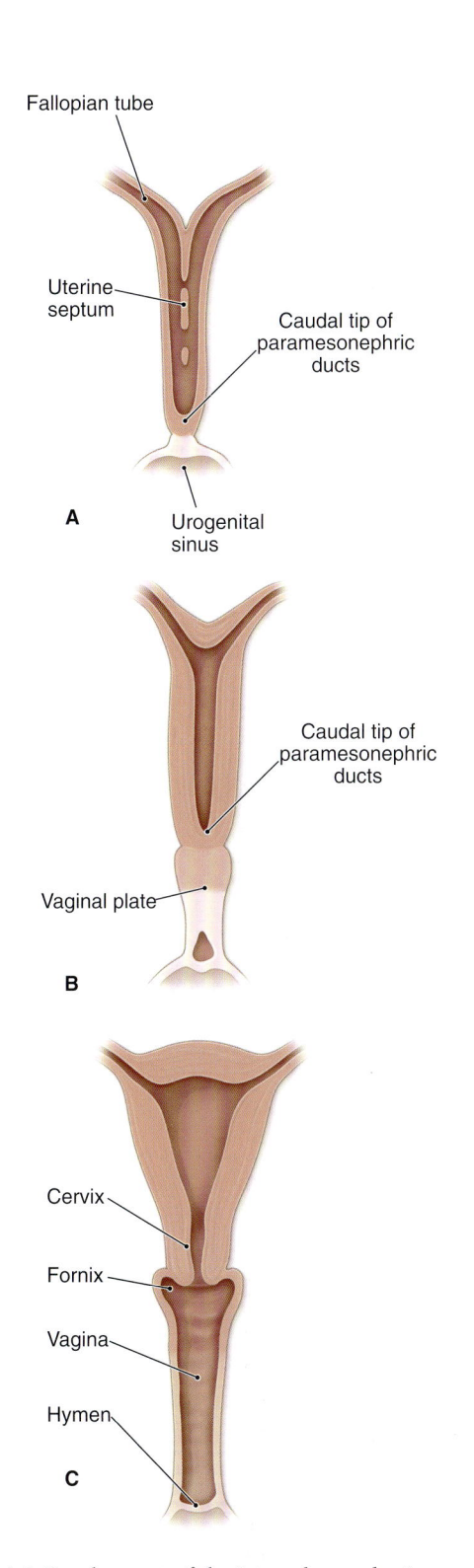

FIGURE 4.4. Development of the internal reproductive organs from the Müllerian ducts in the female embryo. (**A**) Initially, the ducts are separate structures that begin to fuse lengthwise at their caudal ends. (**B**) This fusion creates the lumen of the uterus. Simultaneously, the vagina develops where the urogenital sinus meets the Müllerian ducts, the vaginal plate. (**C**) Eventually, the uterus, cervix, and vagina are formed. (Modified from Sadler TW. *Langman's Medical Embryology*. 10th ed. Baltimore, MD: Lippincott Williams & Wilkins; 2006:246.)

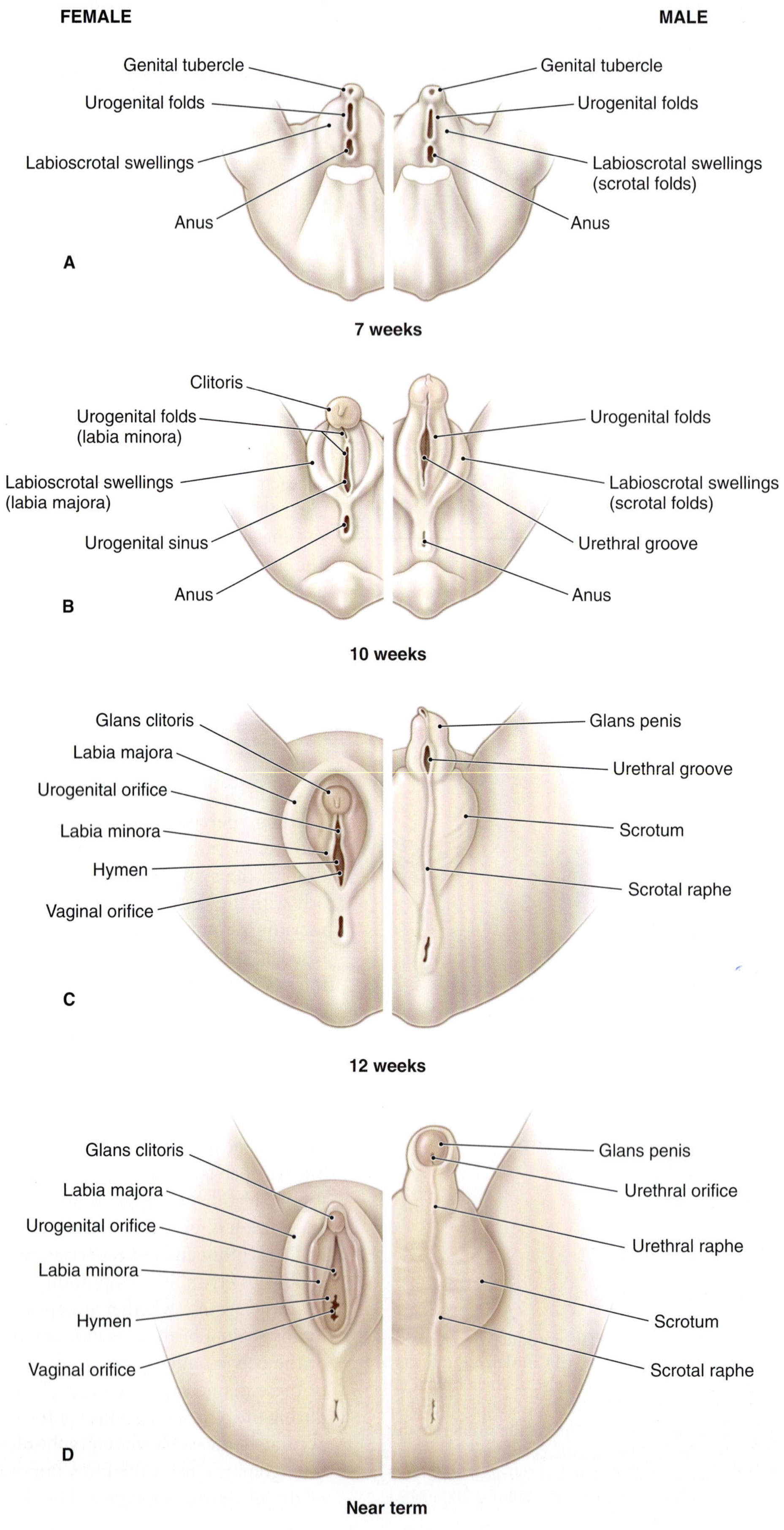

FIGURE 4.5. Comparison of the development of male and female external genitalia. (**A**) Early in gestation, the genital tubercle develops along with labioscrotal swellings and urogenital folds. (**B**) Shortly thereafter, the genital tubercle enlarges in both the male and female fetus. (**C**) The posterior commissure forms, effectively dividing genitals from anus. (**D**) Without the influence of a Y chromosome, the phallus regresses in relative size to form the clitoris.

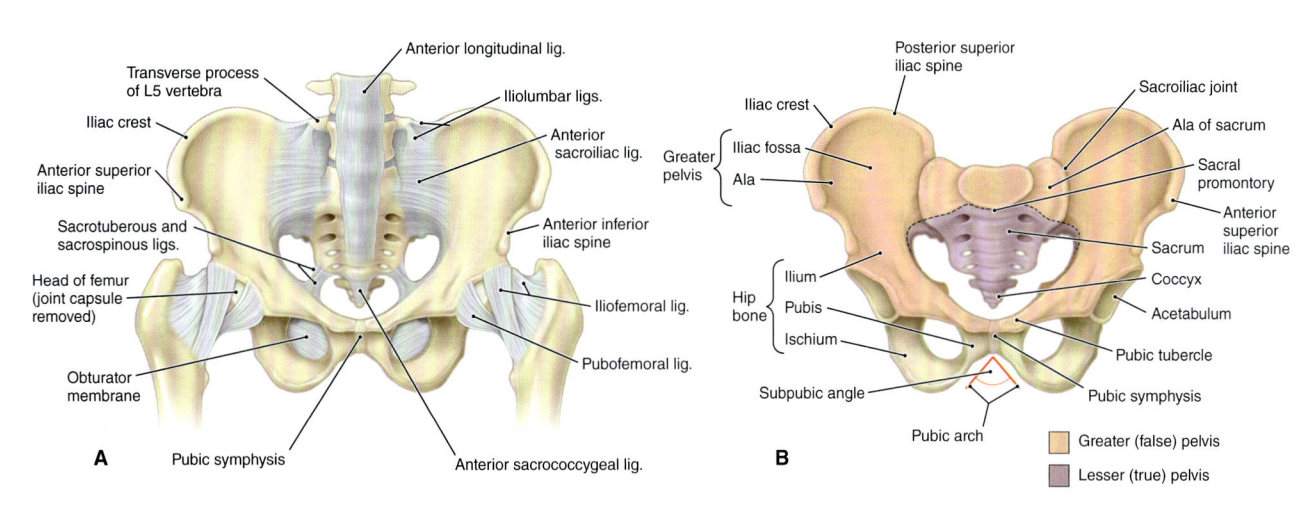

FIGURE 4.6. The bony pelvis. **(A)** Anterior view of the pelvis; the greater and lesser pelves are color-coded. **(B)** The pelvic ligaments are shown in detail. (From Moore KL, Dalley AF. *Clinically Oriented Anatomy*. 5th ed. Baltimore, MD: Lippincott Williams & Wilkins; 2006:Figs. 3.3B and 3.2A.)

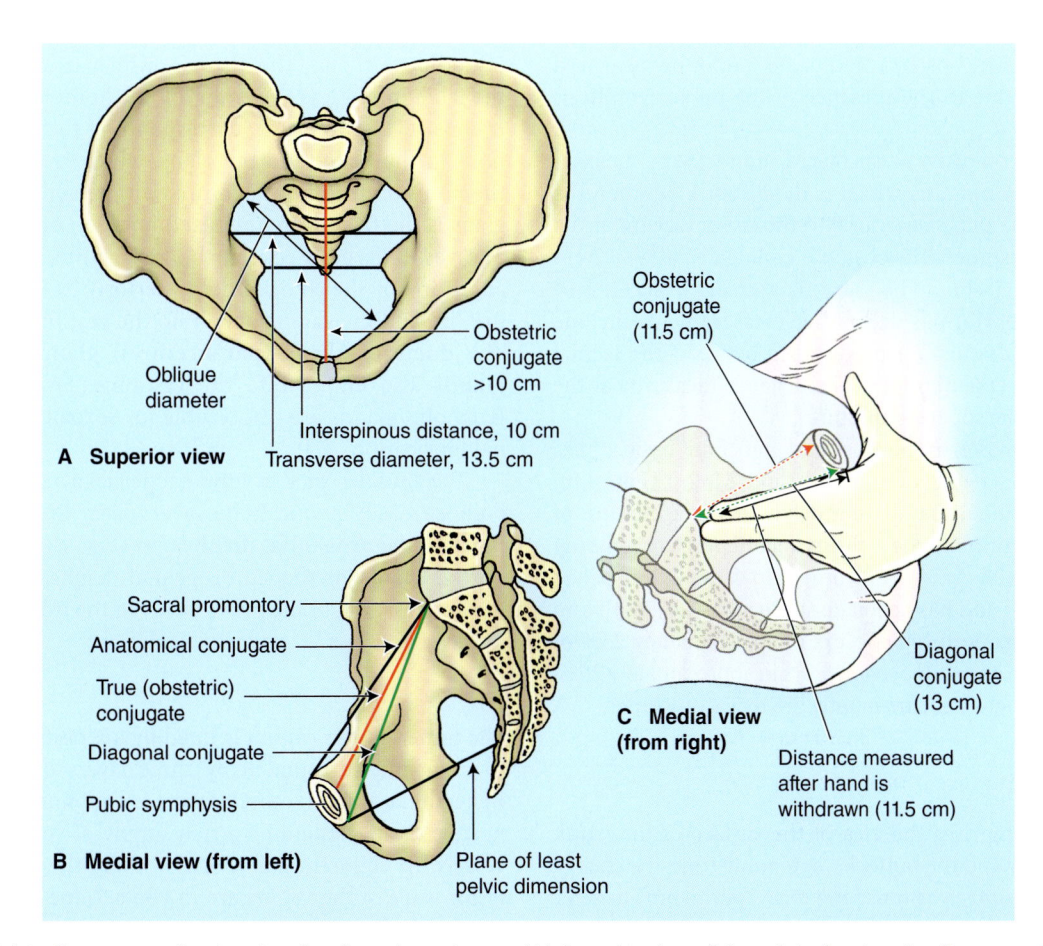

FIGURE 4.7. Pelvic diameters and estimating the obstetric conjugate. **(A)** Superior view of the pelvis showing the diameters that are measured in pelvimetry. **(B)** Medial view of the pelvis demonstrating the diagonal conjugate and the obstetric conjugate. **(C)** Measurement of the obstetric conjugate. The examiner palpates the sacral promontory with the tip of the *middle finger*. The distance between the tip of the *index finger*, which is 1.5 cm shorter than the middle finger, and the place on the hand where the pubic symphysis is felt is measured to yield the obstetric conjugate, which should be at least 11 cm. (From Moore KL, Dalley AF. *Clinically Oriented Anatomy*. 5th ed. Baltimore, MD: Lippincott Williams & Wilkins; 2006:Fig. B3.2.)

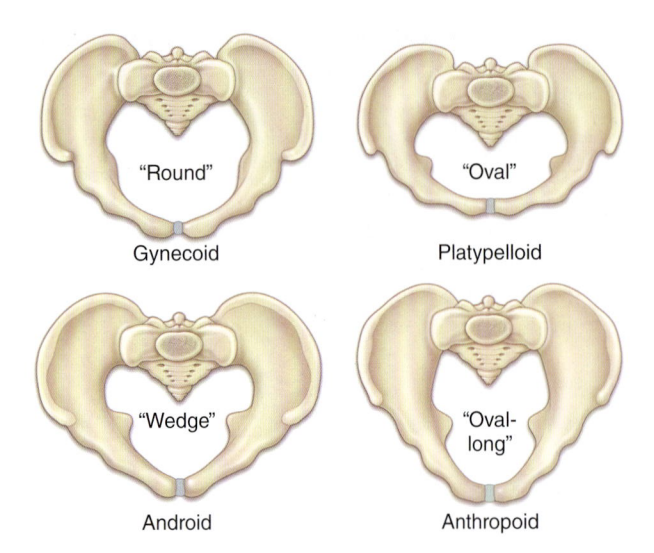

FIGURE 4.8. Caldwell-Moloy pelvic types.

fixed distance through which the fetal head must pass during a vaginal delivery. The obstetric conjugate cannot be measured directly clinically due to the presence of the pubic symphysis and the bladder.

The **obstetric conjugate** is calculated indirectly by measuring the **diagonal conjugate**, which is the distance between the lower border of the pubis anteriorly to the lower sacrum at the level of the ischial spines. The obstetric conjugate is 1.5 to 2 cm shorter. In general, it should be 11.0 cm or greater to accommodate a fetal head of normal size. Other measurements include the **interspinous diameter** (the distance between the ischial spines) and **transverse diameter** (the distance measured at the greatest width of the superior aperture).

The female pelvis may be classified into four basic types, according to the scheme of Caldwell and Moloy (Fig. 4.8), although an individual may have a pelvis that is a mixture of types. The most common type is the **gynecoid pelvis**, occurring in approximately 40% to 50% of women. In general, this pelvic shape is cylindrical and has adequate space along its length and breadth. The **anthropoid** type occurs in approximately 25% of all women, and the **android** pelvis occurs in approximately 20%. The **platypelloid** pelvis occurs in only 2% to 5% of women.

Vulva and Perineum

The **perineum** comprises the area of the surface of the trunk between the thighs and the buttocks, extending from the coccyx to the pubis. Anatomists also use the term "perineum" to refer to the shallow *compartment* that lies deep to this area and inferior to the pelvic diaphragm.

The **vulva** contains the labia majora, labia minora, mons pubis, clitoris, vestibule, and ducts of glands that open into the vestibule (Fig. 4.9). The **labia majora** are folds of skin with underlying adipose tissue, fused anteriorly with the mons pubis and posteriorly at the perineum. The skin of the labia majora contains hair follicles as well as sebaceous and sweat glands. The **labia minora** are narrow skin folds lying inside the

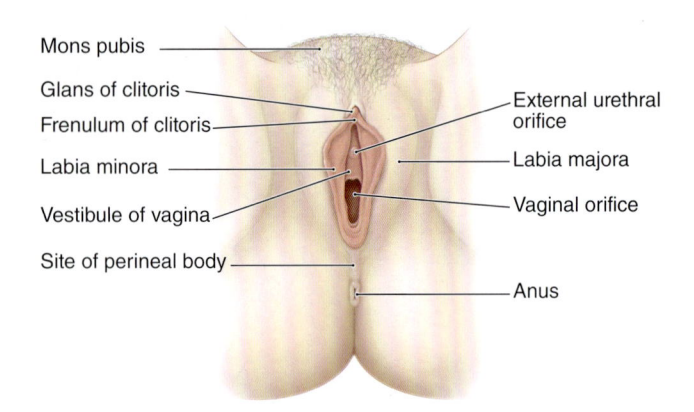

FIGURE 4.9. External female genitalia.

labia majora. The labia minora merge anteriorly with the prepuce and frenulum of the clitoris and posteriorly with the labia majora and the perineum. The labia minora contain sebaceous and sweat glands but no hair follicles, and there is no underlying adipose tissue. The **clitoris**, which is located anterior to the labia minora, is the embryologic homologue of the penis. It consists of two crura (corresponding to the corpora cavernosa in the male) and the glans, which is found superior to the point of fusion of the crura. On the ventral surface of the glans is the **frenulum**, the fused junction of the labia minora. The vestibule lies between the labia minora and is bounded anteriorly by the clitoris and posteriorly by the perineum. The urethra and the vagina open into the vestibule in the midline. The **ducts of Skene (paraurethral) glands** and **Bartholin glands** also empty into the vestibule. Secretions from the Bartholin glands are responsible for sexually stimulated vaginal lubrication.

The muscles of the vulva (superficial transverse perineal, bulbocavernosus, and ischiocavernosus) lie superficial to the fascia of the **urogenital diaphragm** (Fig. 4.10). The vulva rests on the triangular-shaped urogenital diaphragm, which lies in the anterior part of the pelvis between the ischiopubic rami.

The Vagina

The lumen of the **vagina** is lined by a stratified squamous epithelium and surrounded by three layers of smooth muscle. Beneath the smooth muscle layers is a submucosal layer of connective tissue containing a rich supply of veins and lymphatic vessels. In children and young women, the anterior and posterior walls of the vagina are in contact due to the presence of submucosal rugae.

Because the vagina is collapsed, it appears H-shaped in cross section. The underlying rugae connect to the tendinous arch of the pelvic fascia, which is the major support of the walls of the vagina and help maintain its normal architecture. With age and childbirth, the connection between the vaginal walls and the muscular pelvis may weaken or deteriorate, weakening the pelvic floor and causing the surrounding structures (i.e., bladder, rectum, urethra, and uterus) to become less stable.

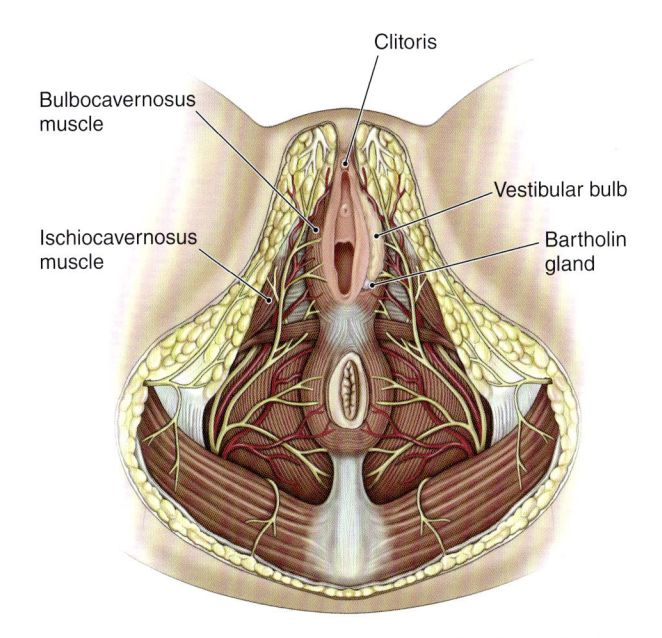

FIGURE 4.10. The urogenital diaphragm with the skin and subcutaneous fat cuts away. The musculature, blood supply, and nerve supply constitute the external part of the pelvic floor.

The **cervix** joins the vagina at an angle between 45° and 90°. The area around the cervix, the fornix, is divided into four regions: the anterior fornix, two lateral fornices, and the posterior fornix. The posterior fornix is in close proximity to the peritoneum that forms the floor of the **posterior pelvic cul-de-sac** (*pouch of Douglas*). The cervical opening to the vagina, the **external os**, is round to oval in women who have not had children but is often a transverse slit after vaginal childbirth. The portion of the cervix that projects into the vagina is covered with stratified squamous epithelium, which resembles the vaginal epithelium. The squamous epithelium of the vaginal aspect of the exocervix changes to the columnar epithelium of the endocervical portion in the **transformation zone**, the most caudal part of which is the original **squamocolumnar junction (SCJ)**. During adolescence and the menstrual years, the SCJ is visible at the upper limit of the transformation zone. As the level of sex steroids falls during menopause, the SCJ passes back up the canal until it is often barely visible, if at all. (The histology of the cervix is discussed in more detail in Chapter 47.)

At its lower end, the vagina traverses the urogenital diaphragm and is then surrounded by the two bulbocavernosus muscles of the vulva. These muscles act as a sphincter. The **hymen**, a fold of mucosa-covered connective tissue, somewhat obscures the external vaginal orifice. The hymen is fragmented into irregular remnants with sexual activity and childbearing. The major blood supply to the vagina is from the **vaginal artery**, a branch of the hypogastric artery, also known as the internal iliac and parallel veins.

Uterus and Pelvic Support

The **uterus** lies between the **rectum** and the **bladder** (Fig. 4.11). Various pelvic ligaments help support the uterus and other pelvic organs. The **broad ligament** overlies the structures and connective tissue immediately adjacent to the uterus. Because it contains the uterine arteries and veins and the ureters, it is important to identify the broad ligament during pelvic surgery. The **infundibulopelvic ligament** connects the ovary to the posterior abdominal wall and is composed mainly of the ovarian vessels. The **uterosacral ligament** connects the uterus at the level of the cervix to the sacrum and is, therefore, its primary support. The **cardinal ligament** is attached to the side of the uterus immediately inferior to the **uterine artery**. The **sacrospinous ligament** connects the sacrum to the iliac spine and is not attached to the uterus. This ligament is frequently used surgically to support the pelvic viscera.

The two major portions of the uterus are the **cervix** and the **body** (**corpus**), which are separated by a narrower isthmus. The length of the cervix is established at puberty. Before puberty, the relative lengths of the body of the uterus and cervix are approximately equal; after puberty, under the influence of increased estrogen levels, the ratio of the body to the cervix changes between 2:1 and 3:1. The junction of the uterus and fallopian tubes is called the **cornu**. The part of the corpus between the cornu is referred to as the **fundus**. In a woman who has had no children, the uterus is approximately 7 to 8 cm long and 4 to 5 cm wide at the widest part. The cervix is relatively cylindrical in shape and is 2 to 3 cm long. The body is generally pear shaped, with the anterior surface flat and the posterior surface convex. In cross section, the lumen of the uterine body is triangular.

The wall of the uterus consists of three layers:

1. The **endometrium**, the inner mucosa, consists of simple columnar epithelium with underlying connective tissue, which changes in structure during the menstrual cycle.
2. The **myometrium**, or middle layer, consists of smooth muscle. This layer becomes greatly distensible during pregnancy; during labor, the smooth muscle in this layer contracts in response to hormonal stimulation.
3. The **serosa**, or outermost layer, consists of a thin layer of connective tissue. It is distinct from the **parametrium**, a subserosal extension of the uterus between the layers of the broad ligament.

The position of the uterus can vary depending on the relationship of a straight axis that extends from the cervix to the uterine fundus to the horizontal. When a woman is in the dorsal lithotomy position, the uterus may be tilted forward (**anteversion**), slightly forward but functionally straight (**midposition**), or tilted backward (**retroversion, RV**). The top of the uterus can also fold forward (**anteflexion**) or backward (**retroflexion, RF**). Five combinations of these configurations are possible (Fig. 4.12). In addition, the uterus may be tilted axially to the right or left. The position of the uterus is clinically important. For example, estimation of gestational age in the late part of the first trimester may be difficult when the uterus is in the retroflexed or retroflexed and retroverted (RVRF or RV) positions. The risk of uterine perforation during procedures such as dilatation and curettage or insertion of an intrauterine device is increased in a woman with a retroflexed or anteflexed uterus.

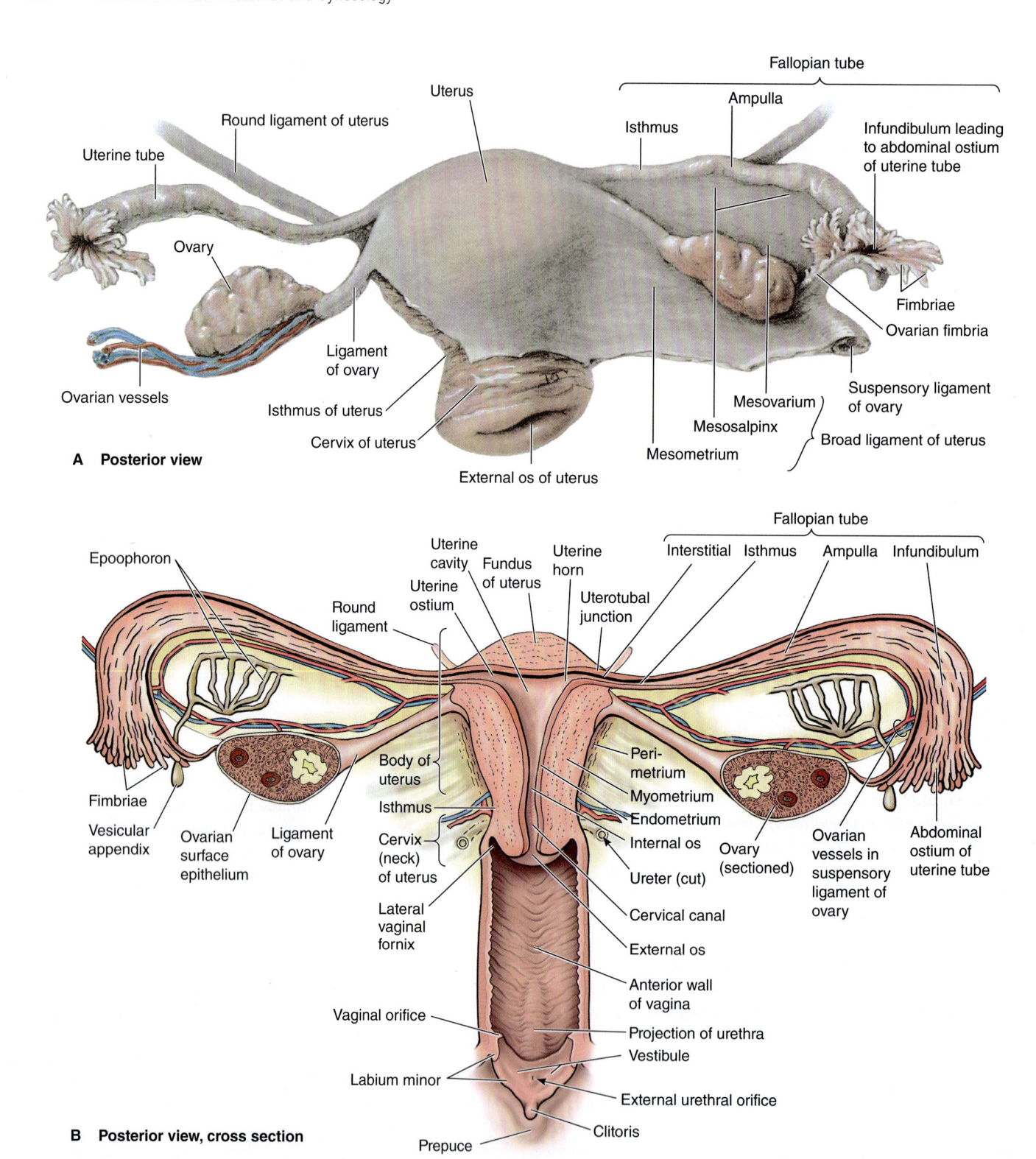

FIGURE 4.11. Internal female reproductive organs. (From Moore KL, Dalley AF. *Clinically Oriented Anatomy*. 5th ed. Baltimore, MD: Lippincott Williams & Wilkins; 2006:Fig. 3.39A&B.)

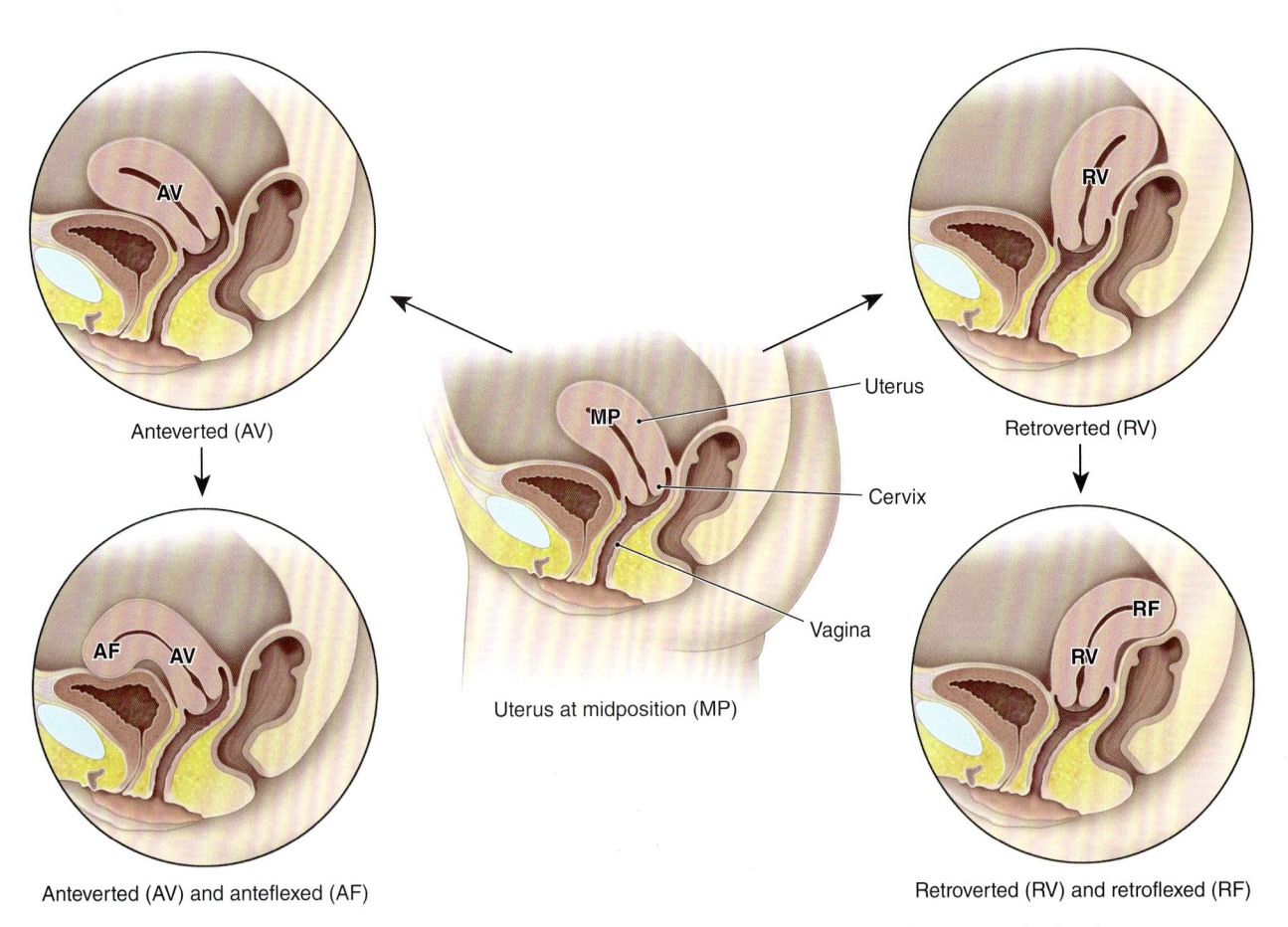

FIGURE 4.12. Positions of the uterus within the pelvis. (From Moore KL, Dalley AF. *Clinically Oriented Anatomy*. 5th ed. Baltimore, MD: Lippincott Williams & Wilkins; 2006:B3.17A-D.)

Applying traction on the cervix to pull the uterine canal into a straight line can greatly reduce this risk.

The blood supply to the uterus comes primarily from the uterine arteries, with a contribution from the ovarian arteries, whereas the venous plexus drains through the uterine vein. Of particular importance in pelvic surgery is the relative position of the uterine arteries to the ureter. The arteries travel in a lateral-to-medial direction at the level of the internal os of the cervix. At the point where they meet the uterus, they overlie the ureter. This proximity can cause inadvertent injury during pelvic surgery. The ureters lie between 1.5 and 3 cm from the uterine sidewall at this point (Fig. 4.13).

Uterine Tubes

The **fallopian (uterine) tubes (oviducts)** are approximately 7 to 14 cm in length and are divided into four portions: the **interstitial** portion of the tube that lies within the wall of the uterus and communicates between the uterine cavity and the next segment of the tube; the **isthmus**, a narrow and straight **segment** that forms the first portion outside the uterine wall; the **ampulla**, a widening central portion; and the **infundibulum**, fringed by the finger-shaped fimbriae that surround the ovary and collect the oocyte at the time of ovulation. The fallopian tubes are supplied by the ovarian and uterine arteries. The epithelial lining of the fallopian tube is ciliated columnar; the cilia beat toward the uterus, assisting in oocyte transport.

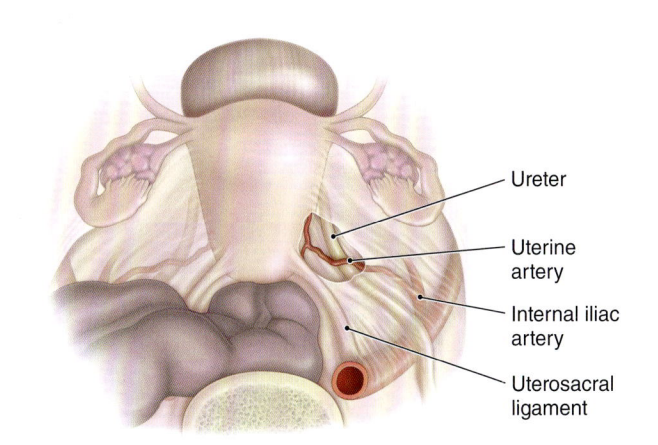

FIGURE 4.13. Relative locations of the ureter and uterine artery. During pelvic surgery, it is important to correctly identify the ureter in order to avoid injury to the uterine artery.

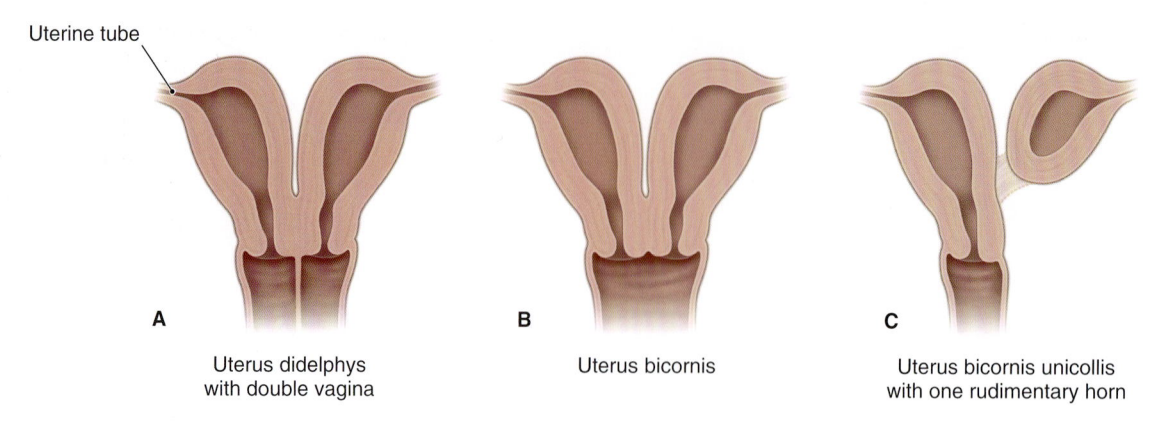

FIGURE 4.14. Uterine and vaginal anomalies. These anomalies result from abnormal or incomplete fusion of the paramesonephric ducts.

Ovaries

Each ovary is approximately 3 to 5 cm long, 2 to 3 cm wide, and 1 to 3 cm thick in the menstrual years. The size decreases by approximately two thirds after menopause, when follicular development ceases. The ovary is attached to the broad ligament by the **mesovarium**, to the uterus by the ovarian ligament, and to the side of the pelvis by the suspensory ligament of the ovary (infundibulopelvic ligament), which is the lateral margin of the broad ligament. The outer ovarian cortex consists of follicles embedded in a connective tissue stroma. Embryologically, this stroma is the medulla that originated as the gonadal ridge, whereas the cortex originated as coelomic epithelium. The medulla contains smooth muscle fibers, blood vessels, nerves, and lymphatics.

The ovaries are mainly supplied by the ovarian arteries, which are direct branches of the abdominal aorta, but there is also a blood supply from the uterine artery, a branch of the hypogastric artery (or internal iliac artery). Venous return via the right ovarian vein is directly into the inferior vena cava and from the left ovary into the left renal vein.

● ANOMALIES OF THE FEMALE REPRODUCTIVE SYSTEM

Anatomic anomalies are infrequent and arise from defects during embryologic development. **Ovarian dysgenesis** or congenital absence is rare except in cases of chromosomal abnormalities. In Turner syndrome (45XO), there are streaks of abnormal ovarian tissues in the pelvis. In the anatomically female patient with a male chromosome compliment (46XY), the gonads only partially descend and can usually be found in the pelvis or even in the inguinal canal.

Much more common are Müllerian (paramesonephric) abnormalities, most of which stem from incomplete or anomalous fusion of the Müllerian ducts. Absence of the uterus occurs when the Müllerian ducts degenerate, a condition called **Müllerian agenesis** (Fig. 4.14). This condition is associated with vaginal anomalies (such as absence of the vagina),

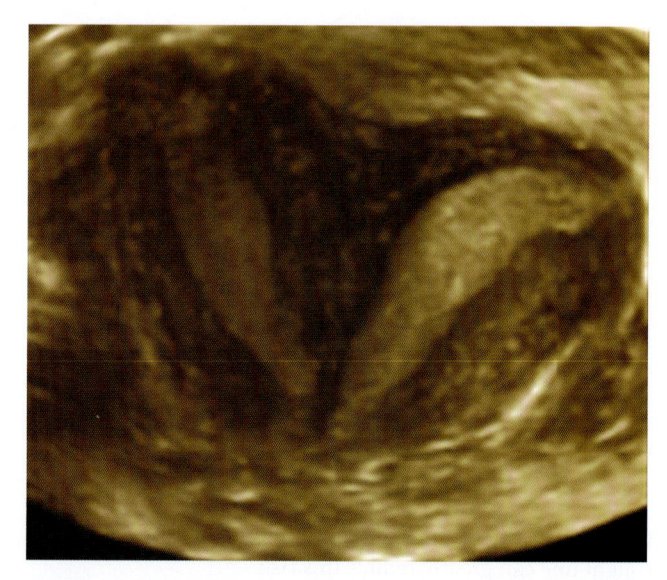

FIGURE 4.15. Reconstructed coronal view of bicornuate uterus.

because vaginal development is stimulated by the developing uterovaginal primordium. Because the vulva and the external portion of the vagina develop from the invagination of the urogenital sinus, the external genitalia can appear normal in these women. A double uterus (**uterus didelphys**) occurs when the inferior parts of the Müllerian ducts do not fuse; this condition may be associated with a double or a single vagina. A **bicornuate uterus** (Fig. 4.15) results when lack of fusion is limited to the superior portion of the uterine body. If one of the ducts is poorly developed, and fusion with the other duct does not occur, the result is a bicornuate uterus with a rudimentary **horn**. This horn may or may not communicate with the uterine cavity.

The mesonephric ducts normally degenerate in the female embryo during development of the reproductive tract. However, remnants of the mesonephric ducts can persist, which can manifest as **Gartner cysts** (Fig. 4.16). These cysts are located along the vaginal wall or within the broad ligament of the uterus.

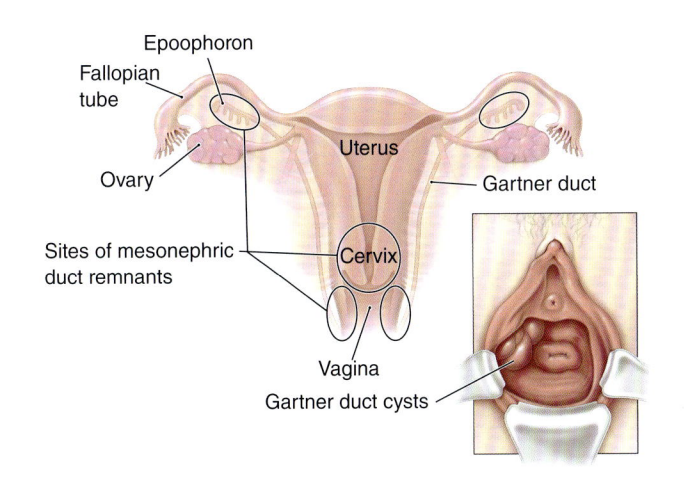

FIGURE 4.16. Gartner cysts. **(A)** These cysts are remnants of the mesonephric ducts that are not completely resorbed during development. **(B)** Gartner cysts are located along the sidewall of the vagina and can be identified during a pelvic examination.

Because the paramesonephric system develops alongside the renal system, when one system is abnormally formed, an abnormality in the other is likewise frequently present. For example, in a woman with renal agenesis on one side, an abnormal fallopian tube is often found. Conversely, despite the functional connection between the ovaries and fallopian tubes, a lack of one does not indicate a probable lack of the other.

CLINICAL FOLLOW-UP

Identification of the uterine arteries guides your surgery, knowing that the arteries travel in a lateral-to-medial direction at the level of the internal os of the cervix. At the point where the arteries meet the uterus, you are aware that they overlie the ureter and that it is at this point that great attention to anatomy is required to avoid inadvertent injury to the ureters. Knowing that the ureters lie between 1.5 and 3 cm from the uterine sidewall at this point, you are guided in your dissection and are able to visually identify the ureters and, thus, protect them during the surgery.

thePoint® Visit http://thePoint.lww.com/activate for an interactive USMLE-style question bank and more!

II Obstetrics

CHAPTER 5
Maternal–Fetal Physiology

This chapter deals primarily with APGO Educational Topic Areas:

TOPIC 8   MATERNAL–FETAL PHYSIOLOGY
TOPIC 13   POSTPARTUM CARE

Students should be able to discuss the normal maternal physiologic and anatomic changes in pregnancy and the postpartum as well as normal fetal physiology. They should understand how these affect common laboratory and radiologic studies.

CLINICAL CASE

You are providing prenatal care for a young couple's first pregnancy that has proceeded without complication through 38 weeks of gestational age. They come to your office for urgent consultation, fearful for the mother's life because of her recently diagnosed heart disease. They request prompt referral to a good cardiologist. Upon taking a careful history, you learn they had traveled to a nearby mountain resort for the weekend, 2,000 feet higher above sea level than here at home. Upon arriving, she had experienced new and very disturbing dyspnea and had been seen in an Urgent Care Clinic where a normal electrocardiogram was obtained, but a chest x-ray was reported as grossly abnormal, with her heart "seriously enlarged and deviated from its normal position" consistent with new, severe heart disease.

● MATERNAL PHYSIOLOGY

Cardiovascular System

The earliest and most dramatic changes in maternal physiology are cardiovascular. These changes improve fetal oxygenation and nutrition.

Anatomic Changes

During pregnancy, the heart is displaced upward and to the left and assumes a more horizontal position as its apex is moved laterally (Fig. 5.1). These position changes are the result of diaphragmatic elevation caused by displacement of abdominal viscera by the enlarging uterus. In addition, ventricular muscle mass increases and both the left ventricle and atrium increase in size parallel with an increase in circulating blood volume. Pregnancy-associated changes in the cardiac position on a chest x-ray may be confused with cardiac pathology until the pregnancy is recognized.

Functional Changes

The primary functional change in the cardiovascular system in pregnancy is a marked increase in **cardiac output**. Overall, cardiac output increases from 30% to 50%, with 50% of that increase occurring by 8 weeks of gestation. In the first half of pregnancy, cardiac output rises as a result of increased stroke volume and, in the latter half of pregnancy, as a result of increased maternal heart rate, whereas the stroke volume returns to near-normal, nonpregnant levels. These changes in stroke volume are due to alterations in circulating blood volume and systemic vascular resistance. Circulating blood volume begins increasing by 6 to 8 weeks of gestation and reaches a peak increase of 45% by 32 weeks of gestation. Systemic vascular resistance decreases because of a combination of the smooth muscle–relaxing effect of progesterone, increased production of vasodilatory substances (e.g., prostaglandins, nitric oxide, and atrial natriuretic peptide), and arteriovenous shunting to the uteroplacental circulation.

However, late in pregnancy, cardiac output may decrease when venous return to the heart is impeded because of vena caval obstruction by the enlarging gravid uterus. At times, in term pregnancy, nearly complete occlusion of the inferior vena cava occurs, especially in the supine position, with venous return from the lower extremities shunted primarily through the dilated paravertebral collateral circulation.

The distribution of the enhanced cardiac output varies during pregnancy. The uterus receives about 2% of the cardiac output in the first trimester, increasing to approximately 20% at term, mainly

43

by means of a relative reduction of the fraction of cardiac output that goes to the splanchnic bed and skeletal muscle. Thus, about one-fifth of the cardiac output goes through the uterus at term increasing the risk from postpartum hemorrhage substantially.

However, the absolute blood flow to these areas does not change, because of the increase in cardiac output that occurs in late pregnancy. During pregnancy, arterial blood pressure follows a typical pattern. When measured in the sitting or standing position, diastolic blood pressure decreases beginning in the 7th week of gestation and reaches a maximal decline of 10 mm Hg from 24 to 26 weeks. Blood pressure then gradually returns to nonpregnant values by term. Resting maternal pulse increases as pregnancy progresses, increasing by 10 to 18 bpm over the nonpregnant value by term. Physiologic changes in blood pressure in midpregnancy may be misunderstood as hypotension unless allowance for gestational age is made.

During labor, at the time of uterine contraction, cardiac output increases approximately 40% above that in late pregnancy, and mean arterial pressure increases by approximately 10 mm Hg. A decline in these parameters following administration of an epidural anesthetic suggests that many of these changes are the result of pain and apprehension. Cardiac output increases significantly immediately after delivery, because venous return to the heart is no longer blocked by the gravid uterus impinging on the vena cava and because extracellular fluid is quickly mobilized.

Symptoms

Although most women do not become overtly hypotensive when lying supine, perhaps 1 in 10 has symptoms that include **dizziness**, **light-headedness**, and **syncope**. These symptoms, often termed the *inferior vena cava syndrome*, may be related to ineffective shunting via the paravertebral circulation when the gravid uterus occludes the inferior vena cava.

Physical Findings

The cardiovascular system is in a hyperdynamic state during pregnancy. Normal physical findings on cardiovascular examination include an **increased second heart sound split with inspiration, distended neck veins,** and **low-grade systolic ejection murmurs**, which are presumably associated with increased blood flow across the aortic and pulmonic valves. Many normal pregnant women have an S_3 gallop, or third heart sound, after midpregnancy. Diastolic murmurs should not be considered normal in pregnancy. Some systolic murmurs may be normal in pregnancy, but diastolic murmurs should always engender evaluation for cardiac pathology.

Diagnostic Tests

Blood pressure assessment is an essential component of each prenatal care visit. These serial blood pressure recordings during pregnancy are influenced by maternal position; therefore, a consistent position should be used during prenatal care, facilitating the recognition of trends in blood pressure during pregnancy and their documentation. Measured blood pressure is highest when a pregnant woman is seated, somewhat lower when supine, and lowest while lying on the side.

In the lateral recumbent position, the measured pressure in the superior arm is about 10 mm Hg lower than that simultaneously measured in the inferior arm. Blood pressures higher than the nonpregnant values for a particular patient should be presumed abnormal pending evaluation.

The normal anatomic changes of the maternal heart in pregnancy can produce subtle, but insignificant, changes in chest radiographs and electrocardiograms (ECGs). In chest radiographs, the cardiac silhouette can appear enlarged, causing a misinterpretation of cardiomegaly. In ECGs, a slight left-axis deviation may be apparent.

Respiratory System

The changes that occur in the respiratory system during pregnancy are necessitated by the increased oxygen demand of the mother and fetus. These changes are primarily mediated by progesterone.

Anatomic Changes

The maternal thorax undergoes several morphologic changes due to pregnancy. The diaphragm is elevated approximately 4 cm by late pregnancy due to the enlarging uterus. In addition, the subcostal angle widens as the chest diameter and circumference increase slightly (see Fig. 5.1).

Functional Changes

Pregnancy is associated with an increase in total body oxygen consumption of approximately 50 mL O_2/minute, which is 20% greater than nonpregnant levels.

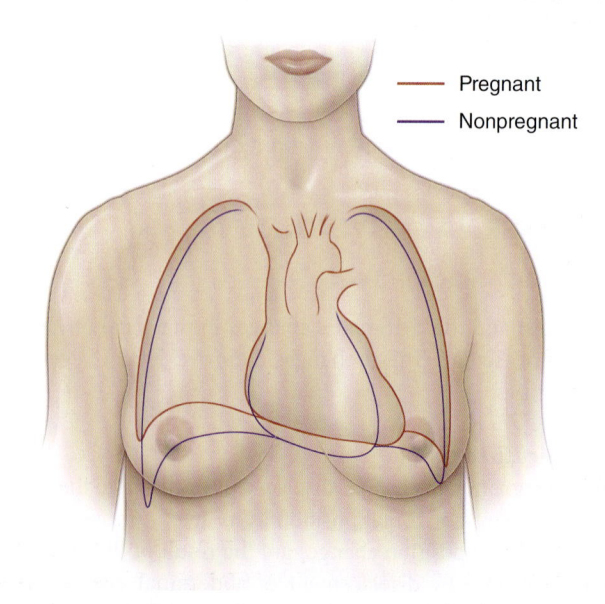

FIGURE 5.1. Changes in the outline of the heart, lungs, and thoracic cage. (Adapted from Bonica JJ, McDonald JS, eds. *Principles and Practice of Obstetric Analgesia and Anesthesia.* 2nd ed. Baltimore, MD: Williams & Wilkins; 1995:47, Fig. 2.)

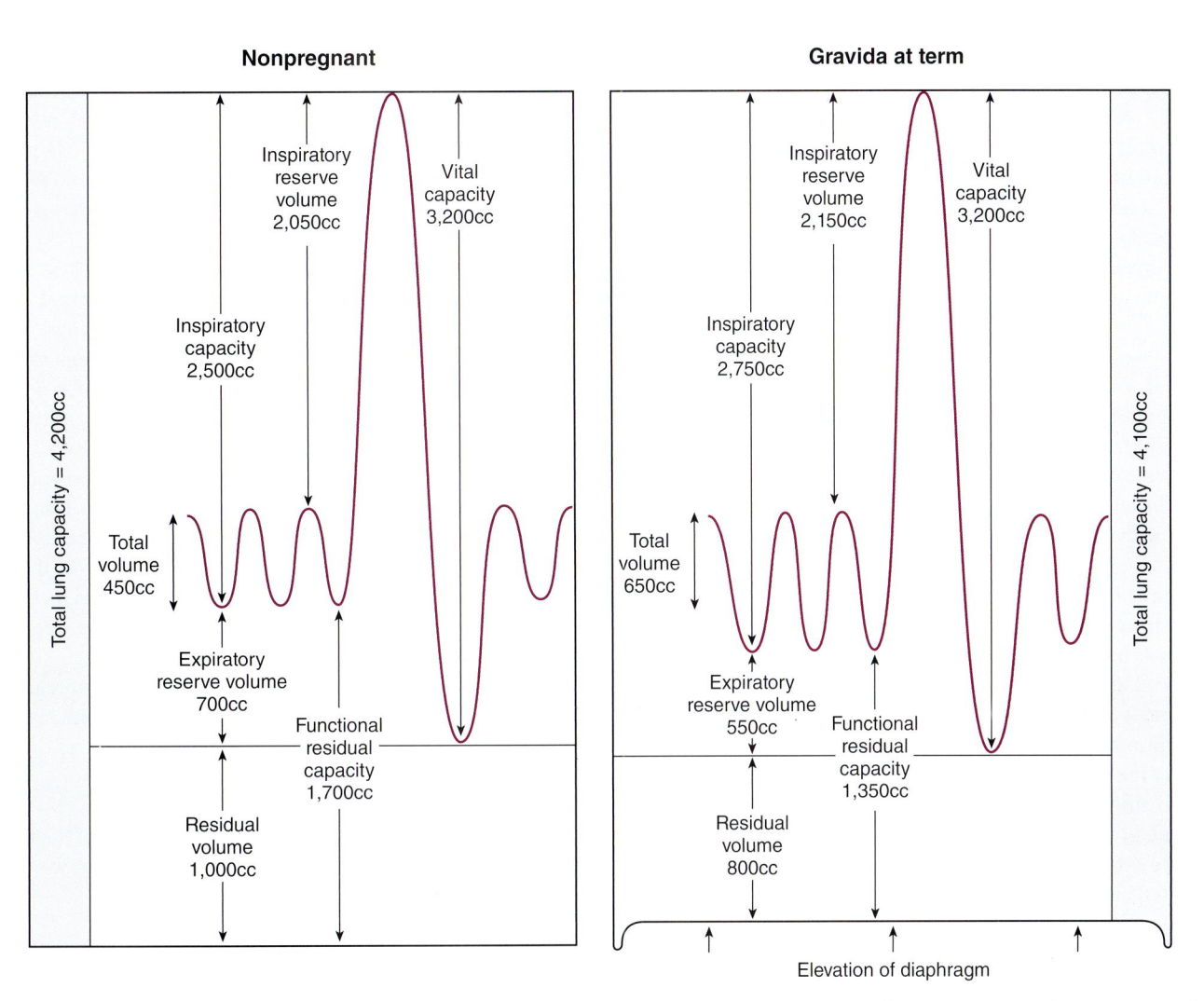

FIGURE 5.2. Pulmonary volumes and capacities in the nonpregnant state and in the gravida at term. Values are given in cubic centimeters (cc). (Adapted from Bonica JJ, McDonald JS, eds. *Principles and Practice of Obstetric Analgesia and Anesthesia*. 2nd ed. Baltimore, MD: Williams & Wilkins; 1995:49, Figs. 2–4.)

Approximately 50% of this increase is consumed by the gravid uterus and its contents, 30% by the heart and kidneys, 18% by the respiratory muscles, and the remainder by the mammary tissues.

Functional adaptations in the pulmonary system enhance oxygen delivery to the lungs. Figure 5.2 lists respiratory volumes and capacities associated with pregnancy. The consequence of diaphragmatic elevation is a 20% reduction in the residual volume and functional residual capacity plus a 5% reduction in total lung volume. Although the maternal respiratory rate is essentially unchanged, there is a 30% to 40% increase in tidal volume due to a 5% increase in inspiratory capacity, resulting in a 30% to 40% increase in minute ventilation.

This significant increase in minute ventilation during pregnancy is associated with important changes in the acid–base equilibrium. Progesterone causes increased central chemoreceptor sensitivity to CO_2, which results in increased ventilation and a reduction in arterial pco_2. The respiratory alkalosis that results from a decreased arterial pco_2 in pregnancy is compensated for by increased renal excretion of bicarbonate, yielding the lower bicarbonate levels normally seen in pregnancy, which means that maternal arterial pH is normal.

Symptoms
Although airway conductance and total pulmonary resistance are reduced in pregnancy, **dyspnea** is common in pregnant women. **Dyspnea of pregnancy** is believed to be a physiologic response to a low arterial pco_2. Dyspnea during pregnancy may be "physiologic" but still requires evaluation insofar as it may also represent coincident respiratory or cardiac illness.

Allergy-like symptoms or chronic colds are also common. Mucosal hyperemia associated with pregnancy results in marked nasal stuffiness and an increased amount of nasal secretions.

Physical Findings
Despite the anatomic and functional changes in the respiratory system during pregnancy, no significant changes in the pulmonary examination are apparent.

Diagnostic Tests

Arterial blood gas assessment during pregnancy normally shows a compensated respiratory alkalosis. Arterial pco_2 levels of 27 to 32 mm Hg and bicarbonate levels of 18 to 31 mEq/L should be considered normal. Maternal arterial pH is maintained at normal levels of 7.40 to 7.45 (Table 5.1).

During normal pregnancy, chest radiography may demonstrate prominent pulmonary vasculature due to the increased circulating blood volume.

Hematologic System

The physiologic adaptations in the maternal hematologic system maximize the oxygen-carrying capacity of the mother to enhance oxygen delivery to the fetus. In addition, they minimize the effects of impaired venous return and blood loss associated with labor and delivery.

Anatomic Changes

The primary anatomic adaptation of the maternal hematologic system is a marked increase in plasma volume, red cell volume, and coagulation factors. Maternal plasma volume begins to increase as early as the sixth week of pregnancy and reaches a maximum at 30 to 34 weeks of gestation, after which it stabilizes. The mean increase in plasma volume is approximately 50% in singleton gestations and greater in multiple gestations. Red cell volume also increases during pregnancy, although to a lesser extent than plasma volume, averaging about 450 mL. Maternal blood volume increases 35% by term.

Adequate iron availability is essential to the increase in maternal red cell volume during pregnancy. The normal pregnant patient requires a total of 1,000 mg of additional iron: 500 mg is used to increase maternal red cell mass, 300 mg is transported to the fetus, and 200 mg is used to compensate for normal iron loss. Because iron is actively transported to the fetus, fetal hemoglobin (Hgb) levels are maintained regardless of maternal iron stores. Supplemental iron use in pregnancy is intended to prevent iron deficiency in the mother not to prevent either iron deficiency in the fetus or to maintain maternal Hgb concentration. To meet maternal iron needs in a woman who is not anemic, 60 mg of elemental iron is recommended daily.

Because iron from dietary sources may not be sufficient, the National Academy of Sciences recommends an iron supplement of 27 mg (present in most prenatal vitamins). In the form of ferrous sulfate, 60 mg of iron is a dosage of 300 mg. Patients who are anemic should receive 60 to 120 mg of iron. Leukocyte count and platelet counts may vary during pregnancy. White blood cell counts typically increase slightly in pregnancy, returning to nonpregnant levels during the puerperium. During labor, the white blood cell count may further increase, primarily from increased granulocytes, presumably linked with stress-associated demargination rather than a true disease-associated inflammatory response. Platelet counts may decline slightly but remain within the normal, nonpregnant range.

The concentration of numerous clotting factors is increased during pregnancy. Fibrinogen (factor I) increases by 50%, as do fibrin split products and factors VII, VIII, IX, and X. Prothrombin (factor II) and factors V and XII remain unchanged. In contrast, the concentration of key inhibitors of coagulation, activated protein C and protein S, decreases.

Functional Changes

During pregnancy, functional adaptations in maternal erythrocytes enable enhanced oxygen uptake in the lungs, allowing increased oxygen delivery to the fetus and promoting co_2 exchange from fetus to mother. The increase in oxygen delivery to the lungs and the amount of Hgb in the blood result in a significant increase in the total oxygen-carrying capacity.

In addition, the compensated respiratory alkalosis of pregnancy causes a shift in the maternal oxygen dissociation curve to the left, a change termed the **Bohr effect**. In the maternal lungs, Hgb affinity for oxygen increases, whereas in the placenta, the CO_2 gradient between fetus and mother is increased, which facilitates transfer of CO_2 from fetus to mother. See pp. 55 to 57 for further discussion.

The risk of thromboembolism doubles during pregnancy, which is considered a **hypercoagulable state**, and increases to 5.5 times the normal risk during the puerperium.

Symptoms and Physical Findings

Some **edema** is normal in pregnancy, and swelling of the hands, face, legs, ankles, and feet may occur. This tends to be worse late in pregnancy and during the summer.

Diagnostic Tests

Pregnancy results in alterations in the normal ranges of several hematologic indices. The disproportionate increase in plasma volume, compared with red cell volume, results in a decrease in Hgb concentration and hematocrit during pregnancy, often referred to as a physiologic anemia. At term, the average Hgb concentration is 12.5 g/dL, compared with approximately 14 g/dL in the nonpregnant state. Values less than 11.0 g/dL are usually due to iron deficiency, but such values should prompt investigation for other kinds of anemia that may occur simultaneously with iron deficiency anemia. Treatment of any anemia should be initiated. The leukocyte count can range from 5,000 to 12,000/L and may increase to as much as 30,000/L during labor and the puerperium. Neither of these higher values is necessarily associated with infection.

The most notable alteration in the coagulation system is increased concentration of fibrinogen, which ranges from 300 to 600 mg/dL in pregnancy, compared with 200 to 400 mg/dL in the nonpregnant state. Despite the prothrombotic state of pregnancy, in vitro clotting times do not change.

Renal System

The renal system is the site of increased functional activity during pregnancy to maintain fluid, solute, and acid–base balance

TABLE 5.1 COMMON LABORATORY VALUES IN EACH TRIMESTER OF PREGNANCY				
	Nongravid	First Trimester	Second Trimester	Third Trimester
Respiratory System				
pH	7.35–7.45	7.40–7.46	—	—
Pao$_2$ (mm Hg)	80–95	75–105	—	—
Paco$_2$ (mm Hg)	35–45	26–32	—	—
HCO^{-3} (mEq/L)	22–26	18–26	—	—
Hematologic System				
Hemoglobin (g/dL)	12–15.5	10.8–14.0	10.0–13.2	10.4–14.0
Hematocrit (%)	36–44	31.2–41.2	30.1–38.5	31.7–40.9
Platelet count (×10^9/L)	140–450	149–357	135–375	121–373
Leukocyte count (×10^9/L)	4.1–11.2	3.9–11.9	5.0–12.6	5.3–12.9
Fibrinogen (g/L)	1.5–4	—	—	3.13–5.53
Renal System				
Sodium (mmol/L)	135–145	131–139	133–139	133–139
Potassium (mmol/L)	3.5–5	3.4–4.8	3.5–4.7	3.7–4.7
Creatinine (μmol/L)	50–100	25–79	25–74	23–93
Urea nitrogen (mmol/L)	6–20	—	6.1–12.1	5.4–15.8
Uric acid (μmol/L)	80–350	75–251	118–250	144–360
Gastrointestinal System				
Albumin, total (g/L)	35–47	33–43	29–37	28–36
Protein, total (g/L)	60–80	58–72	56–64	52–65
Alkaline phosphatase, total (U/L)	41–133	22–91	33–97	73–267
Alanine transaminase	0–35	4–28	4–28	0–28
Aspartate transaminase	0–35	4–30	1–32	2–37
Amylase (U/L)	20–110	11–97	19–92	22–97
Lactate dehydrogenase (U/L)	88–230	217–506	213–525	227–622
Endocrine System				
Thyroxine (T$_4$), total (nmol/L)	64–142	61–153	78–150	59–147
Triiodothyronine (T$_3$), total (nmol/L)	1.5–2.9	1.1–2.7	1.4–3.0	1.6–2.8
Free T$_4$ (pmol/L)	varies by method	8.8–16.8	4.8–15.2	3.5–12.7
Thyrotropin (mU/L)	0.4–6	0–4.4	0–5.0	0–4.2
Cortisol (nmol/L)	140–550	205–632	391–1407	543–1663
Calcium, ionized (mmol/L)	1.1–1.3	1.13–1.33	1.13–1.29	1.14–1.38

Adapted from Gronowski AM. *Handbook of Clinical Laboratory Testing During Pregnancy.* Totowa, NJ: Humana Press; 2004.

in response to the marked activity of the cardiorespiratory systems.

Anatomic Changes
The primary anatomic change of the renal system is enlargement and dilation of the kidneys and urinary collecting system. The kidneys lengthen by approximately 1 cm during pregnancy as a result of greater interstitial volume as well as distended renal vasculature. The renal calyces, pelves, and ureters dilate during pregnancy because of mechanical and hormonal factors. Mechanical compression of the ureters occurs as the uterus enlarges and rests on the pelvic brim. The right ureter is usually more dilated than the left, possibly due to dextrorotation of the uterus and compression from the enlarged right ovarian venous plexus. Progesterone causes relaxation of the smooth muscle of the ureters, which also results in dilation. In addition, because progesterone also decreases bladder tone, residual volume is increased. As the uterus enlarges as pregnancy progresses, bladder capacity decreases.

Functional Changes
The majority of pregnancy-associated functional changes in the renal system are a result of an increase in renal plasma flow. Early in the first trimester, renal plasma flow begins to increase, and, at term, it may be 75% greater than nonpregnant levels. Similarly, the glomerular filtration rate (GFR) increases to 50% over the nonpregnant state. This increase in GFR results in an increased load of various solutes presented to the renal system. Urinary glucose excretion increases in virtually all pregnant patients. A trace of glucose on routine prenatal colorimetric "dipstick" evaluation is normal and is usually not associated with glycemic pathology. However, these serial measurements during routine prenatal visits may show trends suggestive of true glucosuria, hence their importance.

Amino acids and water-soluble vitamins, such as vitamin B12 and folate, are also excreted to a greater extent compared with the nonpregnant state. However, there is no significant increase in urinary protein loss, which means that any proteinuria that occurs during pregnancy should prompt consideration of illness. In addition, sodium metabolism remains unchanged. The potential loss of this electrolyte caused by an increased GFR is compensated for by an increase in renal tubule reabsorption of sodium.

All components of the renin–angiotensin–aldosterone system increase during pregnancy. Plasma renin activity is up to 10 times that of the nonpregnant state, and renin substrate (angiotensinogen) and angiotensin increase approximately 5-fold. Normal pregnant women are relatively resistant to the hypertensive effects of the increased levels of renin–angiotensin–aldosterone, whereas women with hypertensive disease and hypertensive disease of pregnancy are not.

Symptoms
The anatomic changes in the renal system result in a few common symptomatic complaints during pregnancy. Compression of the bladder by the enlarged uterus results in **urinary frequency** that is not associated with urinary tract or bladder infection. Although urinary frequency is a distressing normal finding as pregnancy advances, care must be taken to distinguish such changes from those associated with early urinary tract infection. In addition, 20% of women experience **stress urinary incontinence**, and loss of urine should be considered in the differential diagnosis when rupture of membranes is suspected. Finally, urinary stasis throughout the renal collecting system predisposes to an increased incidence of pyelonephritis in patients with asymptomatic bacteriuria.

Physical Findings
As pregnancy advances, pressure from the presenting part on the maternal bladder can cause edema and protrusion of the bladder base into the anterior vagina. No significant changes in the renal examination are apparent during pregnancy.

Diagnostic Tests
The pregnancy-associated functional changes in the renal system result in a number of alterations in common tests of renal function. Serum levels of creatinine and blood urea nitrogen (BUN) decrease in normal pregnancy. Serum creatinine values fall from a nonpregnant level of 0.8 mg/dL to pregnancy levels of 0.5 to 0.6 mg/dL by term. Creatinine clearance increases 30% above the nonpregnant norms of 100 to 115 mL/min. BUN also falls about 25% to levels of 8 to 10 mg/dL at the end of the first trimester and is maintained at these levels for the remainder of the pregnancy. Because glucosuria is common during pregnancy, quantitative urine glucose measurements are often elevated but may not signify an abnormal blood sugar. By comparison, renal protein excretion is unchanged during pregnancy, and the nonpregnant range of 100 to 300 mg per 24 hours remains valid.

If imaging of the renal system is performed during pregnancy, normal dilation of the renal collecting system resembling hydronephrosis is noted on ultrasound or intravenous pyelogram.

Gastrointestinal System

The anatomic and functional changes in the gastrointestinal (GI) system that occur during pregnancy are due to the combined effect of the enlarging uterus and the hormonal action of pregnancy. These changes produce a number of pregnancy-related symptoms that can range from mild discomfort to severe disability.

Anatomic Changes
The primary anatomic change related to pregnancy is the displacement of the stomach and intestines due to the enlarging uterus. Although the stomach and intestines change in position, they do not change in size. The liver and biliary tract also does not change in size, but the portal vein enlarges due to increased blood flow.

Functional Changes
Functional changes in the GI system are the result of the hormonal action of progesterone and estrogen. Generalized

smooth muscle relaxation mediated by progesterone produces lower esophageal sphincter tone, decreased GI motility, and impaired gallbladder contractility. As a result, transit time in the stomach and small bowel increases significantly—15% to 30% in the second and third trimesters and more during labor. Additionally, the imbalance between the lower intraesophageal pressures and increased intragastric pressures, combined with the lower esophageal sphincter tone, leads to gastroesophageal reflux. However, appropriately changing the maternal recumbent position may ameliorate pregnancy-associated mild gastroesophageal reflux. Reduced gallbladder contractility, in combination with estrogen-mediated inhibition of intraductal transportation of bile acids, leads to an increased prevalence of gallstones and cholestasis of bile salts. Estrogen also stimulates hepatic biosynthesis of proteins such as fibrinogen; ceruloplasmin; and the binding proteins for corticosteroids, sex steroids, thyroid hormones, and vitamin D.

Symptoms

Some of the earliest and most obvious symptoms of pregnancy are noted in the GI system. Although energy requirements vary from person to person, most women increase their caloric intake by about 200 kcal/day. **Nausea and vomiting of pregnancy (NVP)**, or **"morning sickness,"** typically begins between 4 and 8 weeks of gestation and abates by the middle of the second trimester, usually by 14 to 16 weeks. The cause of this nausea is unknown, although it appears to be related to elevated levels of progesterone, human chorionic gonadotropin (hCG), and relaxation of the smooth muscle of the stomach. Severe NVP, which is known as **hyperemesis gravidarum**, can result in weight loss, ketonemia, and electrolyte imbalance.

Many patients report **dietary cravings** during pregnancy. Some may be the result of the patient's perception that a particular food may help with nausea. **Pica** is an especially intense craving for substances such as ice, starch, and clay. Other patients develop dietary or olfactory aversions during pregnancy. **Ptyalism** is perceived by the patient to be the excessive production of saliva but probably represents the inability of a nauseated woman to swallow the normal amounts of saliva that are produced.

Symptoms of **gastroesophageal reflux** typically become more pronounced as pregnancy advances and intra-abdominal pressure increases. **Constipation** is common in pregnancy and is associated with mechanical obstruction of the colon by the enlarging bowel, reduced motility as elsewhere in the GI tract, and increased water absorption during pregnancy. Generalized **pruritus** may result from intrahepatic cholestasis and increased serum bile acid concentrations.

Physical Findings

The two most notable GI pregnancy-related physical findings are **gingival disease** and **hemorrhoids**. Although the incidence of dental caries does not change with pregnancy, the gums become more edematous and soft during pregnancy and bleed easily with vigorous brushing. On occasion, violaceous pedunculated lesions, called *epulis gravidarum*, appear at the gumline. These lesions, which are actually pyogenic granulomas, sometimes bleed very easily, but usually regress within 2 months of delivery. Rarely, excessive bleeding may occur, requiring excision of the granuloma. Hemorrhoids are common in pregnancy and are caused by both constipation and elevated venous pressures resulting from increased pelvic blood flow and the effects of the enlarging uterus.

Diagnostic Tests

Some markers of hepatic function may be altered during pregnancy. Total serum alkaline phosphatase concentration is doubled, mainly due to increased placental production. Serum cholesterol levels increase during pregnancy. Although total albumin increases, serum levels of albumin are lower during pregnancy, primarily due to hemodilution. Levels of aspartate transaminase, alanine transaminase, γ-glutamyl transferase, and bilirubin are largely unchanged or slightly lower. Serum amylase and lipase concentrations are also unchanged.

Endocrine System

Pregnancy influences the production of several endocrine hormones that control the physiologic adaptations in other organ systems.

Thyroid Function

Pregnancy produces an overall **euthyroid** state, despite several changes in thyroid regulation. The thyroid gland enlarges moderately during pregnancy but does not produce thyromegaly or goiter. In the first trimester, hCG, which has thyrotropin-like activity, stimulates maternal thyroxine (T_4) secretion and produces a transient rise in the free T_4 concentration (Fig. 5.3). The

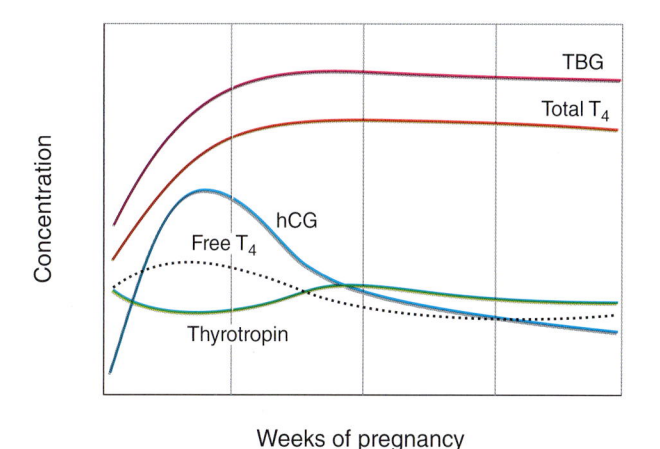

FIGURE 5.3. Changes in maternal thyroid function during pregnancy. The effects of pregnancy on the mother include a marked and early increase in hepatic production of TBG and placental production of hCG. The increase in serum TBG, in turn, increases serum thyroxine (T_4) concentrations; hCG has thyrotropin-like activity and stimulates maternal T_4 secretion. The transient hCG-induced increase in the serum-free T_4 level inhibits maternal secretion of thyrotropin. (Adapted from Burrow GN, Fisher DA, Larsen R. Maternal and fetal thyroid function. *N Engl J Med.* 1994;331(16):1072–1078.)

decline in placental hCG production following the first trimester results in normalization of free T$_4$ concentrations. Beginning early in pregnancy, estrogen induces hepatic synthesis of thyroxine-binding globulin (TBG), resulting in an increase in total T$_4$ and total triiodothyronine (T$_3$) levels. Levels of free T$_4$ and free T$_3$, the active hormones, are unchanged from the normal range for nonpregnant patients.

Adrenal Function

Although pregnancy does not alter the size or morphology of the adrenal gland, it does influence hormone synthesis. As with TBG, estrogen induces hepatic synthesis of cortisol-binding globulin, resulting in elevated levels of serum cortisol. The concentration of free plasma cortisol progressively increases from the first trimester until term. Levels of corticotropin rise in conjunction with serum cortisol. Levels of aldosterone increase markedly due to enhanced adrenal synthesis. Maternal levels of deoxycorticosterone increase as the result of estrogen stimulation of renal synthesis, rather than increased adrenal production. Maternal levels of dehydroepiandrosterone sulfate decrease due to increased hepatic uptake and conversion to estrogen.

Metabolism

Carbohydrate Metabolism

Pregnancy has a diabetogenic effect on maternal carbohydrate metabolism, characterized by reduced tissue response to insulin, hyperinsulinemia, and hyperglycemia. Insulin resistance is primarily due to the action of human placental lactogen (hPL), which increases the resistance of peripheral tissues to the effects of insulin. The hormone hPL is secreted in proportion to placental mass, resulting in increased insulin resistance as pregnancy progresses. Progesterone and estrogen may also contribute to insulin resistance. Hepatic glycogen synthesis and storage is increased, and gluconeogenesis is inhibited. The net effect of these changes is that the maternal response to a glucose load is blunted, producing postprandial hyperglycemia.

Additionally, the fetoplacental unit serves as a constant drain on maternal glucose levels.

Glucose is the primary fuel for the placenta and fetus and, thus, delivery of glucose from the mother to the fetus occurs by facilitated diffusion. As a result, maternal hypoglycemia develops during periods of fasting.

Lipid Metabolism

Pregnancy causes an increase in circulating concentrations of all lipids, lipoproteins, and apolipoproteins. During early pregnancy, fat storage in central tissues predominates. Later in pregnancy, lipolysis predominates, possibly triggered by maternal fasting hypoglycemia. In the absence of glucose, increased plasma concentrations of free fatty acids, triglycerides, and cholesterol provide energy for the mother; this has been characterized as **accelerated starvation**. Following delivery, the concentrations of all lipids return to nonpregnancy levels, a process accelerated by breastfeeding.

Protein Metabolism

Pregnancy is characterized by the intake and utilization of approximately 1 kg of protein above the normal nonpregnant state. At term, 50% of the additional protein is used by the fetus and placenta, and the remainder is shared by the uterus, breasts, maternal Hgb, and plasma proteins.

Other Maternal Systems

Musculoskeletal

As pregnancy advances, a compensatory **lumbar lordosis** (anterior convexity of the lumbar spine) is apparent. This change is functionally useful because it helps keep the woman's center of gravity over the legs; otherwise, the enlarging uterus would shift it anteriorly. However, as a result of this change in posture, virtually all women complain of low back pain during pregnancy. Increasing pressure caused by intra-abdominal growth of the uterus may result in an exacerbation of hernia defects, most commonly seen at the umbilicus and in the abdominal wall (diastasis recti, a physiologic separation of the rectus abdominis muscles). Beginning early in pregnancy, the effects of relaxin and progesterone result in a relative laxity of the ligaments. The pubic symphysis separates at approximately 28 to 30 weeks. Patients often complain of an unsteady gait and should be cautioned about the increased risk of falls during pregnancy that results both from these body habitus changes and an altered center of gravity as pregnancy progresses.

To provide for adequate calcium supplies to the fetal skeleton, calcium stores are mobilized. Maternal serum-ionized calcium is unchanged from the nonpregnant state, but maternal total serum calcium decreases. There is a significant increase in maternal parathyroid hormone, which maintains serum calcium levels by increasing absorption from the intestine and decreasing the loss of calcium through the kidney. The skeleton is well maintained despite these elevated levels of parathyroid hormones. This may be because of the effect of calcitonin. Although the rate of bone turnover increases, there is no loss of bone density during a normal pregnancy if adequate nutrition is supplied.

Skin

Pregnancy induces several characteristic changes in the appearance of the maternal skin. Although the exact etiology of these changes has not been established, hormonal influences appear to predominate.

Vascular spiders (**spider angiomata**) are most common on the upper torso, face, and arms. **Palmar erythema** occurs in more than 50% of patients. Both are associated with increased levels of circulating estrogen and regress after delivery. **Striae gravidarum** occur in more than half of pregnant women and appear on the lower abdomen, breasts, and thighs. Initially, striae can be either purple or pink; eventually, they become white or silvery. These striae are not related to weight gain but are solely the result of the stretching of normal skin. There is no effective therapy to prevent these "stretch marks," and, once they appear, they cannot be eliminated.

Pregnancy may produce a characteristic **hyperpigmentation** believed to be the result of elevated levels of estrogen and **melanocyte-stimulating hormone** and a cross-reaction with the structurally similar hCG. Hyperpigmentation commonly affects the umbilicus and perineum, although it may affect any skin surface. The lower abdomen **linea alba** darkens to become the **linea nigra**. The **"mask of pregnancy,"** or **chloasma** (**melasma**), is also common and may never disappear completely. **Skin nevi** can increase in size and pigmentation but resolve after pregnancy; however, removal of rapidly changing nevi is recommended during pregnancy because of the risk of malignancy. **Eccrine sweating** and **sebum production** increase during normal pregnancy, with many patients complaining of acne.

Hair growth during pregnancy is maintained, although there are more follicles in the **anagen (growth)** phase and fewer in the **telogen (resting)** phase. Late in pregnancy, the number of hairs in telogen is approximately half of the normal 20%, so that postpartum, the number of hairs entering telogen increases; thus, there is significant hair loss 2 to 4 months after pregnancy. Hair growth typically returns to normal 6 to 12 months after delivery. Patients are often concerned about this "hair loss," until they are reassured that it is transient and that hair growth will resume after pregnancy.

Reproductive Tract

The effects of pregnancy on the vulva are similar to the effects on other skin. Because of an increase in vascularity, vulvar varicosities are common and usually regress after delivery. An increase in vaginal transudation as well as stimulation of the vaginal epithelium results in a heavier vaginal discharge, called **leukorrhea of pregnancy**, that some women may mistake as infection or ruptured membranes. The epithelium of the endocervix everts onto the ectocervix, which is associated with a mucus plug.

During pregnancy, the uterus undergoes an enormous increase in weight from the 70-g nonpregnant size to approximately 1,100 g at term, primarily through hypertrophy of existing myometrial cells. After pregnancy, the uterus returns to only a slightly increased size as the actual number of cells comprising it is minimally increased. Similarly, the uterine cavity enlarges to a volume of up to as much as 5 L, compared with less than 10 mL in the nongravid state.

Breasts

The breasts increase in size during pregnancy, rapidly in the first 8 weeks and steadily thereafter. In most cases, the total enlargement is 25% to 50%. The nipples become larger and more mobile and the areola larger and more deeply pigmented, with enlargement of the montgomery glands. Blood flow to the breasts increases as they change to support lactation. Some patients may complain of breast or nipple tenderness and a tingling sensation. Estrogen stimulation also results in ductal growth, with alveolar hypertrophy being a result of progesterone stimulation. During the latter portion of pregnancy, a thick, yellow fluid can be expressed from the nipples. This is **colostrum**, more common in parous women. Ultimately, lactation depends on synergistic actions of estrogen, progesterone, prolactin, hPL, cortisol, and insulin.

Ophthalmic

The most common visual complaint during pregnancy is blurred vision. This visual change is primarily caused by increased thickness of the cornea associated with fluid retention and decreased intraocular pressure. These changes manifest in the first trimester and regress within the first 6 to 8 weeks postpartum. Therefore, changes in corrective lens prescriptions should not be encouraged during pregnancy. Women may be reassured that changes in vision during normal pregnancy are usually transient, not requiring glasses after delivery.

● FETAL AND PLACENTAL PHYSIOLOGY

Placenta

The placenta is an essential and unique "organ of pregnancy," with key functions in respiratory and metabolite exchange and in hormone synthesis and regulation. It is the crucial point of connection between the mother and fetus. The placenta allows the fetus to live and grow until it is mature and able to survive in the outside world.

All gases involved in fetal respiration cross the placenta by simple diffusion. Fetal uptake of O_2 and excretion of CO_2 depend on the blood-carrying capacities of the mother and fetus for these gases and on the associated uterine and umbilical blood flows.

The single primary metabolic substrate for placental metabolism is glucose. It is estimated that as much as 70% of the glucose transferred from the mother is used by the placenta. The glucose that crosses the placenta does so by facilitated diffusion. Other solutes that are transferred from the mother to the fetus depend on the concentration gradient as well as on their degree of ionization, size, and lipid solubility. There is active transport of amino acids, resulting in levels that are higher in the fetus than in the mother. Free fatty acids have very limited placental transfer, resulting in levels that are lower in the fetus than in the mother.

The placenta also produces estrogen, progesterone, hCG, and hPL. These hormones are important for the maintenance of pregnancy, for labor and delivery, and for lactation.

Fetal Circulation

Oxygenation of fetal blood occurs in the placenta rather than in the fetal lungs. This oxygenated blood (80% saturated) is carried from the placenta to the fetus through the umbilical vein, which enters the portal system of the fetus and branches off to the left lobe of the liver (Fig. 5.4). The umbilical vein then becomes the origin of the ductus venosus. Another branch joins the blood flow from the portal vein to the right lobe of the liver. Fifty percent of the umbilical blood supply goes through the ductus venosus. The blood flow from the left hepatic vein is mixed with the blood in the inferior vena cava and is directed

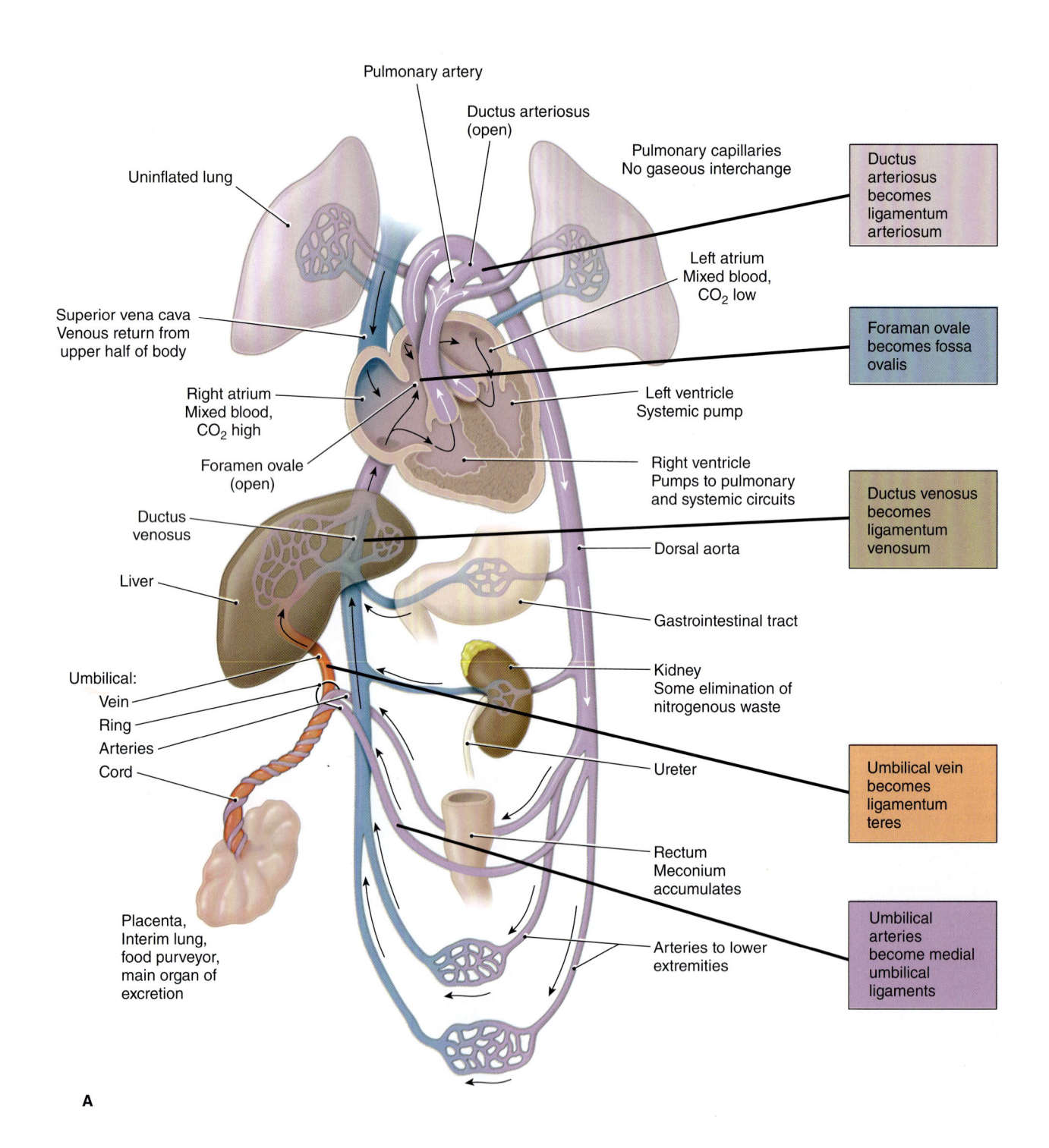

FIGURE 5.4. Fetal circulation at term (**A**) and after delivery (**B**). Note the changes in function of the ductus venosus, foramen ovale, and ductus arteriosus in the transition from intrauterine to extrauterine existence. Red, oxygenated blood; pink/purple, partially oxygenated blood; blue, deoxygenated blood.

Chapter 5: Maternal–Fetal Physiology   53

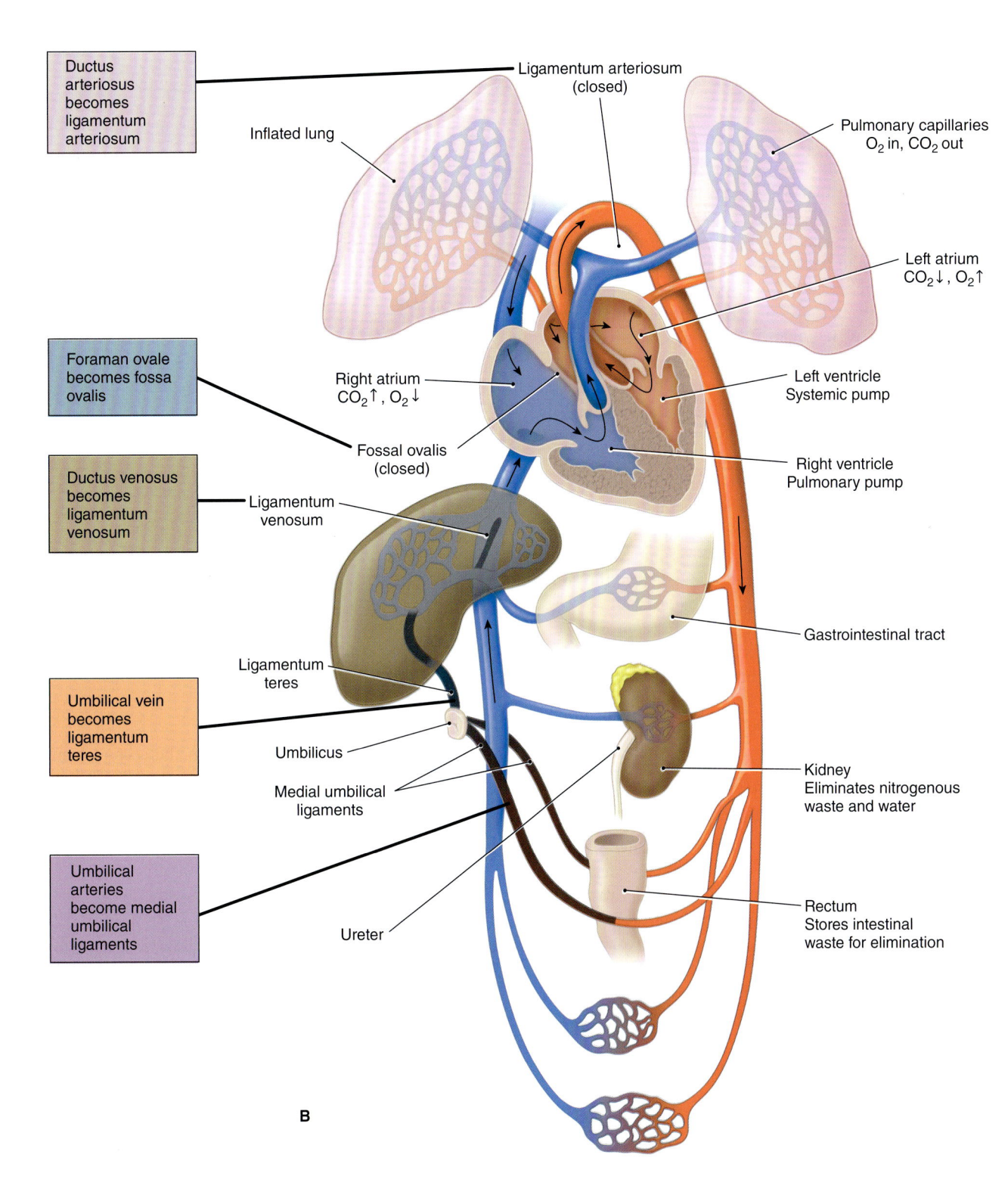

FIGURE 5.4. (*cont.*)

toward the foramen ovale. Consequently, the well-oxygenated umbilical vein blood enters the left ventricle. Less-oxygenated blood in the right hepatic vein enters the inferior vena cava and then flows through the tricuspid valve into the right ventricle. Blood from the superior vena cava also preferentially flows through the tricuspid valve to the right ventricle. Blood from the pulmonary artery primarily flows through the ductus arteriosus into the aorta.

The fetal ventricles work in a parallel circuit, with blood flow from the right and left unequally distributed to the pulmonary and systemic vascular beds. Within a fetal heart rate range of 120 to 180 bpm, the fetal cardiac output remains relatively constant. Overall, less than 10% of right ventricular cardiac output goes to the fetal lungs. The remainder of the right ventricular cardiac output is shunted through the ductus arteriosus to the descending aorta. Output from the left ventricle into the proximal aorta supplies highly saturated blood (65% saturated) to the brain and upper body. Once joined by the ductus arteriosus, the descending aorta then supplies blood to the lower portion of the fetal body, with a major portion of this blood being delivered to the umbilical arteries, which carry deoxygenated blood to the placenta.

The umbilical blood flow represents about 40% of the combined output of both fetal ventricles. In the last half of pregnancy, this flow is proportional to fetal growth (approximately 300 mL/mg/minute), so that umbilical blood flow is relatively constant, normalized to fetal weight. This relationship allows measurement of fetal blood flow to be used as an indirect measure of fetal growth and fetal well-being.

Hemoglobin and Oxygenation

Fetal Hgb, like adult Hgb, is a tetramer composed of two copies of two different peptide chains. But unlike adult **hemoglobin A** (**HgbA**), which is composed of α- and β-chains, fetal Hgb is composed of a series of different pairings of peptide chains that change as embryonic and fetal development progresses. In late fetal life, **hemoglobin F** (**HgbF**), composed of two α-chains and two γ-chains, predominates. The key physiologic difference between adult HgbA and fetal HgbF is that, at any given oxygen tension, HgbF has higher oxygen affinity and oxygen saturation than HgbA. The main reason for this functional difference is that HgbA binds 2,3-DPG (diphosphoglycerate) more avidly than does HgbF.

The Bohr effect modulates the oxygen-binding capacity of Hgb and plays an important role in exchange of O_2 and CO_2 between the maternal and fetal circulations. As maternal blood enters the placenta, the maternal respiratory alkalosis facilitates transfer of CO_2 from the fetal circulation to the maternal circulation. Loss of CO_2 from the fetal circulation causes a rise in the fetal blood pH, shifting the fetal oxygen dissociation curve to the left and resulting in increased oxygen-binding affinity (Fig. 5.5). Conversely, as the maternal circulation takes up CO_2, the blood pH decreases, resulting in a shift in the maternal oxygen dissociation curve to the left, reducing oxygen affinity. Hence, a favorable gradient is created, facilitating diffusion of O_2 from the maternal to the fetal circulation. Therefore, although the partial pressure of oxygen in fetal arterial blood is only 20 to 25 mm Hg, the fetus is adequately oxygenated.

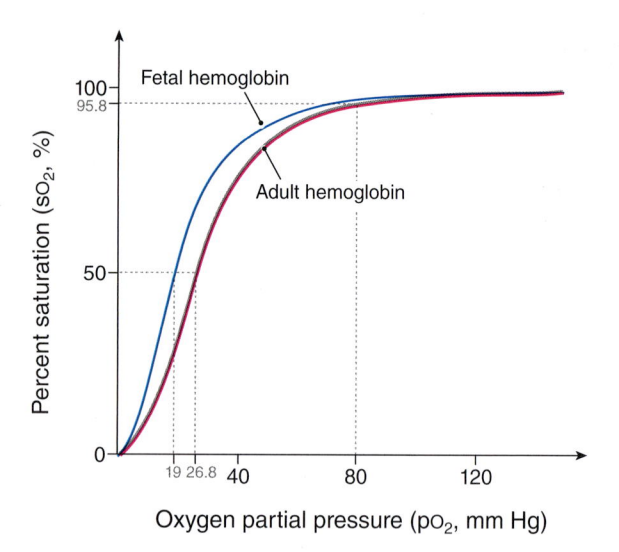

FIGURE 5.5. HgbA vs. HgbF oxygen saturation curve. The oxygen saturation curve for fetal hemoglobin (**blue**) appears left-shifted when compared with adult hemoglobin (**red**), because fetal hemoglobin has a greater affinity for oxygen.

Kidney

The fetal kidney becomes functional in the second trimester, producing dilute, hypotonic urine. The rate of fetal urine production varies with fetal size and ranges from 400 to 1,200 mL/day. Fetal urine becomes the primary source of the amniotic fluid by the middle of the second trimester.

Liver

The fetal liver is slow to mature. The fetal liver capacity for glycogen synthesis and bilirubin conjugation increases with gestational age. As a consequence, during fetal life, bilirubin is primarily eliminated through the placenta. Hepatic production of coagulation factors is deficient and may be attenuated in newborn life due to vitamin K deficiency. Routine neonatal administration of vitamin K prevents newborn hemorrhagic disorders.

Thyroid Gland

The fetal thyroid gland develops without direct influence from the mother, becoming functional by the end of the first trimester, so that, thereafter, levels of fetal T_3, T_4, and TBG increase throughout the rest of gestation. The placenta does not transport the thyroid-stimulating hormone, and only moderate amounts of T3 and T4 cross the placenta. The mother is the primary source of the thyroid hormone for the fetus prior to 24 to 28 weeks of gestation.

Gonads

The primordial germ cells migrate during the eighth week of gestation from the endoderm of the yolk sac to the genital ridge. At this point, the gonads are undifferentiated. Differentiation into the testes occurs 6 weeks after conception, if the embryo is 46, XY. This testicular differentiation appears to depend on the presence of the H–Y antigen and the Y chromosome. If the Y chromosome is absent, however, an ovary develops from the undifferentiated gonad. Development of the fetal ovary begins at approximately 7 weeks. The development of other genital organs depends on the presence or absence of specific hormones and is independent of gonadal differentiation. If the fetal testes are present, testosterone and the Müllerian inhibitory factor inhibit the development of female external genitalia. If these two hormones are not present, the female genitalia develop, with regression of the Wolffian ducts.

IMMUNOLOGY OF PREGNANCY

Although the maternal immune system is not altered in pregnancy, the antigenically dissimilar fetus is able to survive in the uterus without being rejected. The key to this successful fetal allograft appears to be the placenta. The placenta serves as an effective interface between the maternal and fetal vascular compartments by keeping the fetus from direct contact with the maternal immune system. The placenta also produces estrogen, progesterone, hCG, and hPL, all of which may contribute to suppression of maternal immune responses on a local level. In addition, the placenta is the site of origin for blocking and masking antibodies, which alter the immune response.

The mother's systemic immune system remains intact, as evidenced by leukocyte count, B- and T-cell count and function, and immunoglobulin (Ig) levels. Because IgG is the only Ig that can cross the placenta, maternal IgG comprises a major proportion of fetal Ig, both in utero and in the early neonatal period. In this fashion, **passive immunity** is transferred to the fetus.

In this environment, the fetal immune system is afforded the opportunity to gradually develop and mature by term. Fetal lymphocyte production begins as early as 6 weeks of gestation. By 12 weeks of gestation, IgG, IgM, IgD, and IgE are present and are produced in progressively increasing amounts throughout pregnancy. At birth, the newborn fetus is equipped with both passive immunity and a mature immunologic system to defend against infectious diseases.

CLINICAL FOLLOW-UP

Your patient is 20 years old and has a completely negative medical history. On physical examination, her blood pressure and pulse rate are normal as is auscultation of her heart and lungs. After this examination, you explain that shortness of breath (dyspnea) is normal in pregnancy because of a lowered CO_2 level. In her case, it is probable that she had not noted this until her abrupt introduction into a high-altitude environment. You also show her a picture of a chest x-ray during pregnancy, explaining that her heart is quite normal, simply displaced upward, and somewhat sideways by her growing baby. Reassured, they continue prenatal care and subsequently she has a normal vaginal delivery of a healthy daughter 2 weeks after this visit.

---

thePoint® Visit http://thePoint.lww.com/activate for an interactive USMLE-style question bank and more!

CHAPTER 6

Preconception and Antepartum Care

This chapter deals primarily with APGO Educational Topic Area:

TOPIC 9 PRECONCEPTION CARE
TOPIC 10 ANTEPARTUM CARE

Students should be able to describe how medical conditions affect pregnancy outcomes and counsel patients on appropriate interventions to optimize preconception health. They should be able to describe typical care of the pregnant patient, including accurate diagnosis of pregnancy, medication safety, risk factors for poor outcome, assessments for fetal well-being, and nutritional needs.

CLINICAL CASE

A 36-year-old nulliparous woman presents to your office for her first prenatal visit. She is unsure of her last menstrual period as she recently discontinued her birth control pills, but thinks it was 2 months ago. In addition to worrying about her baby having abnormalities related to her age, she is an early elementary school teacher and is concerned about exposure to childhood illnesses. Since she is "older," she is concerned that she may not have other children and really wants to optimize the outcome of this pregnancy. What will you do during her first obstetric visit? What screening will you offer her? How will you counsel her regarding her goal for a healthy pregnancy?

• PRECONCEPTION COUNSELING AND CARE

Preconception counseling and care is intended to optimize a woman's health and knowledge before planning and conceiving a pregnancy, ideally commencing before conception with a preconception visit. During this visit, a thorough family and medical history of both parents is obtained as well as a physical examination of the prospective mother. The goal of this visit is to minimize adverse health effects for the woman and fetus and to promote a healthy pregnancy. Preexisting conditions that may affect conception, pregnancy, or both are identified and addressed. Neural tube defects (NTDs) are associated with folic acid deficiency which may antedate the pregnancy and, therefore, discussion about folic acid supplementation is an essential component of preconception counseling. In addition, women with conditions such as maternal phenylketonuria or diabetes can reduce the risks of adverse fetal effects by establishing strict metabolic control before conception and continuing it throughout the pregnancy. In the absence of preconception metabolic control, establishing control of these conditions early in pregnancy, while of lesser benefit, may minimize morbidity and mortality later in gestation.

All health encounters during a woman's reproductive years, particularly those that are a part of preconception care, should include discussion on a woman's preference for contraception and counseling about appropriate medical care and behaviors to optimize pregnancy outcomes. Women should still be encouraged to seek a specific preconception visit if they are planning a pregnancy. The following maternal assessments may serve as the basis for this counseling:

- Family planning and pregnancy spacing
- Medical, surgical, psychiatric, and neurologic histories
- Obstetric and gynecologic history
- Family history
- Genetic history, appropriate carrier screening, and genetic counseling
- Current medications (prescribed, over-the-counter [OTC], and alternative medicines)
- Substance use (tobacco, alcohol, illicit drugs, OTC drugs such as cold medications, misuse of prescription drugs, and recreational drug use)
- Domestic abuse and violence; bullying; trauma
- Sexual abuse
- Nutrition
- Environmental and occupational exposures
- Immunity and immunization status
- Risk factors for sexually transmitted infections (STIs)
- Physical examination (especially blood pressure with attention to prehypertension and hypertension categories and appropriate weight based on body mass index [BMI])
- Assessment of socioeconomic, education, and cultural context

Ideally, vaccinations should be administered before conception. Live vaccines pose a theoretical risk for the fetus and women who receive a live-virus vaccination should be advised to avoid pregnancy for at least 1 month after vaccination. Vaccinations should be offered to women found to be at risk for or susceptible to rubella, varicella, pertussis, hepatitis A and B, meningococcus, pneumococcus. Human papillomavirus (HPV) is also recommended for women 26 years or younger. All pregnant women should be tested for human immunodeficiency virus (HIV) infection, unless they decline the test. Testing should be offered to women planning a pregnancy.

A number of other tests can be performed for specific indications:

- Screening for STDs
- Testing for maternal diseases based on medical or reproductive history
- Mantoux test with purified protein derivative for tuberculosis by epidermal injection technique and not by the use of "tine" instruments
- Screening for genetic disorders may be based on ethnic, panethnic, or expanded screening strategies. Traditional ethnic screening strategies have included:
  - Sickle hemoglobinopathies (African Americans)
  - β-Thalassemia (individuals of Mediterranean and Southeast Asian descent; African Americans)
  - α-Thalassemia (individuals of Southeast Asian and Mediterranean descent; African Americans)
  - Tay-Sachs disease (Ashkenazi Jews, French Canadians, and Cajuns)
  - Canavan disease and familial dysautonomia (Ashkenazi Jews)
  - Cystic fibrosis (similar to SMA, carrier frequency is higher among Caucasians of European and Ashkenazi descent; however, screening should be made available to all couples)
  - Screening for other genetic disorders on the basis of family history

Patients should be counseled regarding the benefits of the following activities:

- Maintaining good control of any preexisting medical conditions (e.g., diabetes, hypertension, asthma, systemic lupus erythematosus, seizures, thyroid disorders, and inflammatory bowel disease)
- Taking 0.4 mg of folic acid daily while attempting pregnancy and during the first trimester of pregnancy for prevention of NTDs
- Women who have had a prior NTD-affected pregnancy, or using medications that interfere with folate metabolism, should consume 4 mg of folic acid per day in the periconception period (this amount can be achieved by adding a separate supplement to a single multivitamin tablet to provide a total of 4 mg of folic acid while avoiding excessive intake of fat-soluble vitamins, which may have adverse fetal effects if taken in high doses)
- Determining the time of conception by an accurate menstrual history
- Reducing weight before pregnancy, if obese; increasing weight, if underweight
- Exercise
- Avoiding food faddism
- Avoiding pregnancy within 1 month of receiving a live attenuated vaccine (e.g., rubella)
- Preventing HIV transmission if relevant to the patient or partner
- Abstaining from tobacco, alcohol, illicit drug, recreational drug use, and inappropriate use of prescription medicines before and during pregnancy

ANTEPARTUM CARE

Women who receive early and regular antepartum care are more likely to have healthier maternal and infant outcomes. The goals of obstetric care are to 1) provide easy access to care, 2) promote patient involvement, and 3) provide a team approach to ongoing surveillance and education for the patient and about her fetus. High-risk conditions can be identified and a management plan established for any complications that may arise. Routine antepartum care provides an opportunity for screening, periodic assessments, and patient education.

Antepartum surveillance begins with the first prenatal visit. At this time, the health care provider begins to compile an obstetric database of information. The full American College of Obstetricians and Gynecologists Antepartum Record and Postpartum Form is provided in Appendix B.

Complete antepartum care includes the following:

- Diagnosing pregnancy and determining gestational age
- Monitoring the progress of the pregnancy with periodic examinations and appropriate screening tests
- Assessing the well-being of the woman and her fetus
- Providing patient education that addresses all aspects of pregnancy and the postpartum period
- Preparing the patient and her family for her management during labor, delivery, and the postpartum period
- Detecting medical and psychosocial complications and instituting indicated interventions

An important aspect of prenatal/antepartum care is to educate the mother and her family about the value of screening for and managing the unexpected complications that may develop. Specific conditions to which poor maternal and neonatal outcomes are often attributed include preterm labor and preterm delivery, preterm infection, intrauterine growth restriction (IUGR), hypertension and preeclampsia, diabetes mellitus, birth defects, multiple gestation, and abnormal placentation.

DIAGNOSIS OF PREGNANCY

For a woman with regular menstrual cycles, a history of one or more missed periods following a time of sexual activity without effective contraception strongly suggests early pregnancy. Fatigue, nausea/vomiting, and breast tenderness are often associated symptoms.

On physical examination, softening and enlargement of the pregnant uterus becomes apparent 6 or more weeks after the last normal menstrual period. At approximately 12 weeks of gestation (12 weeks from the onset of the last menstrual period [LMP]), the uterus is generally enlarged sufficiently to be palpable in the lower abdomen. Other genital tract findings early in pregnancy include congestion and a bluish discoloration of the cervix and vagina (**Chadwick sign**) and softening of the cervix (**Hegar sign**). Increased pigmentation of the skin and the appearance of circumlinear striae on the abdominal wall occur later in pregnancy and are associated with progesterone effects and physical stretching of the dermis. Palpation of fetal parts and the appreciation of fetal movement and fetal heart tones are diagnostic of pregnancy but at a more advanced gestational age. The patient's initial perception of fetal movement (called **quickening**) is not usually reported before 16 to 18 weeks of gestation and often as late as 20 weeks in first-time mothers.

Pregnancy cannot be diagnosed only on the basis of symptoms and subjective physical findings. A **pregnancy test** is needed to confirm the diagnosis. Once a positive pregnancy test is identified and before fetal heart activity (i.e., a beating fetal heart) is seen on ultrasound, the physician and patient must be aware of signs and symptoms of an abnormal pregnancy, including those associated with spontaneous abortion, ectopic pregnancy, and trophoblastic disease. Several types of urine pregnancy tests are available that measure **human chorionic gonadotropin** (**hCG**) produced in the syncytiotrophoblast of the growing placenta. Because hCG shares an α-subunit with luteinizing hormone (LH), interpretation of any test that does not differentiate LH from hCG must take into account this overlap in structure. The concentration of hCG necessary to evoke a positive test result must therefore be high enough to avoid a false-positive diagnosis of pregnancy. Standard laboratory urine pregnancy tests become positive approximately 4 weeks following the first day of the LMP (i.e., around the time of the missed period). Home urine pregnancy tests have a low false-positive rate but a high false-negative rate (i.e., the test result is negative even though the patient is pregnant). All urine pregnancy tests are best performed on early-morning urine specimens, which contain the highest concentration of hCG.

Serum pregnancy tests are more specific and sensitive because they test for the unique β-subunit of hCG, allowing detection of pregnancy very early in gestation, often before the patient has missed a period. During the first few weeks, the status of a pregnancy may be evaluated by following serial quantitative hCG levels and comparing them to the expected rise derived from normative data for proven normal intrauterine pregnancies. The mean doubling time for hCG in patients with a viable intrauterine pregnancy is approximately 1.5 to 2.0 days.

Such serial studies often allow differentiation of normal and abnormal pregnancy or indicate that further testing, for example ultrasound, is needed for the same purpose.

Detection of fetal heart activity (**fetal heart tones**) is almost always evidence of a viable intrauterine pregnancy. With a traditional, nonelectronic, acoustic fetoscope, auscultation of fetal heart tones is possible at or beyond 18 to 20 weeks of gestational age. The commonly used electronic Doppler devices can usually detect fetal heart tones at approximately 12 weeks of gestation (or perhaps a little later if the mother is obese).

● THE INITIAL PRENATAL VISIT

At the initial prenatal appointment, ideally in the first trimester, a comprehensive history is taken, focusing on past pregnancies, gynecologic history, medical history with attention to chronic medical issues and infections, information pertinent to genetic screening, and information about the course of the current pregnancy. A complete physical examination is performed, including breast and pelvic examinations, as well as routine first-trimester laboratory studies (see Appendix B). Other studies may be performed as indicated. The patient is given instructions concerning routine prenatal care, warning signs of complications, whom to contact with questions or problems, expected course of the pregnancy, risk counseling, and nutritional and social service information.

The initial obstetric pelvic examination also includes a description of the various diameters of the bony pelvis (see Chapter 4), assessment of the cervix (including cervical length, consistency, dilation, and effacement), and uterine size (usually expressed in weeks), shape, consistency (firm to soft), and mobility. When the uterus grows in size so that it exits the pelvis, the fundal height in centimeters represents the gestational age of the fetus from that time to about 36 weeks.

Risk Assessment

Risk assessment is an important part of the initial antenatal evaluation. Questions about history and chronic medical conditions are important in order to identify the pregnant woman who is at risk for maternal and fetal complications and to initiate a management plan at the appropriate time. In addition to understanding the medical risks, it is important to understand each woman's social circumstances, some of which may place her at risk for both physical and emotional complications. Patients should be questioned about the following aspects of their lifestyle that could pose a risk and receive appropriate counseling, if indicated:

- Desire for pregnancy
- Communication barriers
- Depression/anxiety (should be performed at least once during perinatal period)
- Nutrition and weight gain counseling
- Sexual activity
- Exercise
- Tobacco use (smoking, chewed, e-cigarettes)
- Environmental and work hazards
- Alcohol
- Use of any medications (including supplements, vitamins, herbs, or OTC drugs)
- Illicit/recreational drugs/substance use (parents, partner, past, present)
- Domestic violence
- Intimate partner violence
- Seat belt use

Initial Assessment of Gestational Age: Estimated Date of Delivery

Gestational age is the number of weeks that have elapsed between the first day of the LMP (not the presumed time of conception) and the date of delivery. Establishing an accurate estimated gestational age and **estimated date of delivery** (EDD) is an important part of the initial antepartum visit. Issues such as prematurity and post-term pregnancy and their subsequent management as well as the timing of screening tests (i.e., nuchal translucency and maternal serum screening for trisomy 21 and NTDs, and assessment of fetal maturity) are affected by the accuracy of gestational age.

The **Naegele rule** is an easy way to calculate the EDD: add 7 days to the first day of the last normal menstrual flow and subtract 3 months. In a patient with an idealized 28-day menstrual cycle, ovulation occurs on day 14; therefore, the conception age of the pregnancy is actually 38 weeks. The use of the first day of the LMP as a starting point for gestational age is standard, and gestational, not conceptional, age is used. "Normal" pregnancy lasts 40 ± 2 weeks, calculated from the first day of the last normal menses (menstrual or gestational age).

To establish an accurate gestational age, the **date of onset of the last normal menses** is crucial. A light-bleeding episode should not be mistaken for a normal menstrual period. A history of irregular periods or taking medications that alter cycle length (e.g., oral contraceptives, other hormonal preparations, and psychoactive medications) can confuse the menstrual history. If sexual intercourse is infrequent or timed for conception based on assisted reproductive techniques, a patient may know when conception is most likely to have occurred, thus facilitating an accurate calculation of gestational age. However, ultrasound-established dates should take preference over menstrual dates if they differ by more than seven days in the first trimester (less than 14 0/7 weeks).

Ultrasound examination can detect pregnancy early in gestation. With a transabdominal ultrasound, the ultrasound transducer is placed on the maternal abdomen, allowing visualization of a normal pregnancy gestational sac 5 to 6 weeks after the beginning of the last normal menstrual period (corresponding to β-hCG concentrations of 5,000 to 6,000 mIU/mL). **Transvaginal ultrasound** often detects pregnancy at 4 to 5 weeks of gestation (corresponding to β-hCG concentrations of 1,000 to 2,000 mIU/mL) because the probe is placed in the posterior fornix of the vagina only a few centimeters from the uterine cavity, compared with the relatively longer distance from the abdominal wall to the same location. A β-hCG of 1,500 mIU/mL in a singleton pregnancy is often used as the cutoff beyond which an intrauterine gestational sac should be visualized when ruling out an ectopic pregnancy. If the β-hCG concentration is >4,000 mIU/mL, the embryo should be visualized and cardiac activity detected by all ultrasound techniques.

● SUBSEQUENT ANTENATAL VISITS

Regular monitoring of the mother and fetus is essential for identifying complications that may arise during pregnancy and to provide assurance and support for mother and family, especially for first pregnancies or when previous pregnancies have been complicated or had poor outcomes. For a patient with an uncomplicated pregnancy, periodic antepartum visits at 4-week intervals are usually scheduled until 28 weeks, every 2 weeks until 36 weeks, and weekly thereafter. Patients with high-risk pregnancies or those with ongoing complications are usually seen more frequently, depending on the clinical circumstances.

At each visit, patients are asked about how they are feeling and if they are having any problems, such as vaginal bleeding, nausea and vomiting, dysuria, and vaginal discharge. After quickening, patients are asked if they continue to feel fetal movement and if it is the same or less since the last antepartum visit. Decreased fetal movement after the time of fetal viability is a warning sign requiring further evaluation of fetal well-being.

Every prenatal assessment includes the following assessments:

- Blood pressure
- Weight
- Obstetric physical findings

Blood Pressure and Urinalysis

It is important to determine baseline blood pressure and urine protein levels at the first antepartum visit. Blood pressure generally declines at the end of the first trimester and rises again in the third trimester. After 20 weeks of gestation, a persistently elevated systolic pressure greater than or equal to 140 mm Hg or an elevated diastolic pressure greater than or equal to 90 mm Hg without proteinuria suggests **gestational hypertension** (see Chapter 22). Comparison with baseline levels is necessary in order to accurately distinguish preexisting hypertension from hypertension associated with pregnancy.

Weight

Maternal weight is another important parameter to follow through pregnancy, insofar as weight gain recommendations differ for women of differing prepregnancy **BMI**. A total weight gain of 25 to 35 lb is only appropriate for a woman of normal BMI (Table 6.1). The obese pregnant woman with a pregravid BMI ≥ 30 is at an increased risk for multiple complications during pregnancy, including preeclampsia, gestational diabetes, and cesarean delivery. A total gain of 11 to 20 lb over the course of the pregnancy is recommended for women with a BMI ≥ 30. Significant deviation from this trend may require nutritional assessment and further evaluation.

Physical Findings

Obstetric physical findings made at each visit include fundal height measurement, documentation of the presence and rate of fetal heart tones, and determination of the presentation of the fetus. Until 16 to 20 weeks, the uterine size is generally stated as "number-weeks" size, such as "12-week uterus."

Fundal Height Measurement

After 20 weeks of gestation (when the fundus is palpable at or near the umbilicus in a woman of normal body habitus and a singleton

TABLE 6.1 INSTITUTE OF MEDICINE WEIGHT GAIN RECOMMENDATIONS FOR PREGNANCY

Prepregnancy Weight Category	BMI[a] (kg)/[height (m)]^2	Recommended Total Weight Gain Range (lb)	Recommended Rates of Weight Gain[b] Second and Third Trimesters (Mean Range, lb/wk)
Underweight	Less than 18.5	28–40	1 (1–1.3)
Normal weight	18.5–24.9	25–35	1 (0.8–1)
Overweight	25.0–29.9	15–25	0.6 (0.5–0.7)
Obese (includes all classes)	30.0 or greater	11–20	0.5 (0.4–0.6)

[a] BMI, body mass index. To calculate BMI, go to http://www.nhlbisupport.com/bmi.
[b] Calculations assume a 1.1–4.4 lb (0.5–2 kg) weight gain in the first trimester.
Adapted from Preconception and Antepartum Care: In: American Academy of Pediatrics, American College of Obstetricians and Gynecologists. *Guidelines for Perinatal Care.* 7th ed. Elk Grove Village (IL): AAP; Washington, DC: ACOG; 2012, Based on Resource Sheet, Weight Gain During Pregnancy: reexamining the guidelines.

pregnancy in the vertex presentation), the uterine size can be assessed with the use of a tape measure, which is the **fundal height measurement**. In this procedure, the top of the uterine fundus is identified, and the zero end of the tape measure is placed at this uppermost part of the uterus. The tape is then carried anteriorly across the abdomen to the level of the symphysis pubis. From 16 to 18 weeks of gestation until 36 weeks of gestation, the fundal height in centimeters (measured from the symphysis to the top of the uterine fundus) is roughly equal to the number of weeks of gestational age in normal singleton pregnancies in the cephalic presentation within an anatomically normal uterus (Fig. 6.1).

Until 36 weeks in the normal singleton pregnancy, the number of weeks of gestation approximates the fundal height in centimeters. Thereafter, the fetus moves downward into the pelvis beneath the symphysis pubis ("lightening" or engagement of the head into the true pelvis), so that the fundal height measurement is increasingly unreliable.

Fetal Heart Rate
Fetal heart rate should be verified at every visit, by direct auscultation or by the use of a fetal Doppler ultrasound device. The normal fetal heart rate is 110 to 160 bpm, with higher rates found in early pregnancy. The maternal pulse may also be detected with the Doppler device, so simultaneous palpation of maternal pulse and auscultation of fetal pulse may be necessary to differentiate the two. Deviation from the normal rate or occasional arrhythmias must be evaluated carefully.

Uterine Palpation
Several determinations concerning the fetus can be made by **palpation of the pregnant uterus**, such as identifying the presentation, or "presenting part" of the fetus (i.e., what part of the fetus is entering the pelvis first). Before 34 weeks of gestation, breech, oblique, and transverse presentations are not uncommon. The presentation of the fetus may also vary from day to day. At term, more than 95% of fetuses are in the cephalic presentation (head down). Approximately 3.5% are breech (bottom first) and 1% are shoulder first. Unless the fetus is in a transverse lie (the long axis of the fetus is not parallel with the mother's long axis), the presenting part will be either the head (vertex and cephalic) or the buttocks (breech).

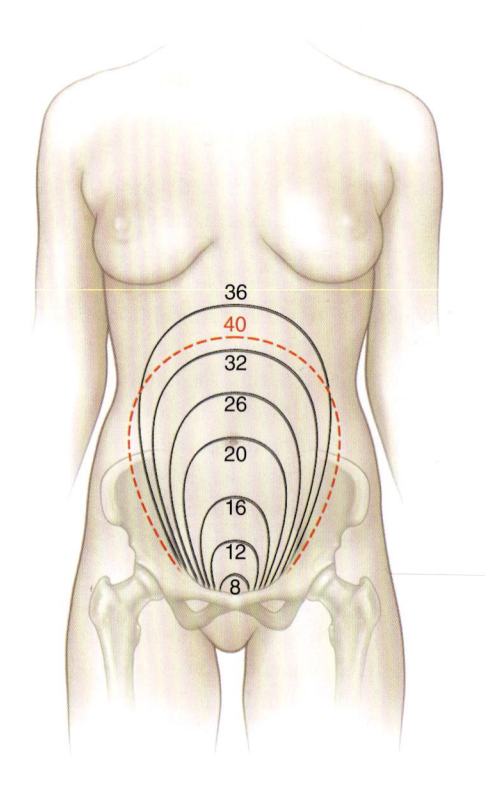

FIGURE 6.1. Fundal height. In a normal singleton pregnancy in the vertex presentation, fundal height roughly corresponds to gestational age between 16 and 36 weeks' gestation. A convenient guideline is 20 weeks equals 20 cm equals fundus at umbilicus in a woman with a normal body habitus. After 36 weeks, the fundal height either grows more slowly or actually decreases as the uterus changes shape and/or the fetal head engages in the pelvis.

Fetal Presentation
The presentation of the fetus can be appreciated on clinical examination with the use of **Leopold maneuvers** (see Fig. 9.7). In the first maneuver, breech presentation can be appreciated by outlining the fundus and determining what part is present. The

head is hard and well defined by ballottement, especially when the head is freely mobile in the fluid-filled uterus; the breech is softer, less round, and, therefore, more difficult to outline. In the second and third maneuvers, the examiner's palms are placed on either side of the maternal abdomen to determine the location of the fetal back and small parts. In the fourth maneuver, the presenting part is identified by exerting pressure over the pubic symphysis. If a breech presentation persists at 36 and 38 weeks, the option of **external cephalic version** should be discussed with the patient. This procedure involves turning the fetus from the breech presentation to a vertex presentation to allow vaginal rather than cesarean delivery. It is contraindicated in the presence of multifetal gestation, fetal compromise, uterine anomalies, and problems of placentation.

● ULTRASOUND

In the United States, approximately 65% of pregnant women have at least one ultrasound examination. In the absence of other specific indications, the optimal timing for a single ultrasound examination is at 18 to 22 weeks of gestation. Ultrasonography in the first trimester may be performed either transabdominally or transvaginally. If a transabdominal examination is inconclusive, a transvaginal or transperineal examination is recommended. First-trimester ultrasonography is used to confirm the presence of an intrauterine pregnancy, estimate gestational age, diagnose or evaluate multiple gestations, confirm cardiac activity, and evaluate pelvic masses or uterine abnormalities (as an adjunct to chorionic villus sampling, embryo transfer, or localization and removal of intrauterine contraceptives). It is also useful for evaluating vaginal bleeding, suspected **ectopic pregnancy**, and pelvic pain.

An ultrasound examination may be targeted to help diagnose chromosomal abnormalities in the first trimester. One such examination is measurement of **nuchal translucency (NT)**, the lucent area behind the head in the **nuchal region**. Use of standardized techniques for measuring NT has resulted in higher detection rates for Down syndrome, trisomy 18, trisomy 13, Turner syndrome, and other anatomic abnormalities such as cardiac defects. Measurement of nuchal translucency alone is less effective for first-trimester screening of the singleton pregnancy than is combined testing (nuchal translucency measurement and biochemical markers). Recent studies demonstrate improved detection of Down syndrome at lower false-positive rates when NT measurement is combined with biochemical markers (see Section "Screening Tests"). This sentence conveys the same information and does not plagiarize ACOG verbatim.

Various types of ultrasound examinations performed during the second or third trimester can be categorized as "standard," "limited," or "specialized." A standard examination is performed during the second or third trimester of pregnancy. It includes an evaluation of fetal presentation and number, amniotic fluid volume, cardiac activity, placental position, fetal biometry, and an anatomic survey. If technically feasible, the uterus and adnexa should be examined as clinically appropriate. A limited examination is performed when a specific question requires investigation. In an emergency, for example, a limited examination can be performed to evaluate heart activity in a bleeding patient. A detailed or targeted anatomic specialized examination is performed when an anomaly is suspected on the basis of history, biochemical abnormalities or clinical evaluation, or suspicious results from either the limited or standard ultrasound examination. Other specialized examinations might include fetal Doppler, biophysical profile (BPP), fetal echocardiography, or additional biometric studies.

Evaluation of placental and cervical abnormalities may be accomplished with ultrasonography. Placental abruption can be identified by ultrasonography in approximately half of all patients who present with bleeding and do not have placenta previa. Grayscale or color-flow Doppler ultrasound assessment is used to identify placenta accreta. Transvaginal ultrasound examination most accurately can visualize the cervix and can also be employed to detect or rule out placenta previa as well as an abnormally shortened cervix (defined as less than 25 mm), which has been correlated with an increased risk of preterm delivery when measured at less than 28 weeks of gestation.

● SCREENING TESTS

In addition to the routine laboratory tests performed at the initial antepartum visit, additional tests are performed at specific intervals throughout the pregnancy to screen for birth defects and other conditions. The specific tests and intervals for each are indicated on the Antepartum Record (see Appendix B). Additional laboratory testing, such as testing for STDs or tuberculosis, is recommended or offered on the basis of the patient's history, physical examination, parental desire, or in response to public health guidelines.

There are several options for screening for fetal aneuploidy (abnormal number of chromosomes) such as trisomies 18 and 21 (see also Chapter 7 for a detailed discussion of each of these markers). Options for aneuploidy screening include the following:

- **First-trimester screening** (10 to 13 weeks' gestation), which includes serum screening for pregnancy-associated plasma protein A (PAPP-A) and β-hCG and an ultrasound assessment of nuchal transparency, and in some cases the presence or absence of the fetal nasal bone.
- **Cell free fetal DNA** which includes evaluation of short segments of fetal DNA found in the maternal blood used to screen for a variety of fetal conditions.
- **Second-trimester screening** (15 0/7-22 6/7 weeks' gestation) consisting of **triple** (maternal serum α-fetal protein [MSAFP], estriol, and hCG) or **quadruple ("quad")** (MSAFP, hCG, unconjugated estriol, and dimeric inhibin A) **screening** tests. The quad screen has a higher sensitivity for the detection of Down syndrome.
- **Combined first- and second-trimester screening**, which includes all of the first-trimester screening tests listed in addition to a PAPP-A test and a quad screen, with or without an ultrasound examination for NTDs, in the second

trimester. Ultrasonographic screening and cell-free DNA screening may also be included.
- **Second trimester ultrasound** which includes identification of existing major structural abnormalities and minor sonographic soft markers of aneuploidy, along with baseline biometry.

Third-trimester screening includes the following:

- Screening for gestational diabetes mellitus. This may include the **glucose challenge test**, a screening test performed for gestational diabetes between 24 and 28 weeks, unless the pregnant patient is obese, has a known impaired glucose metabolism, diabetes, or previous medical history of gestational diabetes mellitus. In these cases, the test should be performed at the first visit; if gestational diabetes mellitus is not diagnosed, blood glucose testing should be repeated at 24 to 28 weeks of gestation. If the test result is abnormal, an oral **glucose tolerance test** is performed to confirm diabetes.
- In addition, the measurement of hemoglobin and hematocrit levels is repeated in the third trimester.
- Repeat screening in the third trimester for antibodies in Rh-negative patients.
- Repeat screening for HIV and other STIs in all patients is commonly recommended based on risk factors, and even required in some regions.
- Universal screening for **group B streptococcus** is performed at 35 to 37 weeks of gestation, and treatment is based on culture results.

• SPECIFIC TECHNIQUES OF FETAL ASSESSMENT

Continued evaluation of the fetus includes techniques for assessment of fetal 1) growth, 2) well-being, and 3) maturity. These tests must be interpreted in light of the clinical context and provide a basis for management decisions.

Assessment of Fetal Growth

Fetal growth can be assessed by fundal height measurement, as the initial measure, and ultrasonography. The increase in fundal height through pregnancy is predictable. If the fundal height measurement is significantly greater than expected (i.e., **large for gestational age**), possible considerations include incorrect assessment of gestational age, multiple pregnancy, macrosomia (large fetus), hydatidiform mole, and excess accumulation of amniotic fluid (polyhydramnios). A fundal height measurement less than expected, or **small for gestational age**, suggests the possibility of incorrect assessment of gestational age, hydatidiform mole, fetal growth restriction, inadequate amniotic fluid accumulation (oligohydramnios), or even intrauterine fetal demise. Deviation in fundal height measurement should be closely evaluated.

Ultrasound is the most valuable tool in assessing fetal growth and has many potential uses for both fetal dating and identifying fetal anomalies. In early pregnancy, determination of the crown-to-rump length correlates closely with gestational age. Later in pregnancy, measurement of the biparietal diameter of the skull, the head circumference, the abdominal circumference, the femur length, and the cerebellar diameter can be used to assess gestational age and, using various formulas, to estimate fetal weight. However, the variability of gestational age estimation increases with advancing pregnancy.

Assessment of Fetal Well-Being

Assessment of **fetal well-being** includes subjective maternal perception of fetal activity and several objective tests using electronic fetal monitoring and ultrasonography. Tests of fetal well-being have a wide range of use, including the assessment of fetal status at a particular time and prediction of future well-being for varying time intervals, depending on the test and the clinical situation.

Evaluation of **fetal activity** is a common indirect measure of fetal well-being. Various methods can be used to quantify fetal activity after viability, including the time necessary to achieve a certain number of movements each day, or counting the number of movements ("**kick counts**") in a given hour. This type of testing is easily performed and involves the patient in her own care. If the mother notices less movement, further evaluation may be needed.

Fetal monitoring tests can provide more objective information about fetal well-being. These tests include the **nonstress test (NST)**, **contraction stress test (CST)** (called the *oxytocin challenge test* [*OCT*] if oxytocin is used), **biophysical profile (BPP)**, and **ultrasonography of umbilical artery blood flow velocity** (also known as umbilical artery Doppler velocimetry). Although there is no optimal time to initiate fetal testing, there are several maternal- and pregnancy-related indications (Box 6.1).

Nonstress Test

The NST measures the fetal heart rate, patterns, and accelerations, which are monitored with an external transducer for at least 20 minutes. The patient may also be asked to note fetal movement, usually accomplished by pressing a button on the fetal monitor, which causes a notation on the monitor strip. The tracing is observed for fetal heart rate accelerations (Fig. 6.2). The results are considered reactive (or reassuring) if two or more fetal heart rate accelerations (peaking 15 beats above the baseline and lasting for 15 seconds) occur in a 20-minute period, with or without fetal movement discernible by the mother. A nonreactive (nonreassuring) tracing is one without sufficient heart rate accelerations in a 40-minute period. A nonreactive NST should be followed with further fetal assessment.

Contraction Stress Test

Whereas the NST evaluates the fetal heart rate response to fetal activity, the CST measures the response of the fetal heart rate to the stress of a uterine contraction. During a uterine contraction, uteroplacental blood flow is temporarily reduced by the contracting myometrium. A healthy fetus is able to compensate for this intermittent decreased blood flow, whereas a fetus that is compromised may be unable to do so. To perform

BOX 6.1 Indications for Fetal Testing

Maternal Conditions
- Antiphospholipid syndrome
- Cyanotic heart disease
- Systemic lupus erythematosus
- Chronic renal disease
- Insulin-treated diabetes mellitus
- Hypertensive disorders
- Hyperthyroidism (poorly controlled)
- Hemoglobinopathies (sickle cell, sickle cell-hemoglobin C, or sickle cell-thalassemia disease)

Pregnancy-Related or Fetal Conditions
- Pregnancy-induced hypertensive disorders
- Decreased fetal movement
- Oligohydramnios and polyhydramnios
- Intrauterine growth restriction
- Late term or post-term pregnancy
- Alloimmunization (moderate to severe)
- Previous fetal demise (unexplained or recurrent risk)
- Multiple gestation (with significant growth discrepancy)
- Monochorionic diamniotic multiple gestation

Used with permission from Preconception and Antepartum Care. American Academy of Pediatrics, American College of Obstetricians and Gynecologists. *Guidelines for Perinatal Care.* 7th ed. Elk Grove Village (IL): AAP; Washington, DC: ACOG; 2012.

a CST, a tocodynamometer is placed on the maternal abdomen along with a fetal heart rate transducer for a baseline tracing for 10 to 20 minutes. If there are no contractions, they are induced by nipple self-stimulation or oxytocin (this test is called an oxytocin contraction test, or *OCT*). The result is negative if there is no change from the baseline fetal heart rate and no fetal heart rate decelerations. If decelerations occur, the results can be considered positive, equivocal, or unsatisfactory, depending on the pattern, frequency, and strength of the deceleration.

These tests of fetal well-being have a significant incidence of false-positive results (i.e., results suggesting that the fetus is in jeopardy, although the fetus is actually healthy). Because of this high incidence of false positives, the results of these tests must be interpreted collectively, and the tests themselves repeated to verify the results. When multiple test results are reassuring, they tend to rule out a problem. When all results are nonreassuring, they tend to signify the presence of a problem.

Biophysical Profile

If an NST is nonreactive, evidence to support fetal well-being, such as that provided by a BPP, is sought. The BPP is a series of five assessments of fetal well-being, each of which is given a score of 0 (absent) or 2 (present), as shown in Table 6.2. The parameters include a reactive NST, the presence of fetal breathing movements, the presence of fetal movement of the body or limbs, the finding of fetal tone (flexed extremities as opposed to a flaccid posture), and an adequate amount of amniotic fluid volume. A total score of 8 out of 10 is considered reassuring. A total score of 6 is equivocal and should prompt further evaluation or delivery if the patient is at early term or beyond. If the patient is preterm, retesting in 24 hours may be appropriate. A score of 4 or less is nonreassuring and usually indicates that delivery is warranted, although further evaluation at pregnancies less than 32 0/7 weeks of gestation may be appropriate. Irrespective of the score, more frequent BPP testing or consideration of delivery may be warranted when oligohydramnios is

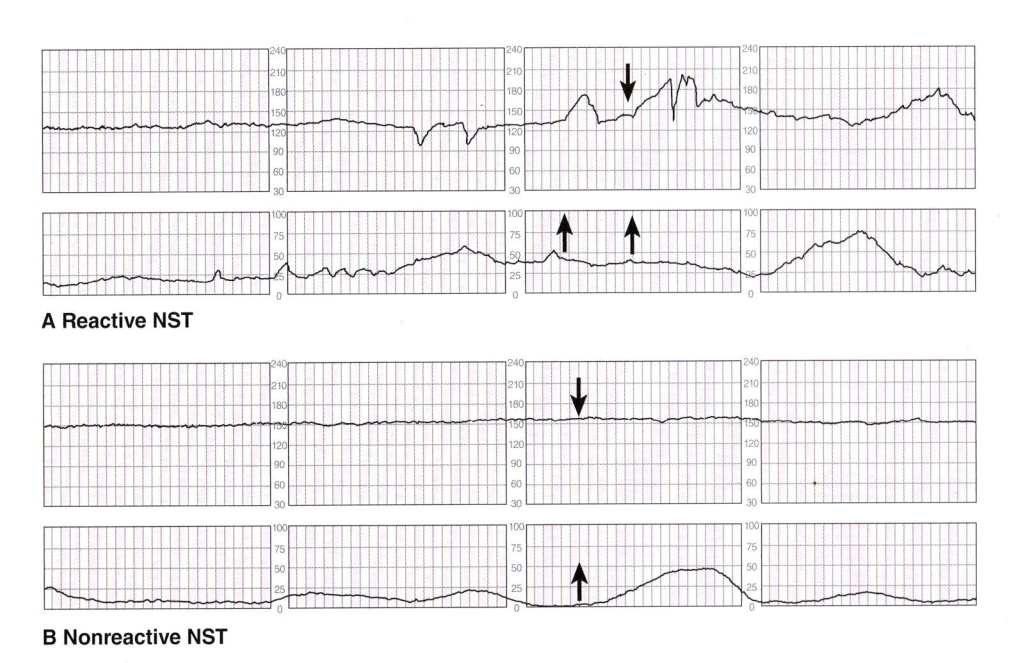

FIGURE 6.2. Nonstress testing. **(A)** Reactive nonstress test (NST); note fetal heart rate acceleration in response to fetal movement. **(B)** Nonreactive NST; note the lack of fetal heart rate acceleration in response to fetal movement.

TABLE 6.2 COMPONENTS OF THE REASSURING BIOPHYSICAL PROFILE

Biophysical Variable	Normal Result
1. Nonstress test (NST)	Because the probability of fetal well-being is identical with scores of 10 out of 10 and 8 out of 10, NST can be omitted if the other four tests are normal
2. Fetal breathing movements	At least one or more episodes of rhythmic fetal breathing movements of 30 seconds or more within 30 minutes
3. Fetal movement	Three or more discrete body or limb movements within 30 minutes
4. Fetal tone	One or more episodes of fetal extremity extension with return to flexion, or opening or closing of hand within 30 minutes
5. Amniotic fluid volume	A pocket of amniotic fluid that measures at least 2 cm in two planes perpendicular to each other

NST, nonstress test; BPP, biophysical profile.
Used with permission from Preconception and Antepartum Care. In: American Academy of Pediatrics, American College of Obstetricians and Gynecologists. *Guidelines for Perinatal Care.* 7th ed. Elk Grove Village (IL): AAP; Washington, DC: American College of Obstetricians and Gynecologists; 2012:149.

present. Management based on the BPP depends not only on the score itself but also on the gestational age of the fetus.

Modified BPP combines the use of an NST and assessment of an amniotic fluid using the deepest vertical pocket sonographically or an amniotic fluid index (AFI). The AFI is a semiquantitative, four-quadrant assessment of amniotic fluid depth. The importance of adequate **amniotic fluid volume** is well established. Diminished amniotic fluid is thought to represent decreased fetal urinary output caused by chronic stress and shunting of blood flow away from the kidneys. The decreased amniotic fluid provides less support for the umbilical cord, which may be more compressed, reducing blood flow. The modified BPP is less cumbersome than the BPP and appears to be as predictive of fetal well-being.

Doppler Ultrasound of Umbilical Artery

Umbilical artery Doppler flow ultrasonography is a noninvasive technique to assess resistance to blood flow in the placenta. It can be used in conjunction with other biophysical tests in high-risk pregnancies associated with suspected IUGR. Umbilical cord Doppler flow velocimetry is based on the characteristics of the systolic blood flow and the diastolic blood flow. The most commonly used index to quantify the flow velocity waveform is the systolic/diastolic ratio. As peripheral resistance increases, diastolic flow decreases and may become absent or reversed, and the systolic/diastolic ratio increases. Reversed end-systolic flow can be seen with severe cases of IUGR secondary to uteroplacental insufficiency and may suggest impending fetal demise.

Assessment of Fetal Lung Maturity

Neonates delivered before their lungs have matured are at risk for **respiratory distress syndrome** (RDS), a serious and life-threatening condition caused by lack of surfactant. RDS in newborns is manifest by signs of respiratory failure—grunting, chest retractions, nasal flaring, and hypoxia—possibly leading to acidosis and death. Management consists of skillful support of ventilation and correction of associated metabolic disturbances until the neonate can ventilate without assistance. Administration of synthetic or semisynthetic surfactant to the neonate has resulted in improved outcomes for infants with RDS.

Results of pulmonary function tests that indicate immaturity do not have a high predictive value for RDS. Because no test indicating maturity can completely rule out the risk of RDS or other neonatal complications, the risk of adverse fetal outcome following delivery must be weighed against the potential risk of allowing the pregnancy to continue.

ANTEPARTUM PATIENT EDUCATION

Plans for the antepartum, intrapartum, and postpartum periods provide an opportunity for patient education and interaction. The Antepartum Record in Appendix B provides a list of the issues to be discussed during antepartum care.

Employment

A woman with an uncomplicated pregnancy can usually continue to work until the onset of labor. It is beneficial to allow moderate activity and to allow for periods of rest and strenuous work (prolonged standing or repetitive, strenuous, and physical lifting) is best avoided.

A period of 4 to 6 weeks generally is required for a woman's physical condition to return to normal. However, the patient's individual circumstances may be a factor in determining when she returns to work. The length of a woman's leave from work can depend on whether there are pregnancy or delivery complications, the work involved, the employer attitude, the rules of the health care system under which the patient receives care, and the wishes of the patient. The Federal Family and Medical Leave Act and state laws should be consulted to determine the family and medical leave that is available.

Exercise

In the absence of either medical or obstetric complications, up to 30 minutes of moderate exercise per day on most if not all days of the week is acceptable (Box 6.2). Each sport should be reviewed for its potential risk, and activities with a high risk of falling or of abdominal trauma should be avoided.

Overly strenuous exercise, especially for prolonged periods, should be avoided. Patients unaccustomed to regular exercise should not undertake vigorous new programs during pregnancy. **Supine exercises** should be discontinued after the first trimester to minimize circulatory changes brought on by pressure of

> **BOX 6.2 Contraindications to Aerobic Exercise during Pregnancy**
>
> **Absolute**
> - Hemodynamically significant heart disease
> - Restrictive lung disease
> - Cervical insufficiency
> - Multiple gestation at risk for premature labor
> - Persistent second-trimester or third-trimester bleeding
> - Placenta previa after 26 weeks of gestation
> - Premature labor during the current pregnancy
> - Ruptured membranes
> - Preeclampsia/gestational hypertension
> - Severe anemia
>
> **Relative**
> - Anemia
> - Unevaluated maternal cardiac arrhythmia
> - Chronic bronchitis
> - Poorly controlled type 1 diabetes
> - Extreme morbid obesity
> - Extreme underweight (BMI < 12)
> - History of extremely sedentary lifestyle
> - Intrauterine growth restriction in current pregnancy
> - Poorly controlled hypertension
> - Orthopedic limitations
> - Poorly controlled seizure disorder
> - Poorly controlled hyperthyroidism
> - Heavy smoker
>
> Used with permission from Physical activity and exercise during pregnancy and the postpartum period. Committee Opinion No. 650. American College of Obstetricians and Gynecologists. *Obstet Gynecol.* 2015;126:e135–42.

> **BOX 6.3 Warning Signs to Terminate Exercise while Pregnant**
>
> - Vaginal bleeding
> - Dyspnea prior to exertion
> - Dizziness
> - Headache
> - Chest pain
> - Muscle weakness
> - Calf pain or swelling (need to rule out thrombophlebitis)
> - Regular painful contractions
> - Amniotic fluid leakage
>
> Used with permission from Physical activity and exercise during pregnancy and the postpartum period. Committee Opinion No. 650. American College of Obstetricians and Gynecologists. *Obstet Gynecol.* 2015;126:e135–42.

the uterus on the vena cava. Any activity should be discontinued if discomfort, significant shortness of breath, or pain in the chest or abdomen appears (Box 6.3). Changes in body contour and balance will alter the advised types of activities; abdominal trauma should be avoided.

Sitting in a hot tub or sauna after exercise is not recommended for pregnant women. Hyperthermia may be teratogenic, particularly in the first trimester. Pregnant women might reasonably be advised to remain in saunas for no more than 15 minutes and in hot tubs for no more than 10 minutes. In a hot tub, if a woman's head, arms, shoulders, and upper chest are not submerged, there is less surface area to absorb heat.

Nutrition and Weight Gain

Concerns about adequate nutrition and weight gain during pregnancy are common. Poor nutrition, obesity, and food faddism are associated with poor perinatal outcome. **Pica**, or an inclination for nonnutritional substances such as ice, food starch, clay, and dirt, is often associated with anemia.

A complete nutritional assessment is an important part of the initial antepartum assessment, including history of dietary habits, special dietary issues or concerns, and weight trends. Anorexia and bulimia increase the risks of associated problems such as cardiac arrhythmias, gastrointestinal (GI) pathology, and electrolyte disturbances. Calculation of BMI is useful because it relates weight to height, allowing for a better indirect measurement of body fat distribution than is obtained with weight alone. Further, because of the "personalized nature" of an individual's BMI, it is often more useful to discuss appropriate weight gain, diet, and exercise with a patient rather than an abstract table.

Recommendations for total weight gain during pregnancy and the rate of weight gain per month appropriate to achieve it may be made based on a BMI calculated for the prepregnancy weight. Pregnant women in their early teens who may still be growing should consider total weight gain in the upper end of these ranges to optimize fetal growth as well. The components that make up the average weight gain in a normal singleton pregnancy are listed in Table 6.3. The maternal component of this weight gain starts in the first trimester and increases linearly after the second trimester. Fetal growth is most rapid in the second half of pregnancy, with the normal fetus tripling its weight in the last 12 weeks.

Published **recommended daily allowances (RDAs)** for protein, minerals, and vitamins are useful approximations. It should be kept in mind, however, that the RDAs are a combination of estimates and values adjusted near the top of the normal ranges to encompass the estimated needs of most women. Thus, many women have an adequate diet for their individual needs, even though it does not supply all the RDAs. Vitamin supplementation is appropriate for specific therapeutic indications, such as a patient's inability or unwillingness to eat a balanced, adequate diet, or clinical demonstration of a specific nutritional risk. Except for iron supplementation in pregnant women with iron deficiency, mineral supplementation in addition to prenatal vitamins is likewise not required in otherwise healthy women.

TABLE 6.3	COMPONENTS OF AVERAGE WEIGHT GAIN IN A NORMAL SINGLETON PREGNANCY WEIGHT	
Organ, Tissue, Fluid	Kilograms (kg)	Pounds (lb)
Maternal		
Uterus	1.0	2.2
Breasts	0.4	0.9
Blood	1.2	2.6
Water	1.7	3.7
Fat	3.3	7.3
Subtotal	7.6	16.7
Fetal		
Fetus	3.4	7.5
Placenta	0.6	1.3
Amniotic fluid	0.8	1.8
Subtotal	4.8	10.6
Total	12.4	27.3

The National Academy of Science recommends 27 mg of iron supplementation (present in most prenatal vitamins). Folic acid is also recommended by the U.S. Public Health Service periconceptionally (one month prior to conception through three months after conception) to prevent neural tube defects. The recommended folic acid supplementation is 400 ug/day for low-risk women, and 4 mg/day for high-risk women.

Financial problems, the inability to get to a grocery store, and foodstuffs unique to a patient's social group that differ in substantial quantitative ways with respect to important nutrients may prevent some women from obtaining adequate nutrition, even if the volume of foodstuffs seems sufficient. The Women, Infants and Children Federal Supplemental Food Program, Food Stamp Programs, and Aid for Families with Dependent Children are resources that may help in these situations.

Breastfeeding

The benefits of **breastfeeding** include the following:

- For the newborn, excellent nutrition and provision of immunologic protection, and lower rates of type 2 diabetes, high blood pressure, and heart disease.
- For the mother, more rapid uterine involution, maternal–child bonding, decreased amount of postpartum bleeding, lower rates of breast and ovarian cancer, and more rapid weight loss associated with extra caloric expenditure (for some women).
- For the preterm infant, lower risk of sudden infant death syndrome, and prevention of short- and long-term health problems.

Contraindications to breastfeeding include certain maternal infections and women who have an infant with galactosemia. Most medications are safe in breastfeeding, with rare exceptions such as cytotoxic chemotherapy drugs. It is important to support each woman's informed decision about whether to initiate or continue breastfeeding. The use of breast pumps and milk storage may allow a mother to continue breastfeeding while continuing to work.

Sexual Activity

Sexual intercourse is not restricted during a normal pregnancy, although advice about more comfortable positions in later pregnancy may be appreciated—for example, side-to-side or the female superior position. Sexual activity may be restricted or prohibited under certain high-risk circumstances, such as known placenta previa, premature rupture of membranes, or history of or current preterm labor (or delivery). Education of the patient (and partner) about safe sex practices is as important in antepartum care as in regular gynecologic care.

Travel

Most airlines allow pregnant women to fly up to 36 weeks, although some airlines may restrict pregnant women from flying earlier in gestation for international flights or other complications. Air travel is not recommended for women who have medical or obstetric complications, such as poorly controlled hypertensive disorder, poorly controlled diabetes mellitus, or sickle cell disease. This recommendation is not due to substantial risk to either mother or fetus but because of the likelihood that labor may ensue away from home and customary health care providers. If a long trip near term is planned, it is useful for the patient to carry a copy of her obstetric record in case she requires obstetric care. When traveling, patients are advised to avoid long periods of inactivity such as sitting. Walking every 1 to 2 hours, even for short periods, promotes circulation, especially in the lower legs, and decreases the risk of venous stasis and possible thromboembolism. Additionally, preventive antiemetic medicine should be considered for pregnant women with increased nausea. Education about the regular use of a seat belt is especially important, with the seat belt worn low on the hip bones, between the protuberant abdomen and the pelvis.

Teratogens

Many patient inquiries concern the teratogenic potential of environmental exposures. Major birth defects are apparent at birth in 2% to 3% of the general population. The possible occurrence of fetal malformations or intellectual disability is a frequent cause of anxiety among pregnant women. Of these, about 5% may be a result of maternal exposure to drugs or environmental chemicals, and only approximately 1% can be attributed to pharmaceutical agents. The most important determinants of the developmental toxicity of an agent are timing, dose, and fetal susceptibility. Many agents have teratogenic effects only if taken while the susceptible fetal organ system is forming.

The health care provider may wish to consult with or refer at-risk patients to health care professionals with special knowledge or experience in teratology and birth defects. The Organization of Teratology Information Services provides information on teratology issues and exposures in pregnancy (www.otispregnancy.org).

Medications

Very few medications have been proven to be true human teratogens (Box 6.4). Most commonly prescribed medications are relatively safe in pregnancy. Until recently, Food and Drug Administration assigned medications a lettered pregnancy risk factor based on information about the medication and its risk/benefit ratio. These pregnancy risk factors helped guide the appropriate use of medications in pregnancy. The FDA has replaced the lettered pregnancy risk factors with four narrative sections for each drug: Pregnancy Exposure Registry, Risk Summary, Clinical Considerations, and Data. For lactation there are three sections: Risk Summary, Clinical Considerations, and Data.

- Section 8.1, Pregnancy (includes labor and delivery), with narrative sections on Pregnancy Exposure Registry, Risk Summary, Clinical Considerations, and Data. This section also includes information for a pregnancy exposure registry.
- Section 8.2, Lactation (includes nursing mothers), with narrative sections on Risk Summary, Clinical Considerations, and Data.
- Section 8.3, Females and Males of Reproductive Potential, includes information about pregnancy testing, contraception recommendations, and infertility.

The new narratives can be accessed on the FDA website (http://www.fda.gov/Drugs/DevelopmentApprovalProcess/DevelopmentResources/Labeling/ucm093307.htm). Table 6.4 provides a summary of the teratogenicity of many common medications. Little data exist about the safety of traditional or folk medications during pregnancy; each physician and patient must consider their use on a case-by-case basis.

Ionizing Radiation

Ionizing radiation exposure is universal; most radiation originates from beyond the earth's atmosphere, from the land, and from endogenous radionuclides. The total radiation exposure from these sources is approximately 125 mrad/y. Although radiation exposure has the potential to cause gene mutations, growth impairment, chromosome damage and malignancy, and fetal death, large doses are required to produce discernible fetal effects. Large doses (10 rad) during the first 2 weeks after fertilization are required to produce a deleterious effect. In the first trimester, 25 rad is required to produce detectable damage, and 100 rad is required later in pregnancy. Diagnostic radiation usually exposes the fetus to much less than 5 rad, depending on the number of radiographs taken and the maternal site examined (Table 6.5). Exposure to less than 5 rad has not been associated with an increase in fetal anomalies or pregnancy loss; therefore, it is recommended to limit accumulated fetal exposure to less than 5 rad during pregnancy.

Methyl Mercury

Industrial pollution is the major source of mercury entry in our ecosystem. Large fish, such as tuna, shark, and king mackerel, retain higher levels of mercury from the smaller fish and organisms they consume. Therefore, women who eat these fish are storing high levels of mercury. Pregnant women should be encouraged to enjoy two to three servings per week (8 to 12 oz total) of a variety of fish that are on the EPA's "best choices" list such as cod, haddock, lobster, salmon, shrimp, and canned tuna; eat only one serving per week of fish from the "good choices" list, such as bluefish, carp, halibut, snapper, and fresh albacore or yellowfin tuna; and avoid the following fish that have high mercury levels: king mackerel, marlin, orange roughy, shark, swordfish, tilefish, and bigeye tuna. Details can be found at https://www.acog.org/About-ACOG/News-Room/Practice-Advisories/ACOG-Practice-Advisory-Seafood-Consumption-During-Pregnancy.

Herbal Remedies

Herbal remedies are not regulated as prescription or OTC drugs; the identity and quantity of their ingredients are unknown, and

---

BOX 6.4 Drugs or Substances Suspected or Proven to Be Human Teratogens

ACE inhibitors[a]	Kanamycin
Aminopterin	Lithium
Androgens	Methimazole
Ang-II antagonists[b]	Methotrexate
Busulfan	Misoprostol
Carbamazepine	Penicillamine
Chlorobiphenyls	Phenytoin
Cocaine	Radioactive iodine
Coumarins	Streptomycin
Cyclophosphamide	Tamoxifen
Danazol	Tetracycline
Diethylstilbestrol	Thalidomide
Ethanol	Tretinoin
Etretinate	Trimethadione
Isotretinoin	Valproic acid

[a] Angiotensin–converting enzyme inhibitors.
[b] Angiotensin–converting enzyme inhibitors.
Adapted from Briggs GG, Freeman RK, Yaffe SJ. *Drugs in Pregnancy and Lactation: A Reference Guide to Fetal and Neonatal Risk.* 8th ed. Philadelphia, PA: Lippincott Williams & Wilkins 2008; Cunningham GF, Leveno KJ, Bloom SL, Hauth JC, Gilstrap LC, Wenstom KD, eds. Williams *Obstetrics.* 22nd ed. New York, NY: McGraw Hill Professional; 2005:T14-1;

TABLE 6.4 SUMMARY OF TERATOGENICITY OF VARIOUS MEDICATIONS

Drug	Effect
Tetracyclines	Yellow-brown discoloration of deciduous teeth has been associated with the use of medications such as doxycycline and minocycline
Sulfonamides	Avoid near delivery due to the risk of hyperbilirubinemia through the displacement of bilirubin from protein-binding sites
Nitrofurantoin	For infants younger than age 1 month and those with a known G6-PD deficiency, nitrofurantoin is contraindicated because of potential hemolysis
Quinolones	Associated with irreversible arthropathies and cartilage erosion in animal studies; no teratogenic effects have been demonstrated in animal studies
Metronidazole	Not teratogenic to fetuses exposed in the first trimester
Warfarin	Highly teratogenic due to their ability to easily cross the placental barrier; if exposed between weeks 6 and 12, the fetus is at risk for developing a warfarin embryopathy—nasal and midface hypoplasia with stippled vertebral and femoral epiphyses; later exposure is associated with hemorrhage-related fetal abnormalities, such as hydrocephalus
Heparin and low-molecular-weight heparins	Anticoagulant of choice for use in pregnancy because the large, polar molecules do not cross the placenta (and, therefore, are not teratogenic); the newer low-molecular-weight heparins are not associated with fetal malformations
Phenytoin	May produce abnormal facies, cleft lip or palate, microcephaly, growth deficiency, and hypoplastic nails and distal phalanges in as many as 10% of exposed offspring
Valproic acid and carbamazepine	Exposure during embryogenesis is associated with a 1%–2% risk of spina bifida and neural tube defects
SSRIs	Paroxetine: Increased risk of ventral and atrial septal cardiac defects All SSRIs: Exposure late in pregnancy associated with a neonatal behavioral syndrome (increased muscle tone, irritability, jitteriness, and respiratory distress)
ACE inhibitors	Associated with numerous fetal anomalies, including growth restriction, limb contractures, and abnormalities in cavarum development
Diuretics	Thiazide diuretics: When given near delivery, the fetus may experience thrombocytopenia with associated bleeding and electrolyte disturbances All: May interfere with breast milk production
β-Blockers	Reported associations with fetal growth restriction and neonatal hypoglycemia; neonates may experience transient mild hypotension with symptomatic β-blockade
Calcium-channel blockers	Generally considered safe during pregnancy
Methyldopa and hydralazine	Generally considered safe during pregnancy
Alkylating agents	Cyclophosphamide: Associated with missing or hypoplastic digits of the hands and feet when the fetus is exposed in the first trimester; second-semester exposure is not associated with defects
Methotrexate	Alters normal folic acid metabolism; high doses can lead to growth restriction, severe limb abnormalities, posteriorly rotated ears, micrognathia, and hypoplastic supraorbital ridges
Androgens	Exposure to exogenous androgens between 7 and 12 weeks can cause full masculinization, with later exposure causing partial masculinization
Testosterone and anabolic steroids	Can result in varying degrees of virilization, including labioscrotal fusion and phallic enlargement, depending on the timing and extent of exposure
Danazol	Dose-related patterns of clitorimegaly, urogenital sinus malformation, and labioscrotal fusion
Aspirin and acetaminophen	Aspirin: Theoretical risk of premature closure of the ductus arteriosus Acetaminophen: Not associated with an increased risk of defect

TABLE 6.4 SUMMARY OF TERATOGENICITY OF VARIOUS MEDICATIONS (Continued)

Drug	Effect
NSAIDs	In general, not teratogenic and can be used short term in the third trimester, with reversible fetal effects Indomethacin: Used as a tocolytic agent; constriction of the fetal ductus arteriosus and neonatal pulmonary hypertension have been associated with the use of indomethacin near delivery
Pseudoephedrine	Retrospective study found an increased risk of gastroschisis (a congenital defect of the anterior abdominal wall characterized by an opening beside the umbilical cord that allows bowel to protrude); should be avoided in the first trimester
Benzodiazepines	Teratogenicity is not clearly defined; exposed neonates should be monitored for transient withdrawal symptoms
Lithium	Associated with an increase in cardiovascular malformations, although evidence for a significant increase has been challenged; limiting exposure until after 8 weeks' gestation to allow the cardiac structures to complete organogenesis is reasonable
Vitamin A	Extremely high doses of vitamin A are associated with congenital anomalies, but categorization is limited by the small number of confirmed cases
Isotretinoin	A potent teratogen; associated with significant fetal loss and malformations with first-trimester use
Tretinoin	Topical retinoid gel; information about teratogenicity is lacking; women should avoid during pregnancy

G6-PD, glucose 6-phosphate dehydrogenase; SSRIs, selective serotonin-reuptake inhibitors; ACE, angiotensin-converting enzyme; NSAIDs, nonsteroidal anti-inflammatory drugs.

TABLE 6.5 ESTIMATED FETAL EXPOSURE FROM SOME COMMON RADIOLOGIC PROCEDURES

Procedure	Fetal Exposure
CT scan of abdomen and lumbar spine	3.5 rad
Barium enema or small bowel series	2–4 rad
Intravenous pyelography (5 views)	686–1,398 milirad[a]
CT scan of head or chest	<1 rad
Spiral CT of the thorax (pitch 1 or greater)	<1 rad
CT pelvimetry	250 milirad
Hip film (2 views)	103–213 milirad
Abdominal film (2 views)	122–245 milirad
Lumbosacral spine film (3 views)	168–359 milirad
Ventilation/perfusion scan with technetium 99m and xenon gas	50 milirad
Mammography (4 views)	7–20 milirad
Chest x-ray (2 views)	0.02–0.07 milirad
Skull films (4 views)	<0.5 milirad
Magnetic resonance imaging	0

CT, computed tomography.
[a] Amount of exposure depends on the number of films obtained.
Modified from the American College of Obstetricians and Gynecologists. *Precis: Obstetrics.* 4th ed. Washington, DC: American College of Obstetricians and Gynecologists; 2010:31.

there are virtually no studies of their teratogenic potential. Because it is not possible to assess their safety, pregnant women should be counseled to consider avoiding these substances. Remedies containing substances with pharmaceutical properties that could theoretically have adverse fetal affects include the following:

- Echinacea—causes fragmentation of hamster sperm at high concentrations
- Black cohosh—contains a chemical that acts like an estrogen
- Garlic and willow barks—have anticoagulant properties
- Ginkgo—can interfere with the effects of monamine oxidase inhibitors; has anticoagulant effects
- Real licorice—has hypertensive and potassium-wasting effects
- Valerian—intensifies the effects of prescription sleep aids
- Ginseng—interferes with the effects of monamine oxidase inhibitors
- Blue cohosh and pennyroyal—stimulate uterine musculature; pennyroyal can also cause liver damage, renal failure, disseminated intravascular coagulation, and maternal death

Alcohol

Alcohol is the most common teratogen to which a fetus is exposed, and alcohol consumption during pregnancy is a leading preventable cause of intellectual disability, developmental delay, and birth defects in the fetus. There is substantial evidence that fetal toxicity is dose related and that the exposure time of greatest risk is the first trimester. There is no established safe level of alcohol use during pregnancy. Women who are pregnant or who are at risk for pregnancy should not drink alcohol. Although consumption of small amounts of alcohol early in pregnancy is unlikely to cause serious fetal problems, patients are best advised to refrain from alcohol entirely.

Fetal alcohol syndrome (FAS) is a congenital syndrome characterized by alcohol use during pregnancy and includes three findings:

1. Growth restriction (which may occur in the prenatal period, the postnatal period, or both)
2. Facial abnormalities, including shortened palpebral fissures, low-set ears, midfacial hypoplasia, a smooth philtrum, and a thin upper lip
3. Central nervous system dysfunction including microcephaly, intellectual disability, and behavioral disorders such as attention deficit disorder

The exact risk incurred by maternal alcohol use is difficult to establish, because the complex pattern of symptoms associated with FAS can make diagnosis difficult. Consumption of eight or more drinks daily throughout pregnancy confers a 30% to 50% risk of having a child with FAS. However, even low levels of alcohol consumption (two or fewer drinks per week) have been associated with increased aggressive behavior in children.

Tobacco Use

The risks of tobacco use (smoked, chewed, ENDS, vaped) during pregnancy have been well established and include risks to the fetus such as IUGR, low birthweight, and fetal mortality. It is important for the obstetrician to take advantage of the prenatal visits to educate patients about the risks of tobacco use for both themselves and their newborns and to coordinate appropriate resources to help patients quit. Counseling programs are available to help patients quit tobacco use. Nicotine replacement products may be considered under close supervision and after careful consideration, although their safety in pregnancy has not been documented.

Substance Abuse

The use of illicit substances by women of childbearing age has led to an increased number of neonates having had in utero exposure and subsequent risk of adverse effects from a variety of drugs. Fetal drug exposure is often unrecognized because of the lack of overt symptoms or structural anomaly following birth.

Illicit drugs may reach the fetus via placental transfer or may reach the newborn through breast milk. The specific effect on the fetus and newborn varies with the respective substances. An opiate-exposed fetus may experience withdrawal symptoms in utero if the woman stops using opiates; when she herself goes through withdrawal, either voluntarily or under supervision; or after birth when opiate delivery by the way of the placenta ceases. For pregnant women with an opioid use disorder, medication-assisted treatment is the recommended therapy and breastfeeding should be encouraged in patients without HIV who are not using additional drugs and who have no other contraindications.

All pregnant women should be asked at their first prenatal visit and throughout pregnancy about past and present use of alcohol; nicotine; and other drugs, including recreational use of prescription and OTC medications. This routine screening should rely on validated screening tools, such as specific questionnaires. Routine screening using biologic specimens of women and newborns for substance abuse is not recommended. A woman who acknowledges the use of these substances should be counseled about the perinatal implications of their use during pregnancy and offered referral to an appropriate drug treatment program if chemical dependence is suspected. Careful follow-up during the postpartum period is also recommended.

• COMMON SYMPTOMS

The normal physiology of pregnancy often results in symptoms that would be considered pathologic were the patient not pregnant. All health care providers caring for pregnant patients should be familiar with what changes are considered normal in pregnancy and be able to educate the patient in that regard.

Headaches

Headaches are common in early pregnancy and may be severe. The etiology of such headaches is not known. Treatment with acetaminophen in usual doses is recommended and is generally adequate. A persistent headache unrelieved by acetaminophen should be further evaluated.

Edema

The presence of significant **edema** in the lower extremities (dependent edema) and/or hands is very common in pregnancy and, by itself, is not abnormal. Fluid retention can be associated with hypertension, however, so that blood pressure as well as weight gain and edema must be evaluated in a clinical context before the findings are presumed to be innocuous.

Nausea and Vomiting

The majority of pregnant women experience some degree of upper GI symptoms in the first trimester of pregnancy. Classically, these symptoms are worse in the morning (the so-called **morning sickness**). However, patients may experience symptoms at other times or even throughout the day. Most mild cases of nausea and vomiting can be resolved with lifestyle and dietary changes, including consuming more ginger, vitamin B_6, or vitamin B_6 with doxylamine. Usually, nausea and vomiting improve significantly by the end of the first trimester, but other pharmacological treatments, such as Diclegis, may be considered for more serious cases. The most severe form of pregnancy-associated nausea and vomiting is **hyperemesis gravidarum**, which occurs in less than 2% of pregnancies. This condition may require hospitalization, with fluid and electrolyte therapy and medications.

Heartburn

Heartburn (gastric reflux) is common, especially postprandially, and is often associated with eating large meals or spicy or fatty foods. Patient education about smaller and more frequent meals and blander foods, combined with not eating immediately before retiring, is helpful. Antacids may be helpful when used judiciously in pregnancy.

Constipation

Constipation is physiologic in pregnancy, associated with increased transit time; increased water absorption; and, often, decreased bulk. Dietary modifications, including increased fluid intake and increased bulk with such foods as fruits and vegetables, are usually helpful. Other useful interventions may include the use of surface-active bowel softeners such as **docusate**, supplemental dietary fibers such as **psyllium hydrophilic mucilloid**, and lubricants.

Fatigue

In early pregnancy, patients often complain of extreme **fatigue** that is unrelieved by rest. There is no specific treatment, other than adjustment of the woman's schedule to the extent possible to accommodate this temporary lack of energy. Patients can be reassured that the symptoms typically disappear in the second trimester.

Leg Cramps

Leg cramps, usually affecting the calves, are common during pregnancy. A variety of treatments, including oral calcium supplement, potassium supplement, and tonic water, have been proposed over the years, none of which are universally successful. Massage and rest are often advised.

Back Pain

Lower back pain is common, especially in late pregnancy. The altered center of gravity caused by the growing fetus places unusual stress on the lower spine and associated muscles and ligaments. Treatment focuses on heat, massage, and limited use of analgesia. A specially fitted maternal girdle may also help, as will not wearing shoes with high heels.

Round Ligament Pain

Sharp groin pain, especially as pregnancy advances, is common, often quite uncomfortable, and disturbing to patients. This pain is often more pronounced on the right side because of the usual dextrorotation of the gravid uterus. The woman should be reassured that the pain represents stretching and spasm of the round ligaments. Modification of activity, especially more gradual movement, is often helpful; analgesics are rarely indicated.

Varicose Veins and Hemorrhoids

Varicose veins are not caused by pregnancy but often first appear during the course of gestation. Besides the disturbing appearance to many patients, varicose veins can cause an aching sensation, especially when patients stand for long periods of time. Support hose can help diminish the discomfort, although it has no effect on the appearance of the varicose veins. Popular brands of support hose do not provide the relief that prescription elastic hose can. **Hemorrhoids** are varicosities of the hemorrhoidal veins. Treatment consists of sitz baths and local preparations. Varicose veins and hemorrhoids regress postpartum, although neither condition may abate completely. Surgical correction of varicose veins or hemorrhoids should not be undertaken for approximately the first 6 months postpartum to allow for the natural involution to occur.

Vaginal Discharge

The hormonal milieu of pregnancy often causes an increase in normal vaginal secretions. These normal secretions must be distinguished from infections, such as vaginitis, which has symptoms of itching and malodor, and bacterial vaginosis, which has been linked to preterm labor. Spontaneous rupture of membranes, which is characterized by leakage of thin, clear fluid, is another possible cause that must be considered.

CLINICAL FOLLOW-UP

The patient is 8 weeks pregnant based on your bedside vaginal sonogram. You perform a thorough history and physical examination, obtaining the appropriate prenatal screening blood work and cervico-vaginal cultures. You discuss available screening for genetic conditions, including fetal chromosome abnormalities, as well as screening for immunity to more common infectious diseases. The patient is educated on the importance of regular prenatal care, appropriate exercise, nutrition, and weight gain, and how to manage common complaints in pregnancy.

CHAPTER 7

Genetics and Genetic Disorders in Obstetrics and Gynecology

This chapter deals primarily with APGO Educational Topic Areas:

TOPIC 9   PRECONCEPTION CARE

TOPIC 32   OBSTETRIC PROCEDURES

Students should be able to identify patients with genetic risk and counsel them regarding that risk as well as genetic screening options. They should also be familiar with the use of amniocentesis, chorionic villus sampling, and ultrasound to evaluate patients with suspected genetic disorders.

CLINICAL CASE

A new obstetric patient presents for her nurse history. She is an only child but reports that she has an aunt and a female cousin who had a great deal of difficulty in school. The aunt also has a son who is mentally retarded and seems to remember at least one other distant cousin with mental retardation. She wants to make sure her baby does not have the same problem. What additional consultations and evaluations will you offer this patient?

● INTRODUCTION

Recent discoveries in the field of genetics have led to the increased use of genetic principles and techniques in all areas of medicine, including obstetrics and gynecology. In obstetrics, prenatal screening is routinely performed to detect genetic disorders, such as Down syndrome and cystic fibrosis. In gynecology, clinicians can offer appropriate genetic testing for women deemed at high risk for genes that increase the risk of breast, bowel, and ovarian cancers. In the future, genetic evaluation may lead to earlier and more accurate diagnosis of conditions such as diabetes. Gene-based therapies may also be used to treat diseases with greater specificity and fewer side effects than conventional treatments.

● BASIC CONCEPTS IN GENETICS

Knowledge of the basic principles of genetics and an understanding of their application are essential in current medical practice. These principles form the basis for screening, diagnosis, and management of genetic disorders.

Genes: Definition and Function

Genes, the basic units of heredity, are segments of deoxyribonucleic acid (**DNA**) that reside on **chromosomes** located in cell nuclei. DNA is a double-stranded helical molecule. Each strand is a polymer of nucleotides made up of three components: 1) a "base," which is either a purine (adenine [A] or guanine [G]) or a pyrimidine (cytosine [C] or thymine [T]); 2) a five-carbon sugar; and 3) a phosphodiester bond. The strands of the DNA helix run in an antiparallel fashion, adenine binding to thymine and cytosine binding to guanine. These base pairs, in their nearly limitless combinations, constitute the **genetic code**.

The information in the DNA must be processed before it can be used by cells. **Transcription** is the process by which DNA is converted to a messenger molecule called **ribonucleic acid** (**RNA**). During transcription, the DNA molecule is "read" from one end (called the *5-prime* [5′] *end*) to the other end (called the *3-prime* [3′] *end*). A **messenger RNA** (**mRNA**) molecule is formed that is exported from the cell nucleus into the cytoplasm. This mRNA contains a translation of the genetic code into **codons**. Transcription is regulated by promoter and enhancer sequences. **Promoter** sequences guide the direction of translation from 5′ to 3′ and are located on the 5′ end. **Enhancer** sequences have the same function but are found further down the 5′-end of the DNA molecule.

After transcription is complete, mRNA is used as a template to construct the amino acids that are the building blocks of proteins. In this process, called **translation**, each codon is matched to its corresponding amino acid. The amino acid strand grows until a "stop" codon is encountered. At this point, the now-completed protein undergoes further processing and is then either used inside the cell or is exported outside the cell for use in other cells, tissues, and organs. Errors in the DNA replication process can occur in a variety of ways and lead to a **mutation**, a change in the normal gene sequence. Most DNA replication errors are rapidly repaired by enzymes that proofread and repair mistakes.

Replication errors are of four basic kinds: 1) **missense** mutations, in which one amino acid is substituted for another; 2) **nonsense** mutations, in which premature stop codons are inserted in a sequence; 3) **deletions**; and 4) **insertions**. An example of a replication error causing a recognized disease is Huntington disease, in which an abnormal number of cytosine–adenine–guanine (CAG) repeats occurs in the Huntington gene. DNA can also be damaged by environmental factors, such as ultraviolet light, ionizing radiation, and chemicals.

Chromosomes

The genetic information in the human genome is packaged as **chromatin**, within which DNA binds with several chromosomal proteins to make **chromosomes**. A **karyotype** reveals the morphology and number of chromosomes. **Somatic cells** are all the cells in the human body that are not gametes (eggs or sperm). **Germ cells**, or gametes, contain a *single set* of chromosomes ($n = 23$) and are described as **haploid** in number. Somatic cells contain *two sets of chromosomes*, for a total of 46 chromosomes. These cells are **diploid**, signifying that they have a $2n$ chromosome complement ($2n = 46$). These chromosome pairs consist of 22 pairs of **autosomes**, which are similar in males and females. Each somatic cell also contains a pair of sex chromosomes. Females have two X sex chromosomes; males have an X and a Y chromosome.

Chromosome Replication and Cell Division

Chromosomes undergo two types of replication, meiosis and mitosis, which are significantly different and produce cell types with crucially different capabilities. **Mitosis** is the replication of chromosomes in somatic cells. It is followed by **cytokinesis**, or cell division, that results in two daughter cells containing the same genetic information as the parent cell. **Meiosis** only occurs in germ cells. It is also followed by cytokinesis; but, in this case, cytokinesis results in four daughter cells with a haploid count.

Somatic cells undergo cell division based on the cell cycle. There are four stages of the cell cycle: G_1, S, G_2, and M. G_1, or gap 1, occurs immediately after mitosis and is a period of inactivity with no DNA replication. During G_1, all the DNA of each chromosome is present in the $2n$ form. The next phase is S, or synthesis, in which the chromosomes double to become two identical sister chromatids with a $4n$ chromosome complement. During G_2, or gap 2, the cells prepare for mitosis. G_1, S, and G_2 are also called **interphase**, which is the period between mitoses.

Mitosis

The goal of mitosis is to form two daughter cells that have a complete set of genetic information. Mitosis is divided into five stages: Prophase, prometaphase, metaphase, anaphase, and telophase. During **prophase** the chromatin swells, or condenses, and the two sister chromatids are in close approximation. The nucleolus disappears, and the mitotic spindle develops. Spindle fibers start to form centrosomes, microtubule-organizing centers that migrate to the poles of the cell. In **prometaphase**, the nuclear membrane vanishes and the chromosomes begin to disperse. They will eventually attach to the microtubules that form the mitotic spindle. **Metaphase** is the stage of maximal condensation. The chromosomes are in a linear formation in the center of the cell, between the two spindle poles. It is during metaphase where cells can most easily be analyzed to obtain a karyotype from an amniocentesis or **chorionic villus sampling** (**CVS**). **Anaphase** is initiated when the two chromatids separate. They form daughter chromosomes that are drawn to opposite poles of the cell by the spindle fibers. Finally, **telophase** is when the nuclear membrane starts to reform around the independent daughter cells, which then go into interphase (Fig. 7.1).

Meiosis

Meiosis differs from mitosis in that a haploid number of cells are initially produced in two successive divisions. The **first division (meiosis I) is termed a reduction division**, because of the resulting decrease in chromosome number from diploid to haploid. Meiosis I is also divided into four stages: Prophase I, metaphase I, anaphase I, and telophase I. **Prophase I** is further divided into five substages: Leptotene, zygotene, pachytene, diplotene, and diakinesis. In prophase I, the chromosomes condense and become shorter and thicker. It is during the pachytene substage that **crossing over** takes place, resulting in four distinct gametes. However, it is during anaphase where most of

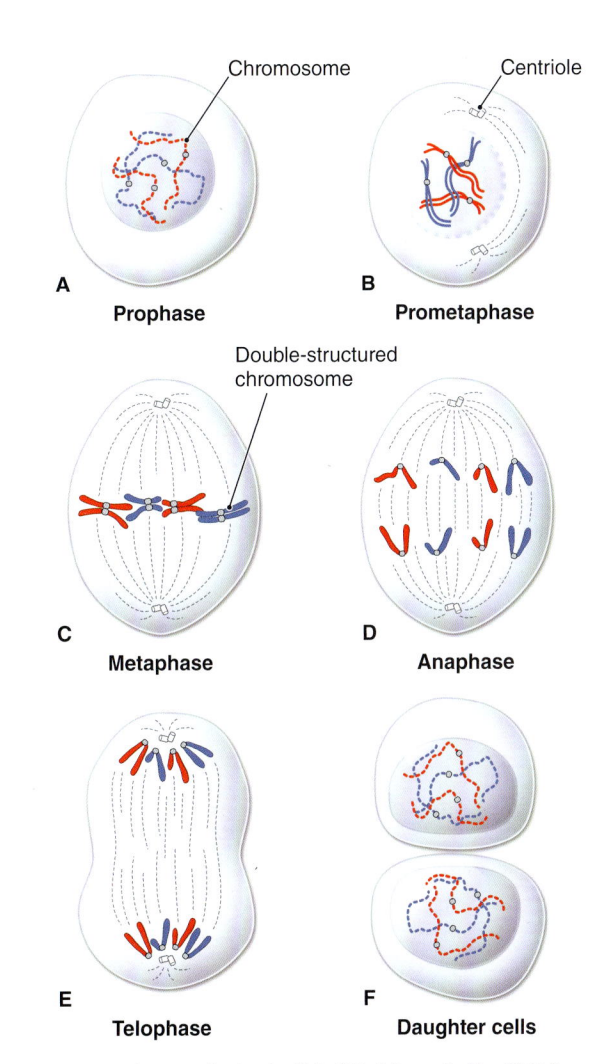

FIGURE 7.1. Stages of mitosis. (Modified from Sadler TW. *Langman's Medical Embryology*. 10th ed. Baltimore, MD: Lippincott Williams & Wilkins; 2006:12.)

the genetic variation occurs. In **anaphase I**, the chromosomes go to opposite poles of the cell by **independent assortment**, signifying that there are 2^{23}, or >8 million, possible variations. Anaphase I is also the most error-prone step in meiosis.

The process of **disjunction**, in which the chromosomes go to opposite poles of the cell, can result in nondisjunction, where both chromosomes go instead to the same pole. Nondisjunction is a common cause of chromosomally abnormal fetuses.

The second meiotic division (meiosis II) is similar to mitosis, except that the process occurs within a cell with a haploid number of chromosomes. Meiosis II is also divided into four stages: Prophase II, metaphase II, anaphase II, and telophase II. The result of meiosis II is four haploid daughter cells. After anaphase II, the possibilities for genetic variation are further increased by $2^{23} \times 2^{23}$, ensuring genetic variation (Fig. 7.2).

Abnormalities in Chromosome Number

Any alteration in the chromosome number is called **heteroploidy**. Heteroploidy can occur in two forms: Euploidy and aneuploidy. In **euploidy**, the haploid number of 23 chromosomes is altered. An example of euploidy is triploidy, in which the haploid number has been multiplied by three. The karyotype is 69,XXX or 69,XXY. Triploidy results from double fertilization of a normal haploid egg or from fertilization by a diploid sperm. Such abnormalities usually result in conceptions of partial hydatidiform moles and end spontaneously in the first trimester.

In **aneuploidy**, the diploid number of 46 chromosomes is altered. The **trisomies** are aneuploidies in which there are three copies of an autosome instead of two. Examples include **trisomy 21 (Down syndrome)**, **trisomy 18 (Edward syndrome)**, **trisomy 13 (Patau syndrome)**, and **trisomy 16**. Most trisomies result from maternal meiotic nondisjunction, a phenomenon that occurs more frequently as a woman ages (Fig. 7.3 and Table 7.1).

Sex chromosome abnormalities occur in 1 of every 1,000 births. The most common are 45,X; 47,XXY; 47,XXX; 47,XYY; and mosaicism (the presence of two or more cell populations with different karyotypes). Numeric sex chromosome abnormalities can result from either maternal or paternal nondisjunction.

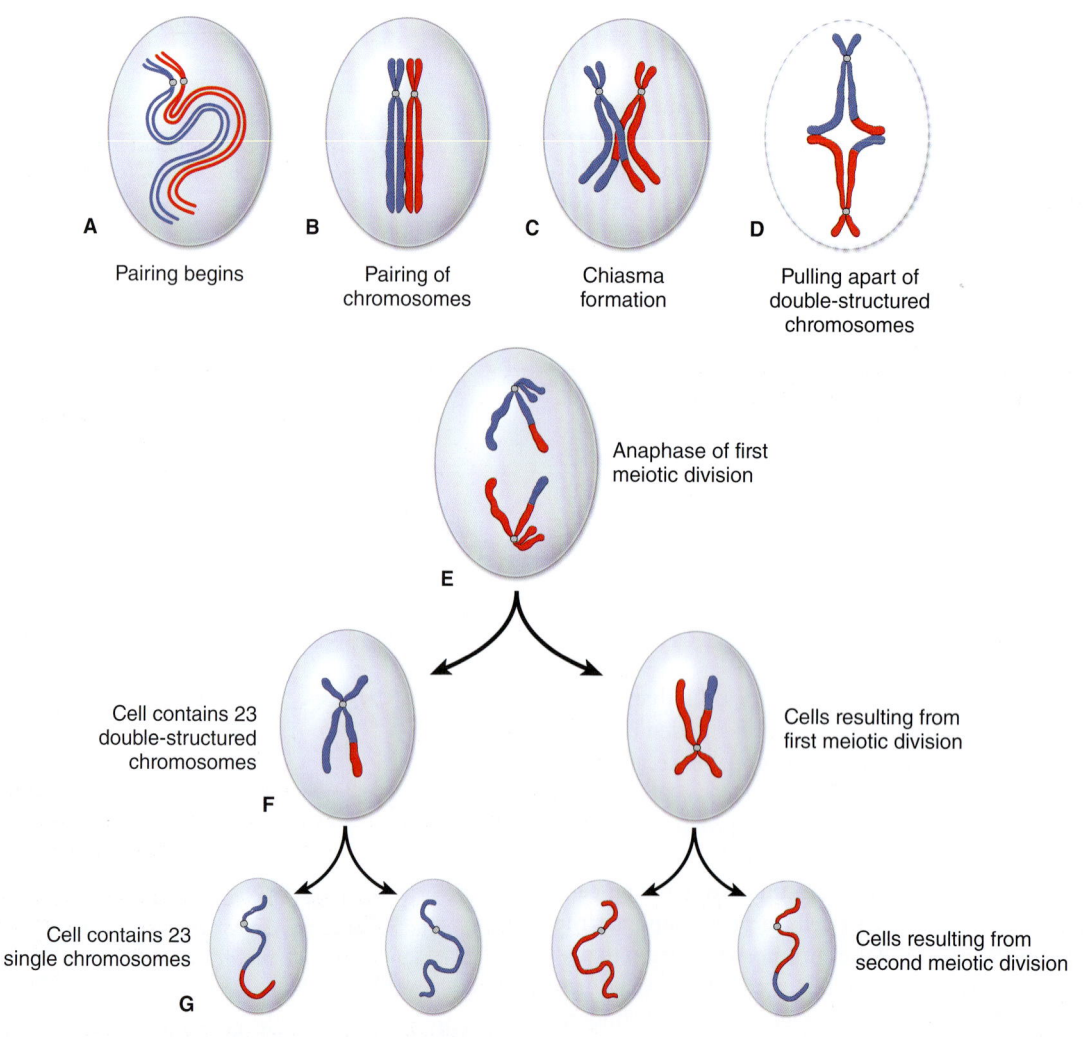

FIGURE 7.2. Stages of meiosis. (Modified from Sadler TW. *Langman's Medical Embryology*. 10th ed. Baltimore, MD: Lippincott Williams & Wilkins; 2006:13.)

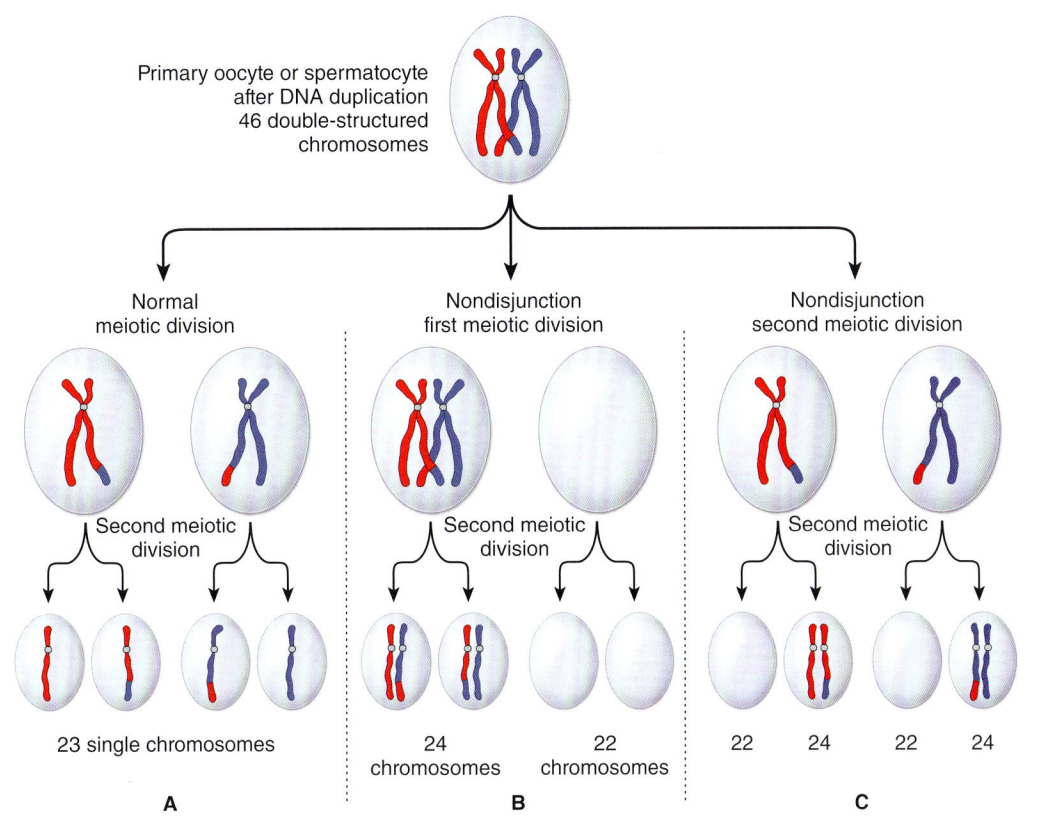

FIGURE 7.3. Comparison of normal and abnormal meiotic divisions. (A) Normal meiotic division. (B) Nondisjunction in the first meiotic division. (C) Nondisjunction in the second meiotic division. (Modified from Sadler TW. *Langman's Medical Embryology*. 10th ed. Baltimore, MD: Lippincott Williams & Wilkins; 2006:15.)

TABLE 7.1 COMMONLY DIAGNOSED CHROMOSOMAL ABNORMALITIES

Chromosome Abnormality	Live Birth Incidence	Characteristics
Trisomy 21 (Down syndrome)	1:800	Moderate-to-severe mental retardation; characteristic facies; cardiac abnormalities; increased incidence of respiratory infections and leukemia; only 2% live beyond age 50 years
Trisomy 18 (Edwards syndrome)	1:6,000	Severe mental retardation; multiple organic abnormalities; less than 10% survive 1 year
Trisomy 13 (Patau syndrome)	1:10,000	Severe mental retardation; neurologic, ophthalmologic, and organic abnormalities; 5% survive 3 years
Trisomy 16	0	Lethal anomaly occurs frequently in first-trimester spontaneous abortions; no infants are known to have trisomy 16
45,X	1:10,000	Occurs frequently in first-trimester (Turner syndrome) spontaneous abortions; associated primarily with unique somatic features; patients are not mentally retarded, although IQs of affected individuals are lower than those of siblings
47,XXX; 47,XYY; 47,XXY (Klinefelter syndrome)	Each approximately 1:500 males	Minimal somatic abnormalities; individuals with Klinefelter syndrome are characterized by a tall, eunuchoid habitus, and small testes; 47,XXX and 47,XYY individuals do not usually exhibit somatic abnormalities, but 47,XYY individuals may be tall
del(5p) (Cri du chat syndrome)	1:20,000	Severe mental retardation, microcephaly, distinctive facial features, characteristic "cat's cry" sound

Abnormalities in Chromosome Structure

Structural alterations in chromosomes are less common than numerical alterations. Structural abnormalities that affect reproduction occur in 0.2% of the population.

Deletions

A **deletion** occurs when a portion of a chromosome segment is lost (Table 7.2). In a **terminal deletion**, the missing portion of the chromosome is appended to the end of the long or short arm. If the missing portion of the chromosome is appended to both the long and short arms of the same chromosome, a **ring chromosome** can result. An **interstitial deletion** occurs when the deleted portion lacks a centromere, or in cases involving chromosomal breakage.

Insertions

Insertions occur when the portion of an interstitially deleted segment is inserted into a nonhomologous chromosome.

Inversions

An **inversion** is the result of faulty repair of a chromosomal breakage. The broken portion is inserted into the chromosome in an inverted fashion. A **paracentric inversion** occurs when both breaks occur on one arm of a chromosome. These types of inversions do not include the **centromere**, the region where the chromosome pairs are joined. Paracentric inversions cannot be identified by a traditional karyotype because the arms appear to be of normal length. **Fluorescence in situ hybridization** (**FISH** see p. 91) with locus-specific probes is used to detect this type of abnormality. A **pericentric inversion** involves a break in each arm. The centromere is included and a notable gain or loss of genetic material can be identified on a karyotype.

For a parent with an inversion, the risk of having an abnormal child depends on the method of detection, the chromosome involved, and the size of the inversion. The observed risk is approximately 5% to 10% if the inversion is identified after the birth of an abnormal child, and 1% to 3% if identified at some other time. An exception is pericentric inversion of chromosome 9, which is not associated with genetic defects in offspring.

Translocations

A **translocation** involves the transfer of two chromosome segments, usually between nonhomologous (nonpaired) chromosomes. They are the most common form of structural rearrangements in humans. A translocation is described as **balanced** when equal amounts of genetic material are exchanged between chromosomes, and **unbalanced** when the chromosomes receive unequal amounts of genetic material. Two types of translocations are possible. A **Robertsonian translocation** only occurs in acrocentric chromosomes—those in which the centromere is located very near one end (chromosomes 13, 14, 15, 21, and 22). Those with Robertsonian translocations are phenotypically normal, but the gametes they produce may be unbalanced. Whether the unbalanced gametes will result in abnormal offspring depends on the type of translocation, the chromosomes involved, and the sex of the carrier parent. The most clinically important Robertsonian translocations are those involving chromosome 21 and another acrocentric chromosome, most commonly chromosome 14. Carriers of these translocations are at increased risk for having a child with trisomy 21. The risk of trisomy 21 is 15% if the translocation is maternal and 2% or less if it is paternal.

Balanced reciprocal translocations may involve any chromosome and are the result of a reciprocal exchange of chromosome material between two or more chromosomes. Like those with Robertsonian translocations, individuals with a balanced reciprocal translocation are also phenotypically normal but they may produce gametes with unbalanced chromosomes. The observed risk of a chromosomal abnormality in an offspring is less than the theoretical risk, because some of these gametes result in nonviable conceptions. In general, carriers of chromosome translocations identified after the birth of an abnormal child have a 5% to 30% risk of having an unbalanced offspring.

Children with an unbalanced chromosome translocation are at increased risk for mental retardation, neurodevelopmental delay, and other congenital abnormalities.

TABLE 7.2 ABNORMALITIES IN CHROMOSOME STRUCTURE

Abnormality in Chromosome Structure	Definition	Clinical Example
Deletion	Loss of a chromosome segment resulting in imbalance	Duchenne muscular dystrophy
Insertion	A segment removed from one chromosome is inserted into another	Hemophilia A
Inversion	A single chromosome has two breaks with reattachment in an inverted fashion	Inv(9); most common; no clinical sequelae
Robertsonian translocation	Loss of the short arm of two acrocentric chromosomes; the acrocentric chromosomes are 13, 14, 15, 21, and 22	t(14q21q); one of the possible causes of Down syndrome
Reciprocal translocation	Breakage of nonhomologous chromosomes with a reciprocal exchange	Common (1 in 600 newborns); usually harmless

Patterns of Inheritance

Single-gene (**Mendelian**) **disorders** display predictable patterns of inheritance related to the location of the gene (autosomal or X-linked) and the expression of the phenotype (dominant or recessive). Although Mendelian disorders were the first type of genetic disorders described, it is now known that there are many genetic and environmental factors that modify these genes, making true single-gene disorders relatively rare. Health care providers should be aware that many single-gene disorders are discovered each year and may be tracked using Internet databases, such as Online Mendelian Inheritance in Man (http://www.nslij-genetics.org/search_omim.html).

Autosomal Dominant

Each gene occupies a specific position, or locus, on a chromosome. At each locus, there are two possible variations of the genes, or two **alleles**. If the phenotype of a disease is based on one allele in a gene pair, the gene is **dominant**. If the gene is located on an autosomal cell, its pattern of inheritance is described as **autosomal dominant**. Individuals with one dominant allele for a disorder (described as being **heterozygous** for the gene) will express disease and transmit the gene to 50% of their offspring (Box 7.1). Examples of genetic disorders with autosomal dominant inheritance include Marfan syndrome, achondroplasia, and Huntington disease.

The phenotypic expression of autosomal dominant genes is not always straightforward and may vary depending on specific characteristics of the gene. **Variable expressivity** is the varying expression of a disease in an affected person. For example, some individuals with **neurofibromatosis** have only a few *café au lait* spots, whereas others have large tumors. Neurofibromatosis, however, demonstrates 100% penetrance. **Penetrance** describes the likelihood that a person carrying the gene will be affected.

Retinoblastoma is an example of incomplete penetrance; not all affected individuals will express any obvious form of disease. **Anticipation** refers to an increase in severity and earlier expression of disease with each subsequent generation. An example of a genetic mutation that shows anticipation is Huntington disease, where an expansion of the trinucleotide CAG repeat leads to earlier expression of the disease in affected offspring.

Autosomal Recessive

An **autosomal recessive** disease is only expressed when the affected individual carries two copies of the gene (described as being **homozygous** for the gene) (see Box 7.1). Individuals who are **heterozygous** for the gene express a normal phenotype. During pregnancy, unless a woman has been screened for a particular disease based on her risk factors (e.g., sickle cell disease and cystic fibrosis), carriers of a recessive gene will not know that they are carriers until they have an affected offspring. Other examples of autosomal recessive disorders include Tay-Sachs disease and phenylketonuria.

X-Linked Inheritance

In **X-linked diseases**, the affected gene is located on the X chromosome. Because males only have one X chromosome, they will manifest the disease if their X chromosome carries the affected gene. The male carrier status is considered **hemizygous**, whereas the female is almost always heterozygous. X-linked recessive diseases are much more common than X-linked dominant diseases (Box 7.2). Some examples of X-linked recessive diseases are hemophilia and color blindness. Hypophosphatemia is an example of an X-linked dominant disease.

BOX 7.1 Patterns of Inheritance

Characteristics of Autosomal Dominant Disorders
- Gene expression rarely skips a generation.
- An affected individual will transmit the gene to progeny 50% of the time.
- There should be equal sex distribution among affected relatives; males should be able to transmit to males and females to females.
- An unaffected first-degree relative will not transmit the gene to his or her progeny.

Characteristics of Autosomal Recessive Disorders
- Gene expression may appear to skip generations.
- Both males and females are affected.
- Neither parent is usually affected; affected individuals usually do not have affected children.
- If one parent is a carrier, half of the offspring will be carriers of the gene. If both parents are carriers, the risk of transmission of the disorder is 25%.
- If the suspected disorder is noted to be rare, consanguinity should be suspected.

BOX 7.2 Differences between X-Linked Recessive and Dominant Disease

X-Linked Recessive Disease
- More common in males than in females.
- An affected male will not pass the disease to his son, but all the daughters will be carriers.
- The disease is transmitted from carrier females to affected males.

X-Linked Dominant Disease
- An affected male will transmit the disease to all of his daughters, but not to any of his sons.
- Heterozygous females will transmit the gene to 50% of their offspring, whereas homozygous females will transmit the gene to all of their offspring.

Fragile X syndrome is an X-linked disorder that causes mental retardation. It is caused by a repeat in the cytosine–guanine–guanine sequence in a specific gene located on the X chromosome. Transmission of the disease-producing genetic mutation to a fetus depends on the sex of the parent and the number of repeats in the parental gene. If the number of repeats is between 61 and 200, the individual is said to have a "premutation." These individuals are phenotypically normal, although women carrying the premutation are at an increased risk for premature ovarian failure. A full mutation is characterized by more than 200 repeats. These individuals display the signs and symptoms of the disorder.

A male may transmit the unexpanded premutation gene to his offspring, but expansion to the full mutation is rare in a male with the premutation gene. A female with a premutation gene may also transmit the gene to her offspring; however, the premutation gene may expand during meiosis and result in a full mutation. Women with a family history of boys with developmental delay, extreme hyperactivity, and speech and language problems should be offered fragile X–carrier testing. Women with ovarian failure or an elevated follicle–stimulating hormone level before age 40 years without a known cause should be screened to determine whether they have the fragile X premutation.

Mitochondrial Inheritance
Mitochondrial inheritance is different from other patterns of inheritance. Mitochondria contain unique DNA (called *mitochondrial DNA*) that differs from the DNA carried in the cell nucleus. Any mutations in this DNA are only transmitted from the mother to all of her offspring, and, if a male fetus is affected, he will not pass it on to any of his offspring.

Multifactorial Inheritance
Multifactorial disorders are caused by a combination of factors, some genetic and some nongenetic (i.e., environmental). Multifactorial disorders recur in families but are not transmitted in any distinctive pattern. Many congenital, single-organ system structural abnormalities are multifactorial, having an incidence in the general population of approximately 1 per 1,000. Examples of multifactorial traits are cleft lip, with or without cleft palate; congenital cardiac defects; neural tube defects (NTDs); and hydrocephalus.

● RISK FACTORS FOR GENETIC DISORDERS

Several factors have been identified that increase the risk of having a child with a chromosomal abnormality, including maternal or paternal age and exposure to certain drugs. Other factors, such as ethnicity or a family history of a disease, may indicate that an individual carries a gene for a Mendelian disorder. The first step in assessing risk is to document information about the patient's family and personal history (see Appendix C). This record is an effective method for obtaining information concerning personal and family medical history, parental exposure to potentially harmful substances, or other issues that may have an impact on risk assessment and management. This information can be collected prior to conception during a preconception office visit or during the first prenatal visit in the first trimester.

Some infectious diseases, including cytomegalovirus, rubella, and sexually transmitted diseases (see Chapter 24), as well as certain drugs (see Chapter 6) have been linked to an increased risk of birth defects. Preexisting diabetes mellitus may also predispose a fetus to a congenital anomaly. Because these defects are not gene based, family history and genetic testing procedures, such as amniocentesis or CVS, cannot be used to detect these abnormalities. Ultrasonography is the mainstay of surveillance for infectious and teratogen-induced congenital abnormalities.

Advanced Maternal Age
Although the risk increases with age, the majority of cases of Down syndrome occur in women younger than age 35 years (Table 7.3). In addition to Down syndrome, other chromosomal abnormalities increase in frequency with advanced maternal age (see Table 7.1).

Previous Pregnancy Affected by Chromosomal Abnormality
Women who have had a previous pregnancy complicated by trisomy 21, 18, or 13 or any other trisomy in which the fetus survived at least to the second trimester are at risk for having another pregnancy complicated by the same or different trisomy. The risk of trisomy recurrence is 1.6 to 8.2 times the maternal age risk, depending on several factors: The type of trisomy, whether the index pregnancy was a spontaneous abortion, maternal age at initial occurrence, and maternal age at subsequent prenatal diagnosis.

Some, but not all, sex chromosome abnormalities carry an increased risk of recurrence. A pregnancy complicated by fetal XXX or XXY increases the recurrence risk by 1.6% to 2.5% the maternal age risk. Turner syndrome (monosomy X; XO) and XYY karyotypes impart a nominal risk of recurrence.

History of Early Pregnancy Loss
At least half of all first-trimester pregnancy losses result from fetal chromosomal abnormalities. The most common are monosomy X; polyploidy (triploidy or tetraploidy); and trisomies 13, 16, 18, 21, and 22.

Advanced Paternal Age
Increasing paternal age, particularly after age 50 years, predisposes the fetus to an increase in gene mutations that can affect X-linked recessive and autosomal dominant disorders, such as neurofibromatosis, achondroplasia, Apert syndrome, and Marfan syndrome.

TABLE 7.3 RISK TABLE FOR CHROMOSOMAL ABNORMALITIES BY MATERNAL AGE AT TERM

Age at Term	Risk for Trisomy 21	Risk for Any Chromosome Abnormality[a]
15	1:1,578	1:454
16	1:1,572	1:475
17	1:1,565	1:499
18	1:1,556	1:525
19	1:1,544	1:555
20	1:1,480	1:525
21	1:1,460	1:525
22	1:1,440	1:499
23	1:1,420	1:499
24	1:1,380	1:475
25	1:1,340	1:475
26	1:1,290	1:475
27	1:1,220	1:454
28	1:1,140	1:434
29	1:1,050	1:416
30	1:940	1:384
31	1:820	1:384
32	1:700	1:322
33	1:570	1:285
34	1:456	1:243
35	1:353	1:178
36	1:267	1:148
37	1:199	1:122
38	1:148	1:104
39	1:111	1:80
40	1:85	1:62
41	1:67	1:48
42	1:54	1:38
43	1:45	1:30
44	1:39	1:23
45	1:35	1:18
46	1:31	1:14
47	1:29	1:10
48	1:27	1:8
49	1:26	1:6
50	1:25	Data not available

[a]Risk for any chromosomal abnormality includes the risk for trisomy 21 and trisomy 18 in addition to trisomy 13, 47,XXY, 47,XYY, Turner syndrome genotype, and other clinically significant abnormalities.
Modified from American College of Obstetricians and Gynecologists. *Screening for Fetal Aneuploidy. Practice Bulletin 163.* Washington, DC: American College of Obstetricians and Gynecologists; May 2016.

Ethnicity

Many mendelian disorders occur more frequently in certain groups. African Americans are at an increased risk for sickle cell disease, the most common hemoglobinopathy in the United States. Approximately 8% of African Americans carry the sickle hemoglobin gene, which is also found with increased frequency in those of Mediterranean, Caribbean, Latin American, and Middle Eastern descent. Caucasians of Northern European descent are at an increased risk for cystic fibrosis, with an estimated carrier percentage of 1 in 22. Tay-Sachs, Gaucher, and Niemann-Pick diseases occur with greater frequency in individuals of Ashkenazi Jewish descent. Other diseases associated with certain ethnic groups are β-thalassemia found at an increased frequency in individuals of Mediterranean origin, and α-thalassemia in individuals of Asian origin.

PRENATAL SCREENING

Obstetricians are responsible for determining if a woman is at an increased risk for fetal abnormalities and for describing and offering appropriate prenatal screening or diagnostic tests. Prenatal genetic diagnostic testing is intended to determine, with as much certainty as possible, whether a specific genetic disorder or condition is present in the fetus. In contrast, prenatal genetic screening is designed to assess whether a patient is at an increased risk of having a fetus affected by a genetic disorder A **screening test** differs from a diagnostic test in that screening tests only assess the risk that a child will have a genetic disease; they cannot confirm or rule out the presence of the disease. A **diagnostic test** is given if a screening test is positive, to assess whether the disease is present or absent in the developing fetus.

Genetic screening tests are routinely offered to all women to detect NTDs, Down syndrome, and trisomy 18. In addition, individuals of certain ethnic groups can be tested to detect whether they carry a gene for a particular disorder.

First-Trimester Screening

First-trimester screening tests are used to assess the risk of Down syndrome, trisomy 18, and trisomy 13 in a developing fetus. An advantage of first-trimester screening is that the tests are performed early enough so that decisions can be made regarding continuing the pregnancy, if necessary (Table 7.4). Disadvantages include the need for specialized training and appropriate ultrasound equipment to achieve optimal NT measurement and the availability of CVS. Detecting pregnancies at high risk for Down syndrome in the first trimester is of low utility if a diagnostic invasive test (i.e., CVS) cannot be performed to verify the findings, or cell-free DNA to increase screening sensitivity and specificity.

Serum Screening

First-semester serum screening for Down syndrome consists of tests for levels of two biochemical markers: Free or total **human chorionic gonadotropin** (**hCG**) and **pregnancy-associated plasma protein A** (**PAPP-A**). An elevated level of hCG (1.98 of the median observed in euploid pregnancies [MoM]) and a decreased level of PAPP-A (0.43 MoM) have been associated with Down syndrome.

Ultrasound Screening

An ultrasonographic marker for Down syndrome is the size of the **nuchal transparency** (**NT**), a fluid collection at the back of the fetal neck that can be seen between 10 and 14 weeks of gestation (Fig. 7.4). An increase in the size of the NT between 10 4/7 and 13 6/7 weeks of gestation is recognized to be an early presenting feature of a variety of chromosomal, genetic, and structural abnormalities. The risk of adverse pregnancy outcome is proportional to the degree of nuchal translucency enlargement. When used alone, NT measurement has a detection rate for Down syndrome of 64% to 70%. Combining NT measurement with the other first-trimester biochemical markers yields an 82% to 87% detection rate of Down syndrome, with

TABLE 7.4 DOWN SYNDROME SCREENING TESTS AND DETECTION RATES (5% POSITIVE SCREEN RATE)

Screening Test	Detection Rate (%)
First Trimester	
NT measurement	64–70[a]
NT measurement, PAPP-A, free or total β-hCG[b]	82–87[a]
Second Trimester	
Triple screen (MSAFP, hCG, unconjugated estriol)	69[a]
Quadruple screen (MSAFP, hCG, unconjugated estriol, inhibin A)	81[a]
First Plus Second Trimester	
Integrated (NT, PAPP-A, quad screen)	96[c]
Serum integrated (PAPP-A, quad screen)	88[c]
Stepwise sequential	95[a]
Contingent sequential	88–94[d]
Cell-free DNA (in patients who receive a result)	99[e]

hCG, human chorionic gonadotropin; MSAFP, maternal serum α-fetoprotein; NT, nuchal translucency; PAPP-A, pregnancy-associated plasma protein A; quad, quadruple.
[a] From the FASTER trial (Malone F, Canick JA, Ball RH, et al. First- and Second-Trimester Evaluation of Risk (FASTER) Research Consortium. First-trimester or second-trimester screening, or both, for Down's syndrome. *N Engl J Med*. 2005;353(1):2001–2011. http://content.nejm.org/cgi/content/full/353/19/2001. Accessed October 20, 2008.)
[b] Also referred to as combined first-trimester screen.
[c] American College of Obstetricians and Gynecologists. *Practice Bulletin 163.*
[d] Modeled predicted detection rates (Cuckle H, Benn P, Wright D. Down syndrome screening in the first and/or second trimester: model predicted performance using meta-analysis parameters. *Semin Perinatol.* 2005;29:252–257.)
[e] From the MELISSA Study Group (Bianchi DW, Platt LD, Goldberg JD, Abuhamad AZ, Sehnert AJ, Rava RP. Genome-wide fetal aneuploidy detection by maternal plasma DNA sequencing. MatErnal BLood IS Source to Accurately diagnose fetal aneuploidy (MELISSA) Study Group [published erratum appears in *Obstet Gynecol* 2012;120:957].
Modified from American College of Obstetricians and Gynecologists. *Screening for Fetal Aneuploidy. ACOG Practice Bulletin 163.* Washington, DC: American College of Obstetricians and Gynecologists; May 2016.

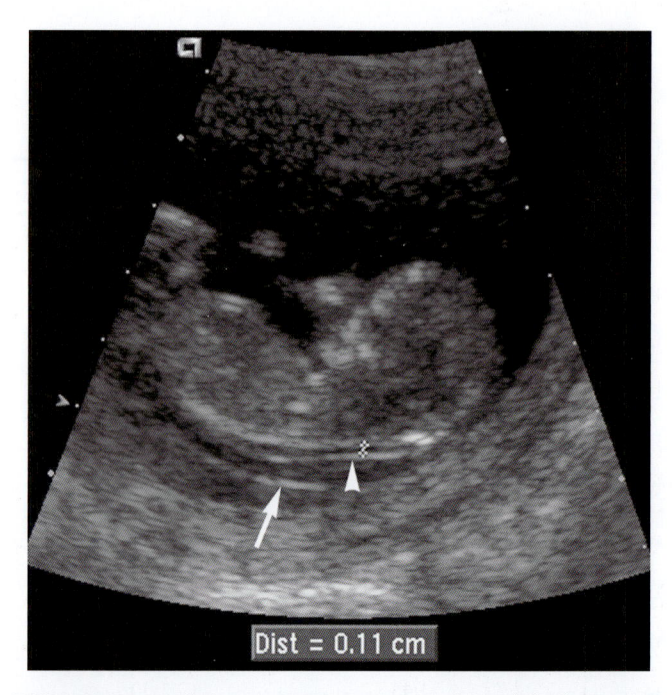

FIGURE 7.4. Nuchal area. Measurement is taken of the lucent area in the posterior neck (*calipers*), with the posterior caliper placed just inside the echogenic skin (*arrowhead*). The amnion (*arrow*) should not be mistaken for the skin. (From Doubilet PM, Benson CB. *Atlas of Ultrasound in Obstetrics and Gynecology*. Philadelphia, PA: Lippincott Williams & Wilkins; 2003:10f.)

a 5% false-positive rate, which is equal to or higher than second-trimester screening tests. Women found to have an increased risk of aneuploidy with first-trimester screening tests should be offered genetic counseling and diagnostic testing by CVS or amniocentesis in the second trimester. Another alternative is the noninvasive cell-free DNA test.

Several other first-trimester ultrasonographic findings have been evaluated as potential markers for aneuploidy in the first and second trimesters. If an enlarged nuchal translucency, an obvious anomaly, or a cystic hygroma is identified on ultrasonography, the patient should be offered genetic counseling and diagnostic testing for aneuploidy as well as follow-up ultrasonography for fetal structural abnormalities. Given the high risk of congenital heart disease in these fetuses, referral for fetal cardiac ultrasonography should be considered. Patients with an enlarged nuchal translucency or cystic hygroma and normal fetal karyotype should be offered an anatomic evaluation in the second trimester, fetal cardiac ultrasonography, and further counseling regarding the potential for genetic syndromes not detected by aneuploidy screening.

Circulating Cell-Free Fetal DNA

Cell-free DNA is found in the maternal plasma and may be used as a screening test for women with an elevated risk of aneuploidy. Screening can be performed from as early as 10 weeks of gestation until term. The sensitivity and specificity for trisomies 21, 18, and 13, and sex chromosome aneuploidy are all greater than 90%. Patients should understand, however, that a negative cell-free DNA does not guarantee the absence of aneuploidy. Likewise, a patient with a positive cell-free DNA result should be offered invasive diagnostic testing prior to a decision for termination or other management. Women with a positive cell-free DNA test or an indeterminate test should be offered genetic counseling and diagnostic testing before deciding on pregnancy termination. Because cell-free DNA is a screening test with the potential for false-positive and false-negative test results, such testing should not be used as a substitute for diagnostic testing.

Second-Trimester Screening

Second-trimester screening may be the only option if a woman is seen for the first time during the second trimester of her pregnancy. Women who have had first-trimester screening for aneuploidy should not undergo independent second-trimester serum screening in the same pregnancy. When these test results are interpreted independently, the false-positive rates are additive, leading to many more unnecessary invasive procedures (11%–17%). After first-trimester screening, subsequent second-trimester Down syndrome screening is not indicated, unless it is being performed as a component of an integrated test (explained later), stepwise sequential test, or contingent sequential test.

Triple and Quadruple Screening Tests

An association between low maternal serum **α-fetoprotein** (**AFP**) levels and Down syndrome was reported in 1984. In the 1990s, hCG and unconjugated estriol were used in combination with maternal serum AFP to improve the detection rates for Down syndrome and trisomy 18. The average maternal serum AFP level in Down syndrome pregnancies is reduced to 0.74 MoM. Intact hCG is increased in affected pregnancies, with an average level of 2.06 MoM, whereas unconjugated estriol is reduced to an average level of 0.75 MoM. When the levels of all three markers (**triple screen**) are used to modify the maternal age-related Down syndrome risk, the detection rate for Down syndrome is approximately 70%; approximately 5% of all pregnancies will have a positive screen result.

Typically, the levels of all three markers are reduced when the fetus has trisomy 18. Adding inhibin A to the triple screen (**quadruple screen**) improves the detection rate for Down syndrome to approximately 80%. The median value of the maternal inhibin A level is increased at 1.77 MoM in Down syndrome pregnancies, but inhibin A is not used in the calculation of risk for trisomy 18. These biochemical screening tests are performed at 15 to 22 weeks of gestation.

Ultrasound Screening

In the second trimester, gross abnormalities, such as cardiac defects, as well as a group of subtle sonographic markers (soft markers), may be associated with an increased risk of Down syndrome in certain women (Box 7.3). Although findings of soft markers do not significantly increase the risk of Down syndrome, they should be considered in the context of first-trimester screening results, patient's age, and history. The significance of ultrasonographic markers identified by a second-trimester ultrasound examination in a patient who has had a negative first-trimester screening test result is unknown. Studies indicate that the highest detection rate is achieved with systematic combination of ultrasonographic markers and gross anomalies, such as thick nuchal fold and cardiac defects. However, an abnormal second-trimester ultrasound finding identifying a major congenital anomaly significantly increases the risk of aneuploidy and warrants further counseling and the offer of a diagnostic procedure.

Screening for Neural Tube Defects

Maternal serum AFP is also used to screen for NTDs, that is, congenital structural abnormalities of the brain and vertebral column. NTDs occur in approximately 1.4 to 2 per 1,000 births

---

BOX 7.3 Some Ultrasonographic "Soft Markers" for Down Syndrome

- Nuchal fold
- Intracardiac echogenic focus
- Mild ventriculomegaly
- Echogenic bowel
- Shortened femur or humerus
- Absent nasal bone
- Pyelectasis

in the United States and are the second most common major congenital abnormality worldwide (cardiac malformations are the most common). Maternal serum AFP evaluation is an effective screening test for NTDs and should be offered to all pregnant women, unless they plan to have amniotic AFP measurement as part of prenatal diagnosis for chromosomal abnormalities or other genetic diseases.

Most affected pregnancies can be identified by an elevated maternal serum AFP level, defined as 2.5 MoM for a singleton pregnancy. Women with a positive screening test should receive an ultrasound examination to detect identifiable causes of false-positive results (e.g., fetal death, multiple gestation, and underestimate of gestational age) and for targeted study of fetal anatomy for NTDs and other defects associated with elevated maternal serum AFP. Approximately 90% of newborns with NTDs are born to women who have no family or medication history that would indicate them to be at increased risk. While routinely offering amniocentesis to all women with an elevated maternal serum AFP before a fetal anatomy sonogram would detect 98% of all neural tube defects, many women would undergo an amniocentesis and incur risk of fetal loss needlessly. **Folic acid** has been shown to prevent recurrence and occurrence of NTDs. Because most individuals at increased risk do not know it until they have an affected child, all women should be advised to take a vitamin that contains at least 0.4 mg of folic acid prior to conception. For women who previously have had a child with an NTD, the recommended dose is 4 mg daily.

Integrated Screening

The results of both first-trimester and second-trimester screening and ultrasound can be combined to increase their ability to detect Down syndrome. This **"integrated"** approach to screening uses both the first-trimester and second-trimester markers to adjust a woman's age-related risk of having a child with Down syndrome. The results are reported only after both first-trimester and second-trimester screening tests are completed. Integrated screening provides the highest sensitivity with the lowest false-positive rate. The lower false-positive rate results in fewer invasive tests and, thus, fewer procedure-related losses of normal pregnancies. Although some patients value early screening, others are willing to wait several weeks if doing so would result in an improved detection rate and less chance that they will need an invasive diagnostic test. Concerns about integrated screening include possible patient anxiety generated by having to wait 3 to 4 weeks between initiation and completion of the screening and the loss of the opportunity to consider CVS if the first-trimester screening indicates a high risk of aneuploidy. Another limitation of integrated screening is nonadherence of the second blood draw.

● PRENATAL DIAGNOSIS OF GENETIC DISORDERS

Prenatal genetic diagnosis should be offered in circumstances in which there is a definable increased risk of a fetal genetic disorder that may be diagnosed by one or more methods. Prenatal screening or diagnosis should be voluntary and informed. In most circumstances, test results are normal and provide patients with a high degree of reassurance that a particular disorder does not affect a fetus, although there is no guarantee that the fetus is normal and with no abnormalities. Early prenatal genetic diagnosis also affords patients the option to terminate affected pregnancies. Alternatively, a diagnosis of a genetic disorder may allow the patient to prepare for the birth of an affected child and, in some circumstances, may be important in establishing a plan for care during pregnancy, labor, delivery, and the immediate neonatal period.

Carrier Testing

Individuals who have a family history of a specific genetic disorder but show no signs of the disorder themselves may undergo carrier testing to determine the risk of passing the disorder on to their offspring. In addition, individuals with certain ethnic backgrounds predisposed to genetic disorders may undergo carrier testing. Information about carrier screening should be provided to every pregnant woman. Carrier screening and counseling ideally should be performed before pregnancy because this enables couples to learn about their reproductive risk and consider the most complete range of reproductive options.

For example, the American College of Obstetricians and Gynecologists (College) recommends that individuals of Ashkenazi Jewish descent should be tested prior to pregnancy or early in pregnancy for Tay-Sachs disease, Canavan disease, cystic fibrosis, and familial dysautonomia. There are also recommendations for other ethnic groups.

Carrier testing involves testing of cells obtained from a saliva or blood sample. Genes responsible for many diseases have been located, and **direct testing** for the presence of a specific mutation can be performed. Examples of diseases for which direct tests exist are Tay-Sachs disease, hemophilia A, cystic fibrosis, sickle cell disease, Canavan disease, familial dysautonomia, and thalassemia. For disorders in which disease-causing mutations have not been delineated, indirect testing is required. **Indirect testing** refers to the process of determining DNA sequences of specific length that are linked to a mutation. These sequences, called **restriction fragment length polymorphisms**, can be tested for by the Southern blot technique. Indirect testing is not as accurate as direct testing.

One partner is usually tested first. If one partner is found to be a carrier of a particular disorder, the other partner is tested as well. If both partners are carriers, genetic counseling should be offered to provide more information regarding the risk of transmitting the disorder.

Fetal Diagnostic Procedures

Prenatal analysis of DNA requires fetal nucleated cells, currently obtained by amniocentesis, CVS, or **percutaneous umbilical blood sampling** (PUBS).

Amniocentesis

Amniocentesis is the withdrawal of 20 to 30 mL of amniotic fluid transabdominally, under concurrent ultrasound guidance, with a 20- or 22-gauge needle. Traditional genetic amniocentesis is usually performed between 15 and 20 weeks of gestation. Direct analysis of the amniotic fluid supernatant is possible for AFP and acetylcholinesterase assays; such analyses permit the detection of fetal NTDs and other fetal structural defects (e.g., omphalocele and gastroschisis).

Studies have confirmed the safety of amniocentesis as well as its cytogenic diagnostic accuracy (>99%). The risk of pregnancy loss is less than 1%. Complications, which occur infrequently, include transient vaginal spotting or amniotic fluid leakage in approximately 1% to 2% of all cases and chorioamnionitis (also known as an intra-amniotic infection) in less than 1 in 1,000 cases. The perinatal survival rate in cases of amniotic fluid leakage following midtrimester amniocentesis is greater than 90%.

Early amniocentesis performed from 11 to 13 weeks of gestation has significantly higher rates of pregnancy loss and complications than traditional amniocentesis as well as significantly more amniotic fluid culture failures. For these reasons, early amniocentesis before 14 weeks of gestation should not be performed.

Chorionic Villus Sampling

CVS was developed to provide prenatal diagnosis in the first trimester. CVS is performed after 10 weeks of gestation by transcervical or transabdominal aspiration of chorionic villi (immature placenta) under concurrent ultrasound guidance. Recent multicenter trials have demonstrated transabdominal CVS to have similar safety and accuracy rates to that of traditional (i.e., performed at or after 15 weeks' gestation) amniocentesis; transcervical CVS carries a higher risk of pregnancy loss. Disorders that require analysis of amniotic fluid, such as NTDs, cannot be diagnosed with CVS. There is also a significant learning curve associated with the safe performance of CVS. The primary advantage of CVS over amniocentesis is that the procedure can be performed earlier in pregnancy and the viable cells obtained by CVS for analysis allow for shorter specimen processing time (5–7 days vs. 7–14 days), so the results are available earlier in pregnancy.

The rate of pregnancy loss associated with CVS appears to approach and may be the same as the loss associated with midtrimester amniocentesis. The most common complication of CVS is vaginal spotting or bleeding, which occurs in up to 32% of patients after transcervical CVS is performed. The incidence after transabdominal CVS is less. There have been reports that CVS performed before 10 weeks of gestation is associated with limb reduction and oromandibular defects. Although these associations are controversial, they should be discussed with the patient during counseling. *Until further information is available, CVS should not be performed before 10 weeks of gestation.*

Percutaneous Umbilical Blood Sampling

PUBS, also known as **cordocentesis,** is usually performed after 20 weeks of gestation and has traditionally been used to obtain fetal blood for blood component analyses (e.g., hematocrit, Rh status, and platelets), as well as cytogenetic and DNA analyses. The indications for PUBS are declining. One major benefit of PUBS is the ability to obtain rapid (18–24 hours) fetal karyotypes. However, with the advent of FISH, the need for a procedure with more potential for complications (i.e., PUBS) has been obviated. The procedure-related pregnancy loss rate of PUBS has been reported to be less than 2%. Cordocentesis is rarely needed but may be useful to further evaluate chromosomal mosaicism discovered after CVS or amniocentesis is performed.

Other prenatal diagnostic procedures include **fetal skin sampling**, **fetal tissue** (muscle and liver) **biopsy**, and **fetoscopy**. These procedures are used only for the diagnosis of rare disorders not amenable to diagnosis by less invasive methods.

Other Tests

Once fetal cells are obtained, a variety of tests and analyses can be performed. A **karyotype** is a photomicrograph of the chromosomes taken during metaphase, when the chromosomes have condensed. A separate image is made of each individual chromosome from this micrograph. The chromosomes are then matched to their homologue, so that the karyotype shows the chromosome pairs. Because most fetal cells in amniotic fluid specimens obtained through amniocentesis are not in metaphase, these cells must first be cultured (grown) in order to perform a karyotype analysis. An advantage of CVS over amniocentesis is that CVS allows for rapid cytogenetic and DNA analyses, because cytotrophoblasts obtained from first-trimester placentas are more likely to be in metaphase than in amniotic fluid cells.

FISH is a technique that involves fluorescent labeling of genetic probes for specific chromosomes, most commonly 13, 18, 21, X, and Y. FISH can identify abnormalities in chromosome number, and results are usually available by 48 hours. Although FISH analysis has been shown to be accurate, false-positive and false-negative results have been reported. Therefore, clinical decision-making should be based on information from FISH along with a traditional karyotype, ultrasound findings, or a positive screening test result. **Spectral karyotyping** (**SKY**) is similar to FISH but can be done for all chromosomes. SKY is useful in detecting translocations.

Comparative genomic hybridization (**CGH**) is an evolving method that identifies submicroscopic chromosomal deletions and duplications. This approach has proven to be useful in identifying abnormalities in individuals with developmental delay and physical abnormalities, when results of traditional chromosomal analysis have been normal. At present, the use of CGH in prenatal diagnosis is limited because of the difficulty in interpreting which DNA alterations revealed through CGH may be normal population variants. Until more data are available, the use of CGH for routine prenatal diagnosis is not recommended.

Genetic Counseling

Many couples at increased risk for having children with genetic disorders can benefit from genetic counseling, in which the primary health care provider, a medical geneticist, or other trained professional provides information and options to individuals or families about genetic disorders and risks. By using a family and genetic history questionnaire such as those found in the ACOG Antepartum Record, the provider may elicit genetic risk factors that prompt a referral to a genetic counselor. Geneticists will commonly complete at least a three-generation pedigree to visualize the mode of inheritance and specific individuals in the family who are at risk for a given genetic condition. Ideally, this counseling takes place before conception. *The key elements in genetic counseling are accurate diagnosis, communication, and nondirective presentation of options.* The counselor's function is not to dictate a particular course of action but to provide information that will allow couples to make informed decisions.

Counseling is directed at helping the patient or family in the following areas:

- Comprehending the medical facts, including the diagnosis, probable course of the disorder, and available management
- Appreciating the way in which heredity contributes to the disorder and the risk of occurrence or recurrence in specific relatives
- Understanding the options for dealing with the risk of recurrence, including prenatal genetic diagnosis
- Choosing the course of action that seems appropriate in view of the risk and the family's goals and act in accordance with that decision
- Making the best possible adjustment to the disorder in an affected family member and to the risk of recurrence in another family member

Genetic counseling may also involve alternative reproductive options (e.g., pregnancy termination, permanent sterilization, selective pregnancy reduction, donor insemination, donor eggs). Patients should also understand that outside parties, such as insurance companies, may be able to obtain the results of genetic testing.

● GENETICS IN GYNECOLOGY: CANCER SCREENING

It is now known that certain breast and ovarian cancers have a genetic predisposition. Genetic tests have been developed for the detection of some of these genes. Gynecologists play a key role in identifying individuals with a genetic disposition for cancer and ensuring that they receive the appropriate screening tests. The most important initial step in identifying women at high risk for hereditary cancers is a thorough family history. Clues to possible hereditary cancers include a history of cancers in first-degree relatives, cancers occurring at young ages, cancers in multiple generations, or many different cancers in one individual. Based on these findings, further testing and genetic counseling may be indicated.

Breast and Ovarian Cancer

The *BRCA1* and *BRCA2* genes have been identified as responsible for the hereditary forms of both breast and ovarian cancers. Clinically important *BRCA* mutations have been found in about 1 in 40 Ashkenazi Jewish women and are estimated to occur in about 1 in 300 to 800 women in the general non-Jewish U.S. population. Criteria developed by the ACOG for *BRCA* testing referral are as follows:

- Women with breast cancer at age 40 years or younger
- Women with ovarian cancer, primary peritoneal cancer, or fallopian tube cancer of high grade, serous histology at any age
- Women with bilateral breast cancer (particularly if the first case of breast cancer was diagnosed at age 50 years or younger)
- Women with breast cancer at age 50 years or younger and a close relative with breast cancer at age 50 years or younger
- Women of Ashkenazi Jewish ancestry with breast cancer at age 50 years or younger
- Women with breast cancer at any age and two or more close relatives with breast cancer at any age (particularly if at least one case of breast cancer was diagnosed at age 50 years or younger)
- Unaffected women with a close relative that meets one of the previous criteria testing for *BRCA* in higher-risk populations is indicated if the following are present:
- Women with a personal history of both breast cancer and ovarian cancer
- Women with ovarian cancer and a close relative with ovarian cancer or premenopausal breast cancer or both
- Women with ovarian cancer who are of Ashkenazi Jewish ancestry
- Women with breast cancer at age 50 years or younger and a close relative with ovarian cancer or male breast cancer at any age
- Women of Ashkenazi Jewish ancestry in whom breast cancer was diagnosed at age 40 years or younger
- Women with a close relative with a known *BRCA1* or *BRCA2* mutation

Other Cancers

In addition to breast cancer, other cancers have been found to have a hereditary component. A hereditary syndrome called **hereditary nonpolyposis colorectal cancer type A (HNPCC type A)**, or **Lynch I syndrome**, increases the risk of developing colon cancer. A family history of colon, endometrial, ureteral, or renal cancers should alert the clinic to screen for the HNPCC-linked genes. **HNPCC type B**, or **Lynch II syndrome**, is an autosomal dominant inherited syndrome that increases the risk of all of the cancers in Lynch I syndrome as well as of ovarian, gastric, and pancreatic cancers. Individuals or families who meet certain criteria can undergo genetic testing to determine whether they have the defective gene. The criteria are as follows:

- Patients with endometrial or colorectal cancer diagnosed before age 50 years

- Patient with endometrial or ovarian cancer with a synchronous or metachronous colon or other Lynch/HNPCC-associated tumor at any age
- Patients with colorectal cancer with tumor-infiltrating lymphocytes, peritumoral lymphocytes, Crohn-like lymphocytic reaction, mucinous/signet-ring differentiation, or medullary growth pattern diagnosed before age 60 years
- Patients with endometrial or colorectal cancer and a first-degree relative† with a Lynch/HNPCC-associated tumor* diagnosed before age 50 years
- Patients with colorectal or endometrial cancer diagnosed at any age with two or more first-degree or second-degree relatives† with Lynch/HNPCC-associated tumors*, regardless of age.

CLINICAL FOLLOW-UP

Your patient's genetic history is suspicious for fragile X syndrome. You explain how this might be inherited in her family and refer her for blood tests. If the result reveals that she might be a carrier, you explain what additional fetal testing is available, along with any potential procedure-related risks to the pregnancy.

thePoint® Visit http://thePoint.lww.com/activate for an interactive USMLE-style question bank and more!

CHAPTER 8

Intrapartum Care

This chapter deals primarily with APGO Educational Topic Area:

TOPIC 11   **INTRAPARTUM CARE**

Students should be able to discuss the management of the laboring patient, including appropriate triage and diagnosis. They should understand the options for pain management and describe deviations from normal labor as well as maternal and fetal monitoring. They should be able to describe how to perform a vaginal delivery and to list indications for cesarean delivery.

CLINICAL CASE

A healthy, 28-year-old patient presents to labor and delivery at 39 weeks of gestation complaining of "crampiness" overnight. Her vital signs are all stable. The fetal heart tracing is reassuring, and there do not appear to be any regular contractions. What are the next steps in evaluation of this patient? If it appears she is in labor, how might you manage this patient?

MATERNAL CHANGES BEFORE THE ONSET OF LABOR

As a patient approaches term, she experiences **uterine contractions** of increasing strength and frequency. Spontaneous uterine contractions, which are not felt by the patient, occur throughout pregnancy. Late in pregnancy they become stronger and more frequent, resulting in the patient's perception of discomfort. These **Braxton Hicks contractions** (false labor) are not associated with dilation of the cervix, however, and do not fit the definition of labor.

It is frequently difficult for the patient to distinguish these often uncomfortable contractions from those of true labor. As a result, it is difficult for the physician to determine the true onset of labor by history alone. Braxton Hicks contractions are typically shorter in duration and less intense than true labor contractions, with the discomfort being characterized as over the lower abdomen and groin areas. It is not uncommon for these contractions to resolve with ambulation, hydration, or analgesia.

True labor is associated with contractions that the patient feels over the uterine fundus, with radiation of discomfort to the low back and lower abdomen. These contractions become increasingly intense and frequent.

Another event of late pregnancy is termed **"lightening,"** in which the patient reports a change in the shape of her abdomen and the sensation that the baby is lighter, the result of the fetal head descending into the pelvis. The patient may also report that the baby is "dropping." The patient often notices that her lower abdomen is more prominent, and she may feel a need to urinate more frequently as the bladder is compressed by the fetal head. The patient may also notice that she is breathing more easily, because there is less pressure on the diaphragm as the uterus becomes smaller.

Patients often report the passage of blood-tinged mucus late in pregnancy. This **"bloody show"** results as the cervix begins thinning (effacement) with the concomitant extrusion of mucus from the endocervical glands and a small amount of bleeding from small vessels in the area. Cervical effacement is common before the onset of true labor, when the internal os is slowly drawn into the lower uterine segment. The cervix is often significantly effaced before the onset of labor, particularly in the nulliparous patient. The mechanism of effacement and dilation and the vectors of the expulsive forces are demonstrated in Figure 8.1.

EVALUATION FOR LABOR

Patients should be instructed to contact their health care provider for any of the following reasons: 1) if their contractions occur approximately every 5 minutes for at least 1 hour, 2) if there is a sudden gush of fluid or a constant leakage of vaginal fluid (suggesting **rupture of membranes** [**ROM**]), 3) if there is any significant vaginal bleeding, or 4) if there is significant decrease in fetal movement.

Initial Evaluation

At the time of initial evaluation, the prenatal records are reviewed to 1) identify complications of pregnancy up to that point, 2) confirm gestational age to differentiate preterm labor from labor in a term pregnancy, and 3) review pertinent laboratory information. A focused history helps in determining the nature and frequency of the patient's contractions, the

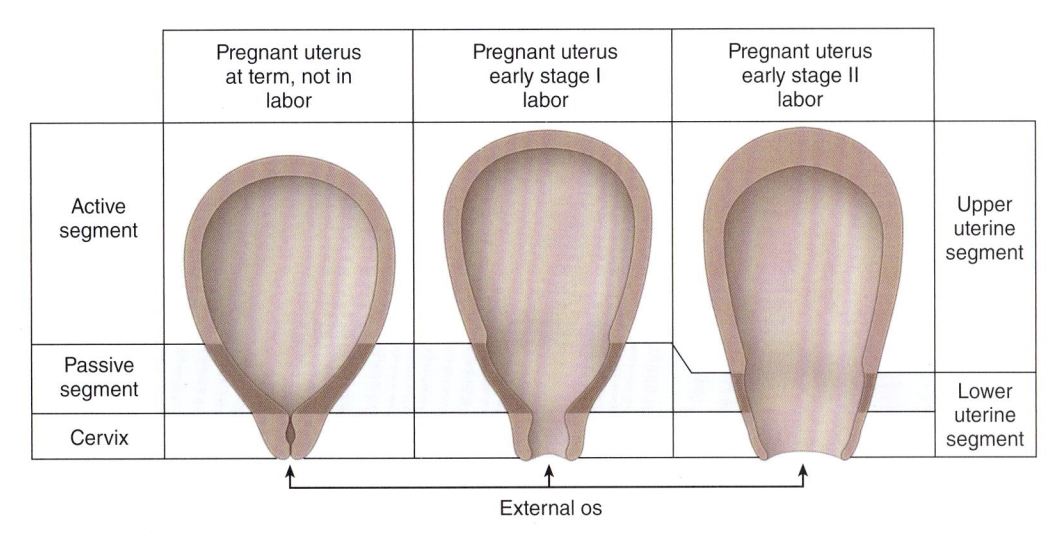

FIGURE 8.1. Mechanism of effacement, dilation, and labor. With continuing uterine contractions, the upper uterus (active segment) thickens, the lower uterine segment (passive segment) thins, and the cervix dilates. In this way, the fetus is moved downward, into, and through the vaginal canal.

possibility of spontaneous ROM or significant bleeding, or changes in maternal or fetal status. A focused review of systems should look for common complications of pregnancy resulting in altered labor management. A limited general physical examination is performed (with special attention to vital signs), along with the abdominal and pelvic examinations. If contractions occur during this physical examination, they may be palpated for intensity and duration by the examining physician. Auscultation of fetal heart tones is also of critical importance, particularly immediately following a contraction, to determine the possibility of any fetal heart rate deceleration. A limited transabdominal ultrasound may also be useful if there is a question of fetal lie, placental location, or decreased amniotic fluid volume or other abnormalities.

Abdominal Examination

The initial examination of the patient's abdomen may be accomplished using **Leopold maneuvers**, a series of four palpations of the uterus and fetus therein through the abdominal wall that helps accurately determine fetal lie, presentation, and position (see Fig. 9.7).

Lie is the relation of the long axis of the fetus to the maternal long axis. It is longitudinal in 99% of cases, occasionally transverse, and rarely oblique (when the axes cross at a 45° angle, usually converting to transverse or longitudinal lie during labor). **Presentation** is determined by the "presenting part," that is, that portion of the fetus lowest in the birth canal, palpated during the examination. For example, in a longitudinal lie, the presenting part is either breech or cephalic. The most common cephalic presentation is the one in which the head is sharply flexed onto the fetal chest such that the occiput or vertex presents. **Position** is the relation of the fetal presenting part to the right or left side of the maternal pelvis (Fig. 8.2).

The four Leopold maneuvers (see Fig. 9.7) include the following, facilitating several obstetric measurements:

1. Determining what occupies the fundus. In a longitudinal lie, the fetal head is differentiated from the fetal breech, the latter being larger and less clearly defined.
2. Determining location of small parts. Using one hand to steady the fetus, the fingers on the other hand are used to palpate either the firm, long fetal spine, or the various shapes and movements indicating fetal hands and feet.
3. Identifying descent of the presenting part. Suprapubic palpation identifies the presenting part as the fetal head, which is relatively mobile, or a breech, which moves the entire body. The extent to which the presenting part is felt to extend below the symphysis suggests the station of the presenting part.
4. Identifying the cephalic prominence. As long as the cephalic prominence is easily palpable, the vertex is not likely to have descended to 0 station.

Palpation of the uterus during a contraction may also be helpful in determining the intensity of that particular contraction. The uterine wall is not easily indented with firm palpation during a true contraction, but it may be indented during a Braxton Hicks "contraction."

Vaginal Examination

A digital vaginal examination allows the examiner to determine the consistency and degree of effacement and degree of dilation of the cervix. This examination should be avoided in women with premature ROM, placenta previa, or vaginal bleeding. **Effacement** is the shortening of the cervical canal from a length of about 2 cm to a mere circular orifice with almost paper-thin edges. Effacement is expressed as a percent of thinning from a perceived uneffaced state (Fig. 8.3).

A cervix that is not effaced, but is softened, is more likely to change with contractions than one that is firm, as it is earlier in pregnancy. If the cervix is not significantly effaced, it may also be evaluated for its relative position, that is, anterior, midposition, or

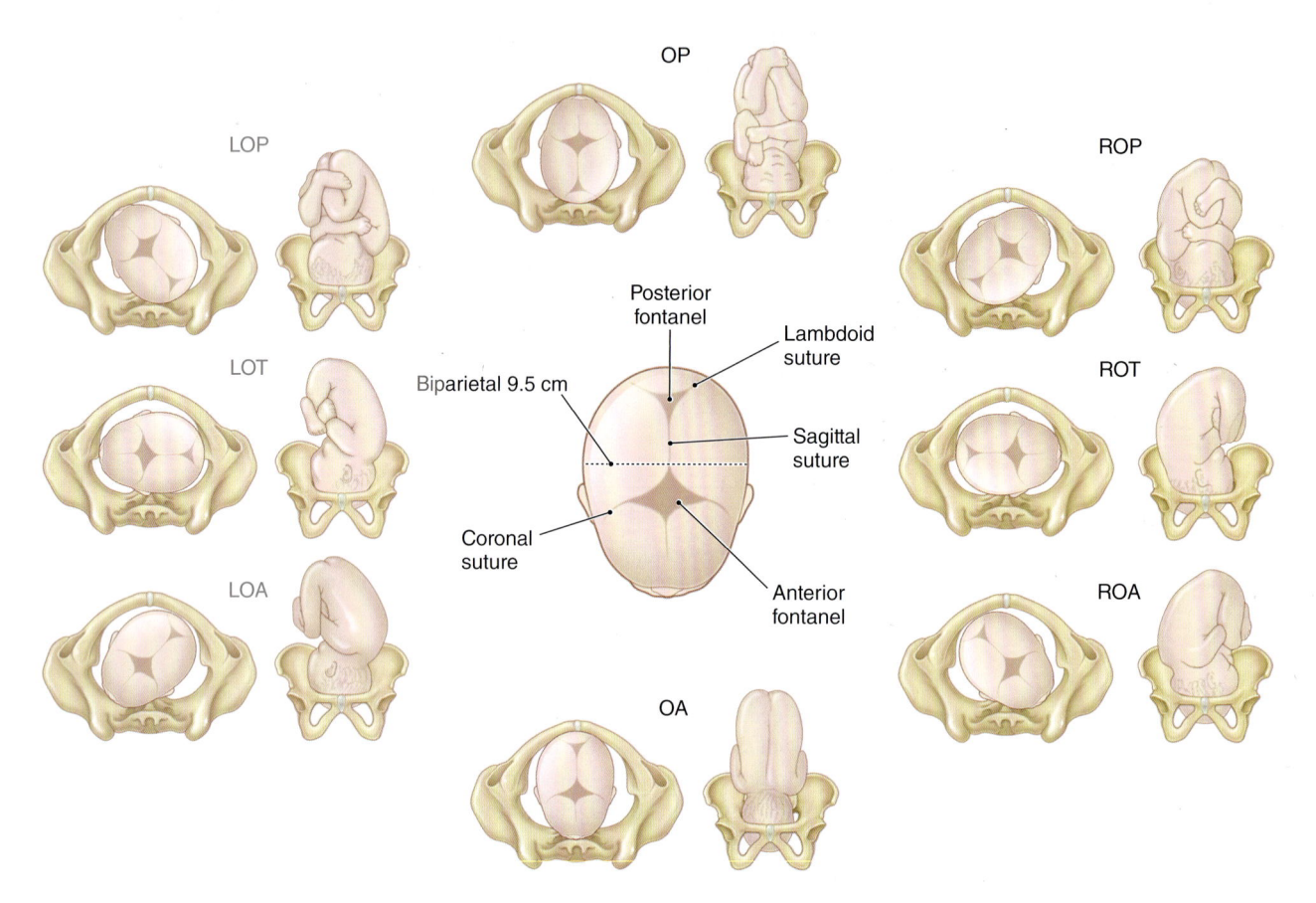

FIGURE 8.2. Various positions in vertex presentation. LOP, left occiput posterior; LOT, left occiput transverse; LOA, left occiput anterior; ROP, right occiput posterior; ROT, right occiput transverse; ROA, right occiput anterior.

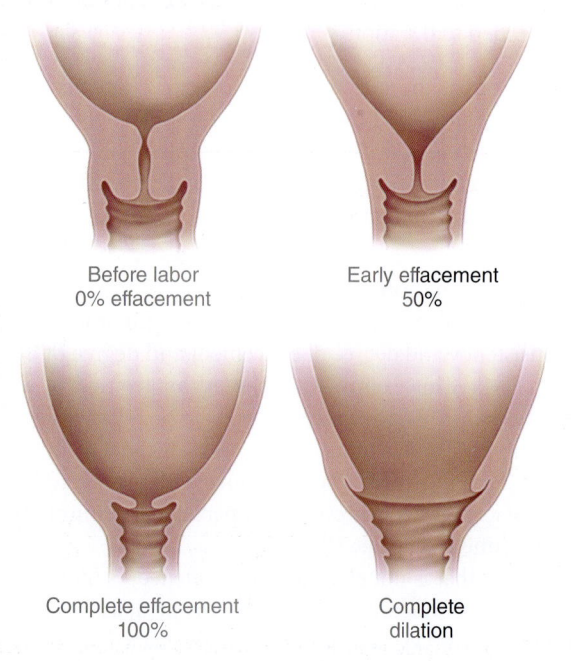

FIGURE 8.3. Effacement and dilation.

posterior in the vagina. A cervix that is palpable anterior in the vagina is more likely to undergo change in labor sooner than one found in the posterior portion of the vagina. This suggests that the presenting part has descended into the pelvis, creating more pressure on the cervix, thereby rotating it anteriorly. With more effective force on the lower uterine segment, contractions would cause a greater change in dilation and effacement of the cervix.

Fetal Station

Fetal station is determined by identifying the level of the fetal presenting part in the birth canal in relation to the ischial spines that are located approximately halfway between the **pelvic inlet** and the **pelvic outlet** (Fig. 8.4). If the presenting part has reached the level of the ischial spines, it is termed "zero station." The distance between the ischial spines to the pelvic inlet above and the distance from the spines to the pelvic outlet below are divided into fifths, and these measurements are used to further define station. These divisions represent centimeters above and below the ischial spines. Thus, as the presenting fetal part descends from the pelvic inlet toward the ischial spines, the designation is −5, −4, −3, −2, −1, then 0 station. The clinical significance of the

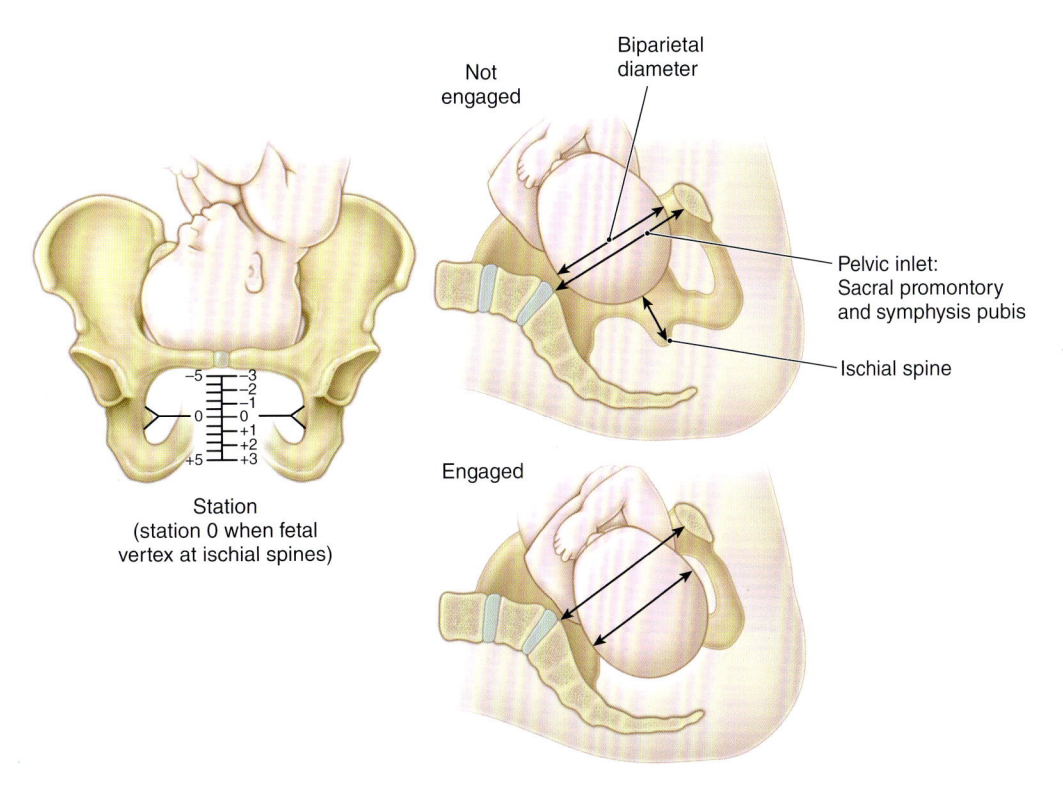

FIGURE 8.4. Station and engagement of the fetal head.

fetal head presenting at 0 station is that the biparietal diameter of the fetal head, the greatest transverse diameter of the fetal skull, is assumed to have negotiated the pelvic inlet. Below the ischial spines, the presenting fetal part passes +1, +2, +3, +4, with +5 station corresponding to the fetal head being visible at the introitus.

The fetal head is said to be engaged at 0 station, a crucial functional "landmark" in the labor path. However, caput succedaneum, cephalohematoma, and molding of the fetal head may mislead the examiner to erroneously describe a more advanced station than has been actually attained.

● STAGES OF LABOR

Although labor is a continuous process, it is divided into four functional stages because each has differing physiological activities and requires differing management.

1. The **first stage of labor** is the interval between the onset of labor and full cervical dilation (10 cm). The first stage is further divided into two phases: 1) The **latent phase** of labor encompasses cervical effacement and early dilation and 2) the **active phase** of labor, during which more rapid cervical dilation occurs, usually beginning at approximately 5 to 6 cm.
2. The **second stage of labor** encompasses complete cervical dilation through the delivery of the infant.
3. The **third stage of labor** begins immediately after delivery of the infant and ends with the delivery of the placenta.
4. The **fourth stage of labor** is defined as the immediate postpartum period of approximately 2 hours after delivery of the placenta, during which time the patient undergoes significant physiologic adjustment.

The stages of labor were first described in the research by Emmanuel Friedman, and Figure 8.5 represents this information graphically, known as the **Friedman curve**. New data, derived since the advent of epidural labor analgesia, suggest that the maximum slope of the normal labor curve during active

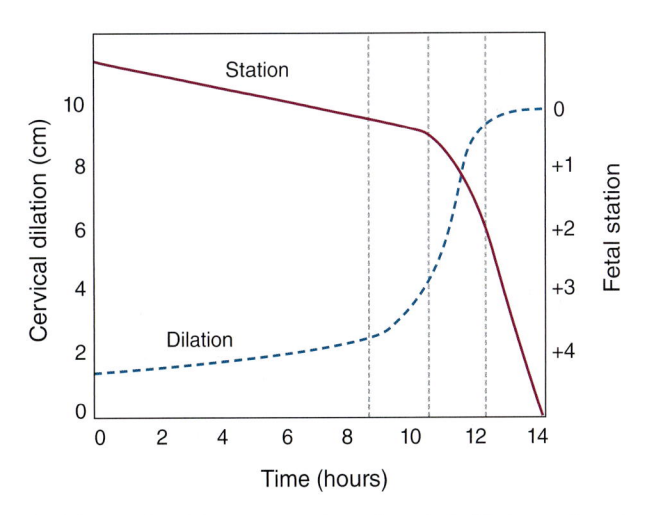

FIGURE 8.5. Graphic representation of cervical dilation and station during the first and second stages of labor.

TABLE 8.1 MEDIAN DURATION OF THE VARIOUS PHASES AND STAGES OF LABOR

Parity	Latent Phase From 4–6 cm (hr)	First Stage From 6–10 cm (hr)	Second Stage (hr)	Second Stage With Epidural (hr)
Nulliparous				
Median	2.1	2.1	0.6	1.1
Upper limit[a]	9.6	7.0	2.8	3.6
Multiparous				
Median	2.2	1.5	0.2	0.4
Upper limit[a]	10.7	5.1	1.3	2.0

[a] 95th percentile.

phase may actually be slightly less steep, and that active labor begins at 5 to 6 cm cervical dilation. Table 8.1 outlines the contemporary duration of the various stages of labor.

MECHANISM OF LABOR

The **mechanisms of labor** (also known as the **cardinal movements of labor**) refer to the changes of the position of the fetus as it passes through the birth canal, as shown in Figure 8.6. The fetus usually descends to where the occipital portion of the fetal head is the lowermost part in the pelvis, and it rotates toward the largest pelvic segment. Because vertex presentation occurs in 95% of term labors, the cardinal movements of labor are defined relative to this presentation. To accommodate to the maternal bony pelvis, the fetal head must undergo several movements as it passes through the birth canal. These movements are accomplished by means of the forceful contractions of the uterus. These **cardinal movements of labor** do not occur as a distinct series of movements but, rather, as a group of movements that overlap as the fetus accommodates and moves progressively through the birth canal.

These movements are as follows:

1. Engagement
2. Flexion
3. Descent
4. Internal rotation
5. Extension
6. External rotation or restitution
7. Expulsion

Engagement is defined as descent of the biparietal diameter of the head below the plane of the pelvic inlet, suggested clinically by palpation of the presenting part below the level of ischial spines (0 station). Engagement commonly occurs days to weeks prior to labor in women who have not delivered a child, whereas in women who have had children, it more commonly happens at the onset of active labor. In any event, the importance of this event is that it suggests that the bony pelvis is adequate to allow significant descent of the fetal head, although it does not always follow that delivery of the fetus through the pelvis will happen during labor. **Flexion** of the fetal head allows for the smaller diameters of the fetal head to present to the maternal pelvis. **Descent** of the presenting part is necessary for the successful completion of passage through the birth canal. The greatest rate of descent occurs during the latter portions of the first stage of labor and during the second stage of labor.

Internal rotation, like flexion, facilitates presentation of the optimal diameters of the fetal head to the bony pelvis, most commonly from transverse to either anterior or posterior. **Extension** of the fetal head occurs as it reaches the introitus. To accommodate the upward curve of the birth canal, the flexed head now extends. **External rotation** occurs after delivery of the head as the head rotates to "face forward" relative to its shoulders. This is known as restitution, followed rapidly by delivery of the body, **expulsion**.

NORMAL LABOR AND DELIVERY

Ideally, a pregnant woman has a principal, designated health care provider or provider team (attending physician and resident team). Beginning with admission to the labor and delivery area, the obstetric team monitors the patient's progress. Once the patient is in active labor, her provider(s) should be readily available.

General Management

Ambulation and Position in Labor and at Delivery

Walking may be more comfortable than being supine during early labor. Women in early labor are confined to bed if they are too uncomfortable to move about safely or if care maneuvers require it. Supine labor is common in the United States. However, this position obstructs venous return, thence cardiac output, leading to hypotension (**supine hypotensive syndrome**). The supine left lateral position keeps the uterus off the inferior vena cava, thereby improving cardiac output. Changing positions to improve maternal comfort and optimize fetal position are encouraged as long as not otherwise

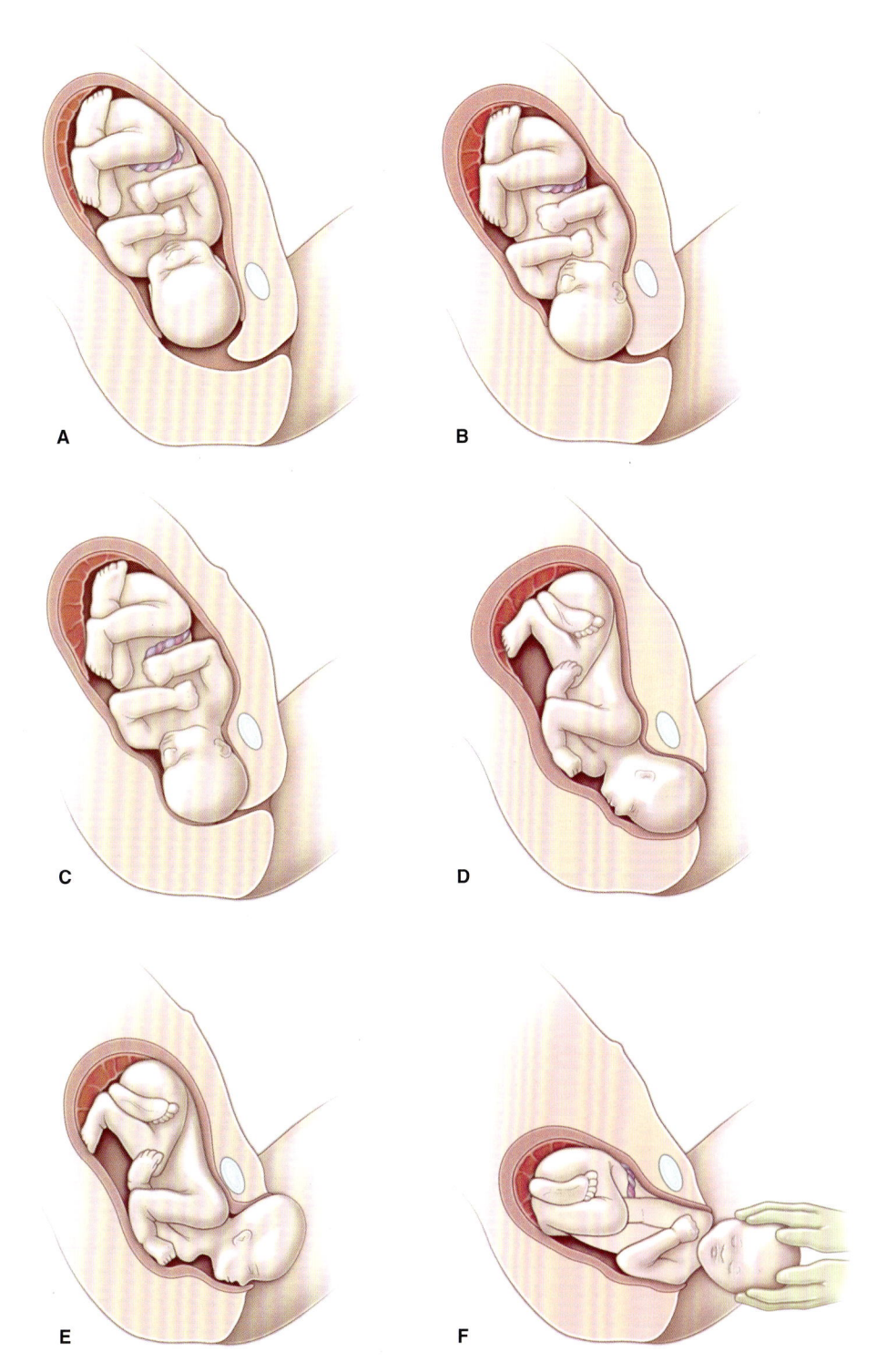

FIGURE 8.6. Cardinal movements of labor: engagement (**A**), flexion (**B**), descent (**C**), internal rotation (**D**), extension (**E**), and external rotation (**F**).

contraindicated by other maternal or fetal conditions. Other laboring positions might include sitting or crouching, and the use of special "birthing chairs," labor balls, or variously configured tubs of warm water. The **dorsal lithotomy position** is most commonly used for spontaneous and operative vaginal delivery in the United States.

Fluid Management and Oral Intake
Because labor is associated with decreased gastrointestinal peristalsis, aspiration during the administration of anesthesia is a concern. Patients in active labor should avoid oral ingestion of anything except moderate intake of clear fluids, occasional ice chips, and preparations for moistening the mouth and lips.

When oral intake is not possible or is insufficient, intravenous therapy with 1/2 normal saline or D5 1/2 normal saline is indicated. Normal saline can be used if increased oncotic pressure is desired, but lactated fluids are generally contraindicated because of the metabolic acid deficit incurred by the lactate administration. Individual patient considerations, clinical considerations, and anticipated duration of labor will guide choice of intravenous therapy.

Evaluation of Fetal Well-Being

Measurement of the **fetal heart rate** and its changes during labor is the primary means of intrapartum assessment of fetal well-being, which may be done by intermittent auscultation with a stethoscope or hand-held Doppler or by the use of electronic fetal monitoring. The method chosen may depend on risk assessment at admission, the preference of the patient and the obstetric staff, and department policy. Risk factors for fetal intolerance of labor may include, but are not limited to, vaginal bleeding, acute abdominal pain, temperature >100.4°F, preterm labor or ROM, hypertension, and nonreassuring fetal heart rate pattern.

In the absence of risk factors on admission, the standard approach to fetal monitoring is to determine, evaluate, and record the fetal heart rate every 30 minutes in the active phase in the first stage of labor, and at least every 15 minutes in the second stage. In the presence of risk factors, fetal surveillance should be performed using either intermittent auscultation or continuous fetal monitoring using the following methods: During the active first stage of labor, auscultation should be performed every 15 minutes, preferably before, during, or after a contraction, and continuous monitoring should be evaluated at least every 15 minutes. During the second stage of labor, the fetal heart rate should be monitored every 5 minutes using either the intermittent or continuous procedure. If electronic fetal monitoring is used, an external tocodynamometer is initially used to assess uterine activity, providing information regarding the frequency and duration of contractions but not their intensity. Electronic fetal monitoring is not necessary for a low-risk term pregnancy.

Pain Control

Management of discomfort and pain during labor is an essential part of good obstetric practice. Some patients tolerate pain by using techniques learned in childbirth preparation programs. It is important that bedside staff be knowledgeable about these pain management techniques and be supportive of the patient's decisions. Unless contraindicated, pain relief to ameliorate pain of contractions should be made available on request to women in labor.

During the first stage of labor, pain results from the contraction of the uterus and dilation of the cervix. This pain travels along the visceral afferents, which accompany sympathetic nerves entering the spinal cord at T10–T12 and L1. As the fetal head descends, there is also distension of the lower birth canal and perineum. This pain is transmitted along somatic afferents that comprise portions of the pudendal nerves that enter the spinal cord at S2–S4. To provide relief from obstetric pain, the following methods of anesthesia and analgesia are used:

- **Epidural block:** Infusion of local anesthetics or narcotics through a catheter into the epidural space. The most effective form of intrapartum pain relief in the United States, it can be used in either vaginal or abdominal deliveries and in postpartum procedures such as tubal ligation. An epidural allows for longer duration of labor analgesia or anesthesia, and may be partially regulated by patient-controlled mechanisms.
- **Spinal anesthesia:** A single injection of anesthetic which affords labor anesthesia for approximately two hours.
- **Combined spinal–epidural:** Combination of the above two techniques.
- **Local block:** Local injection of anesthetic into the perineum or vagina (e.g., **pudendal block**; Fig. 8.7).
- **General anesthesia:** Inhaled or intravenous administration of anesthetic agents that results in a loss of maternal consciousness (reserved only for emergency cesarean deliveries or scenarios in which neuraxial anesthesia cannot be performed or has already failed).

To determine which method of obstetric pain control should be used, the positive and negative aspects of each should be considered. Of the regional modes of analgesia, epidural anesthesia is superior to spinal anesthesia in that it can be left as a continuous source of analgesia and anesthesia during both the labor and delivery process. The advantage of this technique is its ability to provide analgesia during labor as well as excellent anesthesia for delivery, yet is titrated to maintain the patient's sense of touch and motor ability, facilitating participation in the birth process. Spinal anesthesia provides good pain relief for procedures of limited duration, such as cesarean delivery or vaginal delivery when labor is rapidly progressing. Combined spinal–epidural anesthesia has advantages of both techniques, including the ability to titrate medications throughout labor with the epidural catheter and the rapid onset associated with spinal techniques. All of these types of regional anesthesia may be associated with a postdural puncture headache. However, combined spinal–epidural anesthesia greatly decreases the risk of spinal headache in the mother when using newer atraumatic needles and reduces the risk of sympathetic blockade, which could lead to hypotension. There is also less motor blockade than with spinal anesthesia alone. Local block may provide anesthesia for episiotomy and repair of vaginal and perineal lacerations; however, paracervical block may result in fetal bradycardia. General anesthesia is associated with complications such as maternal aspiration and neonatal depression. If properly administered, it is effective for most cesarean deliveries, but regional anesthesia is preferable.

Management of Labor

First Stage

Evaluation of the progress of labor is accomplished by means of a series of pelvic examinations. At the time of each vaginal examination, a sterile lubricant is used. Each examination should identify cervical dilation, effacement, station, position of the presenting part, and the status of the membranes. These findings should be noted graphically on the hospital record, so that abnormalities of labor may be identified.

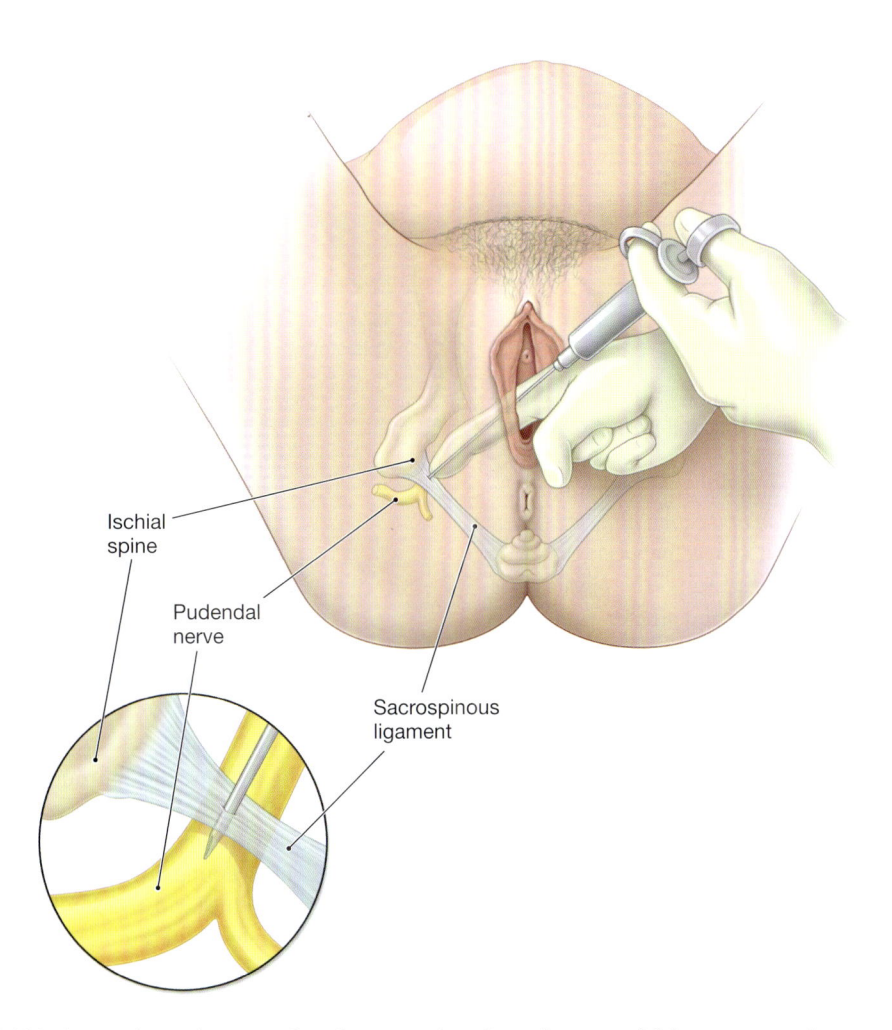

FIGURE 8.7. Pudendal block. Local anesthesia can be administered easily at the time of delivery to provide perineal anesthesia for a vaginal delivery.

During the latter portions of the first stage of labor, patients may report the urge to push, which may indicate significant descent of the fetal head with pressure on the perineum. Pushing should be discouraged at this time in order to avoid traumatic swelling of the cervix caused by the attempt to force the fetus through an incompletely dilated cervix. Should this occur, additional time is needed for the swelling to resolve before complete dilation can be achieved. More frequent vaginal examinations during this time may be necessary. Similarly, if there are significant fetal heart rate decelerations, more frequent examinations may be necessary to determine whether the umbilical cord is prolapsed or if delivery is imminent.

Routine amniotomy is unnecessary if labor is progressing normally and evidence supports the fetus is tolerating labor. If needed, amniotic membranes may be ruptured to insert an intrauterine pressure catheter or a fetal scalp monitor. **Artificial ROM**, known as AROM, may be beneficial in other ways. The presence or absence of meconium (fetal stool) can be identified. However, rupture of the membranes does carry some risk, because the incidence of infection may be increased if labor is prolonged, or umbilical cord prolapse may occur if rupture of the membranes is undertaken before engagement of the presenting fetal part. Spontaneous ROM has similar risks. The fluid should be observed for meconium and blood. Fetal heart tones should be assessed after membranes spontaneously rupture.

Second Stage

Once the **second stage** of labor has been reached (i.e., complete cervical dilation to 10 cm), voluntary maternal effort (**pushing**) can be added to the involuntary contractile forces of the uterus to facilitate delivery of the fetus. With the onset of each contraction, the mother is encouraged to either use open glottis pushing, or perform an extended Valsalva maneuver. This increase in intra-abdominal pressure aids in fetal descent through the birth canal. Alternatively, in low risk women who may not yet have the urge to push, a rest period of 1 to 2 hours may be offered at the onset of the second stage of labor.

During the second stage of labor, the fetal head may undergo further alterations. **Molding** is an alteration in the relation of the fetal cranial bones, even resulting in partial bone overlap (Fig. 8.8). Some minor degree of molding is common as the fetal head adjusts to the bony pelvis. The greater the disparity between

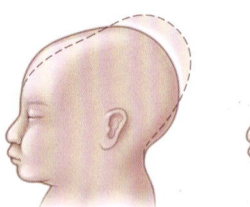

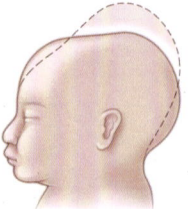

FIGURE 8.8. Molding of head.

the fetal head and the bony pelvis, the greater the amount of molding. **Caput succedaneum** is the edema of the fetal scalp caused by pressure on the fetal head by the cervix. *Molding and caput succedaneum are the two most common causes of overestimation of the amount of descent, that is, of the station of the presenting fetal part.*

When there is a large amount of space "between the back of the fetal head and the curve of the sacrum," the physician is alerted to the possibility that the biparietal diameter of the fetal head is higher than might be thought based upon the physical level to which the presenting part's farthest dimension has reached. An extended second stage may last as long as 2 to 3 hours, and the prolonged resistance encountered by the fetal vertex may prevent appropriate identification of fontanels and sutures. Both caput and molding resolve in the first few days of life. If identified before the second stage of labor, these changes should be noted on the pelvic examination and may indicate a potential problem in negotiation of the birth canal.

Restricted use of **episiotomy** may facilitate delivery by enlarging the vaginal outlet and may be indicated in cases of instrumental delivery and/or protracted or arrested descent; however, there is currently no evidence based indication for use of episiotomy. With progressive labor and control of the fetal head and body at delivery, the risk of obstetric laceration with a normal-sized infant is low, so that the need for episiotomy is minimal. If an episiotomy is needed, it should be performed only after the perineum has been thinned considerably by the descending fetal head. The incision should be somewhat longer on the mucosal surface when compared with the perineal surface of the incision (Fig. 8.9). However, it is important to note that the American College of Obstetricians and Gynecologists (College) recommends that the routine use of episiotomy is not necessary and may lead to an increase in the risk of third-degree and fourth-degree perineal lacerations and a delay in the patient's resumption of sexual activity. Episiotomy should only be done for a specific medical indication. Median episiotomy is associated with higher rates of injury to the anal sphincter and rectum, and mediolateral episiotomy may be preferable to median episiotomy in selected cases.

As the **fetal head crowns** (i.e., distends the vaginal opening), it is delivered by extension to allow the smallest diameter of the fetal head to pass over the perineum. This natural mechanism decreases the likelihood of laceration or extension of an episiotomy.

To support the perineal tissues and facilitate extension of the head, a **modified Ritgen maneuver** is performed (Fig. 8.10). This maneuver involves placing one hand over the vertex while

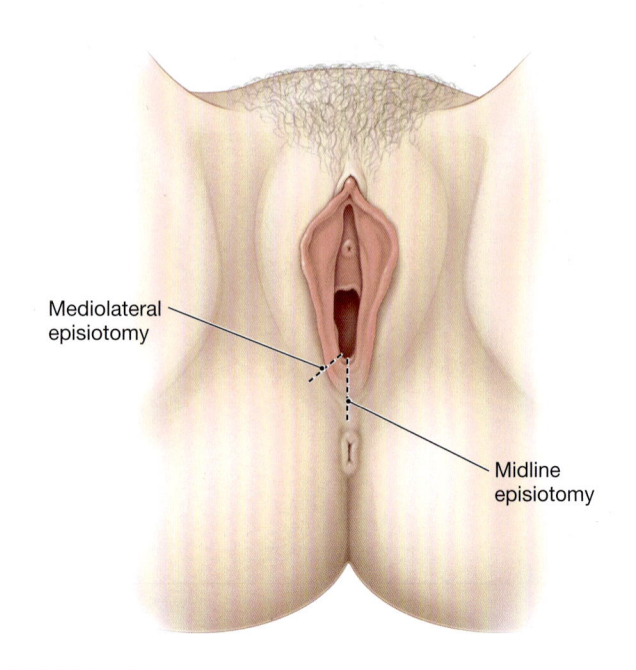

FIGURE 8.9. Episiotomy.

the other hand exerts pressure through the perineum onto the fetal chin. A sterile towel is used to avoid contamination of this hand by contact with the anus. The chin can then be delivered slowly, with control applied by both hands.

After delivery of the head, the shoulders descend and rotate to a position in the anteroposterior diameter of the pelvis. The attendant's hands are placed on either side of the fetal head, applying gentle downward pressure, thus delivering the anterior shoulder. To avoid injury to the brachial plexus, care is taken not to put excessive force on the neck. The posterior shoulder is then delivered by upward traction on the fetal head (Fig. 8.11). Delivery of the body now occurs easily in most cases. Immediately after delivery, the uterus significantly decreases in size. Use of oxytocin immediately after delivery of the infant may shorten the third stage of labor and prevent uterine atony.

Third Stage

Delivery of the placenta is imminent when the uterus rises in the abdomen, becoming globular in configuration, indicating that the placenta has separated and has entered the lower uterine segment; a gush of blood and/or "lengthening" of the umbilical cord also occur. These are the three classic signs of placental separation. Pulling the placenta from the uterus by excessive traction on the cord should be avoided. Inappropriate application of force may result in inversion of the uterus, an obstetric emergency associated with profound blood loss and shock. Instead, it is appropriate to wait for spontaneous extrusion of the placenta, sometimes up to 30 minutes. As the placenta passes into the lower uterine segment, gentle downward traction is applied to the umbilical cord, while the abdominal hand applies gentle suprapubic counterpressure (posterior and cephalad) to secure the uterine fundus and prevent uterine inversion (Fig. 8.12). If necessary, the placenta may be removed

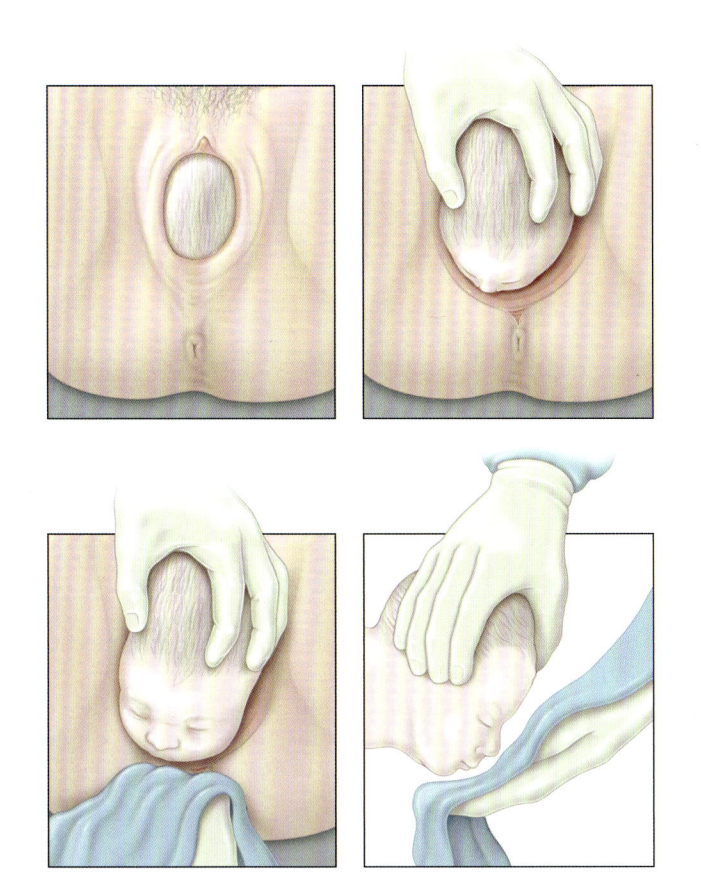

FIGURE 8.10. Vaginal delivery assisted by modified Ritgen maneuver.

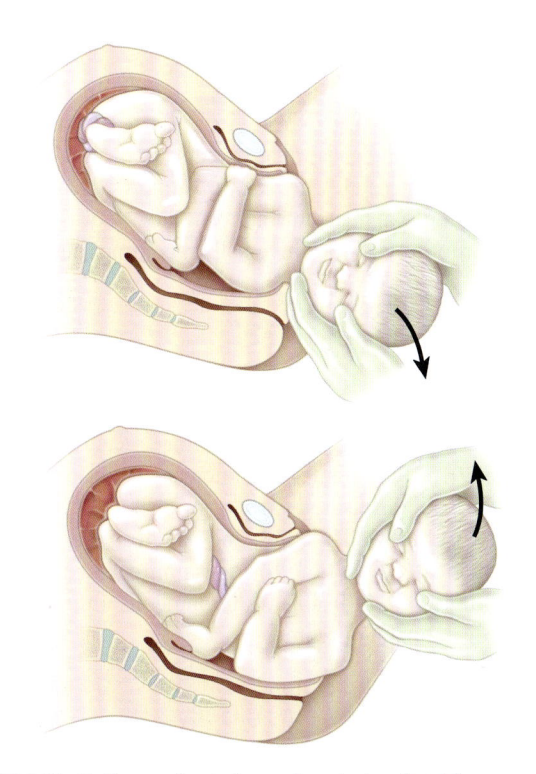

FIGURE 8.11. Delivery of anterior and posterior shoulders.

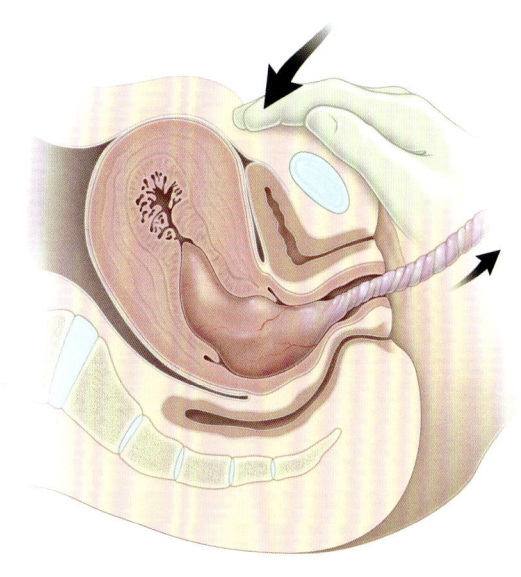

FIGURE 8.12. Delivery of the placenta.

manually. This is accomplished by passing a hand into the uterine cavity and using the side of the hand to develop a cleavage plane between the placenta and the uterine wall. Anesthesia may be required. The umbilical cord should be evaluated for the presence of the expected two umbilical arteries and one umbilical vein.

After the placenta has been removed, the uterus should be palpated to ensure that it has reduced in size and become firmly contracted. Excessive blood loss at this or any subsequent time should suggest the possibility of uterine atony. The use of uterine massage as well as oxytocic agents, such as oxytocin, methylergonovine maleate (methergine), and prostaglandins (carboprost or misoprostol), may be used routinely in the circumstance of excessive postpartum blood loss. Inspection of the birth canal should be performed in a systematic fashion.

The introitus, vagina, perineum, and the vulvar area, including the periurethral area, should be evaluated for lacerations. Ring forceps are commonly used to hold and evaluate the cervix. Lacerations, if present, are most commonly found at the 3 o'clock and 9 o'clock positions of the cervix. Repair of nonhemostatic lacerations are generally accomplished with an absorbable suture. Obstetric lacerations are classified in Table 8.2.

Fourth Stage

For the first hour after delivery, the likelihood of serious postpartum complications is at its greatest. Postpartum uterine hemorrhage occurs in approximately 1% of patients. It is more likely to occur in cases of rapid labor, protracted labor, uterine enlargement (such as from a large fetus, polyhydramnios, and multiple gestation), or intrapartum chorioamnionitis. Immediately after the delivery of the placenta, the uterus is palpated to determine that it is firm. Uterine palpation is done in this period to ascertain uterine tone. Perineal pads are applied, and the amount of blood on these pads and maternal pulse and

TABLE 8.2	CLASSIFICATION OF OBSTETRIC LACERATIONS
Degree of Laceration	Description
First degree	Involves the vaginal mucosa or perineal skin, but not the underlying tissue
Second degree	Involves the underlying subcutaneous tissue, but not the rectal sphincter or rectal mucosa
Third degree	Extends through the rectal sphincter, but not into the rectal mucosa
Fourth degree	Extends into the rectal mucosa

blood pressure are monitored closely for the first several hours after delivery to identify excessive blood loss.

LABOR INDUCTION

Labor can be induced when the benefits to either the woman or the fetus outweigh those of continuing the pregnancy. Labor induction can be achieved with intravenous oxytocin administration, **cervical ripening**, and manipulation of the amniotic membranes.

Oxytocin Administration

The device used to administer oxytocin should permit precise control of the flow rate to ensure accurate, minute-to-minute control. Various regimens exist for stimulation of uterine contractions. These regimens vary in initial dose, amount of incremental dose increase, and interval between dose increases. Lower and less frequent dosage increases are associated with a lower incidence of uterine hyperstimulation. Higher and more frequent dosage increases may result in shorter time in labor and reduce the incidence of chorioamnionitis and the number of cesarean deliveries performed for dystocia (abnormal labor) and also in increased rates of uterine hyperstimulation.

Cervical Ripening

Cervical ripening may be beneficial if the cervix is unfavorable for induction. Several techniques are available. Misoprostol, a prostaglandin E analog, is an effective agent for cervical ripening and induction of labor. It is administered vaginally. Prostaglandin E2 can also be administered vaginally or intracervically. Because of the increased risk of uterine hyperstimulation, both drugs are contraindicated in patients who have had a previous cesarean delivery or previous uterine surgery.

Cervical ripening can also be accomplished with mechanical dilation. One method uses **laminaria**—hygroscopic rods made from the stems of the seaweed *Laminaria japonica* that are inserted into the internal cervical os. As the rods absorb moisture and expand, the cervix is slowly dilated (Fig. 8.13). The risks associated with laminaria use include failure to dilate

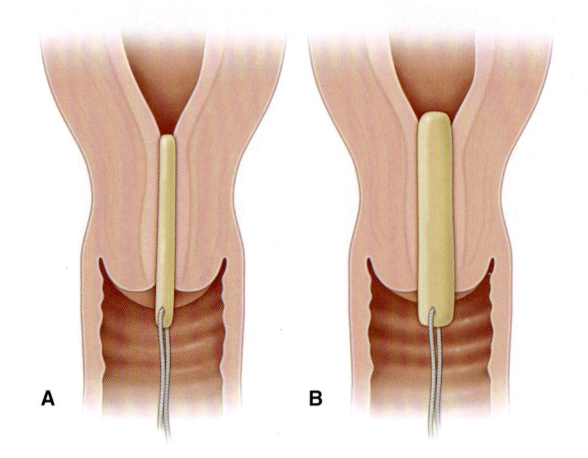

FIGURE 8.13. Use of laminaria. (A) Laminaria properly inserted just beyond the cervical os. (B) Properly placed laminaria that has expanded, causing cervical dilation.

the cervix, cervical laceration, inadvertent ROM, and infection. A synthetic form is also available. Another cervical ripening method is the placement of a 30 mL Foley catheter in the cervical canal, which is lower in cost than other forms of cervical ripening and carries a reduced risk of uterine tachysystole.

Membrane Manipulation

Induction of labor by **"stripping"** or **"sweeping" the amniotic membranes** has associated risks including infection, bleeding from an undiagnosed placenta previa or low-lying placenta, and accidental ROM.

Artificial ROM is another method of labor induction that may be used, particularly when the cervix is favorable. Routine early amniotomy results in a modest reduction in the length of labor but may result in an increased rate of intra-amniotic infection, umbilical cord prolapse, rupture of vasa previa, vertical transmission of HIV in HIV positive women, and cesarean delivery for fetal heart rate abnormalities. For these reasons, routine amniotomy is not universally recommended.

CESAREAN DELIVERY

Cesarean delivery is the most common major operation performed in the United States. Until 1965, the rate of cesarean delivery was stable at less than 5%. More recently, it has risen to 32% in 2015. Reasons for this increase include labor dystocia, nonmedically indicated early term births (37 0/7 to 38 6/7 weeks), use in breech deliveries, and use in situations in which more sophisticated fetal monitoring is nonreassuring. However, evidence does not indicate a simultaneous improvement in maternal or neonatal outcomes.

Decision Making: Mode of Delivery

The decision regarding the mode of delivery should be made by the health care provider together with the patient. Advantages of a successful vaginal delivery include reduced risks of hemorrhage and infection; shorter postpartum hospital stay; and a less painful, more rapid recovery. However, cesarean delivery may be necessary. Examples of indications for cesarean delivery include hemorrhage from placenta previa, abruptio placentae, prolapse of the umbilical cord, and uterine rupture, because these conditions require prompt delivery. Planned vaginal delivery may be a reasonable approach for a fetus in breech presentation but depends on the experience of the health care provider. In such circumstances, women should be informed that the risk of perinatal and neonatal mortality as well as short-term serious neonatal morbidity may be higher with a vaginal delivery than with a cesarean delivery, and the patient's informed consent should be documented.

Cesarean by Maternal Request

An estimated 2.5% of all births in the United States are cesarean delivery on maternal request. This procedure should not be performed before 39 weeks of gestation. It is not recommended for women desiring several children, because the risks of placenta previa, placenta accreta, and gravid hysterectomy increase with each cesarean delivery. In the absence of maternal or fetal indications, a vaginal delivery is safe and should be recommended.

Risk of Maternal Mortality

Decisions regarding cesarean delivery have important ramifications, because the maternal mortality rate associated with cesarean delivery is two to four times that of a vaginal birth (i.e., 1 per 2,500 to 1 per 5,000–10,000 operations). Cesarean delivery can be performed through various incisions in the uterus. An incision through the thin, lower uterine segment allows for subsequent trials of labor after cesarean (**TOLAC**) delivery if the patient has had one to two prior cesarean delivery. An incision through the thick, muscular upper portion of the uterus, a classical cesarean section, carries such a great risk of subsequent uterine rupture that repeat cesarean delivery for these patients is recommended.

TRIAL OF LABOR AFTER CESAREAN DELIVERY

Cesarean deliveries may be performed as repeat procedures. Prior to the mid-1980s, it was believed that a previous cesarean delivery mandated that all subsequent deliveries be abdominal. **TOLAC** has long been referred to as a **vaginal birth after cesarean (VBAC)**. Recently, a distinction has been made between the actual *trial*, or *attempt*, at VBAC versus the successful occurrence of a VBAC. Publication of data suggesting the safety of TOLAC led to a decade-long clinical trend away from the nearly 70-year-old adage, "Once a cesarean, always a cesarean." Success rates of VBAC were found to be 60% to 80%. More recently, the pendulum has again swung, resulting in an increasing trend for patients and their physicians to opt for scheduled elective repeat cesarean delivery. Reasons for this change vary from patient to patient. Avoiding uterine rupture (a small but potentially catastrophic risk) is a worry for many patients. The possibility of a difficult labor without the assurance of a vaginal birth is a concern voiced by many patients. Although the recovery is more prolonged, some patients feel that having a birth experience with which they are familiar makes the repeat cesarean less daunting. The convenience and predictability of a scheduled date for delivery is also attractive to the expectant family.

The risks and benefits of a trial of labor versus repeat cesarean delivery should be discussed with the patient who has had a prior cesarean delivery. Although uterine rupture does occur more often with TOLAC, the frequency is generally less than 1%. The College's guidelines for TOLAC include the availability of a 24-hour blood bank and capability for massive transfusion, continuous electronic fetal heart rate monitoring, a physician and hospital capable of performing an emergency cesarean delivery, and emergently available support services such as anesthesia. Box 8.1 summarizes clinical considerations for TOLAC.

BOX 8.1 **Selected Clinical Factors Associated with Trial of Labor after Previous Cesarean Delivery Success**

Increased Probability of Success (Strong Predictors)
- Prior vaginal birth
- Spontaneous labor

Decreased Probability of Success (Other Predictors)
- Recurrent indication for initial cesarean delivery (labor dystocia)
- Increased maternal age
- Non-white ethnicity
- Gestational age greater than 40 weeks
- Maternal obesity
- Preeclampsia
- Short interpregnancy interval
- Increased neonatal birth weight

Modified from American College of Obstetricians and Gynecologists. Vaginal Birth after Previous Cesarean Delivery. Practice Bulletin No. 115, Washington, DC: American College of Obstetricians and Gynecologists; August 2015:3.

CLINICAL FOLLOW-UP

On examination, the patient appears to be in early labor. You offer her the opportunity to walk around for a couple of hours and then return for reexamination. You explain how you will determine if she is in active labor. She is concerned about pain management in labor and you explain her options.

CHAPTER 9

Abnormal Labor and Intrapartum Fetal Surveillance

This chapter deals primarily with APGO Educational Topic Areas:

TOPIC 22 ABNORMAL LABOR
TOPIC 26 INTRAPARTUM FETAL SURVEILLANCE

Students should be able to distinguish characteristics of normal and abnormal labor using the physical examination as well as fetal monitoring and tocometry. They should understand the indications and options for operative vaginal delivery.

CLINICAL CASE

After walking for 2 hours, your patient returns to Labor and Delivery, where she is reexamined and found to be 5 cm dilated with regular uterine contractions. She is admitted, given an epidural for pain management, and, after 6 hours, has not progressed past 6 cm dilated. How will you manage her labor at this time? What further evaluation of the patient and fetus might assist in determining the proper management of her labor?

ABNORMAL LABOR

Abnormal labor, or labor **dystocia** (literally, "difficult labor or childbirth"), is characterized by the abnormal progression of labor. Dystocia is the leading indication for primary cesarean delivery in the United States. Despite the high prevalence of labor disorders, considerable variability exists in the diagnosis, management, and criteria for dystocia that requires intervention. Because dystocia can rarely be diagnosed with certainty, the relatively imprecise term "failure to progress" has been used, which includes lack of progressive cervical dilation or lack of descent of the fetal head or both.

Factors That Contribute to Normal Labor—the Three Ps

Labor is the occurrence of uterine contractions of sufficient intensity, frequency, and duration to bring about demonstrable effacement and dilation of the cervix. Dystocia results from what have been categorized classically as abnormalities of the "power" (uterine contractions or maternal expulsive forces), "passenger" (position, size, or presentation of the fetus), or "passageway" (pelvis or soft tissues).

Uterine Contractions: "Power"

Uterine activity can be monitored by palpation, by external **tocodynamometry**, or by using **intrauterine pressure catheters [IUPCs]** (Fig. 9.1). A tocodynamometer is an external strain gauge that is placed on the maternal abdomen. It records the frequency of uterine contractions and relaxations as well as the duration of each contraction. An IUPC, in addition to recording contraction frequency and duration, also directly measures the pressure generated by uterine contractions via a catheter inserted into the uterine cavity. The catheter is attached to a gauge that measures intrauterine pressure in mmHg.

Recent studies suggest that the use of an IUPC instead of external tocodynamometry does not affect the outcome in cases of abnormal labor. However, an IUPC may be useful in specific situations, such as maternal obesity and other factors that may prevent accurate clinical evaluation of uterine contractions.

For cervical dilation and fetal descent to occur, each uterine contraction must generate at least 25 mmHg of peak pressure. Optimal intrauterine pressure is 50 to 60 mm Hg. The frequency of uterine contractions is also important in generating a normal labor pattern: the optimal frequency of uterine contractions is a minimum of three contractions in a 10-minute interval, often described as "adequate." Uterine contractions that are too frequent are not optimal, because they prevent intervals of uterine relaxation. During this "rest interval," the fetus receives unimpeded uteroplacental blood flow for oxygen and waste transport. Without these rest periods, fetal oxygenation may be compromised.

Another unit of measure commonly used to assess contractile strength is the **Montevideo unit** (**MVU**). This unit is the number of uterine contractions in 10 minutes times the average intensity (above the resting baseline intrauterine pressure). Normal progress of labor is usually associated with 200 or more MVU.

Fetal Factors: "Passenger"

Evaluation of the passenger includes clinical estimation of fetal weight and clinical evaluation of fetal lie, presentation, position, and attitude. If a fetus has an estimated weight

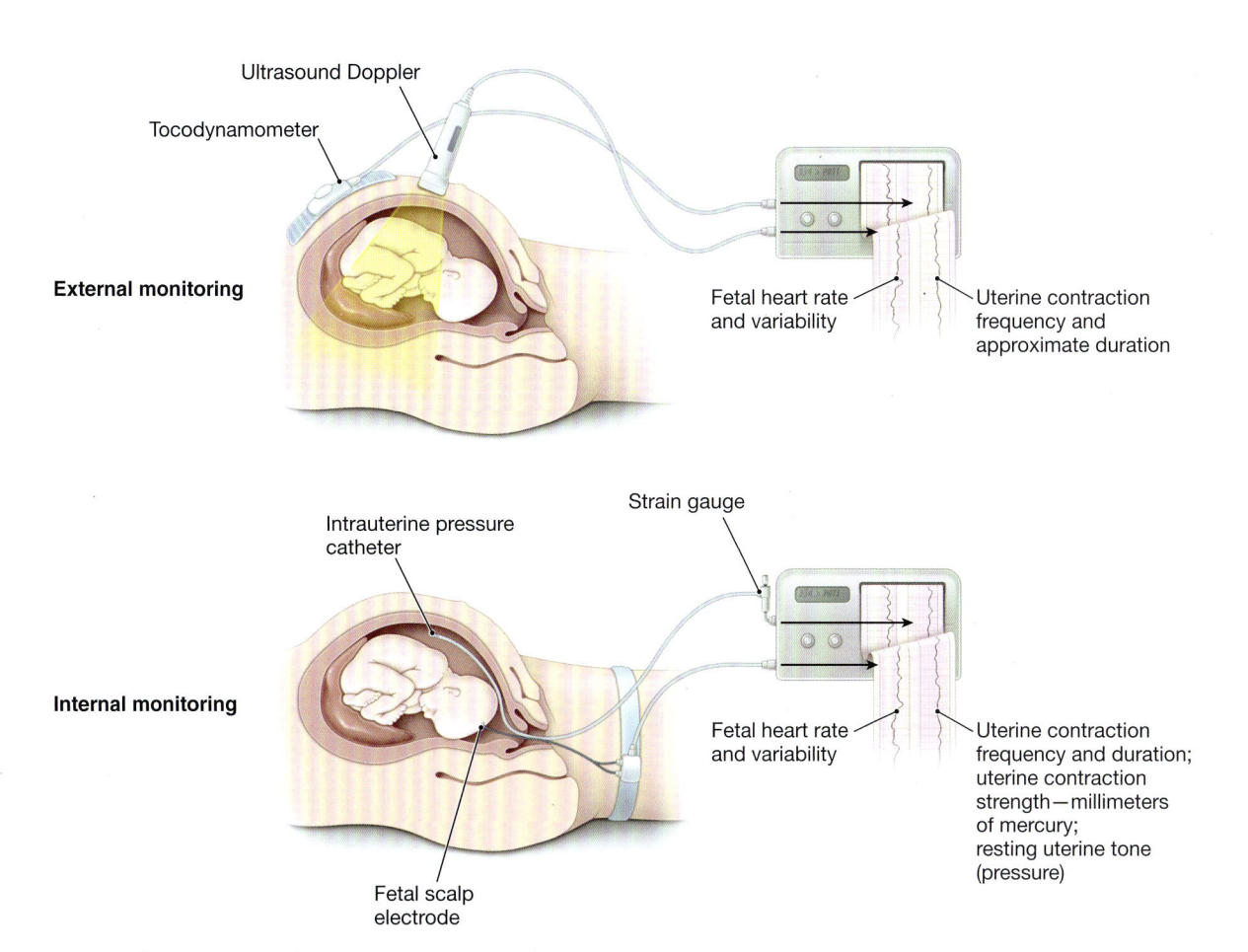

FIGURE 9.1. Tocodynamometer and intrauterine pressure catheter.

greater than 4,000 to 4,500 g, the risk of dystocia, including shoulder dystocia and fetopelvic disproportion, is greater. Because ultrasound estimation of fetal weight is often inaccurate by as much as 500 to 1,000 g when the fetus is near term (40 weeks of gestational age), this information must be used in conjunction with other parameters when making management decisions.

Fetal attitude, presentation, and lie also play a role in the progress of labor (Fig. 9.2). If the fetal head is turned to one side (**asynclitism**) or extended (**extension**), a larger cephalic diameter is presented to the pelvis, thereby increasing the possibility of dystocia. A **brow presentation** (about 1 in 3,000 deliveries) typically converts to either a vertex or face presentation, but, if persistent, may cause dystocia requiring cesarean delivery. Likewise, a **face presentation** (about 1 in 600–1,000 deliveries) requires cesarean delivery in most cases. However, a **mentum anterior face presentation** (chin toward mother's abdomen) may be delivered vaginally if the fetal head undergoes flexion, rather than the normal extension.

A persistent **occipitoposterior position** is also associated with longer labors (approximately 1 hour in multiparous patients and 2 hours in nulliparous patients). In **compound presentations**, when one or more limbs prolapse alongside the presenting part (about 1 in 700 deliveries), the extremity usually retracts (either spontaneously or with manual assistance) as labor continues. When it does not, or in the 15% to 20% of compound presentations associated with umbilical cord prolapse, cesarean delivery is required.

Fetal anomalies, such as hydrocephaly and soft tissue tumors, may also cause dystocia. The routine use of prenatal ultrasound for other causes has allowed identification of these situations, significantly reducing the incidence of unexpected dystocia of this kind.

Maternal Factors: "Passage"

A number of maternal factors are associated with dystocia. Dystocia can result from maternal skeletal or soft tissue anomalies that obstruct the birth canal. **Cephalopelvic disproportion**, in which the size of the maternal pelvis is inadequate to the size of the presenting part of the fetus, may impede fetal descent into the birth canal. Clinical, radiographic, and computed tomography (CT) measurements of the bony pelvis are poor predictors of successful vaginal delivery, due to the inaccuracy of these measurements as well as case-by-case differences in fetal accommodation and mechanisms of labor.

Clinical pelvimetry, the manual evaluation of the diameters of the pelvis, is also a poor predictor of successful vaginal birth, except in rare circumstances when the pelvic diameters are so

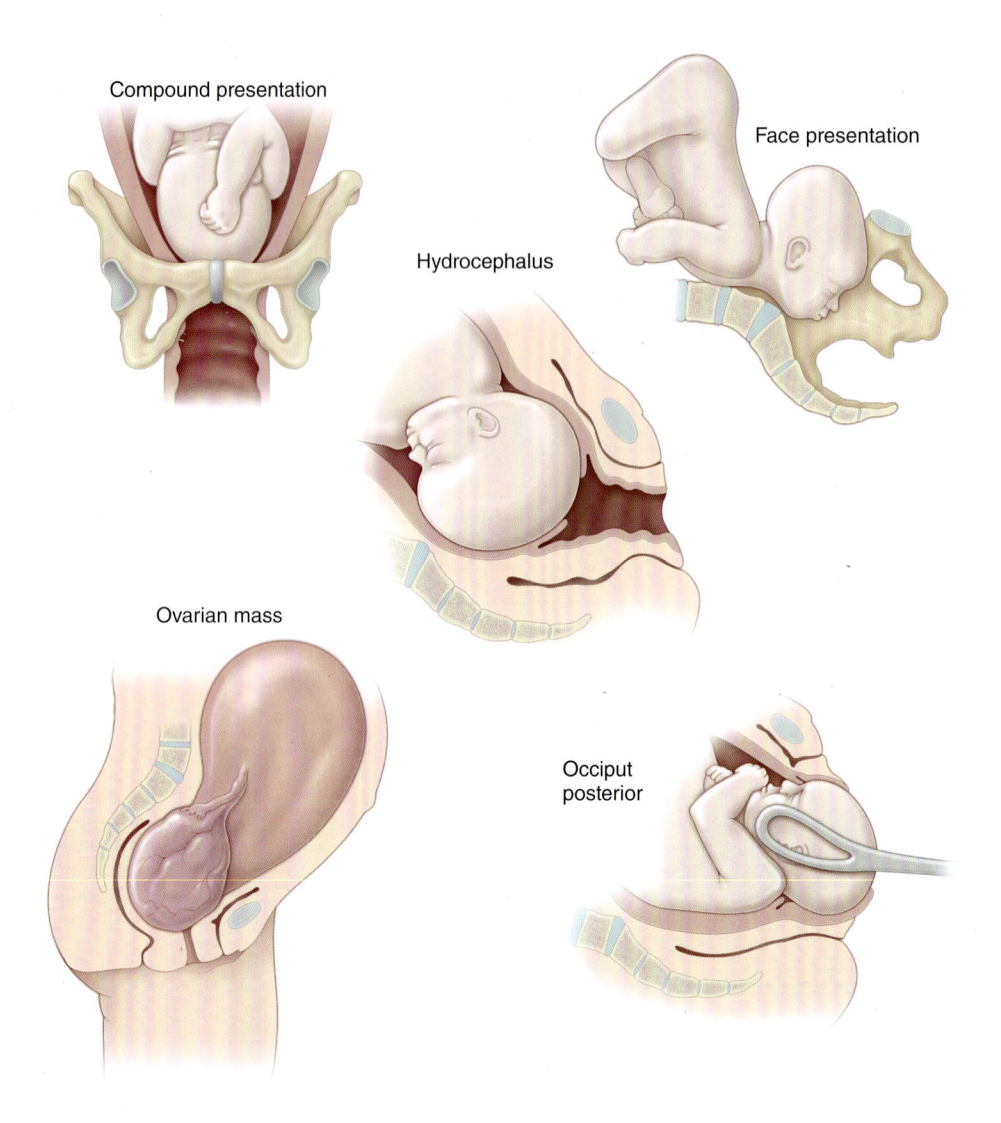

FIGURE 9.2. Some of the fetal factors associated with dystocia.

small as to render the pelvis "completely contracted." Although radiographic and CT pelvimetry can be helpful in some cases, the progress of descent of the presenting part in labor is the best test of pelvic adequacy.

Soft tissue causes of dystocia include abnormalities of the cervix, tumors or other lesions of the colon or adnexa, distended bladder, uterine fibroids, an accessory uterine horn, and morbid obesity. Epidural anesthesia may contribute to dystocia by decreasing the tone of the pelvic floor musculature.

Risks

Dystocia may be associated with serious complications for both the woman and the fetus. Infection (chorioamnionitis) is a consequence of prolonged labor, especially in the setting of ruptured membranes. Fetal infection and bacteremia, including pneumonia caused by aspiration of infected amniotic fluid, is linked to prolonged labor. In addition, there are the attendant risks of cesarean or operative delivery, such as maternal soft tissue injury to the lower genital tract and fetal trauma.

Diagnosis and Management of Abnormal Labor Patterns

Graphic documentation of progressive cervical dilation and effacement facilitates assessing a patient's progress in labor and identifying abnormal labor patterns. The Friedman curve (see Chapter 8) is commonly used for this purpose. Labor abnormalities can be categorized into two general types: **protraction disorders**, in which labor is slow to progress, and **arrest disorders**, in which labor ceases to progress (Table 9.1). Protraction can occur during both the latent and active phases of labor, whereas arrest is recognized only in the active phase. Although the definition of the **latent phase** of labor is controversial, in general it can be defined as the phase in which the cervix effaces but undergoes minimal dilation (see Chapter 8).

TABLE 9.1	ABNORMAL LABOR PATTERNS	
Stage	Protraction Disorder	Arrest Disorder
First stage		
Latent phase		
Nulliparous	Duration of >20 hours	
Multiparous	Duration of >14 hours	
Active phase		
Nulliparous	Cervical dilation rate of <1 cm/hour	No cervical dilation for more than 2 hours for both multiparous and nulliparous
		With regional anesthesia, no cervical dilation for more than 4 hours
Multiparous	Cervical dilation rate of <1.2–1.5 cm/hour	
Second stage		
Nulliparous and multiparous	With regional anesthesia: Duration of >3 hours	No descent after 1 hour of pushing
	No regional anesthesia: Duration of >2 hours or if fetus descends at a rate of <1 cm/hour	

From Shields SG, Ratcliffe SD, Fontain P, Leeman L. Dystocia in nulliparous women. *Am Fam Physician*. 2007;75:1671–1678.

Management of abnormal labor encompasses a wide range of options, from observation to operative or cesarean delivery. Management choice depends on several factors:

- Adequacy of uterine contractions
- Fetal malposition or cephalopelvic disproportion
- Other clinical conditions, such as nonreassuring fetal status or chorioamnionitis

Management decisions should be balanced between ensuring a positive outcome for mother and fetus and avoiding the concomitant risks of operative and cesarean delivery.

First-Stage Disorders

A **prolonged latent phase** is one that exceeds 20 hours in a nulliparous patient or 14 hours in a multiparous patient. A prolonged latent phase does not necessarily predict an abnormal active phase of labor. Some patients who have initially been diagnosed as having a prolonged latent phase are subsequently found to have been in false labor. A prolonged latent phase does not in itself pose a danger to the mother or fetus. Options for management of women with a prolonged latent phase of labor include observation and sedation. With either of these options, the patient may stop having contractions, in which case she is not in labor; may go into active labor; or may continue experiencing prolonged labor into the active phase. In the latter case, other interventions as described below may be administered to augment uterine contractions.

Once the patient is in active labor, the first stage is considered prolonged when the cervix dilates less than 1 cm/hour in nulliparous women, and less than 1.2 to 1.5 cm/hour in multiparous women. Management options for a prolonged first stage include observation, augmentation by amniotomy or oxytocin, and continuous support. Cesarean delivery is usually warranted if maternal or fetal status becomes nonreassuring.

Augmentation

Augmentation refers to stimulation of uterine contractions when spontaneous contractions have failed to result in progressive cervical dilation or descent of the fetus. Augmentation can be achieved with **amniotomy** (artificial rupture of membranes [ROM]) and oxytocin administration. Augmentation should be considered if the frequency of contractions is less than 3 contractions per 10 minutes, the intensity of contractions is less than 25 mmHg above the baseline, or both. Before augmentation, the maternal pelvis and cervix as well as fetal position, station, and well-being should be assessed. If there is no evidence of disproportion and fetal well-being is reassuring, oxytocin can be used if uterine contractions are judged to be inadequate. Contraindications to augmentation are similar to those for labor induction (see Chapter 8).

If the membranes have not ruptured, amniotomy may enhance progress in the active phase and negate the need for oxytocin augmentation. Amniotomy allows the fetal head, rather than the otherwise intact amniotic sac, to be the dilating force. It may also stimulate the release of prostaglandins, which could aid in augmenting the force of contractions.

Amniotomy is usually performed with a thin, plastic rod with a sharp hook on the end. The end is guided to the open cervical os with the examiner's fingers, and the hook is used to snag and disrupt the amniotic sac. Risks of amniotomy include fetal heart rate (FHR) decelerations due to cord compression and an increased incidence of chorioamnionitis. For these reasons, amniotomy should not be routine and should be used for women with prolonged labor. The **FHR** should be evaluated both before and immediately after ROM.

It has been shown that amniotomy combined with oxytocin administration early in the active stage reduces labor by up to 2 hours, although there is no change in the rate of cesarean delivery with this treatment protocol. The goal of oxytocin administration is to effect uterine activity sufficient to produce cervical change and fetal descent while avoiding uterine tachysystole (defined as more than five contractions in a 10-minute period, averaged over 30 minutes). Typically, a goal of a maximum of five contractions in a 10-minute period with resultant cervical dilation is considered adequate. Uterine activity >200

MVUs may also be defined as adequate when utilizing an IUPC to monitor contractions. Oxytocin may be administered in low-dose or high-dose regimens. Low-dose regimens are associated with a decreased incidence and severity of uterine hyperstimulation. High-dose regimens are associated with decreased labor times, incidence of chorioamnionitis, and cesarean delivery for dystocia.

Continuous Labor Support

Continuous support during labor from caregivers (e.g., nurses, midwives, and lay individuals) may have a number of benefits for women and their newborns. Continuous care has been associated with reduced need for pain relief and oxytocin administration, lower rates of cesarean and operative deliveries, decreased incidence of 5-minute Apgar scores lower than 7, and increased patient satisfaction with the labor experience. However, there are insufficient data comparing differences in benefits on the basis of level of training of support personnel—that is, whether the caregivers are nurses, midwives, or doulas. There is no evidence of harmful effects from continuous support during labor.

Second-Stage Disorders

A second-stage protraction disorder should be considered when the second stage exceeds 3 hours if regional anesthesia has been administered, 2 hours if no regional anesthesia is used, or if the fetus descends at a rate of less than 1 cm/hour if no regional anesthesia is used. **Second-stage arrest** is diagnosed when there is no descent after 1 hour of pushing. In the past, the fetus was thought to be at increased risk for morbidity and mortality when the second stage exceeded 2 hours. Currently, more intensive intrapartum surveillance provides the ability to identify the fetus that may not be tolerating labor well. Thus, the length of the second stage of labor is not in itself an absolute to immediately proceed with an operative or cesarean delivery; however, prolonged second stage may be considered an indiction for an operative delivery.

As long as heart tones continue to be reassuring and cephalopelvic disproportion has been ruled out, it is considered safe to allow the second stage to continue. If uterine contractions are inadequate, oxytocin administration can be initiated or the dosage increased if already in place.

Bearing-down efforts by the patient in conjunction with uterine contractions help bring about delivery. Labor positions other than the dorsal lithotomy position (e.g., knee–chest, sitting, squatting, and sitting in a birthing chair) may bring about subtle changes in fetal presentation and facilitate vaginal delivery. Fetal accommodation may also be facilitated by allowing the effects of epidural analgesia to dissipate. The absence of epidural analgesia may increase the tone of the pelvic floor muscles, thereby facilitating the cardinal movements of labor and restoring the urge to push. In some cases of fetal malpresentation, manual techniques can facilitate delivery. If the fetus is in the occipitoposterior position and does not spontaneously convert to the normal position, rotation can be performed to turn the fetus to the anterior position (Fig. 9.3).

The decision to perform an operative delivery in the second stage versus continued observation should be made on the basis of clinical assessment of the woman and the fetus and the skill and training of the obstetrician. Nonreassuring status of the fetus or mother is an indication for operative or cesarean delivery.

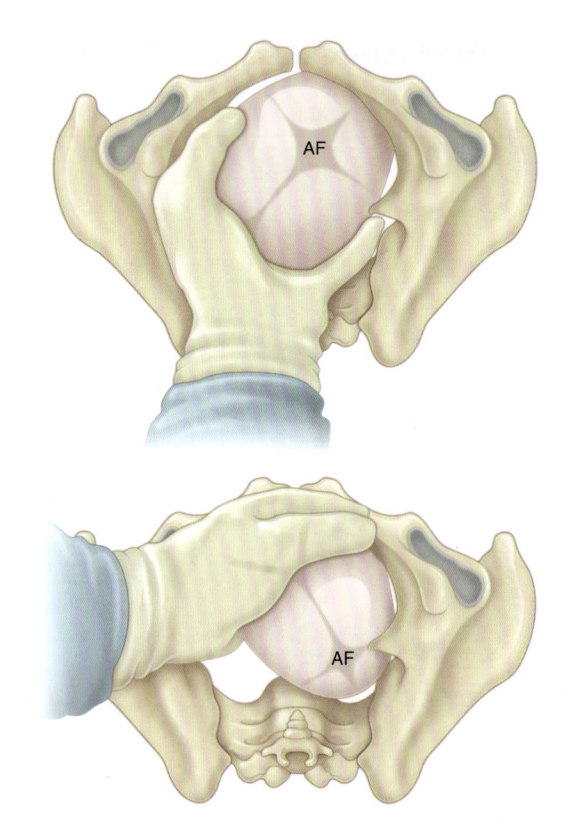

FIGURE 9.3. Manual rotation of a fetus in the occipitoposterior position to the occipitoanterior position. (A) The physician's hand is placed palm upward into the vagina. (B) The hand serves as a wedge to flex the fetal head while the fingers exert a rotating force to bring the occiput to anterior. *AF,* anterior fontanel. (Adapted from Shields SG, Ratcliffe SD, Fontain P, Leeman L. Dystocia in nulliparous women. *Am Fam Physician.* 2007;75(11):1675.)

● OPERATIVE DELIVERY

Operative vaginal deliveries are accomplished by applying direct traction on the fetal skull with forceps or by applying traction to the fetal scalp by means of a vacuum extractor. The prevalence of operative vaginal delivery in the United States in 2015 was approximately 3%. Although considered safe in appropriate circumstances, operative vaginal delivery has the potential for maternal and neonatal complications.

Operative vaginal delivery should be performed only by experienced individuals with privileges for such procedures and in settings in which personnel are readily available to perform a cesarean delivery in the event the operative vaginal delivery is unsuccessful. However, the incidence of intracranial hemorrhage is highest among infants delivered by cesarean delivery following a failed vacuum or forceps delivery. The combination of vacuum and forceps has a similar risk of intracranial hemorrhage. Therefore, an operative vaginal delivery should not be attempted when the probability of success is very low.

Classification

For both forceps and vacuum extraction deliveries, the type of delivery depends on the fetal station—the relationship between the leading portion of the fetal head and the level of the maternal ischial spines. **Outlet operative vaginal delivery** is the application of forceps or vacuum under the following conditions:

1. The scalp is visible at the introitus without separating labia.
2. The fetal skull has reached pelvic floor.
3. The sagittal suture is in anteroposterior diameter or right or left occiput anterior or posterior position.
4. The fetal head is at or on the perineum.
5. Rotation does not exceed 45°.

Low operative vaginal delivery is the application of forceps or vacuum when the leading point of the fetal skull is at station +2 or more and is not on the pelvic floor. This type of operative vaginal delivery has two subtypes:

1. Rotation of 45° or less (left or right occiput anterior to occiput anterior, or left or right occiput posterior to occiput posterior)
2. Rotation greater than 45°

Midpelvis operative vaginal delivery is the application of forceps or vacuum when the fetal head is engaged but the leading point of the skull is above station +2. Under very unusual circumstances, such as the sudden onset of severe fetal or maternal compromise, application of forceps or vacuum above station +2 may be attempted while simultaneously initiating preparation for a cesarean delivery in the event that the operative vaginal delivery is unsuccessful.

Indications and Contraindications

No indication for operative vaginal delivery is absolute. The following indications apply when the fetal head is engaged and the cervix is fully dilated:

- Prolonged or arrested second stage of labor
- Suspicion of immediate or potential fetal compromise
- Shortening of the second stage for maternal benefit

In certain situations, operative vaginal delivery should be avoided or, at the least, carefully considered in terms of relative maternal and fetal risks. Most authorities consider vacuum extraction inappropriate in pregnancies before 34 weeks of gestation because of the risk of fetal intraventricular hemorrhage. Operative delivery is also contraindicated if a live fetus is known to have a bone demineralization condition (e.g., osteogenesis imperfecta) or a bleeding disorder (e.g., alloimmune thrombocytopenia, hemophilia, and von Willebrand disease), and if the fetal head is unengaged or the position of the fetal head is unknown.

Forceps and vacuum extractors have low risk of complications and are acceptable for operative vaginal delivery. The choice of whether to use vacuum or forceps and which specific instrument to use are defined by the clinical circumstances and operator preference based on experience and training. Both types of instruments can be effective in delivering the fetus and shortening the time to delivery. Vacuum extraction may be used when asynclitism prevents proper forceps placement. Use of forceps provides a more secure application and is appropriate for rotation of the fetal head to occiput anterior or occiput posterior position.

Forceps

Forceps are primarily used to apply traction to the fetal head to augment the expulsive forces, when the mother's voluntary efforts in conjunction with uterine contractions are insufficient to deliver the infant (Fig. 9.4). Occasionally, forceps are used to rotate the fetal head before applying traction to complete vaginal delivery. Forceps may also be used to control delivery of the fetal head, thereby avoiding precipitous delivery. Different types of forceps are available for the different degrees of molding of the fetal head.

Maternal complications of forceps delivery include perineal trauma, hematoma, and pelvic floor injury. Neonatal risks include injuries to the brain and spine, musculoskeletal injury, and corneal abrasion if the forceps are mistakenly applied over the neonate's eyes. The risk of **shoulder dystocia**, in which the fetus' anterior shoulder becomes lodged against the pubic symphysis, is increased in forceps deliveries of infants weighing over 4,000 g.

Vacuum Extraction

In **vacuum extraction**, a soft vacuum cup is applied to the fetal head and suction is exerted by means of a mechanical pump (Fig. 9.5). Vacuum extraction is associated with less maternal trauma than forceps but as with forceps delivery carries potential neonatal risks. Although the amount of traction applied to the fetal skull is less than that applied with forceps, it is still substantial and can cause serious fetal injury. Neonatal risks include intracranial hemorrhage, subgaleal hematomas, scalp lacerations (if torsion is excessive), hyperbilirubinemia, and retinal hemorrhage. In addition, separation of the scalp from the underlying

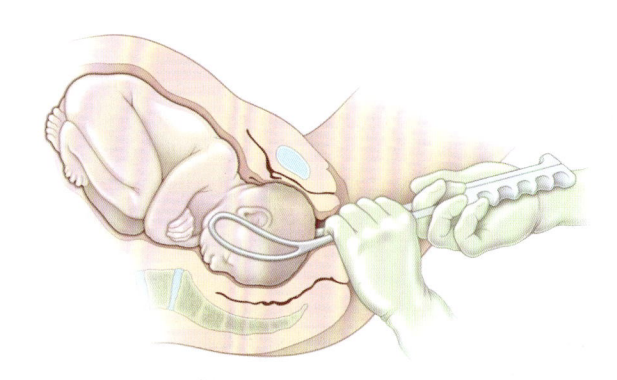

FIGURE 9.4. Forceps delivery. (From Bofill JA. *Forceps in Obstetrics*, [Slide presentation]. Washington, DC: American College of Obstetricians and Gynecologists; 2001.)

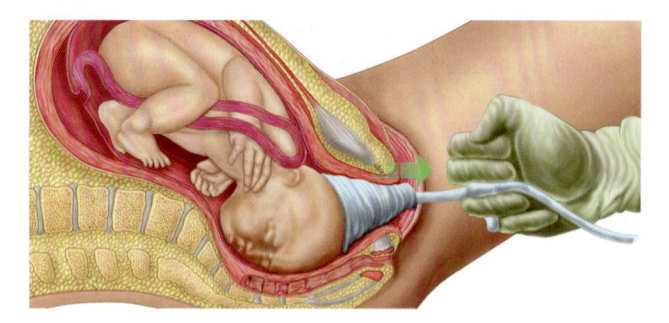

FIGURE 9.5. Illustration of a vacuum extraction.

structures can lead to cephalohematoma. It is recommended that rocking movements or torque should not be applied to the device and that only steady traction in the line of the birth canal should be used. Neonatal care providers should be made aware of the mode of delivery in order to observe for potential complications associated with operative vaginal delivery.

● BREECH PRESENTATION

Breech presentation occurs in about 3% to 4% of singleton deliveries at term and more frequently in the early third and second trimesters. In addition to prematurity, other conditions associated with breech presentation include multiple pregnancy, polyhydramnios, hydrocephaly, anencephaly, aneuploidy, uterine anomalies, and uterine tumors. The three kinds of breech presentation—**frank, complete,** and **incomplete** (**footling**) **breech** (Fig. 9.6)—are diagnosed by a combination of Leopold maneuvers, pelvic examination, ultrasonography, and other imaging techniques (Fig. 9.7).

The morbidity and mortality rates for mother and fetus, regardless of gestational age or mode of delivery, are higher in the breech than in the cephalic presentation. This increased risk to the fetus comes from associated factors such as fetal anomalies, prematurity, and umbilical cord prolapse as well as birth trauma.

External cephalic version (**ECV**) involves applying pressure to the mother's abdomen to turn the fetus in either a forward or backward somersault to achieve a vertex presentation prior to labor (Fig. 9.8). The goal of ECV is to increase the proportion of vertex presentations among fetuses that were formerly in the breech position near term. Once a vertex presentation is achieved, the chances for a vaginal delivery increase. This maneuver is successful in approximately half of the properly selected cases. Patients who have completed 36 weeks of gestation are preferred candidates for ECV for several reasons. First, if spontaneous version is going to occur, it is likely to have taken place by 36 completed weeks of gestation. Second, the risk of a spontaneous reversion is decreased after ECV at term compared with earlier gestations. Selection criteria include a normal fetus with reassuring fetal heart tracing, adequate amniotic fluid, presenting part not having descended into the birth canal, and absence of mullerian duct anomalies, placental abruption, or previa. The risks include premature ROM, placental abruption, cord accident, and uterine rupture. External version is more often successful in parous women. Existing evidence

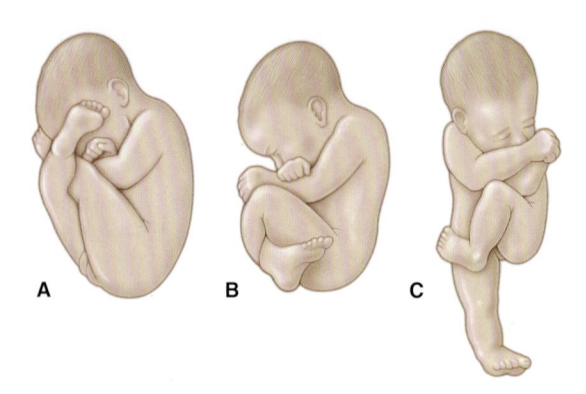

FIGURE 9.6. Types of breech presentations. (A) Frank breech, in which the feet are near the head; (B) complete breech, in which the legs are crossed; (C) incomplete (footling) breech, in which one or both feet are extended.

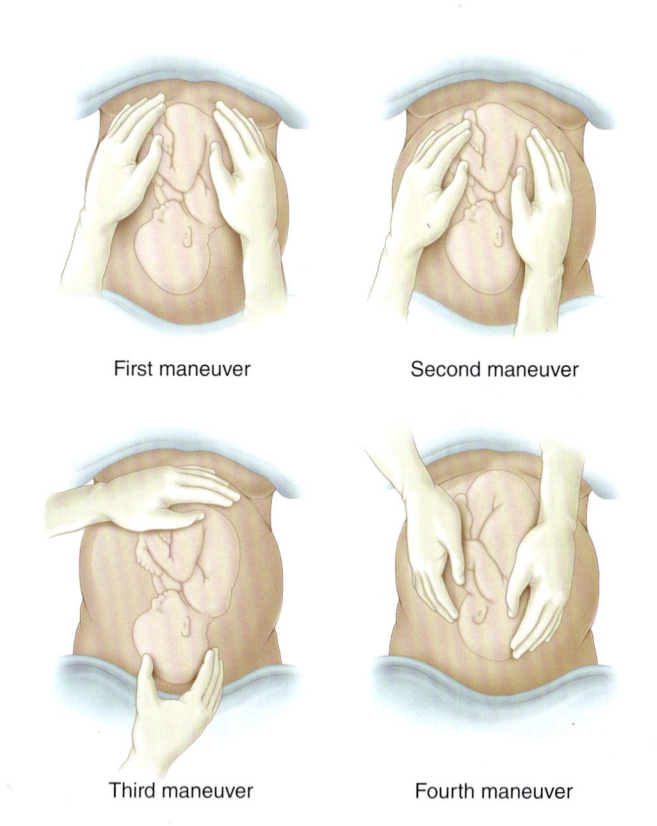

FIGURE 9.7. Leopold maneuvers. The maneuvers are used to determine fetal position: 1) determination of what is in the fundus; 2) evaluation of the fetal back and extremities; 3) palpation of the presenting part above the symphysis; and 4) determination of the direction and degree of flexion of the head.

may support the use of a tocolytic agent (i.e., a drug that stops uterine contractions) during ECV attempts, particularly in nulliparous patients. Administration of anti-D immunoglobulin to Rh-negative women is recommended.

In light of studies that clarify the long-term risks of vaginal breech delivery, the decision regarding the mode of delivery should depend on the experience of the health care provider. Cesarean delivery will be the preferred and safest mode for most, in part due to diminishing expertise in vaginal breech

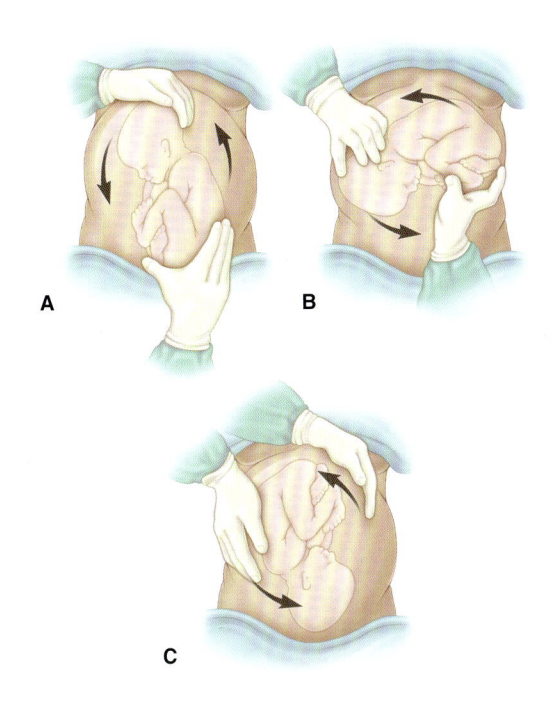

FIGURE 9.8. External cephalic version. In this maneuver, the fetus is converted from a breech to a vertex presentation.

delivery. Planned vaginal delivery of a term singleton breech fetus may be reasonable under hospital-specific protocol guidelines for both eligibility and labor management. The following criteria have been suggested for vaginal breech delivery:

- Normal labor curve
- Gestational age greater than 37 weeks
- Frank or complete breech presentation (because of the risk of umbilical cord prolapse, vaginal delivery of a fetus in the footling breech position is not recommended)
- Absence of fetal anomalies on ultrasound examination
- Adequate maternal pelvis
- Estimated fetal weight between 2,500 and 4,000 g
- Documentation of fetal head flexion (hyperextension of the fetal head occurs in about 5% of term breech fetuses, requiring cesarean delivery to avoid head entrapment)
- Adequate amniotic fluid volume (defined as a 3-cm vertical pocket)
- Availability of anesthesia and neonatal support

If a vaginal breech delivery is planned, the woman should be informed that the risk of perinatal or neonatal mortality or short-term serious neonatal morbidity may be higher than in a cesarean delivery, and the patient's informed consent should be documented.

SHOULDER DYSTOCIA

Shoulder dystocia may sometimes arrest expulsion. Shoulder dystocia cannot be predicted or prevented, because accurate methods for identifying which fetuses will experience this complication do not exist. Antepartum conditions associated with shoulder dystocia include increased birth weight, maternal diabetes, and a previous history of shoulder dystocia. Although fetal macrosomia increases the risk of shoulder dystocia, elective induction of labor or elective cesarean delivery for all women suspected of carrying a fetus with macrosomia is not appropriate.

Diagnosis of shoulder dystocia has a subjective component, especially in less severe forms. The delivered fetal head may retract against the maternal perineum (**turtle sign**) and, if so, may assist in the diagnosis. Interventions that may be used to facilitate delivery include the **McRoberts maneuver** (hyperflexion of the mother's legs tight to the abdomen) and the application of suprapubic pressure to assist in dislodging the impacted shoulder (Fig. 9.9). In contrast, fundal pressure may further worsen impaction of the shoulder and may also result in uterine rupture.

Controversy exists as to whether episiotomy is necessary, because shoulder dystocia is typically not caused by obstructing soft tissue. The use of episiotomy should be based on clinical circumstances and is primarily reserved for cases in which additional access is needed to perform maneuvers to effect delivery of the fetus. Direct fetal manipulation with either rotational maneuvers or delivery of the posterior arm may also be used. In severe cases, more aggressive interventions, such as the **Zavanelli maneuver** (in which the fetal head is flexed and reinserted into the vagina to reestablish umbilical cord blood flow and delivery performed through cesarean section) and intentional fracture of the fetal clavicle, may be performed. Regardless of the procedures used, brachial plexus injury is associated with shoulder dystocia; incidence ranges from 10% to 20%. However, most cases resolve without permanent disability. Fewer than 10% of all cases of shoulder dystocia result in a persistent brachial plexus injury.

INTRAPARTUM FETAL SURVEILLANCE

Evidence suggesting a **nonreassuring fetal status** during labor occurs in 5% to 10% of pregnancies. **Intrapartum fetal surveillance** is the indirect measurement of indicators of fetal status, such as FHR, blood gases, pulse rate, amniotic fluid volume, and fetal stimulation responses, during labor. The goal of intrapartum fetal surveillance is to recognize changes in fetal oxygenation that could result in serious complications. However, it is now recognized that many neurologic conditions previously attributed to **birth asphyxia** (defined as *a process of* marked impairment of gas exchange leading, to progressive hypoxemia, hypercapnia, and significant metabolic acidosis) are in fact attributable to other causes not associated with labor, such as maternal infection, coagulation disorders, autoimmune disorders, genetic causes, and low birthweight. Intrapartum fetal surveillance is a tool for detection of events that occur during labor that could compromise fetal oxygenation and, in rare cases, lead to permanent neurologic disability.

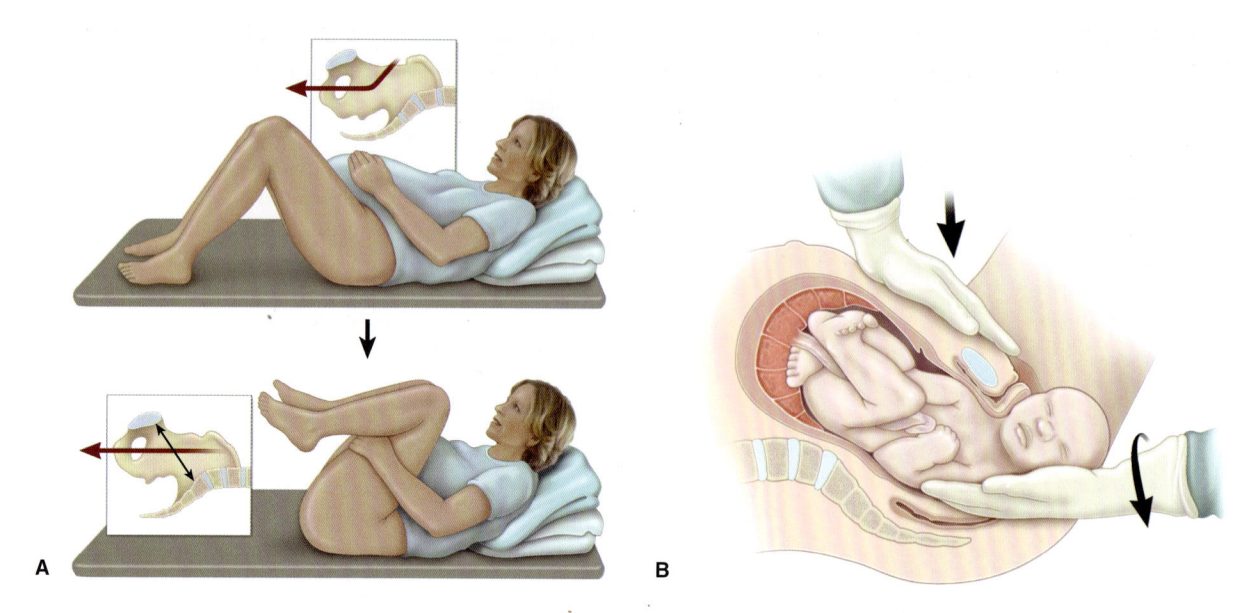

FIGURE 9.9. Procedures used to relieve shoulder dystocia. (A) McRoberts maneuver. Hyperflexion and abduction of the hips cause cephalad rotation of the symphysis pubis and flattening of the lumbar lordosis that frees the impacted shoulder. (B) Suprapubic pressure directed downward on the anterior shoulder and laterally toward the baby's sternum.

Pathophysiology

The **uteroplacental unit** provides oxygen and nutrients to the fetus while receiving carbon dioxide and wastes, the products of the normal aerobic fetal metabolism. **Uteroplacental insufficiency** occurs when the uteroplacental unit is compromised. Initial fetal responses include fetal hypoxia (decreased blood oxygen levels); shunting of blood flow to the fetal brain, heart, and adrenal glands; and transient, repetitive, late decelerations of the FHR. If hypoxia continues, the fetus will eventually switch over to anaerobic glycolysis and develop metabolic acidosis. Lactic acid accumulates, and progressive damage to vital organs occurs, especially the fetal brain and myocardium. If intervention is not timely, serious and possibly permanent damage and sometimes death can result.

Neonatal Encephalopathy

Neonatal encephalopathy is a clinically defined syndrome of disturbed neurologic function in the earliest days of life in the term infant, manifested by difficulty with initiating and maintaining respiration, depression of tone and reflexes, subnormal level of consciousness, and sometimes seizures. Neonatal encephalopathy is not always associated with permanent neonatal neurologic impairment. **Hypoxic-ischemic encephalopathy (HIE)** is a subtype of neonatal encephalopathy for which the cause is considered to be the limitation of oxygen and blood flow near the time of birth. Historically, it has been assumed that most cases of neonatal encephalopathy were HIE, but epidemiologic studies have established that this assumption is incorrect. Approximately 70% of cases of neonatal encephalopathy are caused by factors that were present before the onset of labor. It is estimated that the incidence of neonatal encephalopathy caused by intrapartum hypoxia is approximately 1.6/10,000, in the absence of any other coincident preconceptual or antepartum abnormalities. HIE is, thus, one among the larger category of encephalopathies that may result from conditions such as prenatal stroke, prenatal infection, genetic abnormalities, and neonatal cerebral malformation. The criteria sufficient to suggest that an encephalopathy is associated with an acute intrapartum event are presented in Box 9.1.

Cerebral Palsy

Cerebral palsy is a chronic disability of the central nervous system (CNS) characterized by aberrant control of movement and posture appearing early in life and not as a result of progressive neurologic disease. Only one type of cerebral palsy, **spastic quadriplegia**, is associated with antepartum or intrapartum interruption of the fetal blood supply. Disorders not associated with intrapartum or peripartum asphyxia include dyskinetic or ataxic cerebral palsy (which commonly has a genetic origin) and epilepsy, mental retardation, or attention-deficit hyperactivity disorders.

Intrapartum Fetal Heart Rate Monitoring

FHR monitoring is a modality intended to determine if a fetus is well oxygenated. The majority of neonates (approximately 85%) born in the United States are assessed with **electronic fetal monitoring (EFM)**, making it the most common obstetric procedure. **Intermittent auscultation** of the FHR after a contraction is also used to assess intrapartum fetal well-being. Beginning in the 1980s, EFM became more common; the rates of its use have doubled over the past 35 years.

EFM may be performed externally or internally. Most external monitors use a Doppler device with computerized logic to interpret and count the Doppler signals. Internal FHR monitoring is accomplished with a fetal electrode, which is a spiral wire placed directly on the fetal scalp or other presenting part.

BOX 9.1 Criteria to Define an Acute Intrapartum Hypoxic Event as Sufficient to Cause Cerebral Palsy

I. Essential criteria (must meet all four) are as follows:
   1. Fetal metabolic acidosis demonstrated from umbilical cord arterial blood gas measurement (pH < 7 and base deficit ≥12 mmol/L)
   2. Early-onset severe or moderate neonatal encephalopathy in newborn of ≥34 weeks of gestational age
   3. Spastic or, less commonly, dyskinetic cerebral palsy
   4. Exclusion of other identifiable causes (trauma, coagulopathy, infection, or genetic anomaly)

II. Criteria nonspecific to asphyxial insult, but suggestive of intrapartum timing (close proximity to labor and delivery, within 48 hours)
   1. Sentinel hypoxic event immediately before or during labor
   2. Fetal heart rate monitor patterns consistent with an acute peripartum or intrapartum event
   3. Apgar scores of 0 to 4 at five and ten minutes
   4. Onset of multisystem illness (e.g., acute bowel injury, renal failure, hepatic failure, cardiac damage, and hematologic abnormalities) within 72 hours of birth consistent with hypoxic-ischemic encephalopathy
   5. Early cerebral imaging with evidence of acute brain injury on brain magnetic resonance imaging or magnetic resonance spectroscopy consistent with hypoxia–ischemia
   6. No evidence of other proximal or distal contributing factors

Adapted from ACOG Task Force on Neonatal Encephalopathy and Cerebral Palsy. Neonatal Encephalopathy and Cerebral Palsy: Defining the Pathogenesis and Pathophysiology. Washington, DC: American College of Obstetricians and Gynecologists; 2003, p.74.; Based on MacLenna, A., A template for defining a causal relation between acute intrapartum events and cerebral palsy: international consensus statement. BMJ. 1999; 319:1054–1059, Box 2.

FHRs by EFM are described in terms of baseline rate, variability, presence of accelerations, periodic or episodic decelerations, and the changes in these characteristics over time (Table 9.2) and classified by a three-tier FHR interpretation system (Box 9.2).

The goal of FHR monitoring is to detect signs of fetal jeopardy in time to intervene before irreversible damage occurs. Despite the liberal use of continuous EFM in both high-risk and low-risk patients, there has been no consistent decrease in the frequency of cerebral palsy in the past two decades. Fetuses who are severely asphyxiated during the intrapartum period will have abnormal heart rate patterns. However, most patients with nonreassuring FHR patterns give birth to healthy infants. In addition, the false-positive rate of EFM for predicting adverse outcomes is high. Guidelines for intrapartum FHR monitoring are given in Table 9.3.

Fetal Heart Rate Patterns

The normal baseline FHR is 110 to 160 beats per minute (bpm). An FHR less than 110 bpm is considered **bradycardia**. Fetal bradycardia between 100 and 110 bpm can usually be tolerated for long periods when it is accompanied by normal FHR variability. An FHR between 80 and 100 bpm is nonreassuring. An FHR that persists below 80 bpm is an ominous sign and may presage fetal death.

An FHR above 160 bpm is considered **tachycardia**. The most common cause of fetal tachycardia is chorioamnionitis, but it may also be due to maternal fever, thyrotoxicosis, medication, and fetal cardiac arrhythmias. Fetal tachycardia between 160 and 200 bpm without any other abnormalities in FHR is usually well tolerated when accompanied by normal FHR variability.

Fetal Heart Rate Variability

FHR variability refers to the fluctuations in the FHR of two cycles or more, visually quantified as the amplitude of peak to trough in bpm. FHR is graded according to amplitude range (Fig. 9.10; also see Table 9.2). Moderate variability is a reassuring sign that reflects adequate fetal oxygenation and normal brain function. In the presence of normal FHR variability, regardless of what other FHR patterns exist, the fetus is not experiencing cerebral tissue asphyxia.

Decreased variability is associated with fetal hypoxia, acidemia, drugs that may depress the fetal CNS (e.g., maternal narcotic analgesia), fetal tachycardia, fetal CNS and cardiac anomalies, prolonged uterine contractions (uterine hypertonus), prematurity, and fetal sleep.

Periodic Fetal Heart Rate Changes

The FHR may vary with uterine contractions by slowing or accelerating in periodic patterns. These **periodic FHR changes** are classified as accelerations or decelerations, based on whether they increase or decrease in the FHR and on their magnitude (in bpm).

Accelerations

Accelerations of the FHR are visually apparent increases (onset to peak in less than 30 seconds) in the FHR from the most recently calculated baseline (see Table 9.2). Accelerations are generally associated with reassuring fetal status and an absence

TABLE 9.2 ELECTRONIC FETAL MONITORING DEFINITIONS

Pattern	Definition
Baseline	• The mean FHR rounded to increments of 5 bpm during a 10-minute segment, excluding periodic or episodic changes; periods of marked FHR variability; segments of baseline that differ by more than 25 bpm • The baseline must be for a minimum of 2 minutes in any 10-minute segment, or the baseline for that time period is indeterminate. In this case, one may refer to the prior 10-minute window for determination of baseline • Normal FHR baseline: 110–160 bpm • Tachycardia: FHR baseline is greater than 160 bpm • Bradycardia: FHR baseline is less than 110 bpm
Baseline variability	• Fluctuations in the baseline FHR that are irregular in amplitude and frequency • Variability is visually quantitated as the amplitude of peak to trough in bpm: absent, amplitude range undetectable; minimal, amplitude range detectable but 5 bpm or fewer; moderate (normal), amplitude range 6–25 bpm; marked, amplitude range greater than 25 bpm
Acceleration	• A visually apparent abrupt increase (onset to peak in less than 30 seconds) in the FHR • At 32 weeks gestation and beyond, an acceleration has a peak of 15 bpm or more above baseline, with a duration of 15 seconds or more but less than 2 minutes from onset to return • Before 32 weeks gestation, an acceleration has a peak of 10 bpm or more above baseline, with a duration of 10 seconds or more but less than 2 minutes from onset to return • Prolonged acceleration lasts 2 minutes or more but less than 10 minutes in duration • If an acceleration lasts 10 minutes or longer, it is a baseline change
Early deceleration	• Visually apparent usually symmetrical gradual decrease and return of the FHR associated with a uterine contraction • A gradual FHR decrease is defined as from the onset to the FHR nadir of 30 seconds or more • The decrease in FHR is calculated from the onset to the nadir of the deceleration • The nadir of the deceleration occurs at the same time as the peak of the contraction • In most cases, the onset, nadir, and recovery of the deceleration are coincident with the beginning, peak, and ending of the contraction, respectively
Late deceleration	• Visually apparent usually symmetrical gradual decrease and return of the FHR associated with a uterine contraction • A gradual FHR decrease is defined as from the onset to the FHR nadir of 30 seconds or more • The decrease in FHR is calculated from the onset to the nadir of the deceleration • The deceleration is delayed in timing, with the nadir of the deceleration occurring after the peak of the contraction • In most cases, the onset, nadir, and recovery of the deceleration occur after the beginning, peak, and ending of the contraction, respectively
Variable deceleration	• Visually apparent abrupt decrease in FHR • An abrupt FHR decrease is defined as from the onset of the deceleration to the beginning of the FHR nadir of less than 30 seconds • The decrease in FHR is calculated from the onset to the nadir of the deceleration • The decrease in FHR is 15 bpm or greater, lasting 15 seconds or greater, and less than 2 minutes in duration • When variable decelerations are associated with uterine contractions, their onset, depth, and duration commonly vary with successive uterine contractions
Prolonged deceleration	• Visually apparent decrease in the FHR below the baseline • Decrease in FHR from the baseline that is 15 bpm or more, lasting 2 minutes or more but less than 10 minutes in duration • If a deceleration lasts 10 minutes or longer, it is a baseline change
Sinusoidal pattern	• Visually apparent, smooth, sine wave–like undulating pattern in FHR baseline with a cycle frequency of 3–5 per minute which persists for 20 minutes or more

FHR, fetal heart rate; bpm, beats per minute.
Macones GA, Hankins GD, Spong CY, Hauth J, Moore T. The 2008 National Institute of Child Health and Human Development workshop report on electronic fetal monitoring: update on definitions, interpretation, and research guidelines. *Obstet Gynecol*. 2008;112:661–666.

BOX 9.2 — Three-Tier Fetal Heart Rate Interpretation System

Category I
Category I fetal heart rate (FHR) tracings include all of the following:
- Baseline rate: 110 to 160 bpm
- Baseline FHR variability: moderate
- Late or variable decelerations: absent
- Early decelerations: present or absent
- Accelerations: present or absent

Category II
Category II FHR tracings include all FHR tracings not categorized as category I or category III. Category II tracings may represent an appreciable fraction of those encountered in clinical care. Examples of category II FHR tracings include any of the following:

Baseline Rate
- Bradycardia not accompanied by absent baseline variability
- Tachycardia

Baseline FHR Variability
- Minimal baseline variability
- Absent baseline variability not accompanied by recurrent decelerations
- Marked baseline variability

Accelerations
- Absence of induced accelerations after fetal stimulation

Periodic or Episodic Decelerations
- Recurrent variable decelerations accompanied by minimal or moderate baseline variability
- Prolonged deceleration ≥2 minutes but <10 minutes
- Recurrent late decelerations with moderate baseline variability
- Variable decelerations with other characteristics, such as slow return to baseline, "overshoots," and "shoulders"

Category III
Category III FHR tracings include either:
- Absent baseline FHR variability and any of the following:
  ▸ Recurrent late decelerations
  ▸ Recurrent variable decelerations
  ▸ Bradycardia
- Sinusoidal pattern

From Macones GA, Hankins GDV, Spong CY, Hauth J, Moore T. The 2008 National Institute of Child Health and Human Development Workshop Report on Electronic Fetal Monitoring: Update on Definitions, Interpretation and Research Guidelines. Obstet Gynecol. September 2008;112(3):661–666.

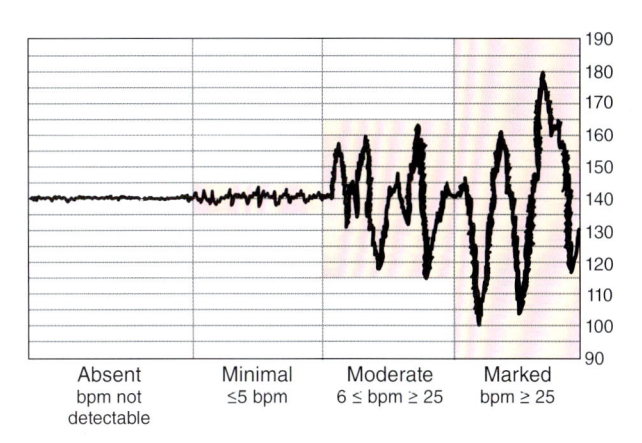

FIGURE 9.10. Fetal heart rate (FHR) variability. *bpm, beats per minute.*

of hypoxia and acidemia. Stimulation of the fetal scalp by digital examination usually causes heart rate acceleration in the normal fetus with an arterial fetal pH > 7.20 if delivery were to occur at the time of measurement. For this reason, fetal scalp stimulation is sometimes used as a test of fetal well-being. External vibration stimulation, also termed **vibroacoustic stimulation**, elicits the same response and is also used for this purpose (see Section "Ancillary Tests").

Decelerations
FHR **decelerations** are visually apparent decreases in FHR from the baseline. They can be either gradual (onset to nadir in 30 seconds or more) or abrupt (onset to nadir in less than 30 seconds). **Early decelerations** are associated with uterine contractions: the nadir of the deceleration occurs at the same time as the peak of the uterine contraction and, thus, is a "mirror image" of the contraction (Fig. 9.11). Early decelerations are the result of pressure on the fetal head from the birth canal, digital examination, or forceps application that causes a reflex response through the vagus nerve with acetylcholine release at the fetal sinoatrial node. This response may be blocked with vagolytic drugs such as atropine. Early FHR decelerations are considered physiologic and are not a cause of concern.

Late FHR decelerations are visually apparent decreases in the FHR from the baseline FHR, associated with uterine contractions. The onset, nadir, and recovery of the deceleration occur, respectively, after the beginning, peak, and end of the contraction. Late decelerations are considered significantly nonreassuring, especially when repetitive and associated with decreased variability. Repetitive late decelerations are defined as occurring after 50% or more of contractions in a 20-minute period. Late decelerations are associated with uteroplacental insufficiency, as a result of either decreased uterine perfusion or decreased placental function, and, thus, with decreased intervillous exchange of oxygen and carbon dioxide and progressive fetal hypoxia and acidemia.

Variable FHR decelerations are abrupt, visually apparent decreases in the FHR below the baseline FHR. These variable

TABLE 9.3 GUIDELINES FOR INTRAPARTUM FETAL MONITORING

	Auscultation		Continuous Electronic Monitoring	
	Low Risk	High Risk	Low Risk	High Risk
Active phase of first stage	Evaluate and record FHR every 30 minutes after a contraction	Evaluate and record FHR every 15 minutes, preferably after a contraction	Evaluate tracing at least every 30 minutes	Evaluate tracing at least every 15 minutes
Second stage	Evaluate and record FHR every 15 minutes	Evaluate and record FHR at least every 5 minutes	Evaluate tracing at least every 15 minutes	Evaluate tracing at least every 5 minutes

FHR, fetal heart rate.

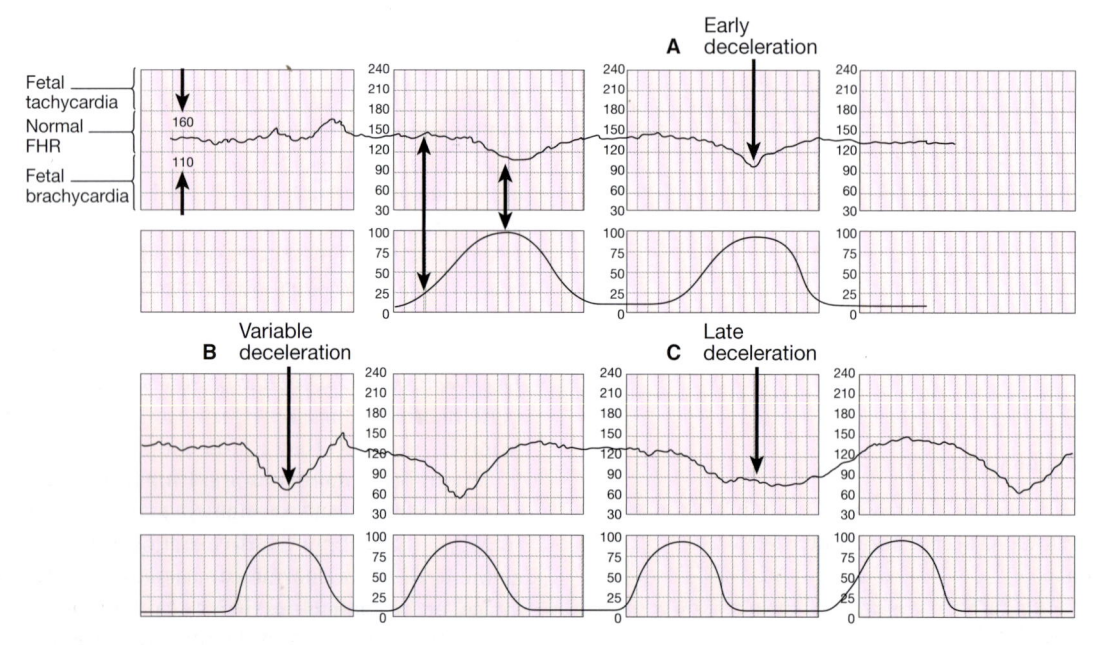

FIGURE 9.11. Fetal heart rate decelerations: (A) Early deceleration. Notice how the nadir of the deceleration occurs at the same time as the peak of the uterine contraction; they are mirror images of each other. (B) Variable deceleration. These decelerations may start before, during, or after a uterine contraction starts. (C) Late deceleration. The onset, nadir, and recovery of the deceleration occur, respectively, after the beginning, peak, and end of the contraction.

decelerations may start before, during, or after uterine contraction starts, hence the term "variable." Variable decelerations are also mediated through the vagus nerve, with sudden and often erratic release of acetylcholine at the fetal sinoatrial node, resulting in their characteristic sharp deceleration slope. They are usually associated with umbilical cord compression, which may result from wrapping of the cord around parts of the fetus, fetal anomalies, or even knots in the umbilical cord. They are also commonly associated with oligohydramnios, in which the buffering space for the umbilical cord created by the amniotic fluid is lost. Variable decelerations are the most common periodic FHR pattern. They are often correctable by changes in the maternal position to relieve pressure on the umbilical cord. Infusion of fluid into the amniotic cavity (**amnioinfusion**) to relieve umbilical cord compression in cases of oligohydramnios or when ROM has occurred has been shown to be effective in decreasing the rate of decelerations and cesarean delivery.

Ancillary Tests

Because the rate of false-positive diagnosis of EFM is high, attempts have been made to find ancillary tests that help confirm a nonreassuring FHR tracing.

Fetal Stimulation

In the case of an EFM tracing with decreased or absent variability without spontaneous accelerations, an effort should be made to elicit one. Four techniques are available to stimulate the fetus: 1) fetal scalp sampling, 2) Allis clamp scalp stimulation, 3) digital scalp stimulation, and 4) vibroacoustic stimulation. Each of the first three techniques involves accessing the fetal scalp through the dilated cervix. In vibroacoustic stimulation, the fetus is stimulated when the device is placed on the maternal abdomen over the area of the fetal head. In digital scalp stimulation, the physician uses his or her finger to gently stroke the scalp.

Each of these tests is a reliable method to exclude acidosis if accelerations are noted after stimulation. Because vibroacoustic stimulation and scalp stimulation are less invasive than the other two methods, they are the preferred methods. When there is an acceleration following stimulation, acidosis is unlikely and labor can continue.

Determination of Fetal Blood pH or Lactate

When a nonreassuring FHR tracing persists without spontaneous or stimulated accelerations, a scalp blood sample for the determination of pH or lactate can be considered (Fig. 9.12). However, the use of scalp pH has decreased, and it may not be available at some tertiary hospitals. Furthermore, the positive predictive value of a low scalp pH to identify a newborn with HIE is only 3%.

Pulse Oximetry

The use of pulse oximetry has been suggested as a modality to reduce the false-positive diagnosis of a nonreassuring FHR. However, research has demonstrated that neither the overall rate of cesarean delivery nor the rate of umbilical arterial pH less than 7 decreased when pulse oximetry was used in association with EFM in cases of nonreassuring fetal status. Because of the uncertain benefit of pulse oximetry and concerns about falsely reassuring fetal oxygenation, use of the fetal pulse oximeter in clinical practice cannot be supported at this time.

Diagnosis and Management of a Persistently Nonreassuring Fetal Heart Rate Pattern

A reassuring FHR pattern (category I) may include a normal baseline rate, moderate FHR variability, persistence of accelerations, and absence of decelerations. Patterns believed to be predictive of current or impending fetal asphyxia (category III) include absence of FHR variability and recurrent late decelerations, recurrent severe variable decelerations, and sustained bradycardia. An indeterminate FHR pattern (category II) is one that falls between these two extremes.

In the presence of an indeterminate (category II) or nonreassuring (category III) FHR pattern, the etiology should be determined, if possible, and an attempt should be made to correct the pattern by addressing the primary problem. If the pattern persists, initial measures include placing the patient in the left lateral position, administering oxygen, correcting maternal hypotension, and discontinuing oxytocin, if appropriate. Where the pattern does not respond to change in position or oxygenation, the use of tocolytic agents has been suggested to abolish uterine contractions and prevent umbilical cord compression. Uterine tachysystole can be identified by evaluating uterine contraction frequency and duration and can be treated with β-adrenergic drugs. Amnioinfusion may also be used to prevent umbilical cord compressions. Awaiting vaginal delivery is appropriate if it has been determined that delivery is imminent. If it is not, and there is evidence of progressive fetal hypoxia and acidosis, cesarean delivery is warranted.

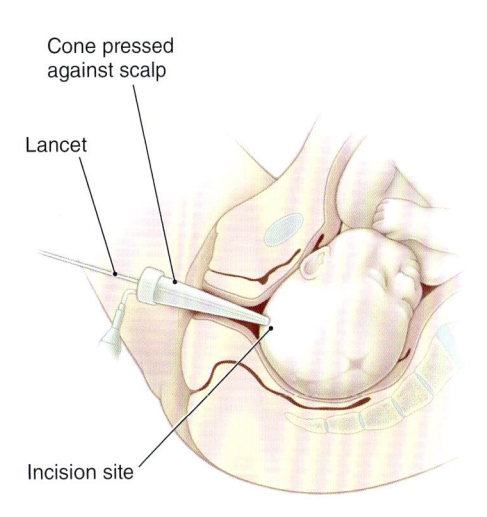

FIGURE 9.12. Fetal scalp sampling.

MECONIUM

Meconium is a thick, black, tarry substance that is present in the fetal intestinal tract. It is composed of amniotic fluid, **lanugo** (the fine hair that covers the fetus), bile, and fetal skin and intestinal cells. The neonate's first stool consists of meconium. However, the fetus may pass the meconium in utero, which is a sign of fetal stress. Meconium passage is detected during labor when the amniotic fluid is stained dark green or black. Meconium-stained amniotic fluid is present in about 10% to 20% of births, and most meconium-stained neonates do not develop problems.

Meconium aspiration syndrome, a condition caused by inhalation of meconium-stained amniotic fluid by the fetus, occurs in about 6% of births in which meconium is present. Severe cases of this syndrome may cause pneumonitis, pneumothorax, and pulmonary artery hypertension.

When there is thick meconium at delivery, interventions to prevent or decrease meconium aspiration syndrome should be considered. *Because meconium passage may predate labor, amnioinfusion should not be used as a preventive measure for meconium aspiration syndrome.* Suctioning of the upper airway on the perineum does not prevent or alter the course of meconium aspiration syndrome. In the presence of meconium-stained amniotic fluid, routine suctioning or intubation is no longer recommended; however, a credentialed neonatal resuscitation team should be available in case endotracheal intubation is needed.

CLINICAL FOLLOW-UP

The fetal heart rate is a category I, and your patient previously delivered an 8-lb infant vaginally. You decide to artificially rupture her membranes, and, if her contractions do not subsequently become adequate, you plan to augment her labor with oxytocin. You evaluate the estimated fetal weight and position of the fetal vertex in the pelvis prior to augmenting her labor.

CHAPTER 10

Immediate Care of the Newborn

This chapter deals primarily with APGO Educational Topic Area:

TOPIC 12 IMMEDIATE CARE OF THE NEWBORN

Students should be able to discuss techniques for care and assessment of the newborn and to recognize more acute situations requiring more immediate intervention or resuscitation. Students should understand the risks and benefits of circumcision.

CLINICAL CASE

You are attending the birth of the much awaited child of a young couple. The father and both sets of grandparents are in the delivery room looking forward with anticipation of the baby boy being handed into his mother's arms. The labor had been unremarkable except for mild meconium staining of the amniotic fluid until the last minutes of the second stage when descent to delivery seemed beyond the expulsive efforts of the exhausted patient, and deep variable decelerations are noted. Prenatal clinical pelvimetry had been judged as gynecoid and normal. The estimated fetal weight was 6 lb, and the vertex was occiput-anterior and just at the level of the perineum. The cervix, of course, was fully dilated and effaced. It was suggested to the parents that a vacuum-assisted vaginal delivery would be prudent, and, with explanation, they gave consent for the operative obstetric procedure.

● INITIAL CARE OF THE WELL NEWBORN

Delivery Room Assessment of the Newborn

In accordance with the American Heart Association (AHA) and the American Academy of Pediatrics (AAP), at least one person skilled in neonatal assessment and resuscitation should be available at every delivery to care for the newborn. Thus, every delivering physician should know the initial assessment, resuscitation, and care of a newborn infant and, if not able to perform all the tasks of resuscitation, should strive to have someone who is proficient in these skills immediately available at delivery.

The preterm newborn has special needs; these complications are discussed in Chapter 15.

Immediately following delivery, the newborn infant should be first assessed to decide whether resuscitation is necessary. Three characteristics define a newborn that requires no additional resuscitation:

1. A full-term infant
2. Spontaneous breathing and crying
3. Good muscle tone

Ballard Scoring System

In an effort to predict which newborns will require more intensive resuscitation, the gestational age should be estimated as accurately as possible before delivery. This allows the appropriate neonatal team to be present and prepared for resuscitation. It is also possible to assess the infant gestational age after delivery using the **Ballard scoring system**. The Ballard scoring system uses a specified set of physical examinations of neuromuscular and physical maturity which, when scored, yields an estimated gestational age (Fig. 10.1).

Apgar Scoring System

The **Apgar scoring system** is commonly used as an objective means to assess the newborn's condition (Table 10.1). Five signs are given scores of 0, 1, or 2, for a total of up to 10. Scores are assigned at 1 and 5 minutes, and at every 5 minutes until 20 minutes thereafter if the 5-minute Apgar score is less than 7. Although these continued assessments are not part of the original Apgar scoring system, many clinicians find them to be of value in evaluating how an infant is responding to resuscitation. In the term and late-preterm infant, a 5-minute Apgar score of 7 to 10 is reassuring; a 5-minute score of 4 to 6 is considered indicative of a mildly to moderately depressed infant; and a 5-minute score of less than 4 is suggestive of a severely depressed infant. The Apgar score should not be used to define **birth asphyxia**, because it is not designed to do so and, indeed, does not provide such information. The term asphyxia should not be loosely used in relation to Apgar scores. This term is well defined and is addressed in Section "Umbilical Cord Blood Gases."

Although a low 1-minute Apgar score identifies the newborn that requires particular attention, it does not predict any

Neuromuscular maturity

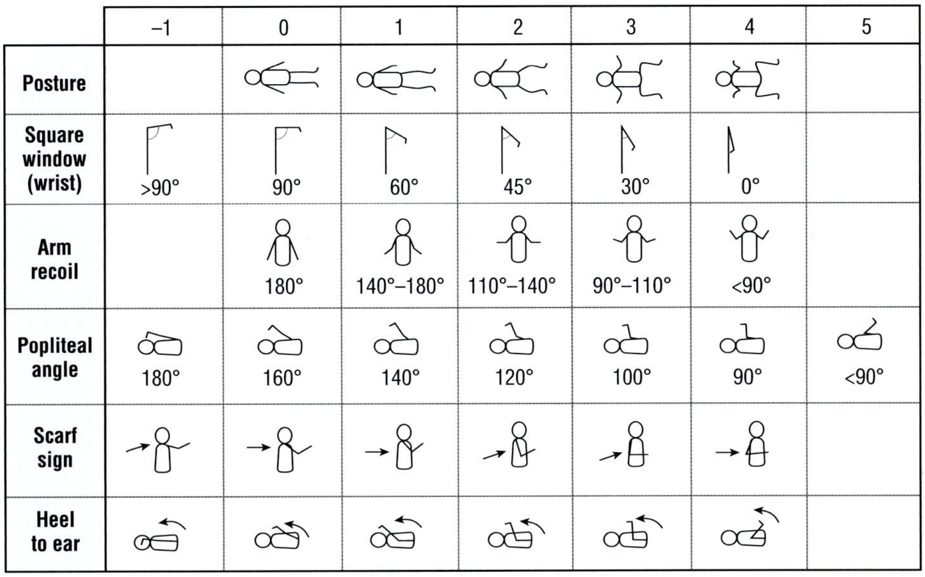

	−1	0	1	2	3	4	5
Posture							
Square window (wrist)	>90°	90°	60°	45°	30°	0°	
Arm recoil		180°	140°–180°	110°–140°	90°–110°	<90°	
Popliteal angle	180°	160°	140°	120°	100°	90°	<90°
Scarf sign							
Heel to ear							

Physical maturity

Skin	Sticky friable, transparent	Gelatinous red, translucent	Smooth pink, visible veins	Superficial peeling or rash or both, few veins	Cracking pale areas, rare veins	Parchment deep cracking, no vessels	Leathery, cracked, wrinkled
Lanugo	None	Sparse	Abundant	Thinning	Bald areas	Mostly bald	
Plantar surface	Heel-toe 40–50 mm: −1 <40 mm: −2	<50 mm, no crease	Faint red marks	Anterior transverse crease only	Creases on anterior 2/3	Creases over entire sole	
Breast	Imperceptible	Barely perceptible	Flat areola—no bud	Stripped areola, 1–2 mm bud	Raised areola, 3–4 mm bud	Full areola, 5–10 mm bud	
Eye/ear	Lids fused loosely (−1) tightly (−2)	Lids open, pinna flat, stays folded	Slightly curved pinna, soft, slow recoil	Well curved pinna, soft but ready recoil	Formed and firm, instant recoil	Thick cartilage, ear stiff	
Genitals male	Scrotum flat, smooth	Scrotum empty, faint rugae	Testes in upper canal rare rugae	Testes descending, few rugae	Testes down, good rugae	Testes pendulous deep rugae	
Genitals female	Clitoris prominent, labia flat	Prominent clitoris, small labia minora	Prominent clitoris, enlarged minora	Majora and minora equally prominent	Majora large, minora small	Majora cover clitoris and minora	

A Measurements

Maturity rating

Score	Weeks
−10	20
−5	22
0	24
5	26
10	28
15	30
20	32
25	34
30	36
35	38
40	40
45	42
50	44

B Scanning to estimate age in weeks

FIGURE 10.1. (A) The Ballard score. The Ballard scoring system uses points assigned to observations about neuromuscular maturity and physical maturity. (B) The points are summed, yielding a score used to arrive at an estimated age in weeks. (*Guidelines for Perinatal Care*. 6th ed. Washington, DC: American College of Obstetricians and Gynecologists; 2007:216–217. Original source: Ballard JL, Khoury JC, Wedig K, Wang L, Eilers-Walsman BL, Lipp R. New Ballard Score expanded to include extremely premature infants. *J Pediatr*. 1991;119(3):417–423.)

TABLE 10.1	APGAR SCORING SYSTEM			
Sign	0	1	2	
Color	Blue or pale	Acrocyanotic	Completely pink	
Heart rate	Absent	<100 bpm	>100 bpm	
Reflex activity response to stimulation	No response	Grimace	Cry or active withdrawal	
Muscle tone	Limp	Some flexion	Active motion	
Respirations	Absent	Weak cry; hypoventilation	Good, crying	

bpm, beats per minute.

individual infant's outcome. The 5-minute Apgar score can be used to evaluate the effectiveness of any resuscitative efforts that have been undertaken or to identify an infant who needs continuing evaluation and management. It too should not be used to predict neurologic outcome in term infants.

Routine Care

Basic routine care is necessary for all newborn infants, regardless of the need for resuscitative efforts. For infants who do not require resuscitation at birth, routine care is performed immediately following delivery. It is important for the delivery team to remember to perform these tasks at a later time for newborns that require resuscitation.

Delayed cord clamping after 30 seconds is generally recommended for both term and preterm infants, although immediate cord clamping may be warranted of certain maternal (e.g., hemorrhage, hemodynamic instability, abnormal placentation) and fetal (e.g., placental circulation not intact, need for immediate resuscitation) conditions. There is insufficient evidence to recommend an approach to cord clamping for infants who require resuscitation at birth. In infants who do not require resuscitation, delayed cord clamping is associated with less intraventricular hemorrhage, higher blood pressure and blood volume, less need for transfusion after birth, and less necrotizing enterocolitis. The only adverse consequence found was a slightly increased level of bilirubin in term infants, associated with more need for phototherapy.

Warming

First, the newborn infant is thoroughly dried to maintain appropriate body temperature. Warm blankets, skin-to-skin contact with the mother, or a radiant warmer can all accomplish this task.

For healthy, vigorous, term neonates, skin-to-skin contact promotes maternal–infant bonding and initiation of breastfeeding in the first hour of life.

Premature infants have more difficulty maintaining their body temperature and are more susceptible to cold stress. These infants require warming pads, heated towels, and a preheated radiant warmer to stay warm. The infant's temperature must be monitored closely because overheating has been described when plastic wrap is used in combination with an exothermic mattress. The goal should be an axillary temperature of approximately 36.5°C (97.7°F).

Umbilical Cord Care

Second, after the **umbilical cord** is clamped and cut, it is left exposed to air to facilitate drying and separation. Local application of antimicrobial agents (e.g., triple-dye, iodophor ointment, and hexachlorophene powder) is common, although it has no advantage over dry umbilical cord care in reducing the incidence of omphalitis in developed countries. However, these agents may reduce neonatal morbidity and mortality in low-resource settings.

The umbilical cord loses its bluish-white appearance within the first 24 hours after delivery. After a few days, the blackened, dried stump sloughs, leaving a granulating wound. If cord blood banking has been requested, the sample should be obtained and stored at the time of delivery. It is important to note that delayed cord clamping will significantly decrease the volume and total nucleated cell counts of cord blood

Vital Signs

Another essential component of routine care is the assessment of vital signs. An infant's temperature, heart and respiratory rate, core and peripheral color, level of alertness, tone, and activity should be monitored at delivery and every 30 minutes thereafter until these measures are stable for at least 2 hours.

Practices to Promote Breastfeeding

Maternity care practices can influence breastfeeding success and the obstetrician is in a unique position to effect changes in postpartum care to positively affect change through encouragement during pregnancy and especially postpartum. Many hospitals are also facilitating breastfeeding success by incorporating the World Health Organization's "Ten Steps to Successful Breastfeeding," an evidence-based set of health care practices that support breastfeeding physiology, including early skin-to-skin care, rooming-in, and feeding on demand (see Box 10.1). Randomized controlled studies have demonstrated that skin-to-skin care in the first hour of life increased the duration of breastfeeding by over 42 days.

Transitional Care

Following the initial assessment and routine care of a healthy neonate, continued close observation is necessary for the subsequent stabilization–transition period (the first 6 to 12 hours after birth) to identify any problems that may arise. The following findings should raise concern and result in closer observation: temperature instability; change in activity, including refusal of feeding; unusual skin coloration; abnormal cardiac or respiratory activity; abdominal distention; bilious vomiting; excessive lethargy or sleeping; delayed or abnormal stools; and delayed voiding.

> **BOX 10.1 Ten Hospital Practices to Encourage and Support Breastfeeding**
>
> 1. Have a written breastfeeding policy that is routinely communicated to all health care staff.
> 2. Train all health care staff in the skills necessary to implement the policy.
> 3. Inform all pregnant women about the benefits and management of breastfeeding.
> 4. Help women initiate breastfeeding within 1 hour of birth.
> 5. Show women how to breastfeed and how to maintain lactation, even if they are separated from their newborns.
> 6. Give newborns no food or drink other than breast milk, unless medically indicated.
> 7. Practice rooming-in – allow mothers and newborns to remain together 24 hours a day.
> 8. Encourage breastfeeding on demand.
> 9. Give no pacifiers or artificial nipples to breastfeeding infants.*
> 10. Foster the establishment of breastfeeding support groups and refer to them on discharge from the hospital or birth center.
>
> Data from Baby-Friendly USA. (2012). The Ten Steps to Successful Breastfeeding. Retrieved from https://www.babyfriendlyusa.org/about-us/baby-friendly-hospital-initiative/the-ten-steps
> * The American Academy of Pediatrics endorsed the UNICEF-WHO Ten Steps to Successful Breastfeeding but does not support a categorical ban on pacifiers because of their role in reducing the risk of sudden infant death syndrome and their analgesic benefit during painful procedures when breastfeeding cannot provide the analgesia.

Antimicrobial ophthalmic prophylaxis is recommended for all neonates soon after delivery but may be delayed until after the initial breastfeeding in the delivery room. Every newborn should also receive a parenteral dose of natural **vitamin K1 oxide** (phytonadione, 0.5–1 mg) following delivery to prevent vitamin K–dependent hemorrhagic disease of the newborn. This form of administration is efficacious, and no commercial oral vitamin K preparation is approved for use in the United States at this time. This measure also can be delayed for up to 1 hour to allow breastfeeding in the first hour of life.

A newborn infant's voiding pattern and bowel movements should be closely observed within the first 24 hours following birth. Concern about an obstruction or congenital defect of the urinary tract is appropriate if voiding has not occurred within the first day of life. Ninety percent of newborns pass stool within the first 24 hours. A congenital abnormality such as **imperforate anus** should be considered if this does not occur. For the first 2 or 3 days of life, the stool is greenish brown and tar-like in consistency. With the ingestion of milk, the stool becomes yellow in color and semisolid.

Jaundice

Jaundice, which occurs in most newborns, is usually benign, but because of the potential toxicity of bilirubin, all newborns should be assessed prior to hospital discharge to identify those at high risk for severe **hyperbilirubinemia**. Two methods of assessment can be used: 1) predischarge measurement of total serum bilirubin or transcutaneous bilirubin levels plotted on an hour-specific nomogram to determine the risk of subsequent hyperbilirubinemia and 2) application of clinical risk factors for predicting severe hyperbilirubinemia. Late preterm (34 to 37 weeks of gestation) infants are at higher risk for hyperbilirubinemia than are term infants. Bilirubin-induced neurologic dysfunction (BIND) is the constellation of neurologic sequelae following milder degrees of neonatal hyperbilirubinemia than are seen with kernicterus, which is associated with total serum bilirubin levels greater than 30 mg/dL in term and late preterm infants.

If possible, the cause of the hyperbilirubinemia should be determined. Breastfeeding has a significant effect on unconjugated hyperbilirubinemia (breast milk jaundice and inadequate intake). Jaundice that persists for 2 weeks requires further investigation, including measurement of both total and direct serum bilirubin concentrations. Elevation of the direct serum bilirubin concentration always requires further investigation and possible intervention, which includes phototherapy or exchange transfusion.

INITIAL CARE OF THE ILL NEWBORN

Although most deliveries are uncomplicated, requiring only basic neonatal care, **resuscitation** may be necessary in up to 10% of all deliveries; 1% of these require major resuscitative efforts. The need for these efforts increases in circumstances such as premature birth, low-birthweight infants, prolonged labor, and nonreassuring measures of fetal well-being. Not all deliveries occur in a setting with intensive pediatric care immediately available. In the absence of such staff and facilities, maternal transport to a facility with a greater capacity to provide appropriate care should be attempted before delivery. Alternatively, the transport of a neonatal team from a tertiary care center to the primary care site is a possible option.

Neonatal Resuscitation

The normal newborn breathes within seconds of delivery and usually has established regular respirations within 1 minute of delivery. If the neonate is having difficulty breathing, ventilation, chest compression, and epinephrine should be instituted,

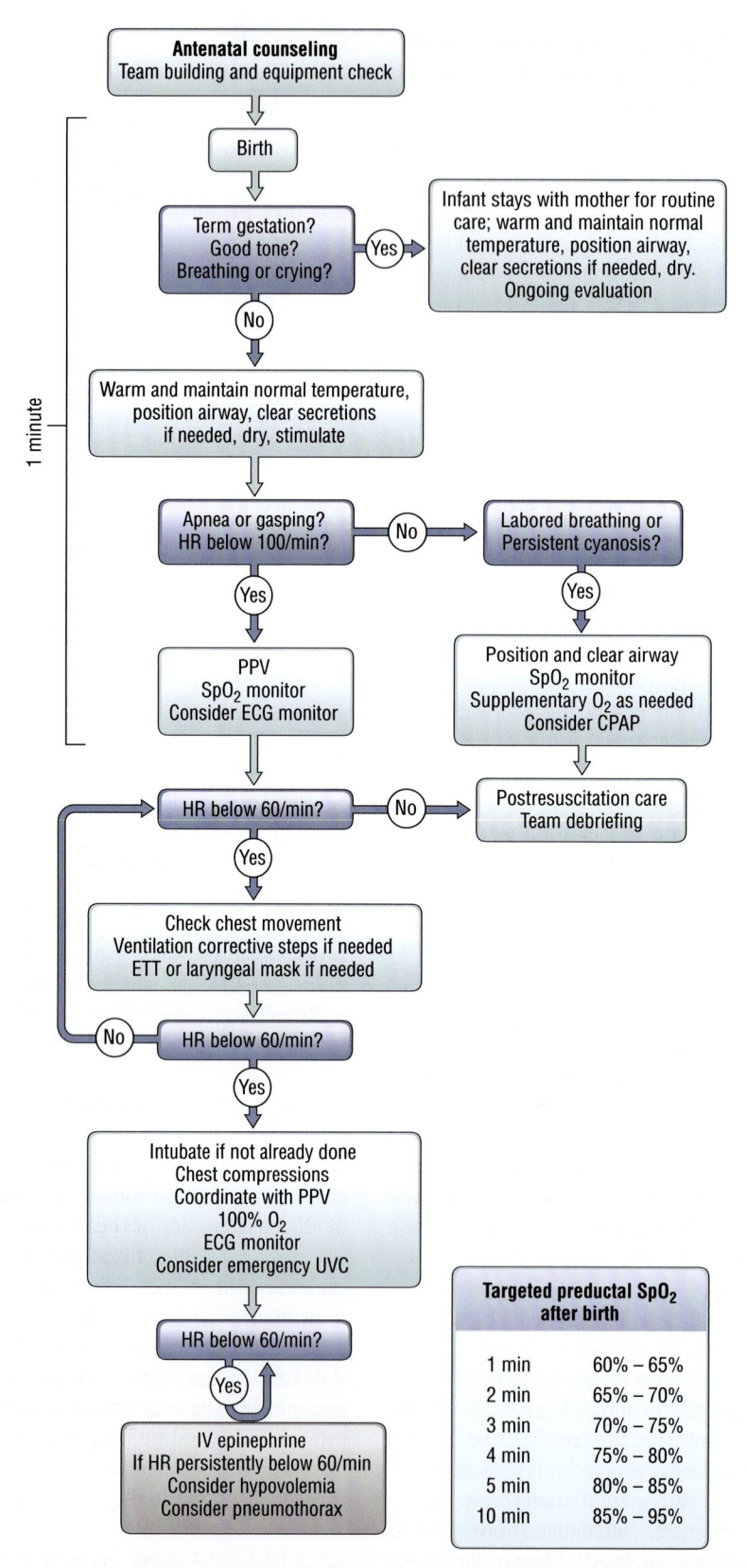

FIGURE 10.2. Algorithm for neonatal resuscitation. Source: Wyckoff, Myra H, Khalid Aziz, Marilyn B Escobedo, Vishal S Kapadia, John Kattwinkel, Jeffrey M Perlman, Wendy M Simon, Gary M Weiner, and Jeanette G Zaichkin. 2015. "Part 13: Neonatal Resuscitation 2015 American Heart Association Guidelines Update for Cardiopulmonary Resuscitation and Emergency Cardiovascular Care." In, 132:S543–60. doi:10.1161/CIR.0000000000000267.

as shown in the protocol in Figure 10.2. If an infant does not respond to epinephrine, hypovolemic shock should be considered, especially if there is evidence of blood loss. In this case, intravenous **normal saline** at 10 mL/kg should be given. A newborn who is apneic or gasping and has a heart rate of less than 100 bpm usually requires positive pressure ventilation, which may be done with a face mask after clearing the airway.

The same principles of adult resuscitation (airway, breathing, and circulation) apply to neonatal resuscitation (Fig. 10.3).

First, the newborn is transported to a radiant warming unit to be thoroughly dried. When drying the infant, it is important to remove wet towels to minimize the effect of evaporation that would otherwise lead to a rapid drop in core body temperature. The nose and oropharynx are suctioned to ensure an open airway as the infant is placed in the supine position. The head should be positioned with the neck slightly extended—the "**sniffing position**"—to allow for maximal air entry. Drying and suctioning, along with providing mild stimulation by rubbing the back or soles of the feet—or flicking the soles of the feet—help to stimulate the infant to breathe and cry.

Respiratory distress may occur as a consequence of situations such as preterm delivery, blockage of the newborn's airway, or maternal narcotic administration during labor. **Narcotic antagonists** such as naloxone are not recommended for initial newborn resuscitation with respiratory depression because of concerns about the possible exposure of the infant to maternal narcotic analgesia and the risk of life-threatening withdrawal in the infant born of a narcotic-addicted mother.

Umbilical Cord Blood Gases

During the resuscitation process, the metabolic well-being of an ill newborn is most accurately assessed using **umbilical cord blood gases.** Cord blood gases should be obtained in cases for which fetal metabolic status is in question, such as cesarean delivery for fetal compromise, a low 5-minute Apgar score, severe growth restriction, abnormal fetal heart rate tracing, maternal thyroid disease, intrapartum fever, and multifetal gestations. A segment of the umbilical cord is double-clamped and cut. Efforts should be made to obtain and analyze the blood sample expeditiously to assess pH, pO_2, pCO_2, HCO_3^-, and base deficit. It should be remembered that, in the fetus, freshly oxygenated blood from the placenta travels to the fetus through the umbilical vein and blood metabolized by the fetus travels back to the placenta through two umbilical arteries. *The most meaningful assessment of metabolic status of the infant at the time of delivery is through analysis of* **umbilical artery blood gases.** Analysis of paired arterial and venous specimens should prevent debate over whether a true arterial specimen was obtained. Therefore, where possible, obtaining both venous and arterial samples (paired specimen) is recommended. Normal values for umbilical arterial and venous samples are given in Table 10.2.

The terms acidemia, acidosis, and asphyxia should be used carefully when applied to the newborn condition, because each term defines a series of changes that may or may not represent true metabolic compromise. A**cidemia** describes the state of low blood pH. A**cidosis** describes the processes leading to these states. However, the terms are often used interchangeably. Acidemia is generally accepted as an increase in hydrogen ion concentration in an umbilical arterial sample resulting in a pH of <7.20. **Fetal asphyxia** is defined as a condition of impaired blood gas exchange leading to progressive hypoxemia and hypercapnia with a significant metabolic acidosis (base deficit ≥12 mmol/L).

Umbilical artery pH and base deficit may provide an index of fetal acid–base status at the time of delivery. A pH less than 7.0–7.1 or a base deficit of 12–16 mmol/L is associated with increased neonatal morbidity and mortality including multisystem organ failure and long-term neurologic disability.

Umbilical Cord Blood Banking

Umbilical cord blood banking is not part of routine obstetric care and is not medically indicated. Because cord blood contains potentially life-saving hematopoietic stem cells, it can be used for possible adult transplant for the correction of inborn errors of metabolism, hematopoietic malignancies, and genetic disorders of the blood and immune system.

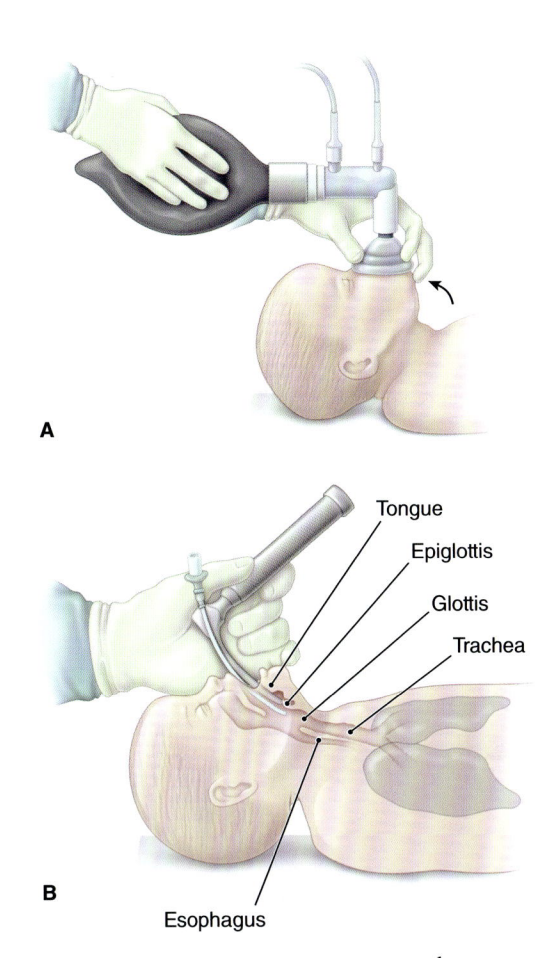

FIGURE 10.3. Airway management in newborn resuscitation. (A) Management with mask and Ambu bag. Most newborns can be safely and effectively managed with a face mask, elevating the chin [1] so that the airway is pulled up and opened [2] into the "sniffing position." (B) Management with endotracheal intubation. Intubation should only be performed by trained personnel to avoid iatrogenic injury.

However, use of one's own stem cells is contraindicated in certain instances. If a patient requests information on umbilical cord banking, balanced and accurate information regarding the advantages and disadvantages of public or private banking should be provided. The remoteness of the chance of an autologous unit of umbilical cord blood being used for a child or a family member (approximately 1 in 2,700 individuals) should also be disclosed.

TABLE 10.2	NORMAL UMBILICAL CORD BLOOD GAS VALUES	
	Arterial	Venous
pH	7.25–7.30	7.30–7.40
pCO_2 (mmHg)	50	40
pO_2 (mmHg)	20	30
HCO_3^- (mEq/hours)	25	20

Male Circumcision

Circumcision is the surgical removal of a distal portion of the foreskin of the penis, exposing the underlying glans penis. It is usually performed within the first 2 days of life on healthy male term infants using a variety of instruments specific to the surgery (Fig. 10.4). Local anesthesia should always be used for circumcision, for example, by ring block or by dorsal penile block (Fig. 10.5). Complications from circumcision are rare and include local infection and bleeding.

Male circumcision is an elective procedure usually performed for cultural or religious reasons. It is estimated that 1.2 million newborn males are circumcised annually in the United States. In some communities, the pediatrician performs the procedure, whereas in others, it is under the purview of the obstetrician. In a policy statement published in 2012, the American Academy of Pediatrics states that evidence shows that the health benefits of circumcision outweigh its risks. These benefits include a decrease in urinary tract infections, especially in newborns; a decrease in cancer of the penis; and lower risk of transmission of sexually transmitted infections, including

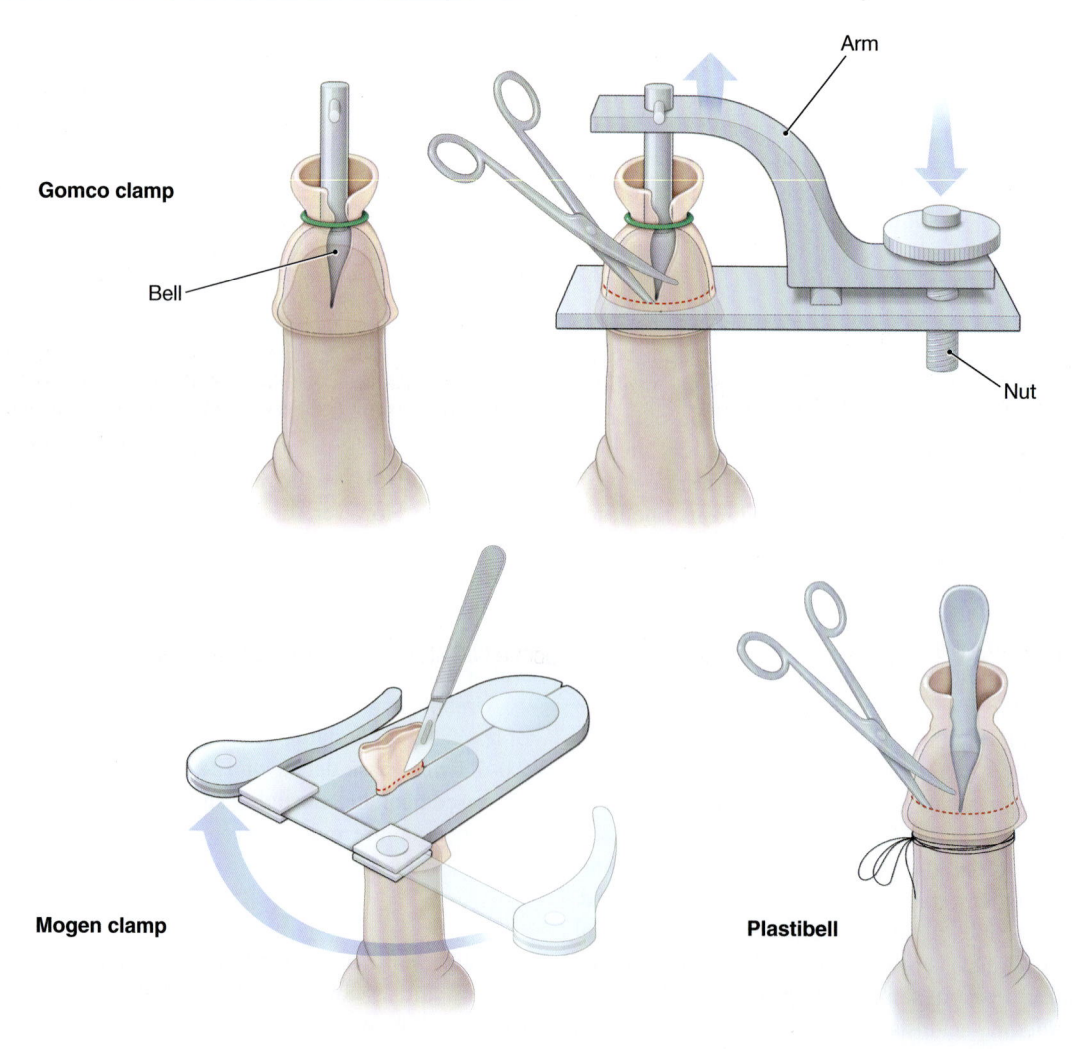

FIGURE 10.4. Instruments used for circumcision include the Gomco clamp, Plastibell, and Mogen clamp. Local anesthesia is requisite from, for example, a dorsal penile block.

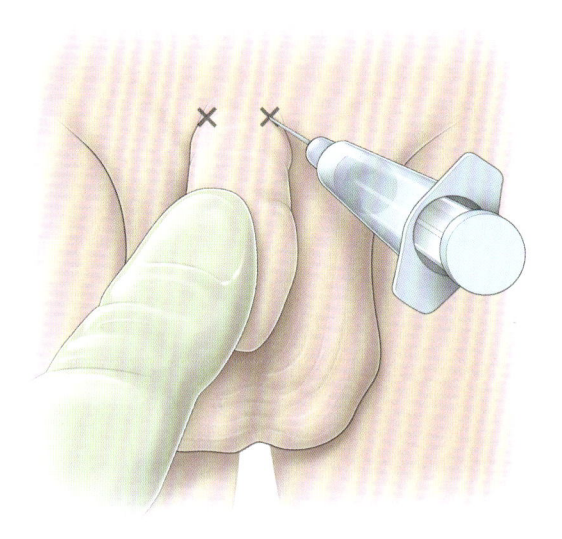

FIGURE 10.5. Dorsal block local anesthesia for circumcision.

human papillomavirus and human immunodeficiency virus. Because male circumcision is an entirely elective procedure, parents should be given accurate and impartial information about the procedure and its complications as well as the controversy over potential benefits. Parents should be allowed to ask questions and should be given full and complete answers prior to providing informed consent for the performance of the procedure. If the family decides against circumcision, gentle washing of the genital area while bathing is sufficient for normal hygiene of the uncircumcised penis, and the foreskin should not be forcibly retracted. This discussion is an excellent example of how the power of empathic communication enhances patient–physician communication and the quality of shared decision making.

Newborn Screening

Newborn screening programs, which are mandated programs that should be available to all newborns, include tests designed to detect infants with specific conditions who may benefit from early diagnosis and treatment. These conditions include disorders of metabolism, endocrinopathies, hemoglobinopathies, hearing loss, and cystic fibrosis. The tests may also identify parents who are carriers of inherited conditions.

To obtain a sample for testing, heelstick-derived blood is collected and placed onto filter paper. Newborn screening specimens are ideally collected between 24 and 48 hours of age. If the initial sample is collected before 24 hours after delivery, a second sample should be collected at 10 to 14 days of age to decrease the probability that phenylketonuria and other disorders with metabolite accumulation are missed as a result of early testing.

Each state has a system in place for notification, timely follow-up, and evaluation of any infant with a positive screening result. Positive results are usually reported to the newborn's primary care provider who in turn contact the parents.

CLINICAL FOLLOW-UP

A soft plastic vacuum extractor was easily applied at the first attempt. Traction assistance was provided with each maternal contraction (occurring about every 2½ minutes), with delivery of the head on the third expulsive effort followed rapidly by completion of the delivery. At this time, a true knot was noted in the umbilical cord, and examination of the newborn revealed acrocyanosis, a heart rate of 80 bpm, limp muscle tone with absent reflex responsiveness, and a weak cry. The planned "handoff" to the new mother was replaced by immediate full neonatal resuscitation. These findings were consistent with a 1-minute Apgar score of 4. There was a rapid positive response with Apgar scores of 8 and 9 at 5 and 10 minutes, respectively, the incident attributed to the tightening of an unknown true umbilical knot during the vacuum-assisted vaginal birth.

thePoint® Visit http://thePoint.lww.com/activate for an interactive USMLE-style question bank and more!

CHAPTER 11
Postpartum Care

This chapter deals primarily with APGO Educational Topic Areas:

TOPIC 13 POSTPARTUM CARE
TOPIC 14 LACTATION
TOPIC 29 ANXIETY AND DEPRESSION

Students should be able to list the normal anatomic and physiologic changes in the postpartum period and describe the key components of routine postpartum care including patient counseling regarding contraception, breastfeeding, and perinatal mood disorders. They should be able to outline a basic approach for evaluation and management of common breast complaints in the breastfeeding patient and be able to describe common challenges and barriers to breastfeeding as well as benefits of breastfeeding. They should be able to perform medication reconciliation for breastfeeding patients. They should be able to identify risk factors for perinatal mood disorders and outline a basic approach to their evaluation and management.

CLINICAL CASE

Following a normal term pregnancy and spontaneous vaginal delivery, your new mother elects to breastfeed after an explanation of the benefits of breastfeeding for the baby as well as herself. She experiences moderately heavy, bloody vaginal discharge for the first 2 postpartum days and, during the next 3 days, progressively lighter bleeding to cessation of bleeding. She returns to your office at 3 weeks, however, complaining of a whitish non–foul-smelling vaginal discharge. She is concerned that she may have a postpartum infection although she has no fever, chills, or discomfort.

● INTRODUCTION

The **puerperium** is the 6- to 8-week period following birth during which the reproductive tract returns to the nonpregnant state. Some of the physiologic changes of pregnancy have returned to normal within 1 to 2 weeks postpartum. An initial comprehensive postpartum examination should be completed within 6 weeks after delivery, although earlier follow-up is recommended for high risk women. Patients with hypertension, perinatal depression, cesarean or perineal wound infections or other conditions may warrant follow-up as early as 72 hours postpartum and again 7 to 10 days postpartum as indicated.

● PHYSIOLOGY OF THE PUERPERIUM

Involution of the Uterus

The uterus weighs approximately 1,000 g and has a volume of 5,000 mL immediately after delivery, compared with its nonpregnant weight of approximately 70 g and capacity of 5 mL. Immediately after delivery, the fundus of the uterus is easily palpable halfway between the pubic symphysis and the umbilicus.

The immediate reduction in uterine size is a result of delivery of the fetus, placenta, and amniotic fluid. Further uterine involution is caused by autolysis of intracellular myometrial protein, resulting in a decrease in cell size but not in cell number. As a result of these changes, the uterus returns to the pelvis by 2 weeks postpartum and is at its normal size by 6 weeks postpartum. Immediately after birth, uterine hemostasis is maintained by contraction of the smooth muscle of the arterial walls and compression of the vasculature by the uterine musculature.

Lochia

As the myometrial fibers contract, the blood clots from the uterus are expelled, and the thrombi in the large vessels of the placental bed undergo organization. Within the first 3 days, the remaining decidua differentiates into a superficial layer, which becomes necrotic and sloughs, and a basal layer adjacent to the myometrium, which had contained the fundi of the endometrial glands. This basal layer is the source of the new endometrium.

The subsequent discharge, called **lochia**, is fairly heavy at first and rapidly decreases in amount over the first 2 to 3 days postpartum, although it may last for several weeks. Lochia is classically described as (1) **lochia rubra**, menses-like bleeding in the first several days, consisting mainly of blood and necrotic decidual tissue; (2) **lochia serosa**, a lighter discharge with considerably less blood in the next few days; and (3) **lochia alba**, a whitish discharge that may persist for several weeks. Lochia alba may be misunderstood as illness by some women, requiring explanation and reassurance. In women who breastfeed, the lochia seems to resolve more rapidly, possibly because of a more rapid involution of the uterus caused by uterine contractions associated with breastfeeding. In some patients, there is an increased amount of lochia 1 to 2 weeks after delivery, because the eschar that developed over the site of placental attachment

120

has been sloughed. By the end of the third week postpartum, the endometrium is reestablished in most patients.

Cervix and Vagina

Within several hours of delivery, the cervix has reformed, and by 1 week, it usually admits only one finger (i.e., it is approximately 1 cm in diameter). The round shape of the nulliparous cervix is usually permanently replaced by a transverse, fish mouth–shaped external os, the result of laceration and dilation during delivery. Vulvar and vaginal tissues return to normal over the first several days, although the vaginal epithelium reflects a hypoestrogenic state if the woman breastfeeds, because ovarian function is suppressed during breastfeeding. The muscles of the pelvic floor gradually regain their tone. Vaginal muscle tone may be strengthened by the use of **Kegel exercises**, consisting of repetitive contractions of these muscles.

Return of Ovarian Function

Prolactin levels remain elevated in lactating women, suppressing ovulation, whereas prolactin levels return to normal by 3 weeks postpartum in nonlactating women. The average time to ovulation in nonlactating women is 45 days. Women who breastfeed exclusively may expect amenorrhea for up to 6 months. Estrogen levels fall immediately after delivery in all patients, but begin to rise approximately 2 weeks after delivery if breastfeeding is not initiated. The likelihood of ovulation increases as the frequency and duration of breastfeeding decreases.

Abdominal Wall

Return of the elastic fibers of the skin and the stretched rectus muscles to normal configuration occurs slowly and is aided by exercise. The silvery **striae gravidarum** seen on the skin usually lighten in time. **Diastasis recti**, separation of the rectus muscles and fascia, also usually resolves over time.

Cardiovascular System

Pregnancy-related cardiovascular changes return to normal 2 to 3 weeks after delivery. Immediately postpartum, plasma volume is reduced by approximately 1,000 mL, caused primarily by blood loss at the time of delivery. During the immediate postpartum period, there is also a significant shift of extracellular fluid into the intravascular space. The increased cardiac output seen during pregnancy also persists into the first several hours of the postpartum period. The elevated pulse rate that occurs during pregnancy persists for approximately 1 hour after delivery, but then decreases. These cardiovascular events may contribute to the decompensation that sometimes occurs in the early postpartum period in patients with heart disease. Immediately after delivery, approximately 5 kg of weight is lost as a result of diuresis and the loss of extravascular fluid. Further weight loss varies in rate and amount from patient to patient.

Hematopoietic System

The **leukocytosis** seen during labor persists into the early puerperium for several days, thus minimizing the usefulness of identifying early postpartum infection by laboratory evidence of a mild-to-moderate elevation in the white cell count. There is some degree of autotransfusion.

Renal System

Glomerular filtration rate represents renal function and remains elevated in the first few weeks postpartum, then returns to normal. Therefore, drugs with renal excretion should be given in increased doses during this time. Ureter and renal pelvis dilation regress by 6 to 8 weeks.

There may be considerable edema around the urethra after vaginal delivery, resulting in transitory urinary retention. About 7% of women experience urinary stress incontinence, which usually regresses by 3 months. Urinary incontinence persisting more than 90 days may indicate a need for evaluation for other causes of incontinence.

● MANAGEMENT OF THE IMMEDIATE POSTPARTUM PERIOD

Hospital Stay

In the absence of complications, the postpartum hospital stay ranges from 48 hours after a vaginal delivery to 96 hours after a cesarean delivery, excluding day of delivery. Shortened hospital stays are appropriate when the infant does not require continued hospitalization, both the mother and the obstetric provider desire a shortened hospital stay, and certain criteria are met to ensure the health of the mother and baby such as normal vital signs; normal amount of lochia and color appropriate for the duration of recovery; absence of any abnormal physical, laboratory, or emotional findings; and ability of the mother to perform activities such as walking, eating, drinking, self-care, and care for the newborn.

In addition, the mother should have adequate support in the first few days following discharge and should receive instructions about postpartum activity, exercise, and common postpartum discomforts and relief measures.

During the hospital stay, the focus tends to be on preparation of the mother for newborn care, infant feeding including the special issues involved with breastfeeding, and required newborn laboratory testing. However, one must not forget to initiate discussions about expressing and storing milk in preparation for return to work, postpartum weight retention, sexuality, physical activity, nutrition, contraception, and signs and symptoms of perinatal depression. Any intrapartum complications should be outlined along with the need for follow-up. When patients are discharged early, a home visit or follow-up telephone call by a health-care provider within 48 hours of discharge is recommended. If early discharge of the mother is being considered, there should be communication with the pediatric provider about the safety of early discharge for the infant.

Maternal–Infant Bonding

Shortly after delivery, the parents will likely become totally engrossed in the events surrounding the newborn infant. The mother should have sustained skin-to-skin contact with her infant as soon as possible. Obstetric units should be organized to facilitate these interactions by providing an environment of patient-centered and family-centered care. Nursing staff can observe the interactions between the infant and the new parents and provide additional support or care when necessary.

Postpartum Complications

Infection occurs in approximately 5% of patients and may be evidenced by fever and/or uterine tenderness on palpation. Significant immediate or **primary postpartum hemorrhage** occurs in approximately 4% to 6% of patients (see Chapter 12) and is primarily prevented by the routine administration of uterotonics at the time of delivery. Immediately after the delivery of the placenta, the uterus is palpated bimanually to ascertain that it is firm. Uterine palpation through the abdominal wall is repeated at frequent intervals during the immediate postpartum period to prevent and/or identify uterine atony. Uterine tenderness may also help identify early infection. Perineal pads are applied, and the amount of blood on these pads as well as the patient's pulse and pressure are monitored closely for the first several hours after delivery to detect excessive blood loss.

Bleeding that persists more than 24 hours and up to 12 weeks is called **secondary postpartum hemorrhage** and occurs in less than 1% of cases. The etiology of uterine atony with or without infection may indicate retained products of conception but may also include endometritis or a bleeding disorder. Treatment should focus on the underlying etiology and may include uterotonic agents such as intravenous (IV) oxytocin, ergot derivatives, and prostaglandins as well as antibiotics. Most of these women do not have retained placental tissue; therefore, sharp curettage, which was a standard practice in the past, should be reserved for persistent bleeding or failures of medical management as it may actually worsen the bleeding by traumatizing the implantation site. PPH is covered in detail in Chapter 12.

Some patients will experience an episode of increased vaginal bleeding between days 8 and 14 postpartum, most likely associated with the separation and passage of the placental eschar. This is self-limited and needs no therapy other than reassurance.

Analgesia

Analgesic medication may be necessary to relieve perineal or episiotomy pain and facilitate maternal mobility after vaginal delivery,. This is best addressed by administering the drug on an as-needed basis according to postpartum orders. Most mothers experience considerable pain in the first 24 hours after cesarean delivery. Analgesic techniques include spinal or epidural opiates, patient-controlled epidural or IV analgesia, and potent oral analgesics. Regardless of the route of administration, opioids can cause respiratory depression and decrease intestinal motility. Adequate supervision and monitoring should be ensured for all postpartum patients receiving these drugs.

Ambulation

Postpartum patients should be encouraged to begin ambulation (with assistance as needed) as soon as they feel able to do so. Early ambulation may help avoid urinary retention, puerperal venous thrombosis and pulmonary emboli.

Breast Care

Breast engorgement in women who are not breastfeeding occurs in the first few days postpartum and gradually abates over this period. If the breasts become painful, they should be supported with a well-fitting brassiere. Ice packs and analgesics may also help relieve discomfort. Women who do not wish to breastfeed should be encouraged to avoid nipple stimulation and should be cautioned against continued manual expression of milk.

A plugged duct (**galactocele**) and mastitis may also result in an enlarged, tender breast postpartum (Table 11.1). **Mastitis**, or infection of the breast tissue, most often occurs in lactating women and is characterized by sudden-onset fever and localized pain and swelling. Mastitis is associated with infection by *Staphylococcus aureus*, group A or B streptococci, β *Haemophilus* species, and *Escherichia coli*. Treatment includes continuation of breastfeeding or emptying the breast with a breast pump and the use of appropriate antibiotics. Breast milk remains safe for the full-term, healthy infant; in fact, cessation of breastfeeding will increase engorgement and delay resolution of the infection as well as worsen the pain associated with mastitis.

Breastfeeding is safe when postpartum mastitis occurs. If symptoms continue, however, evaluation for a postpartum **breast abscess** is often indicated. Symptoms of a breast abscess are similar to those of mastitis, but a fluctuant mass is also present. Persistent fever after starting antibiotic therapy for mastitis may also suggest an abscess. Treatment requires surgical drainage of the abscess in addition to antibiotic therapy.

Immunizations

Women who are identified as susceptible to **rubella** or varicella infection should receive the appropriate vaccine before discharge. The **tetanus–diphtheria–acellular pertussis vaccine** should be administered to the mother immediately postpartum if she did not receive it during pregnancy. During the flu season, women who were not vaccinated antepartum should be offered the seasonal flu vaccine before discharge. Breastfeeding is not a contraindication to receiving any of these vaccinations. If the woman is D-negative, is unsensitized, and has given birth to a D-positive or weak-D-positive infant, 300 μg of **anti–immunoglobulin D** should be administered postpartum, ideally within 72 hours of giving birth, even when anti–immunoglobulin D has been administered in the antepartum

TABLE 11.1 DIFFERENTIAL DIAGNOSIS OF AN ENLARGED, TENDER BREAST POSTPARTUM

Finding	Engorgement	Mastitis	Plugged Duct
Onset	Gradual	Sudden	Gradual
Location	Bilateral	Unilateral	Unilateral
Swelling	Generalized	Localized	Localized
Pain	Generalized	Intense, localized	Localized
Systemic symptoms	Feels well	Feels ill	Feels well
Fever	No	Yes	No

period. Note that this dose may be inadequate in circumstances in which there is a potential for greater-than-average fetal-to-maternal hemorrhage, such as placental abruption, placenta previa, intrauterine manipulation, and manual removal of the placenta (see Chapter 23).

Universal immunization with hepatitis B surface antigen (HBsAg1) is recommended for all medically stable newborns weighing more than 2,000 g whose mother is HBsAg negative. If the mother is HBsAg positive, hepatitis B immune globulin (HBIG) and hepatitis B vaccine should be administered to all infants, regardless of birth weight, at different sites within 12 hours of birth. In addition, all newborns receive a full range of screening tests.

Bowel and Bladder Function

It is common for a patient not to have a bowel movement for the first 1 to 2 days after delivery, because they have often not eaten for a long period. Stool softeners may be prescribed, especially if the patient has had an obstetric anal sphincter injury. Although postpartum constipation may be alleviated by stool softener, it may be aggravated by opioid postpartum analgesics.

Hemorrhoids are varicosities of the hemorrhoidal veins. Surgical treatment should not be considered for at least 6 months postpartum to allow for natural involution. Sitz baths, stool softeners, and local preparations are useful, combined with reassurance that resolution is the most common outcome.

Periurethral edema after vaginal delivery may cause transitory urinary retention. Patients' urinary output should be monitored for the first 24 hours after delivery. If catheterization is required more than twice in the first 24 hours, placement of an indwelling catheter for 1 to 2 days is advisable.

Care of the Perineum

During the first 24 hours, perineal pain can be minimized using oral analgesics, topical anesthetic sprays or creams, application of an ice bag to minimize swelling, baths, and rectal suppositories. Local anesthetics, such as witch hazel pads or benzocaine spray, may be beneficial. Beginning 24 hours after delivery, moist heat in the form of a warm sitz bath may reduce local discomfort and promote healing. Severe perineal pain unresponsive to the usual analgesics may signify the development of a **hematoma**, which requires careful examination of the vulva, vagina, and rectum.

Infection of an episiotomy or laceration is rare (<0.1%) and usually is limited to the skin and responsive to broad-spectrum antibiotics. **Dehiscence** (rupture of the incision) is uncommon, with repair individualized on the basis of the nature and extent of the wound.

Contraception

Approximately 15% of non-nursing women are fertile at 6 weeks postpartum; therefore, postpartum care in the hospital should include a discussion of **contraception.** Ideally, the conversation was initiated during pregnancy. Although combined estrogen–progestin oral contraceptives should not be initiated for the first 3 weeks after delivery, progestin-only oral contraceptives may be initiated any time postpartum, including immediately postpartum, regardless of whether the mother is breastfeeding or not. Chapter 26 includes a discussion of immediate postpartum long-acting reversible contraception (LARC) to reduce unintended and short-interval pregnancy by bypassing barriers to interval placement (6-week postpartum visit) of LARC. The contraceptive rod or an intrauterine device may be inserted any time before hospital discharge including in the delivery room. Since 40% of patients do not attend the 6-week postpartum visit, patients should be counseled during pregnancy about the availability of these methods. Those who are interested in LARC but missed the opportunity for immediate postpartum placement should be informed about placement at the time of the 6-week postpartum visit and arrangements should be made to make the devices available at that time.

Postpartum Sterilization

Postpartum sterilization can be performed at the time of cesarean delivery or after a vaginal delivery and should not extend the patient's hospital stay. Ideally, postpartum minilaparotomy is performed before the onset of significant uterine involution but following a full assessment of maternal and neonatal well-being (see Chapter 27). Postpartum minilaparotomy may be performed using local anesthesia with sedation, regional anesthesia, or general anesthesia. However, hysteroscopic techniques are not indicated for sterilization after delivery. Postpartum sterilization requires counseling and informed consent before labor and delivery.

Consent should be obtained during prenatal care, when the patient can make a considered decision, review the risks and benefits of the procedure, and consider alternative contraceptive methods. In all cases of intrapartum or postpartum medical or obstetric complications, the physician should consider postponing sterilization to a later date. The federal and state regulations that address the timing of consent are also important to consider.

Sexual Activity

Coitus may be resumed when the patient is comfortable, after healing of the perineum, and when bleeding has decreased; however, the risks of hemorrhage and infection are minimal at approximately 2 weeks postpartum. Women should be counseled, especially if breastfeeding, that coitus may initially be uncomfortable because of a lack of lubrication due to low estrogen levels, and that the use of exogenous, water-soluble lubrication is helpful. The lactating patient may also be counseled to apply topical estrogen or a lubricant to the vaginal epithelium to minimize the dyspareunia caused by coital trauma to the hypoestrogenic tissue. The female-superior position may be recommended, as the woman is thereby able to control the depth of penile penetration.

Patient Education

Patient education at the time of discharge should not be solely focused on postpartum and contraceptive issues—it is also a good opportunity to reinforce the value and need for health care of both mother and infant. To optimize postpartum care and improve outcomes for women, infants, and families, it is essential that the care team help the patient develop a postpartum care plan, ideally during the antepartum period. Such a plan would clearly identify the care team, establish importance and timing of postpartum visits based on the patient's needs, outline an infant feeding plan, and discuss the patient's reproductive life plan and contraceptive options. Furthermore, it would include an explanation of any pregnancy complications and chronic health problems along with recommended follow-ups, as well as a discussion of the management of mental health issue and other postpartum problems. See Table 11.2.

Weight Loss

Maternal postpartum weight loss can occur at a rate of 2 lb per month without affecting lactation. On average, a woman will retain 2 lb more than her prepregnancy weight at 1 year postpartum. Evidence supports associations between excessive gestational weight gain and postpartum weight retention.

Residual postpartum retention of weight gained during pregnancy that results in obesity is a concern. Special attention to lifestyle, including exercise and eating habits, will help these women return to a normal BMI.

TABLE 11.2 SUGGESTED COMPONENTS OF THE POSTPARTUM CARE PLAN

Element	Components
Care team	Name, phone number, office, or clinic address for each member of care team
Postpartum visits	Time, date, and location for postpartum visit(s); phone number to call to schedule or reschedule appointments
Infant feeding plan	Intended method of infant feeding, resources for community support (e.g., Lactation Warm Lines, Mothers' groups), return-to-work resources
Reproductive life plan	Desired number of children and timing of next pregnancy
Contraceptive plan	Method of contraception, instructions for when to initiate, effectiveness, potential adverse effects, and care team member to contact with questions
Pregnancy complications	Pregnancy complications and recommended follow-up or test results (e.g., glucose screening for gestational diabetes, blood pressure check for gestational hypertension)
Mental health	Management recommendations for women with anxiety, depression, or other psychiatric issues identified during pregnancy or in the postpartum period
Postpartum problems	Recommendations for management of postpartum problems (i.e., pelvic floor exercises for stress urinary incontinence, water-based lubricant for dyspareunia)
Chronic health problems	Treatment plan for ongoing health conditions and the care team member responsible for follow-up

WIC = Special Supplemental Nutrition for Women, Infants, and Children.
Used with permission from Optimizing postpartum care. Committee Opinion No. 666. American College of Obstetricians and Gynecologists. *Obstet Gynecol.* 2016;127:e187–92.

Lactation and Breastfeeding

Because breast milk is the ideal source of nutrition for the neonate, it is recommended that women breastfeed exclusively for the first 6 months and continue breastfeeding for as long as mutually desired. Neonatal benefits of breastfeeding include multiple health, nutritional, immunologic, developmental, psychological, social, economic, and environmental benefits. Breast milk may also reduce the risk of necrotizing enterocolitis in premature infants. Maternal benefits to full or nearly full breastfeeding may include improved maternal–child attachment, and reduced incidence of some hormonally sensitive cancers such as breast cancer, diabetes, hypertension, and heart disease.

Contraindications

There are few contraindications to breastfeeding. Women with HIV should not breastfeed due to the risk of vertical transmission. Women with active, untreated tuberculosis should not have close contact with their infants until they have been treated and are noninfectious; their breast milk may be expressed and given to the infant, except in the rare case of tuberculosis mastitis. Mothers undergoing chemotherapy, receiving antimetabolites, or who have received radioactive materials should not breastfeed until the breast milk has been cleared of these substances. Infants with galactosemia should not be breastfed due to their sensitivity to lactose. While breastfeeding should be encouraged in women who are stable on their opioid agonists, mothers who use illegal drugs should not breastfeed their infants.

Drugs in the breast milk are a common concern for the breastfeeding mother. Less than 1% of the total dosage of any medication appears in breast milk. This should be considered when any medication is prescribed by a physician or when any over-the-counter medications are contemplated by the patient. Specific medications that would contraindicate breastfeeding include lithium carbonate, tetracycline, bromocriptine, methotrexate, and any radioactive substance. All substances of misuse are included as well, such as amphetamine, cocaine, heroin, marijuana, and phencyclidine.

Prolactin Release

At the time of delivery, the decrease in estrogen levels and other placental hormones is a major factor in removing the inhibition of the action of prolactin. Also, suckling by the infant stimulates release of oxytocin from the neurohypophysis. The increased levels of oxytocin in the blood result in contraction of the myoepithelial cells and emptying of the alveolar lumen of the breast. The oxytocin also increases uterine contractions, thereby accelerating involution of the postpartum uterus. Prolactin release is also stimulated by suckling, with resultant secretion of fatty acids, lactose, and casein. **Colostrum** is produced in the first 5 days postpartum and is slowly replaced by maternal milk. Colostrum contains more minerals and protein but less fat and sugar than maternal milk, although it does contain large fat globules, the so-called *colostrum corpuscles*, which are probably epithelial cells that have undergone fatty degeneration. Colostrum also contains immunoglobulin A, which may offer the newborn some protection from enteric pathogens. Subsequently, on approximately the third to sixth day postpartum, milk is produced. Thus, colostrum is steadily replaced by milk around the fifth postpartum day, providing some nutrition as well as helping the newborn with immunologic response to enteric pathogens. To maintain breastfeeding, the alveolar lumen must be emptied on a regular basis.

For milk to be produced on an ongoing basis, there must be adequate insulin, cortisol, and thyroid hormone as well as adequate nutrients and fluids in the mother's diet. The minimal caloric requirement for adequate milk production in a woman of average size is 1,800 kcal/day. In general, an additional 500 kcal of energy daily is recommended throughout lactation.

Vitamin K may be administered to the infant to prevent hemorrhagic disease of the newborn (see Chapter 10). A vitamin-mineral supplement is not routinely needed but mothers at nutritional risk may benefit from a multivitamin supplement with calcium, Vitamin b12 and Vitamin D.

Lactational Amenorrhea

The natural contraceptive effect of exclusive breastfeeding (elevated prolactin levels and associated anovulation) may be used to advantage in what is known as the **lactational amenorrhea** method. Note that breastfeeding will only prevent ovulation in the woman who is fully or nearly fully breastfeeding and there is continued amenorrhea. Therefore, relying on breastfeeding as a contraceptive method is not recommended. Regardless if the mother is exclusively breastfeeding or not, it is prudent to counsel the mother on additional methods of contraception (see Chapter 26).

Nipple Care

Nipple care is also important during breastfeeding. The nipples should be washed with water and exposed to air for 15 to 20 minutes after each feeding. A water-based cream such as lanolin or A and D ointment may be applied if the nipples are tender. Fissuring of the nipple may make breastfeeding extremely difficult. Temporary cessation of breastfeeding, manual expression of milk, and use of a nipple shield will aid in recovery.

PERINATAL DEPRESSION

Although pregnancy and childbirth are usually joyous times, depression is actually common in the postpartum period affecting one in seven women. Clinicians should screen women for depression and anxiety symptoms using a standardized, validated tool at least one during the perinatal period. Women with current anxiety or depression, a history of mood disorders or risk factors for perinatal mood disorders as outlined in Box 11.1 should be closely monitored.

Perinatal depression often goes unrecognized since the signs and symptoms can often be attributed to the normal changes of pregnancy and the postpartum period. Anxiety and insomnia are very common symptom of perinatal mood disorders and it may be beneficial to inquire about intrusive, frightening thoughts and about inability to sleep even when the infant is resting. The use of screening questionnaires that have been

> **BOX 11.1** Risk Factors for Perinatal Depression

Depression during Pregnancy
- Maternal anxiety
- History of depression
- Life stress
- Lack of support system
- Unintended pregnancy
- Medicaid insurance
- Domestic violence
- Lower income
- Lower education
- Smoking
- Single status
- Poor relationship quality

Postpartum Depression
- Depression during pregnancy
- Anxiety during pregnancy
- Experiencing stressful life events during pregnancy
- Experiencing stressful life events in the early postpartum period
- Traumatic birth experience
- Preterm birth/infant admission to neonatal intensive care
- Low levels of social support
- Previous history of depression
- Breastfeeding problems

validated for pregnancy cannot be overemphasized. The 10 question Edinburgh Postpartum Depression Scale takes less than 5 minutes to complete. In addition, it includes anxiety symptoms, but excludes constitutional symptoms that are common in pregnancy that may otherwise reduce its specificity.

Screening by itself is not enough to improve clinical outcomes. The clinician must include follow-up and treatment where indicated along with appropriate referrals.

THE POSTPARTUM VISIT

At the time of the postpartum visit(s), the Postpartum Care Plan should be reviewed with inquiries into the birth experience, the status of breastfeeding or infant feeding, return of menstruation, resumption of coital activity, use of contraception, interaction of the newborn with the family, and resumption of other physical activities such as return to work. The patient should be provided instructions for pelvic muscle exercise/kegel, milk expression, weight retention, birth spacing, exercise, nutrition as indicated. Efforts should be made to facilitate the placement of long acting reversible contraception in patients who expressed an interest while in hospital. Patients should be reminded about pregnancy complications that may affect their future health or complicate subsequent pregnancies. Follow-up glucose screening and cardiometabolic risks should be discussed with patients with gestational diabetes or hypertension. Observation about and appropriate questions concerning sadness and depression, anxiety, the parents' concerns about infant care, and the relationship of mother and her partner are also part of the first postpartum visit. A validated instrument such as the Edinburgh Postnatal Depression Scale (http://www.fresno.ucsf.edu/pediatrics/downloads/edinburghscale.pdf) may be useful. Screening by itself is insufficient to improve clinical outcomes. It must be coupled with appropriate follow-up and treatment when indicated.

CLINICAL FOLLOW-UP

No infection is discovered on pelvic examination with wet preparation, and you are confident to reassure the new mother that she has experienced a normal lochia rubra and then lochia serosa (explaining each kind of normal lochia), and that she is now experiencing lochia alba. You explain that this may persist as long as a few weeks and is simply a longer expression of the end of a normal birth process. She is reasonably reassured but more so when the lochia alba ceases in the following week.

CHAPTER 12
Postpartum Hemorrhage

This chapter deals primarily with APGO Educational Topic Area:

TOPIC 27   POSTPARTUM HEMORRHAGE

Students should be able to list the risk factors for postpartum hemorrhage (PPH) and to outline a basic approach to evaluation and management of immediate and delayed PPH.

CLINICAL CASE

After a prolonged labor, a 22-year-old patient delivers her second child at term. Her infant is healthy, with good Apgar scores. Soon after her delivery, and before the placental expulsion occurs, sudden, profuse hemorrhage is noted.

INTRODUCTION

It is estimated that, worldwide, 140,000 women die of **postpartum hemorrhage** (**PPH**) each year—one every 4 minutes. More than half of all maternal deaths occur within 24 hours of delivery. In addition to death, serious morbidity may follow PPH. Sequelae include adult respiratory distress syndrome, coagulopathy, shock, loss of fertility, and pituitary necrosis (Sheehan syndrome).

The prevalence of PPH is about 4%. It can be sudden and profuse, or blood loss can occur more insidiously. PPH has been traditionally defined as a delivery-associated blood loss in excess of 500 mL for vaginal delivery and 1,000 mL for cesarean birth; however, these estimates actually represent the average blood loss for each mode of delivery, respectively. The estimation of blood loss is subjective, introducing wide variance and inaccuracy.

Additionally, the same absolute volume loss for a patient weighing 50 kg may have vastly different effects than it would for someone weighing 75 kg or for a patient with triplets versus a singleton. Thus, it is likely more appropriate and meaningful to use physiologic and objective criteria in defining clinical hemorrhage. Criteria in use include a 10% drop in hematocrit, need for transfusion, and signs and symptoms along the spectrum of physiologic effects of blood loss, described below. More recently, the ACOG Revitalize program has recommended a single definition of PPH regardless of route of delivery: a cumulative blood loss of ≥1000 mL or blood loss accompanied by signs and symptoms of hypovolemia within 24 hours following delivery.

For descriptive purposes, PPH is termed "primary" (also called *immediate* or *early*) if it occurs within 24 hours of delivery and "secondary" (*delayed* or *late*) if it occurs between 24 hours and (usually) 12 weeks after delivery. Primary PPH is of much greater importance, insofar as secondary PPH is less common and generally much less serious in nature.

RECOGNITION AND EARLY DETECTION

PPH is not a diagnosis but, rather, a critically important sign that often occurs without warning and in the absence of risk factors. When present, however, these factors warrant heightened awareness about the risk of PPH (Box 12.1). Maternal hemodynamic responses to blood loss should also be monitored, *insofar* as these responses are indicators of well-being, volume deficit, and prognosis. The loss of 10% (500 mL for an

BOX 12.1   **Risk Factors for Postpartum Hemorrhage**

- Prolonged labor
- Augmented labor
- Rapid labor
- History of postpartum hemorrhage
- Episiotomy, especially mediolateral
- Preeclampsia
- Overdistended uterus (macrosomia, multiple gestation, and hydramnios)
- Prior uterine surgery and other risk factors for abnormal placentation
- Operative delivery
- Asian or Hispanic ethnicity
- Chorioamnionitis

average patient with a singleton pregnancy) of blood volume may be tolerated with no signs or symptoms. As blood loss approaches 15% to 20%, the first signs of intravascular depletion manifest, including **tachycardia, tachypnea**, and **delayed capillary refill**, followed by **orthostatic changes** and **narrowed pulse pressure** (due to elevated diastolic pressure secondary to vasoconstriction with maintenance of systolic pressure). Beyond approximately 30% volume loss, breathing and heart rate further increase, and overt hypotension develops. Finally, with profound blood loss above 40% to 50%, oliguria, shock, coma, and death may occur.

The source and etiology of bleeding should be identified as soon as possible, and targeted interventions applied in order to minimize morbidity and prevent mortality. The most common cause of PPH is uterine atony, representing about 80% of cases. Retained placenta, genital tract trauma, lacerations, and coagulation disorders are other causes. Hematomas can occur anywhere in the lower genital tract. Ruptured uterus and inverted uterus are rare but serious causes of PPH.

● GENERAL MANAGEMENT OF PATIENTS

PPH is an unequivocal emergency; all available resources should be mobilized immediately upon its recognition. A general approach to management is outlined in Box 12.2. Because most cases of PPH are caused by **uterine atony**, the uterus should be palpated abdominally, seeking the soft, "boggy" consistency of the relaxed uterus. If this finding is confirmed, oxytocin infusion should be increased and either methylergonovine maleate or prostaglandins administered if excessive bleeding continues.

Other questions that may help direct assessment include the following:

- Was expulsion of the placenta spontaneous and apparently complete? (Think: retained placental fragment?)
- Were forceps or other instrumentation used in delivery? (Think: laceration?)
- Was the baby large or the delivery difficult or precipitous? (Think: uterine atony?)
- Were the cervix and vagina inspected for lacerations?
- What was the admission or baseline hematocrit?
- Is the blood clotting? (Think: coagulopathy?)

While the cause of the hemorrhage is being identified, general supportive measures should be initiated (see Box 12.2). Such measures include large-bore intravenous access; rapid crystalloid infusions; type, cross-match, and administration of blood or blood components as needed; periodic assessment of hematocrit and coagulation profile; and monitoring of urinary output. The judicious use of blood component therapy is key to management. There has been a shift in philosophy regarding transfusion of blood products in the setting of active hemorrhage, with greater willingness to intervene earlier and prevent coagulopathy rather than to delay treatment until coagulopathy is diagnosed. The mainstay of blood replacement therapy is packed red blood cells (PRBCs), with other components used as indicated

BOX 12.2 Management of the Patient with Postpartum Hemorrhage

General Measures
- Evaluate excessive bleeding immediately
- Assess overall patient status
- Notify other members of obstetrics team (i.e., obtain help!)
- Monitor and maintain circulation
  ▸ Establish intravenous (IV) access: two large bore
  ▸ Type and cross-match blood
  ▸ Begin/increase crystalloid infusion
  ▸ Assess for clotting or check coagulation profile
- Review clinical course for probable cause
  ▸ Any difficulty removing placenta?
  ▸ Were forceps used?
  ▸ Other predisposing factors?
- Have operating room (OR) and personnel on standby

Evaluation: Perform in Rapid Succession
- Assess hemodynamic status
- Bimanual examination: assess for atony
  ▸ May palpate for retained placental fragments
  ▸ May palpate uterine wall for rupture
- Inspect perineum, vulva, vagina, and cervix
  ▸ Identify lacerations, hematomas, inversions
  ▸ Recruit assistance for exposure
  ▸ You or assistant may re-inspect placenta
- Assess clotting

Targeted Interventions
Atony
- Immediate bimanual massage
- Administer uterotonics (with requisite precautions)
  ▸ Oxytocin—IV: 10 to 40 units/1 L normal saline or lactated Ringer solution, continuous
  ▸ Methylergonovine—intramuscular (IM): 0.2 mg IM; may repeat in 2 to 4 hours
  ▸ 15-Methyl PGF$_{2\alpha}$—IM 0.25 mg every 15 to 90 minutes for up to 8 doses
  ▸ Dinoprostone—Suppository: rectal; 20 mg every 2 hours
  ▸ Misoprostol—600 to 1,000 μg orally or rectally; one dose
  ▸ Intrauterine tamponade—Bakri balloon, packing

Operative Measures
- Uterine compression sutures
- Sequential arterial ligation or selective arterial embolization
- Hysterectomy

Retained Placenta
- Manual removal; manage atony as above
- Ultrasound assessment/guidance to assure complete removal
- Suction curettage—ideally performed with ultrasound guidance in OR

- Maintain suspicion for accreta—additional intervention required

Genital Tract Lacerations and Hematomas
- Repair lacerations immediately
- Exposure critical—get assistance, move to OR
- No blindly placed sutures
- Packing may be necessary
- Observe stable, asymptomatic hematomas

Coagulopathy
- Appropriate factor replacement
- Identify underlying cause
- Hemorrhage, infection, amniotic fluid embolism, other

for various disorders of the clotting cascade. Depending on the clinical scenario, the use of laboratory measurements to guide transfusion of plasma, cryoprecipitate, and platelets may be reasonable. However, in the setting of severe, ongoing hemorrhage (4 or more units of PRBCs needed over 1 hour or 10 or more units over 12–24 hours), the current recommendation is to transfuse blood products in a 1:1 ratio (i.e., for each unit of PRBCs transfused, 1 unit of fresh frozen plasma and 1 unit of random donor platelets should also be transfused). The recent recommendation to avoid transfusion in stable, asymptomatic hospitalized patients with a hemoglobin >7 to 8 mg/dl does not apply in the setting of postpartum hemorrhage. See Table 12.1 for an outline of blood products and their effects.

The management of PPH is greatly facilitated if patients at high risk are identified and preliminary preparations are made before the bleeding episode. Box 12.3 reviews such preliminary, precautionary measures.

MAJOR CAUSES OF PPH AND THEIR MANAGEMENT

Uterine Atony

Ordinarily, the uterine corpus contracts promptly after delivery of the placenta, constricting the spiral arteries in the newly created placental bed, which prevents excessive bleeding. This muscular contraction, rather than coagulation, prevents excessive bleeding from the placental implantation site. When contraction does not occur as expected, the resulting **uterine atony** leads to PPH.

Conditions that predispose to uterine atony include those in which there is extraordinary enlargement of the uterus (e.g., hydramnios and multiple fetuses), abnormal labor (both precipitous and prolonged or augmented by oxytocin), and conditions that interfere with contraction of the uterus (e.g., uterine leiomyomata and magnesium sulfate). The clinical diagnosis of atony is based largely on the tone of the uterine muscle on palpation. Instead of the normally firm, contracted uterine corpus, a softer, more pliable—often called "boggy"—uterus is found. The cervix is usually open. Frequently, the uterus contracts briefly when massaged, only to become relaxed again when the manipulation ceases. Because hemorrhage can occur in the absence of atony, other etiologies must be sought in the presence of a firm fundus.

Management of Uterine Atony

Management of uterine atony is both preventive and therapeutic. Active management of the third stage of labor (the interval between the delivery of the fetus and delivery of the placenta) has been shown to reduce the incidence of PPH by as much as 70%. The protocol for management of the third stage includes oxytocin infusion (usually 20 units in 1 L of normal saline infused at 200 to 500 mL/hour) initiated immediately following delivery of the infant or its anterior shoulder, gentle cord traction, and uterine massage. Some physicians do not begin oxytocin infusion until after delivery of the placenta to avoid placental entrapment; however, there is no firm evidence that the rates of entrapment are higher with active management than with other strategies. Immediate breastfeeding may also enhance uterine contractility and, thus, reduce blood loss. In low resource settings, 10 units IM oxytocin may be given if there is no IV access, or 600 μg misoprostol may be given orally if no oxytocin is available.

Once uterine atony is diagnosed, management can be categorized as medical, manipulative, or surgical. Management must be individualized in cases of severe uterine atony, taking

TABLE 12.1 BLOOD COMPONENT THERAPY

Product	Contents	Volume (mL)	Effect
Packed RBCs	RBCs, WBCs, plasma	240	Increase Hct 3%/unit, hemoglobin by 1 g/dL
Platelets	Platelets, RBCs, WBCs, plasma	50	Increase platelet count 5,000–10,000/mm^3 per unit
Fresh frozen plasma	Factors V and VIII, fibrinogen, antithrombin III	250	Increase fibrinogen by 10 mg/dL
Cryoprecipitate	Factors VIII and XIII, fibrinogen, vWF	40	Increase fibrinogen by 10 mg/dL

Hct, hematocrit; RBC, red blood cell; vWF, von Willebrand factor; WBC, white blood cell.

BOX 12.3 Precautionary Measures to Prevent or Minimize Postpartum Hemorrhage

Before Delivery
- Baseline hematocrit
- Blood type and screen (cross-match for very high risk)
- Intravenous access
- Obtain baseline coagulation studies and platelet count, if indicated
- Identify risk factors

In Delivery Room
- Avoid excessive traction on umbilical cord
- Use forceps and vacuum judiciously
- Inspect placenta for complete removal
- Perform digital exploration of uterus (if indicated)
- Active management of the third stage
- Visualize cervix and vagina
- Remove all clots in uterus and vagina before transfer to recovery area

In Recovery Area
- Closely observe patient for excessive bleeding
- Continue uterotonic agents
- Frequently palpate uterus with massage
- Determine vital signs frequently

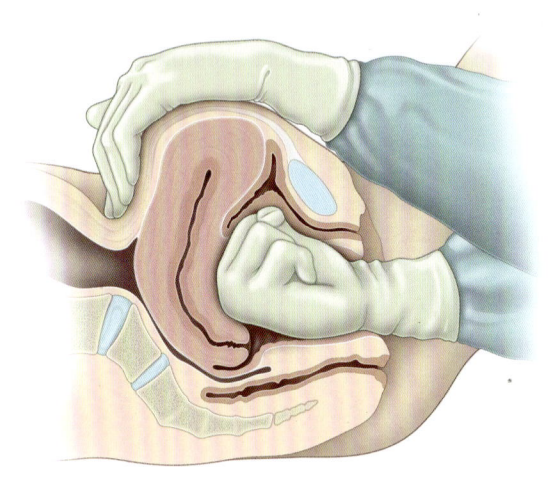

FIGURE 12.1. Management of uterine atony with manual massage. One hand gently compresses the uterus through the abdominal wall. The other is inserted so that the pressure can be placed against the anterior lower uterine segment.

into account the extent of hemorrhage, the overall status of the patient, and her future childbearing desires (see Box 12.2). Bimanual uterine massage alone is often successful in causing uterine contraction, and this should be done while preparations for other treatments are under way (Fig. 12.1).

Uterotonic Agents

Uterotonic agents include oxytocin, methylergonovine maleate, misoprostol (an analogue of prostaglandin E_1), dinoprostone (an analogue of prostaglandin E_2), and 15-methyl prostaglandin $F_{2\alpha}$, administered separately or in combination. **Methylergonovine maleate** is a potent uterotonic agent that can cause uterine contractions within several minutes. It is always given intramuscularly, because rapid intravenous administration can lead to dangerous hypertension, and its use is often avoided in those with hypertensive disorders. Although it should be avoided or used with extreme caution in those with cardiac, pulmonary, liver, or renal diseases, **15-methyl prostaglandin $F_{2\alpha}$** may be given intramuscularly or directly into the myometrium. **Dinoprostone** may be given by rectal suppository. More recently, **misoprostol** has been used for treatment and prevention of PPH. These prostaglandins result in strong uterine contractions. Typically, oxytocin is given prophylactically, as noted previously; if uterine atony occurs, the infusion rate is increased, and additional agents are given sequentially. Uterotonic agents are only effective for uterine atony. If the uterus is firm, the use of these agents is not necessary and other causes of bleeding should be explored.

Occasionally, uterine massage and uterotonic agents are unsuccessful in bringing about adequate uterine contraction, and other measures must be used. Some practitioners use intrauterine compression with in utero packing or placement of a balloon compression device (e.g., Bakri, BT-cath, and Foley catheters) as a means of halting blood loss while preserving the uterus.

Surgical Management

Surgical management of uterine atony may include uterine compression sutures (B-Lynch or multiple squares), sequential arterial ligation (ascending or descending branches of the uterine, utero-ovarian, then internal iliac arteries), selective arterial embolization, and hysterectomy (Fig. 12.2). Very high success rates have been noted with surgical compression techniques, with consequent decreases in the use of hysterectomy and iliac artery ligations, both of which are associated with high rates of morbidity. Additional advantages of compression techniques include rapid execution and preservation of fertility.

As in other clinical circumstances, recombinant factor VIIa is reserved for life-threatening hemorrhage despite virtually all other therapies. Extremely expensive, such therapy also increases the likelihood of subsequent and serious thrombosis.

Lacerations of the Lower Genital Tract

Lacerations of the lower genital tract are far less common than uterine atony as a cause of PPH, but they can be serious and require prompt surgical repair. Predisposing factors include instrumented delivery, manipulative delivery such as a breech extraction, precipitous labor, presentations other than occiput anterior, and macrosomia.

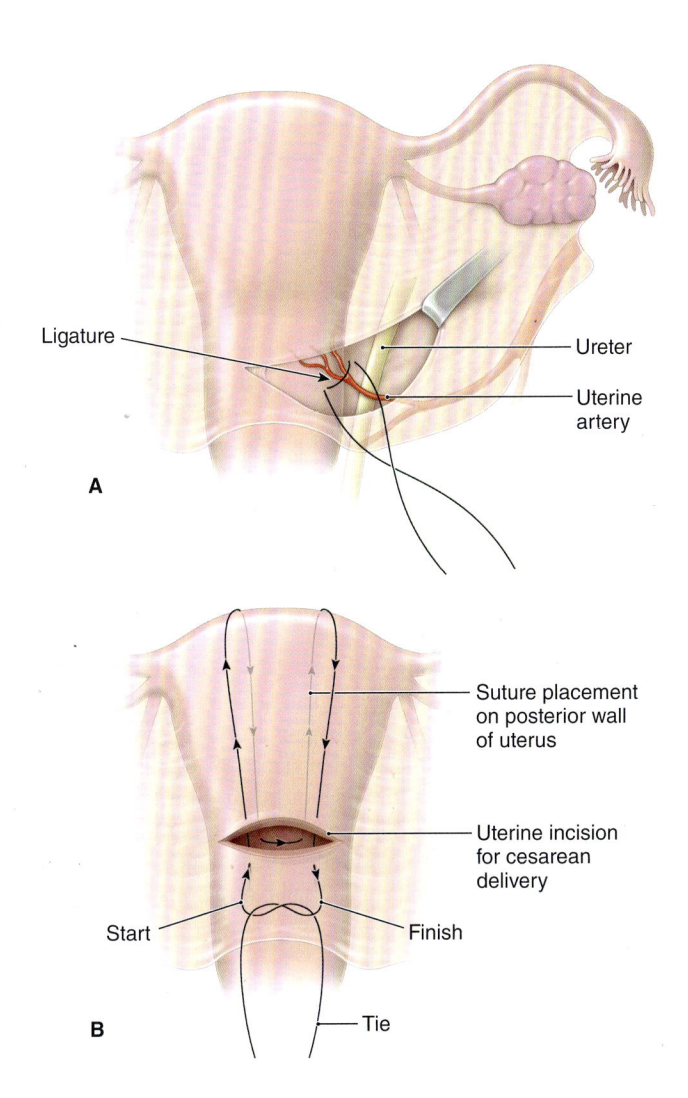

FIGURE 12.2. Surgical treatment of atonic uterine hemorrhage. **(A)** Ligation of the uterine artery. The artery crosses over the ureter and is ligated beyond this point at the uterine corpus. **(B)** "B-Lynch" suture.

Although minor lacerations to the cervix are common in delivery, extensive lacerations and those that are actively bleeding usually require repair. To minimize blood loss caused by significant cervical and vaginal lacerations, all patients with any predisposing factors and any patient in whom blood loss soon after delivery appears to be excessive despite a firm and contracted uterus should have a careful repeat inspection of the lower genital tract. This vaginal examination may require assistance to allow adequate visualization. As a rule, repair of these lacerations is usually not difficult, if adequate exposure is provided.

Lacerations of the vagina and perineum (first-degree through fourth-degree vaginal and periurethral lacerations) are not common causes of substantial blood loss, although the continued steady loss of blood, which may come from deeper lacerations, may become so significant that their timely repair is requisite. Periurethral lacerations may be associated with sufficient edema to occlude the urethra, causing urinary retention; a Foley catheter for 12 to 24 hours usually alleviates this problem.

Retained Placenta

Normally, separation of the placenta from the uterus occurs because of cleavage between the **zona basalis** and the **zona spongiosa** facilitated by uterine contraction. Once separation occurs, expulsion is caused by strong uterine contractions. **Retained placenta** can occur when either the process of separation or the process of expulsion is incomplete. Predisposing factors to retained placenta include a previous cesarean delivery, uterine leiomyomata, prior uterine curettage, and accessory (succenturiate) placental lobe.

Placental tissue remaining in the uterus can prevent adequate contractions, leading to atony and excessive bleeding. After expulsion, every placenta should be inspected to detect missing placental cotyledons, which may remain in the uterus.

Sheared or abruptly ending surface vessels may indicate an accessory, or **succenturiate**, placental lobe. If retained placenta is suspected—either because of apparently absent cotyledons or because of excessive bleeding—it can often be removed by inserting two fingers through the cervix into the uterine cavity and manipulating the retained tissue downward into the vagina. If this is unsuccessful, or if there is uncertainty regarding the cause of hemorrhage, an ultrasound examination of the uterus can be helpful. Curettage with a suction apparatus and/or a large, sharp curette may be used to remove the retained tissue. Care must be exercised to avoid perforation through the uterine fundus. An additional concern is that overly vigorous curettage can lead to **Asherman syndrome**, in which intrauterine adhesions can lead to a variety of complications, including menstrual irregularities, infertility, and future pregnancy loss.

Abnormal Placental Separation

Placental tissue may also remain in the uterus because separation of the placenta from the uterus may not occur normally. At times, placental villi penetrate the uterine wall to varying degrees, collectively called placenta accreta. Risk factors for placenta accreta include placenta previa with and without prior uterine surgery, previous myomectomy, prior cesarean delivery, prior endometrial ablation, Asherman's syndrome, submucous leiomyomata and maternal age greater than 35 years. More specifically, abnormal adherence of the placenta to the superficial lining of the uterus is termed **placenta accreta**, penetration into the uterine muscle itself is called **placenta increta**, and complete invasion through the thickness of the uterine muscle is termed **placenta percreta**. If this abnormal attachment involves the entire placenta, no part of the placenta separates. Much more commonly, however, attachment is not complete, with a portion of the placenta separating and the remainder attached. Major, life-threatening hemorrhage can ensue.

More recently, the term *morbidly adherent placenta* has been used to collectively describe placenta accreta, increta, and percreta. As the rate of cesarean delivery increases in the United States, the number of repeat cesarean deliveries increases as well.

In a large prospective study of cesarean delivery without labor, the rate of morbidly adherent placenta increased with increasing number of cesarean sections; 0.2% with the first cesarean delivery, 0.3% with the second, 0.6% with the third, 2% with the fourth, and almost 7% with six or more cesarean deliveries. If the current pregnancy is complicated by placenta previa, the rate of morbidly adherent placenta is even higher; 3% with the first cesarean section, 11% with the second, 40% with the third, and greater than 60% with four or more cesarean deliveries. See Chapter 16 on Third-Trimester Bleeding for more details on diagnosis and management of placenta previa and the morbidly adherent placenta.

If a portion of the placenta separates and the remainder stays attached, hysterectomy is often required; however, an attempt to separate the placenta by curettage or other means of controlling the bleeding (such as surgical compression or sequential arterial ligation) may be appropriate in trying to avoid a hysterectomy in a woman who desires more children.

Other Causes

Hematomas

Hematomas can occur anywhere from the vulva to the upper vagina as a result of delivery trauma. Hematomas may also develop at the site of episiotomy or perineal laceration. Hematomas may occur without disruption of the vaginal mucosa such as when the fetus or forceps causes shearing of the submucosal tissues without mucosal tearing.

Vulvar or vaginal hematomas are characterized by exquisite pain with or without signs of shock. Hematomas that are ≤5 cm in diameter and are not enlarging can usually be managed expectantly by frequent evaluation of the size of the hematoma and close monitoring of vital signs and urinary output. Application of ice packs can also be helpful. Larger and enlarging hematomas must be managed surgically. If the hematoma is at the site of episiotomy, the sutures should be removed, and a search made for the actual bleeding site, which is then ligated. If it is not at the episiotomy site, the hematoma should be opened at its most dependent portion and drained; the bleeding site identified, if possible; and the site closed with interlocking hemostatic sutures. Often, specific sources of bleeding cannot be identified. If this is the case, surgical management involves "oversewing" the mucosal edges of the vaginal wall with interlocking suture. Drains and vaginal packs are often used to prevent reaccumulation of blood. It should be noted that large amounts of blood can dissect and accumulate along tissue planes, especially into the ischiorectal fossa, precluding easy identification. This may be seen in those with trauma involving the vaginal side walls and sulci. Thus, careful monitoring of hemodynamic status is important in identifying those with occult bleeding.

Coagulation Defects

Virtually, any congenital or acquired abnormality in blood clotting can lead to PPH. Abruptio placentae, amniotic fluid embolism, acute fatty liver, sepsis, and severe preeclampsia are obstetric conditions associated with disseminated intravascular coagulopathy. The treatment of **coagulation disorders** involves correction of the coagulation defect with appropriate factor replacement.

It also should be recalled that profuse hemorrhage itself can lead to coagulopathy, thus creating a vicious cycle of bleeding.

Amniotic Fluid Embolism

Amniotic fluid embolism is a rare, sudden, and sometimes fatal obstetric complication thought to be caused primarily by entry of amniotic fluid into the maternal circulation. Significant biochemical, as well as physical, mediators are thought to be involved in the development of the clinical scenario, which unfolds as five findings that occur in sequence: 1) respiratory distress, 2) cyanosis, 3) cardiovascular collapse, 4) hemorrhage, and 5) coma. Amniotic fluid embolism also often results in severe coagulopathy. Treatment is directed toward total support of the cardiovascular and coagulation systems.

Uterine Inversion

Uterine inversion is a rare condition in which the uterus literally turns inside out, with the top of the uterine fundus extending through the cervix into the vagina and sometimes even past the introitus (Fig. 12.3). Hemorrhage with uterine inversion is characteristically severe and sudden. Treatment includes manual replacement, which frequently requires administration of an agent that causes uterine relaxation (e.g., sublingual nitroglycerin, terbutaline, magnesium sulfate, and halogenated general anesthetics). If manual replacement fails, surgery is required.

Uterine Rupture

Uterine rupture should be distinguished from dehiscence of a low transverse incision, insofar as the clinical connotations are quite different. A **uterine rupture** is a frank opening between the uterine cavity and the abdominal cavity. A **uterine dehiscence**

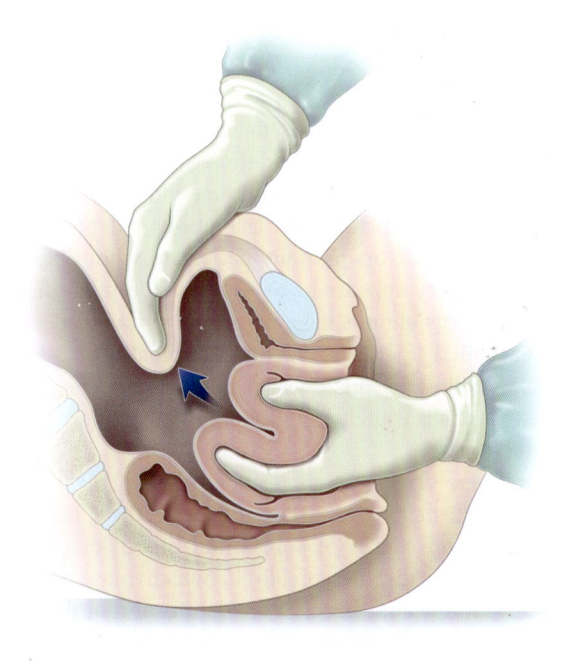

FIGURE 12.3. Manual replacement of an inverted uterus.

is a "window" covered by the visceral peritoneum. Significantly higher rates of maternal and fetal morbidity, and even maternal and fetal mortality, occur in cases of overt rupture.

Rupture can occur at the site of a previous cesarean delivery or other surgical procedure involving the uterine wall—from intrauterine manipulation or trauma, from congenital malformation (e.g., small uterine horn), or spontaneously. Abnormal labor, operative delivery, and placenta accreta can lead to rupture. Surgical repair is required, with the specific approach tailored to reconstruct the uterus, if possible. Care depends on the extent and site of rupture, the patient's current clinical condition, and her desire for future childbearing. Rupture of a previous cesarean delivery scar often can be managed by revision of the edges of the prior incision, followed by primary closure. In addition to the myometrial disruption, consideration must be given to the neighboring structures, such as the broad ligament, parametrial vessels, ureters, and bladder. Regardless of the patient's wishes for the avoidance of hysterectomy, this procedure may be necessary in a life-threatening situation. Careful assessment in the face of maternal hemodynamic changes and monitoring other signs, such as acute abdominal pain, change in abdominal contour, nonreassuring fetal heart patterns, and loss of fetal station, are critical in early detection and intervention in such cases.

● PREVENTION

Several preventive strategies can help curtail the incidence of delivery-associated hemorrhage, and many are quite effective. Active management of the third stage of labor, which involves gentle traction on the umbilical cord with uterine massage to expedite expulsion of the placenta and the administration of a uterotonic agent, has been shown to reduce the incidence of hemorrhage. In addition to preventing many cases of uterine atony, manual removal of the placenta as part of active management of the third stage of labor, will also reduce the incidence of uterine inversion although the risk of postpartum infection is slightly increased. The incidence of retained placenta is not increased with these techniques.

Finally, all obstetric units and practitioners must have the facilities, personnel, and equipment in place to manage PPH properly. Clinical drills to enhance the management of patients with maternal hemorrhage are also helpful. Checklists or algorithms for the management of postpartum hemorrhage posted in the labor and delivery unit and obstetric operating rooms may also be helpful in reducing the negative consequences of suboptimal treatment for or unrecognized postpartum hemorrhage.

CLINICAL FOLLOW-UP

Postpartum hemorrhage is a serious complication seen in obstetrics. Clinicians must have a systematic plan for management. Diagnosis and treatment typically are generally simultaneous. A team approach, involving obstetricians, nurses, and anesthesia, is necessary to minimize morbidity for the patient.

---

thePoint® Visit http://thePoint.lww.com/activate for an interactive USMLE-style question bank and more!

CHAPTER 13
Multifetal Gestation

This chapter deals primarily with APGO Educational Topic Area:

TOPIC 20 MULTIFETAL GESTATION

Students should be able to distinguish different types of multifetal gestation based on embryologic development and ultrasound findings. They should be able to describe the appropriate management and possible complications of multifetal gestation.

CLINICAL CASE

At the time of a gestational dating ultrasound examination at 12 weeks of pregnancy, a twin pregnancy is noted. While initially excited with this news, your patient and her partner have a number of questions and concerns about pregnancy and delivery.

INTRODUCTION

The overall incidence of multiple gestations in the United States is 3.5%, but these pregnancies account for a disproportionate share of perinatal morbidity and mortality. The natural rate of twinning is approximately 1 in 80 and is slightly higher in African Americans than in whites. The incidence of multifetal gestations in the United States has increased dramatically over the past several decades. The multiple birth rate is rising as a result of an increase in maternal age and the more frequent use of assisted reproductive technologies (ARTs) and ovulation induction agents. From 1980 to 2009, the twin birth rate rose 76%; since 2009 there has been a more modest increase of 2% to 3%. The triplet and higher-order birth rate rose 400% from 1980 to 1998. It is estimated that 43% of triplet and higher order gestations result from ART procedures and 38% from ovulation induction; spontaneous conception accounts for the remainder. Although the exact mechanism is not known, monozygotic twinning is also higher in pregnancies conceived using ART. Since 1998, the triplet and higher-order birth rate has decreased by more than 40%, with an average annual decrease of approximately 4%. This decline in triplet and higher-order births is linked to changes in ART procedures and guidelines by the American Society for Reproductive Medicine and the Society for Assisted Reproductive Technology specifically aimed at reducing the risk of higher-order multifetal gestations.

Twin gestations can be characterized as dizygotic (fraternal) or monozygotic (identical). **Dizygotic twins** occur when two separate ova are fertilized by two separate sperms. **Monozygotic twins** result from the division of the fertilized ovum after conception. There is a marked difference in the incidence of twinning in various populations, almost exclusively the result of the incidence of dizygotic twinning. The incidence of monozygotic twinning is fairly constant around the world, at approximately 1 in 250 pregnancies. Increasing maternal age and increasing parity are independent risk factors for dizygotic twinning, and rates are higher among mothers of families with twins.

NATURAL HISTORY

Zygosity refers to the genetic make-up of the pregnancy as described above. *Chorionicity* refers to the placental make-up of the pregnancy. Since dizygotic twins are formed from two separate ova and two separate sperms, they always have two separate placentas (although they can appear "fused" on late-trimester ultrasound if close to each other). The following describes the various developmental sequences and placental compositions possible when the monozygotic conceptus separates into twins (**chorionicity**), as shown in Figure 13.1:

- **Diamnionic/dichorionic**: If division of the conceptus occurs within 3 days of fertilization, each fetus will be surrounded by an amnion and chorion. There may be two separate placentas or one "fused" placenta.
- **Diamnionic/monochorionic**: If division occurs between the fourth and eighth day following fertilization, the chorion has already begun to develop, whereas the amnion has not. Therefore, each fetus will later be surrounded by an amnion, but a single chorion will surround both fetuses.
- **Monoamnionic/monochorionic**: In 1% of monozygotic gestations, division occurs between days 9 and 12, after development of both the amnion and the chorion, and the twins will share a common sac.
- Division thereafter is incomplete, resulting in the development of **conjoined twins**. The fetuses may be fused in a

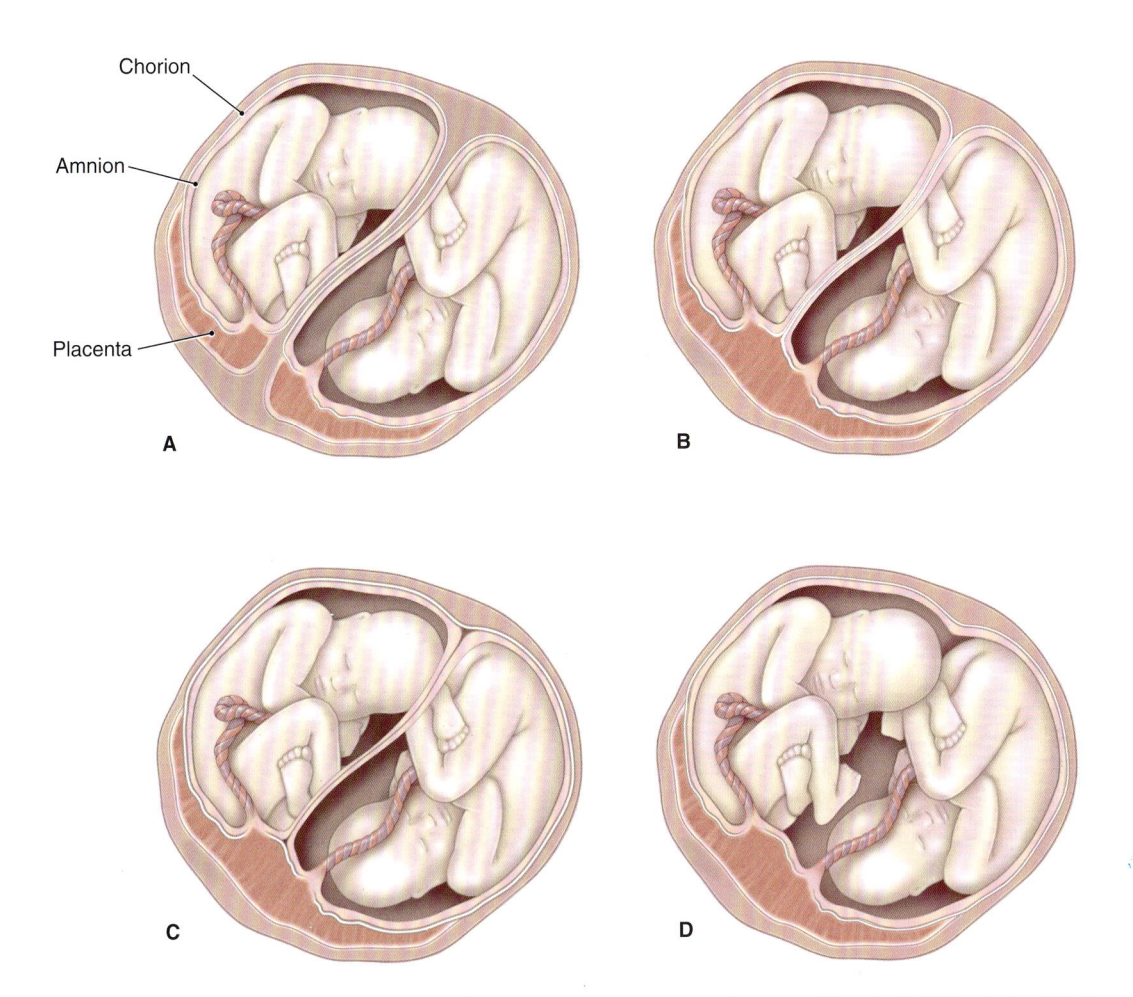

FIGURE 13.1. Chorionicity in twin pregnancies. **(A)** Two placentas, two amnions, two chorions: diamniotic/dichorionic. **(B)** One placenta, two amnions, two chorions: diamniotic/dichorionic. **(C)** One placenta, two amnions, one chorion: diamniotic/monochorionic. **(D)** One placenta, one amnion, one chorion: monoamniotic/monochorionic. (Based on American College of Obstetricians and Gynecologists. Patient Education Pamphlet AP092. Washington, DC: ACOG; 2004.)

number of ways, with the most common involving the chest and/or abdomen. This rare condition is seen in approximately 1 in 70,000 deliveries. This condition is associated with a mortality rate of greater than 50%.

During routine prenatal evaluation, it is not possible to distinguish dizygotic twins of the same gender from diamnionic/dichorionic monozygotic twins. Early determination of chorionicity is very important since the risks associated with monochorionic twins are much higher and must be managed differently from dichorionic twins.

• RISKS OF MULTIFETAL GESTATION

Multifetal pregnancies are associated with increased perinatal morbidity. The most significant cause of neonatal morbidity is preterm labor and delivery. Multifetal gestations are associated with increased risk of fetal and infant morbidity and mortality. There is an approximate fivefold increased risk of stillbirth and a sevenfold increased risk of neonatal death, which primarily is due to complications of prematurity. Women with multifetal gestations are 6 times more likely to give birth preterm and 13 times more likely to give birth before 32 weeks of gestation than women with singleton gestations.

Compared with singleton pregnancies, which are delivered at an average gestational age of 39 weeks, twins are delivered at an average of 35 weeks, triplets at 32 weeks, and quadruplets at an average of 30 weeks. Thus, with each additional fetus, the length of gestation is decreased by approximately 2 to 3 weeks (Table 13.1).

Other associated maternal and fetal/neonatal morbidities include hyperemesis, anemia, intrauterine growth restriction, hydramnios (in approximately 10% of multiple gestations, predominantly monochorionic gestations), preeclampsia (three times more frequent in twin gestations), gestational diabetes mellitus, congenital anomalies, cesarean delivery, postpartum hemorrhage, placental abruption, umbilical cord accidents, and postpartum depression. Both spontaneous abortions and congenital anomalies are approximately twice as common in multiple gestations. Neonatal death and neurodevelopmental impairments including cerebral palsy are also more common in multiple gestations when compared to singletons (Table 13.2).

TABLE 13.1 PREMATURITY AND MULTIFETAL GESTATIONS

Characteristic	Singleton	Twin	Triplets	Quadruplets
Mean birth weight[a]	3296 g	2336 g	1660 g	1291 g
Mean gestational age[a]	38.7 weeks	35.3 weeks	31.9 weeks	29.5 weeks
Percentage <32 weeks gestation[b]	1.2	10.6	39.3	72
Percentage <37 weeks gestation[b]	7.7	58.7	98.4	98

[a] The American College of Obstetricians and Gynecologists. Multifetal gestations: twin, triplet and higher-order multifetal pregnancies. Practice Bulletin No. 169. American College of Obstetricians and Gynecologists. *Obstet Gynecol*. 2016;128:e131–146.
[b] Hamilton BE, Martin JA, Osterman MJK, Curtin SC, Matthews TJ. Births: final data for 2014 *Natl Vital Stat Rep*. 2015;64(12):1–63.

TABLE 13.2 MORBIDITY AND MORTALITY IN MULTIFETAL GESTATIONS

Characteristic	Singleton	Twin	Triplets	Quadruplets
Overall rate of cerebral palsy (per 1000 live births)[a]	1.6	7	28	—
Overall infant mortality rate (per 1000 live births)[a]	5.4	23.6	52.6	96.3[d]
Percentage death before discharge among ELBW infants[b]	25.1	32.1	26.3[c]	—
Percentage neurodevelopmental impairment among ELBW infants[b]	36.1	41.1	39.1[c]	—
Percentage cerebral palsy among ELBW infants[b]	5	6.9	5.6[c]	—

ELBW = extremely low birth weight (401–1000g)
[a] The American College of Obstetricians and Gynecologists. Multifetal gestations: twin, triplet and higher-order multifetal pregnancies. Practice Bulletin No. 169. American College of Obstetricians and Gynecologists. *Obstet Gynecol*. 2016;128:1e131–146.
[b] Wadhawan R, Oh W, Vohr BR, Wrage L, Das A, Bell EF, Laptock AR, Shankaran S, Stoll BJ, Walsh MC, Higgins RD for the Eunice Kennedy Striver NICHD Neonatal Research Network. Neurodevelopmental outcomes of triplets and higher-order extremely low birth weight infants. *Pediatrics* 2011;127:e654–e660.
[c] Triplet and higher-order gestation.
[d] Quadruplet and quintuplet data combined.

Because of the higher rates of multiple gestation, particularly higher-order multiple births (more than two), counseling for infertility treatment should include a discussion of the risks associated with multiple gestation and the option of **multifetal pregnancy reduction**. This procedure is defined as a first-trimester or early second-trimester termination of one or more fetuses in a multifetal gestation, to increase the chances of survival of the remaining fetuses and decrease long-term morbidity for the delivered infants. Of course, the primary approach to this problem is to try to prevent higher-order multiple births. Physicians providing infertility treatment should follow guidelines designed to limit the risk of multiple gestation in the setting of ART or ovulation induction.

Twin-Twin Transfusion Syndrome

As development of a monochorionic gestation progresses, various vascular anastomoses between the fetuses can develop that, in turn, can lead to a condition known as **twin–twin transfusion syndrome (TTTS)**. This condition complicates approximately 10% to 15% of monochorionic-diamniotic pregnancies. Through arteriovenous anastomoses, there is net flow from one twin to another, often with untoward pregnancy outcomes. The so-called *donor twin* can have impaired growth, anemia, hypovolemia, and other problems. The *recipient twin* can develop hypervolemia, hypertension, polycythemia, and congestive heart failure as a result of this preferential transfusion. A secondary manifestation involves amniotic fluid dynamics. The hypervolemia in the recipient twin leads to an increase in urinary output and, in turn, to an increase in amniotic fluid volumes (hydramnios). The opposite effect may occur in the donor twin—hypovolemia leads to decreased urinary output and, possibly, a decrease in amniotic fluid volume (oligohydramnios). Hydramnios in the one twin compounds the risk of preterm labor already present for multifetal pregnancies.

Traditionally, serial removal of amniotic fluid from the sac of the recipient twin has been the only treatment option associated with improved survival. However, endoscopic intrauterine laser ablation of the vascular anastomoses has met with greater success in treating this difficult problem, especially in more severe cases. When available, fetoscopic laser photocoagulation has largely replaced serial amnioreduction as first-line therapy for TTTS. Other vascular abnormalities include the absence of one umbilical artery, which may be associated in 30% of cases with other congenital problems, especially renal agenesis. A single umbilical artery is seen in approximately 3% to 4% of twins, compared with 0.5% to 1% of singletons.

Monoamniotic Twins

In 1% of monozygotic twins, division occurs between 9 and 12 days following fertilization, resulting in both fetuses occupying a single sac composed of inner amnion and outer chorion. The risk of entanglement of the umbilical cords, with subsequent fetal death, is considerable. Traditionally, arbitrary cesarean delivery (after steroids) at approximately 32 weeks of gestation was the usual management. Recent management, involving hospitalization at 24 to 26 weeks, steroid administration, and fetal heart rate monitoring several times daily, has allowed for the prediction of impending difficulty with cord entanglement. Delivery is still recommended early, at 32 to 34 weeks (after steroids), by cesarean delivery. The historic perinatal mortality rate for monoamniotic twins was >50%. Although the optimal management of these complicated pregnancies is not certain, the perinatal mortality rate (excluding pregnancies with congenital anomalies) is now <10% with current management as described above.

Death of One Fetus

Multiple gestations, especially high-order gestations, are at increased risk for losing one or more fetuses remote from delivery. As summarized by the American College of Obstetricians and Gynecologists, no fetal monitoring protocol has been shown to predict most of these losses. Consensus about the preferred antepartum surveillance method and management once demise has occurred has not been reached. Whereas some advocate immediate delivery of the remaining fetus(es), if the death was the result of an abnormality of the fetus itself (i.e., rather than maternal or uteroplacental pathology) and the pregnancy is remote from term, expectant management may be appropriate.

The most difficult cases are those in which the fetal demise occurs in one fetus of a monochorionic twin pair. Because virtually 100% of monochorionic placentas contain vascular anastomoses that link the circulations of the two fetuses, the surviving fetus is at significant risk for sustaining damage caused by the sudden, severe, and prolonged hypotension that occurs at the time of the demise or by embolic phenomena that occur later. By the time the demise is discovered, the greatest harm has most likely already been done, and there may not be any benefit in immediate delivery, especially if the surviving fetus(es) are very preterm and otherwise healthy. In such cases, allowing the pregnancy to continue may provide the most beneficial outcome.

DIAGNOSIS

Most multifetal pregnancies are diagnosed using ultrasound. On a clinical basis, twin pregnancy should be suspected when the uterine size is large for the calculated gestational age. A difference of 4 cm or more between the weeks of gestation and the measured fundal height should prompt evaluation with ultrasound to detect the cause (e.g., inaccurate gestational age, multiple gestation, hydramnios, gestational trophoblastic disease, and pelvic tumor). Serial ultrasound assessments have shown that only 50% of twin pregnancies detected in the first trimester result in the delivery of viable twins. The other 50% of cases deliver a single fetus because of intrauterine demise and ultimate resorption of one embryo/fetus (**vanishing twin syndrome**).

During the first ultrasonographic examination that confirms a twin gestation, chorionicity should be determined because, as mentioned above, the potential morbidity and mortality associated with a monochorionic gestation is different from that of a dichorionic gestation. Chorionicity can be determined by ultrasound with almost 100% certainty as early as 8 to 9 weeks of gestational age. The optimal timing for determination of chorionicity is in the first trimester or early second trimester. Findings that indicate dichorionic twins include the twin peak (or lambda) sign (Fig 13.2), a thick dividing membrane (>2 mm), and discordant genders.

ANTENATAL MANAGEMENT

Once the diagnosis of twin pregnancy has been made, and chorionicity has been assigned, subsequent antenatal care addresses each of the potential concerns for mother and fetus. Although the maternal blood volume is greater with a twin gestation than with a singleton pregnancy, the anticipated blood loss at delivery is likewise also greater. Anemia is more common in these patients, and a balanced diet during pregnancy, which includes increased intake of iron, folate, and other micronutrients, is important.

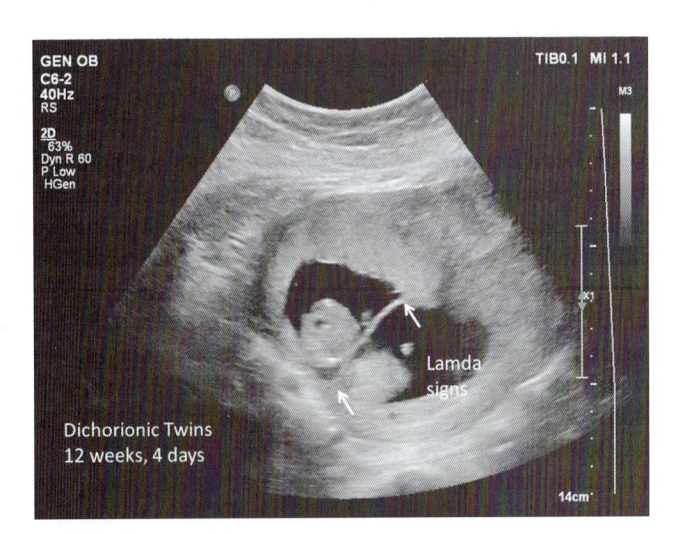

FIGURE 13.2. Twin peak or lambda sign in a dichorionic twin pregnancy at 12 weeks', 4 days' gestation.

TABLE 13.3	BODY MASS INDEX-SPECIFIC WEIGHT GAIN GOALS IN TWINS	
Pre-pregnancy Weight Category	BMI (kg/m^2)*	Recommended Total Weight Gain Range (lb)
Underweight	<18.5	Insufficient data
Normal Weight	18.5–24.9	37–54
Overweight	25–29.9	31–50
Obese (all classes)	30 or greater	25–42

*BMI, body mass index, to calculate BMI go to https://www.nhlbi.nih.gov/health/educational/lose_wt/BMI/bmicalc.htm
From the National Academy of Sciences/Institute of Medicine, Weight Gain During Pregnancy: Reexamining the Guidelines, 2009; 1995 WHO BMI categories (endorsed by NIH/NHLBI, 1998).

The maternal resting energy expenditure (an indicator of basal metabolic rate) is increased in multiple gestations and results in an increased need for caloric intake. Although there are no established nutritional guidelines for mothers carrying twins, the Society for Maternal-Fetal Medicine recommends increased daily caloric consumption based on pre-pregnancy body mass index (BMI): 4000 kcal/day for underweight women (BMI <19.8 kg/m^2), 3000 to 3500 kcal/day for normal weight women (BMI 19.8 to 26 kg/m^2), 3250 kcal/day for overweight women (BMI 26.1 to 29 kg/m^2) and 2700 to 3000 kcal/day for obese women (BMI >29 kg/m^2). The dietary intake should be derived from 20% protein, 40% from low-glycemic index carbohydrates, and 40% from fat. The BMI-specific weight gain recommendations for twins are listed in Table 13.3.

Because of the increased risk of preterm labor in multiple gestations, careful attention to detection of uterine contractions is important, and the patient should be cautioned about signs and symptoms of preterm labor, such as abdominal pain, low back pain, a thin or increase in vaginal discharge, and vaginal bleeding. If there are symptoms of preterm labor, cervical examination should be performed. The use of **transvaginal ultrasound assessment for cervical length screening** in multiple gestations is controversial, largely due to the lack of proven interventions to prevent preterm birth if a short cervix is found. **Cervical cerclage** for short cervix in twins has been associated with an increased risk for preterm birth and is not recommended. **Progesterone** treatment does not appear to reduce the risk for preterm birth in unselected women with twin or triplet gestations and is not recommended. The finding of a short cervix may be an indication for work or activity modification (not complete bed rest). There are ongoing studies of **pessary** placement to reduce the risk of preterm birth in women with twins and a short cervix. Based on available evidence, the use of prophylactic cervical pessary is not recommended in multifetal pregnancies. There is no role for the **prophylactic administration of tocolytics** in women with multifetal gestations, including the prolonged use of betamimetics for this indication. Likewise, in women with uncomplicated multifetal pregnancies, there is no evidence of benefit with routine bed rest with or without hospitalization; this is not recommended and may be associated with harm including increased risk of thrombosis and deconditioning.

Although assessment of **fetal fibronectin** may aid in predicting preterm delivery in women, it has limited predictive value and is not recommended in multifetal gestations. At each visit, blood pressure should be evaluated, and, if elevated, urine protein should be assessed. Beginning at 30 to 32 weeks, daily fetal kick counts are usually begun to help assess fetal well-being.

ULTRASONOGRAPHY

With dichorionic twin gestations, there are no evidence-based recommendations regarding the frequency of fetal growth scans after 20 weeks of gestation. However, it is reasonable to perform periodic ultrasonographic examination every 4 to 6 weeks after 20 weeks. If there is evidence of fetal growth restriction or other pregnancy complications, the frequency should be increased appropriately. Due to the increased risk for the complication of TTTS, monochorionic pregnancies should be monitored earlier and more frequently (every 2 weeks from 16 to 28 weeks, if normal growth and no evidence TTTS, every 3 to 4 weeks thereafter). At the initial evaluation, special attention is given to identification of fetal anomalies, and this is especially so in monochorionic gestations, among which such abnormalities are more frequently seen. A careful ultrasound examination to identify fetal anomalies is performed at 16 to 20 weeks, at which time fetal size permits such diagnoses. At each subsequent examination, growth of each fetus is assessed, and an estimate of amniotic fluid volume is made. **Discordant growth** is defined as a 20% or greater difference in the estimated fetal weight between the larger and smaller fetus (ratio calculated by determining the difference in the estimated fetal weight between the two fetuses, divided by the weight of the larger fetus). Additional antenatal surveillance, such as the nonstress test or biophysical profile, is often used when there is growth restriction of one or more fetuses, discordant growth, or another high-risk situation such as maternal medical comorbidity.

INTRAPARTUM MANAGEMENT

Not surprisingly, the average duration of pregnancy is inversely related to the number of fetuses. The average length of pregnancy in twin gestations is about 36 weeks. Many consider the optimal time for uncomplicated dichorionic-diamniotic twins to be delivered as between 38.0 and 38.6 weeks. Induction of labor or cesarean delivery is usually scheduled because the risk of perinatal mortality increases at 39 weeks and beyond. Women with uncomplicated monochorionic-diamniotic twins are typically delivered between 34.0 weeks and 37.6 weeks. The special case of monochorionic-monoamniotic twins was discussed earlier (delivery at 32–34 weeks). Intrapartum management is largely determined by the presentation of the twins. In general, if the first (presenting) twin is in the cephalic (vertex) presentation, labor is allowed to progress to vaginal delivery, whereas if the presenting twin is in a position other than cephalic, cesarean delivery is often performed. During labor, the heart rate of both fetuses is monitored separately. Approaches to the delivery of twins vary, depending on gestational age or estimated fetal weight, presentation of the twins, and the experience of the attending physician. Monochorionic-monoamniotic twins should be delivered by cesarean due to the risk for umbilical cord complications.

Regardless of the delivery plan, access to full obstetric, anesthetic, and pediatric services is mandatory because cesarean delivery may be required on short notice. About 40% of all twin pairs enter labor with both in the cephalic presentation. After delivery of the first twin, if the second fetus remains cephalic, vaginal delivery of the second twin generally proceeds smoothly. With proper monitoring of the second twin, there is no urgency in accomplishing the second delivery.

Delivery Maneuvers

If the second twin is presenting in any way other than cephalic (40% of all twin deliveries), there are two primary manipulations that may affect vaginal delivery. The first is **external cephalic version**. Using ultrasonographic visualization, the fetus is gently guided into the cephalic presentation by abdominal massage and pressure (Fig. 13.3A). The second maneuver is **breech extraction**, in which the physician reaches a hand into the uterine cavity, grasps the lower extremities of the fetus, and gently delivers the infant via breech delivery (see Fig. 13.3B). Delivering the second twin via cesarean delivery is another management option but is usually reserved for cases in which there is an inability to safely deliver the second twin vaginally (including an obstetrician without experience in vaginal breech extraction).

Complications

The possibility of a prolapsed umbilical cord must always be borne in mind when delivery of twins is to be accomplished. Twin gestations in which the first twin is in the breech presentation (20% of all twin deliveries) are most often delivered via cesarean delivery. Some clinicians and their patients plan for cesarean delivery unless both fetuses are in a cephalic presentation.

For patients with three or more fetuses, because of the potential for presentation of different fetal parts, delivery is accomplished by planned cesarean delivery in most cases.

Postpartum, the overdistended uterus may not contract normally, leading to uterine atony and postpartum hemorrhage (see Chapter 12).

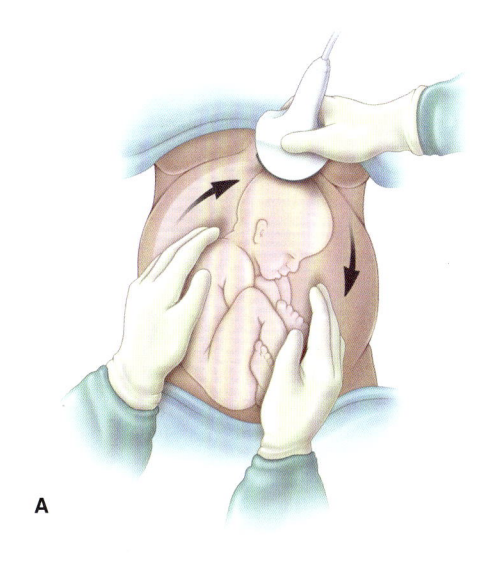

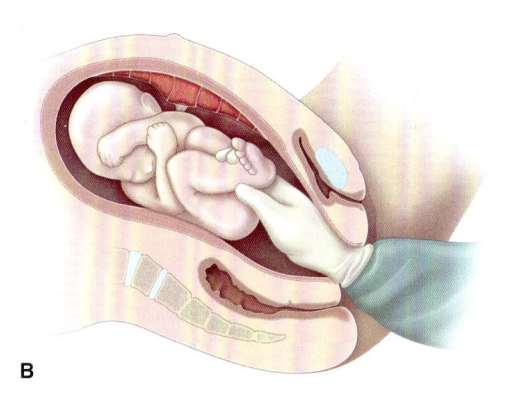

FIGURE 13.3. Delivery of second twin. **(A)** External cephalic version. **(B)** Breech extraction (internal podalic version).

CLINICAL FOLLOW-UP

After the diagnosis of multiple fetuses is made, it is important to carefully review the management of pregnancy and delivery with your patient and her partner. Management of patients with a multiple gestation requires considerable planning and close follow-up, and they should be made aware of the differences in caring for a patient with multiple fetuses versus those with one fetus. Although outcome is generally favorable, a close relationship and more frequent visits are necessary. You should encourage your patient and her partner to ask questions and express concerns throughout her pregnancy.

thePoint® Visit http://thePoint.lww.com/activate for an interactive USMLE-style question bank and more!

CHAPTER 14

Fetal Growth Abnormalities: Intrauterine Growth Restriction and Macrosomia

This chapter deals primarily with APGO Educational Topic Area:

TOPIC 31   FETAL GROWTH ABNORMALITIES

Students should be able to list the various fetal growth abnormalities, discuss possible etiologies, and describe possible complications. They should be able to outline a basic approach to evaluation and management of fetal growth abnormalities.

CLINICAL CASE

A 26-year-old G2P1001 female has been receiving routine prenatal care. Her previous pregnancy and delivery were uncomplicated. She is of average height and weight. When seen for her visit at a well-dated gestational age of 29 weeks, her fundal height is noted to be 24 cm, which is less than the 28 to 29 cm you would expect at this time. Fetal heart tones are normal. Based on the fact that her uterine size is less than the expected for her gestational age, you suspect intrauterine growth restriction (IUGR). Such a situation as described is reasonably common in obstetrics, and care providers must have a good understanding of the possible etiologies and management of patients with IUGR. Likewise, an estimated fetal size and weight significantly above that expected poses additional challenges for those caring for such patients.

INTRAUTERINE GROWTH RESTRICTION

"Fetal growth restriction" describes infants whose weights are much lower than expected. Population-based norms are used to categorize abnormal growth (Table 14.1). A fetus or infant whose weight is less than the 10th percentile of a specific population at a given gestational age is designated as having **IUGR**. Therefore, careful assignment of gestational age is crucial to the diagnosis and management of patients with IUGR.

The term **small for gestational age** (**SGA**) is used to describe an infant with a birth weight at the lower extreme of the normal birth weight distribution. In the United States, the most commonly used definition of SGA is a birth weight below the 10th percentile for gestational age. The use of the terms "small for gestational age" and "intrauterine growth restriction" has been confusing, and the terms are often used interchangeably. In this chapter, SGA will be used only in reference to the infant and IUGR to the fetus.

The use of gestational age percentiles remains limited for a number of reasons. First, by definition, the prevalence of IUGR will be 9%, but not all such neonates are pathologically small. Second, any percentile cutoff fails to take into account an individual's growth potential. Also, a simple percentile cannot take into account growth rate. The change in percentile over time or change in specific measurements may be more important. Finally, the time when the growth restriction is found may be a factor in morbidity and mortality: growth restriction at earlier gestational ages has greater effects on morbidity and mortality.

Significance

The goal of recognizing neonates with growth abnormalities is to identify infants at risk for increased short-term and long-term morbidity or mortality. In the short term, the growth-restricted fetus potentially lacks adequate reserves to continue intrauterine existence, to undergo the stress of labor, and to fully adapt to neonatal life. These conditions make the infant vulnerable to intrauterine fetal death, asphyxia, acidemia, and intolerance to labor. Neonatal complications include low Apgar scores, polycythemia, hyperbilirubinemia, hypoglycemia, hypothermia, apnea, respiratory distress, seizures, sepsis, meconium aspiration, and neonatal death.

Alterations in fetal growth may have lifelong implications. The antenatal response or fetal adaptation to the intrauterine nutritional and metabolic environment may predict or dictate the response to an extrauterine environment. Increasing evidence supports the concept of fetal origins for adult diseases and the association between birth size and long-term health. Associations have been reported between birth weight and adult obesity, cardiovascular disease (e.g., coronary heart disease, hypertension, and stroke), insulin resistance, and dyslipidemia. Therefore, intrauterine growth may reflect the foundation of many aspects of lifelong physiologic function.

In general, the smaller the fetus with IUGR, the greater its risk for morbidity and mortality. Perinatal morbidity and

TABLE 14.1 DEFINITION OF COMMONLY USED FETAL GROWTH DESCRIPTORS

Fetal Growth Descriptor	Definition
Intrauterine growth restriction	<10% for gestational age
Suspected macrosomia	>4,500 g
Large for gestational age	>90% for gestational age

mortality are significantly increased; risk of fetal death is 1.5% for fetal weights less than the tenth percentile for gestational age (twice the background rate for a normally grown fetus) and 2.5% for fetal weights less than the fifth percentile. One study found that 26% of all were SGA. Thus, it is important to identify such infants in utero so that management maximizes the quality of their intrauterine environment, permits planning and implementation of delivery using the safest means possible, and provides necessary care in the neonatal period.

Pathophysiology

For a fetus to thrive in utero, an adequate number of fetal cells and cells that differentiate properly are both requisite. In addition, nutrients and oxygen must be available via an adequately functioning uteroplacental unit to allow an increase in the number of cells and in cell size. Early in pregnancy, fetal growth occurs primarily through **cellular hyperplasia**, or cell division, and early-onset IUGR may lead to an irreversible diminution of organ size and, perhaps, function. Early-onset IUGR is also more commonly associated with genetic factors, immunologic abnormalities, chronic maternal disease, fetal infection, and multiple pregnancies. Later in pregnancy, fetal growth depends increasingly on **cellular hypertrophy** rather than hyperplasia alone, so that delayed-onset IUGR may also result in decreased cell size, which may be more amenable to restoration of fetal size with adequate nutrition. The normal fetus grows throughout the pregnancy, but the rate of growth decreases after 37 weeks of gestational age as the fetus depletes fat for cellular growth.

The **placenta** grows early and rapidly compared with the fetus, reaching a maximum surface area of about 11 m² and weight of 500 g at approximately 37 weeks of gestational age. Thereafter, there is a slow but steady decline in placental surface area (and, hence, function), primarily because of microinfarctions of its vascular system. Late-onset growth restriction may, therefore, be primarily related to decreased function and nutrient transport of the uteroplacental unit, a condition termed **uteroplacental insufficiency**. In addition, because there is a close relationship between placental surface area and fetal weight, factors that act to decrease placental size are also associated with decreased, that is, restricted, growth. Abnormal placentation that results in poor placental perfusion (i.e., placental insufficiency) is the most common pathology associated with fetal growth restriction.

Etiology

IUGR is a descriptive term for a condition that has numerous potential causes. Determining the specific diagnosis is important for optimal management. Although a number of causes of IUGR have been recognized, a definite etiology of IUGR cannot be identified in approximately 50% of all cases. In addition, because the utilization of a percentile cutoff of 10% alone will result in a high proportion of false positives, two thirds or more of such fetuses categorized as IUGR will be simply constitutionally small and otherwise healthy.

Factors that affect fetal growth are extensive and include maternal, fetal, and placental causes; these are listed in Box 14.1.

Maternal Factors

Maternal factors associated with IUGR include viral infections, such as rubella, varicella, and cytomegalovirus, which are associated with high rates of growth restriction, particularly if infection occurs early in pregnancy. Although these infections may manifest in the mother only as mild "flu-like" illnesses, injury to the fetus during organogenesis can result in a decreased cell number, resulting in diminished growth with or without multiple congenital anomalies. Other infections associated with IUGR include malaria, toxoplasmosis and syphilis. It is estimated that intrauterine infection is the primary cause for approximately 5% to 10% of cases of IUGR.

Maternal substance abuse affects fetal growth, and almost all infants with fetal alcohol syndrome will be growth restricted.

BOX 14.1 Risk Factors Associated with Intrauterine Growth Restriction

- Maternal medical conditions
  - Pregestational diabetes mellitus
  - Renal insufficiency
  - Autoimmune disease (e.g., systemic lupus erythematosus)
  - Cyanotic cardiac disease
  - Pregnancy-related hypertensive diseases of pregnancy (e.g., chronic hypertension, gestational hypertension, or preeclampsia)
  - Antiphospholipid antibody syndrome
- Substance use and abuse (e.g., tobacco, alcohol, cocaine, or narcotics)
- Multiple gestation
- Teratogen exposure (e.g., cyclophosphamide, valproic acid, or antithrombotic drugs)
- Infectious diseases (e.g., malaria, cytomegalovirus, rubella, toxoplasmosis, or syphilis)
- Genetic and structural disorders (e.g., trisomy 13, trisomy 18, congenital heart disease, or gastroschisis)
- Placental disorders and umbilical cord abnormalities

American College of Obstetricians and Gynecologists. Fetal Growth Restriction. ACOG Practice Bulletin 134. *Obstet Gynecol.* 2013;121: 1122–1133. Used with permission.

Women who smoke during pregnancy deliver babies 200 g smaller on average than do women who do not smoke; moreover, the rate of growth restriction is three- to fourfold greater among babies born to women who smoke during pregnancy. Women who use narcotics, heroin, methadone, or cocaine also have rates of growth-restricted babies ranging from as much as 30% to 50%. Medications known to be associated with IUGR include certain antiepileptic medications (e.g., valproic acid), warfarin, and some antineoplastic agents (e.g., folic acid antagonists and cyclophosphamide). Altitude may also affect fetal growth.

Other maternal factors that affect fetal growth and body composition include demographic factors and medical conditions. Extremes in maternal age (age younger than 16 years and older than 35 years) are associated with an increased risk of fetal growth restriction. Medical conditions that alter or affect placental function such as any chronic disorder associated with vascular disease (hypertensive disorders, chronic renal disease, and pregestational diabetes) may also be causative factors.

Although one common pathway has not been clearly identified, many of these disorders occur together. Women with a history of prior obstetric complications have an increased risk of growth abnormalities. Maternal metabolism and body composition are two of the strongest regulators of fetal growth. Nutritional deficiencies and inadequate weight gain, particularly in teens or in underweight women, may result in IUGR.

Fetal Factors

The inherent growth potential of the individual is determined genetically. Female fetuses are at greater risk for IUGR than males. In addition, up to 5% of growth-restricted fetuses have a chromosomal abnormality, a number that rises to 20% if both IUGR and structural abnormalities are present. At least 50% of fetuses with trisomy 13 or trisomy 18 have fetal growth restriction. In addition, single-gene mutations, such as the glucokinase gene mutation, and structural malformations (with or without genetic abnormalities), such as gastroschisis, congenital cardiac disease, and renal agenesis, can also result in abnormalities of growth. Finally, multifetal pregnancies are at increased risk for growth restriction.

Placental Factors

The placenta is critical for nutrient regulation and transportation from mother to fetus. Abnormalities in placentation or defective trophoblast invasion and remodeling may contribute to fetal growth restriction as well as other disorders of pregnancy. In addition, uterine anomalies (uterine septum or fibroids) may limit placental implantation and development and, consequently, nutrient transport, resulting in inadequate nutrition for the developing fetus. Finally, the genetic composition of the placenta is important, and abnormalities such as confined placental mosaicism are associated with growth delay.

Diagnosis

Assessment of gestational age is critically important in early pregnancy, because dating becomes increasingly imprecise as gestational age advances. Antenatal recognition of IUGR depends upon the recognition of risk factors and the clinical assessment of uterine size, followed by biometric measurements.

Physical Examination

Physical examination is limited in usefulness in making a specific diagnosis of IUGR, but it is an important screening test for abnormal fetal growth. Maternal size and weight gain throughout pregnancy also have limited value, but access to such information is readily available; a low maternal weight or little or no weight gain during pregnancy may suggest increased risk for IUGR. Serial measurements of **fundal height** are commonly used as a screening test for IUGR but have high rates of false-negative and false-positive predictive values. Between 24 and 38 weeks of gestation, fundal height should increase approximately 1 cm/week, consistent with gestational age in weeks (Fig. 14.1). A discrepancy may be related to constitutional factors, but a significant discrepancy of more than 3 cm may indicate IUGR and the need for an ultrasound examination. Clinical estimations of fetal weight alone are not helpful in diagnosing IUGR, except when fetal size is grossly diminished.

Ultrasonography

If IUGR is suspected based on risk factors and/or clinical assessment, ultrasonography should be performed to assess fetal size and growth. Specific **fetal biometry measurements** are compared with standardized tables that reflect normal growth at a certain gestational age. The four standard fetal measurements include the (1) biparietal diameter, (2) head circumference, (3) abdominal circumference (AC), and (4) femur length. Conversion of individual morphologic measurements to fetal weight using published equations or ratios of measurements can provide useful estimations of fetal size. An AC within the normal range reliably excludes growth restriction, with a false-negative rate of less than 10%. A small AC or fetal weight estimate below the 10th percentile suggests the possibility of growth restriction, with the likelihood increasing as the percentile rank decreases.

Direct Studies

Direct invasive studies of the fetus are useful in selected patients with IUGR, particularly those with midtrimester onset of IUGR or structural abnormalities concerning for chromosomal or genetic disorders or fetal infection. Fetal karyotyping and viral cultures and/or polymerase chain reaction can be performed on fluid obtained by amniocentesis. Rarely, **chorionic villus sampling** (biopsy of placenta) or direct blood sampling (**percutaneous umbilical blood sampling**) may be necessary for specific studies.

Doppler Velocimetry

Doppler velocimetry of fetal vessels provides further insight into the fetal response to altered growth and has become part of the standard assessment of the fetus once IUGR is diagnosed. Doppler velocimetry has been shown to both reduce interventions and improve fetal outcome in pregnancies at risk for IUGR. The rate of perinatal mortality is reduced by 29%

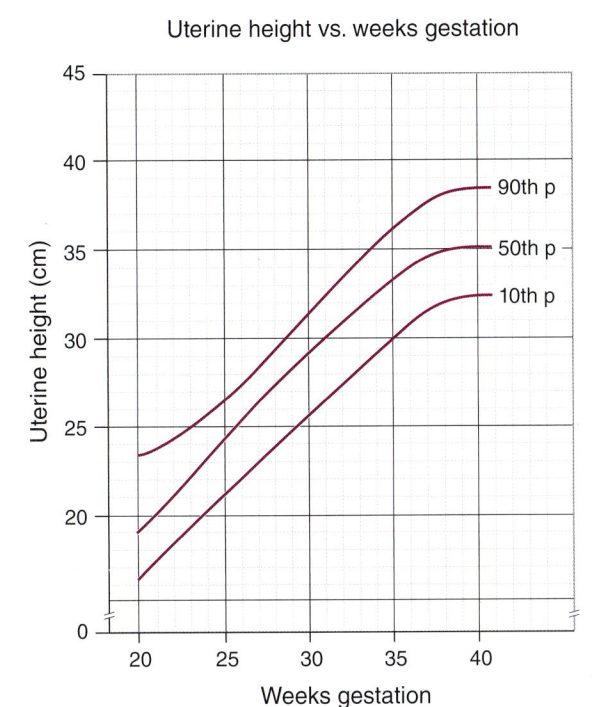

FIGURE 14.1. Fundal height evaluation as a screening test for intrauterine growth restriction. *p*, percentile. (Reprinted with permission from Scott JR, Di Saia PJ, Hammond CB, et al. *Danforth's Obstetrics and Gynecology*. 8th ed. Baltimore, MD: Williams & Wilkins; 1999.)

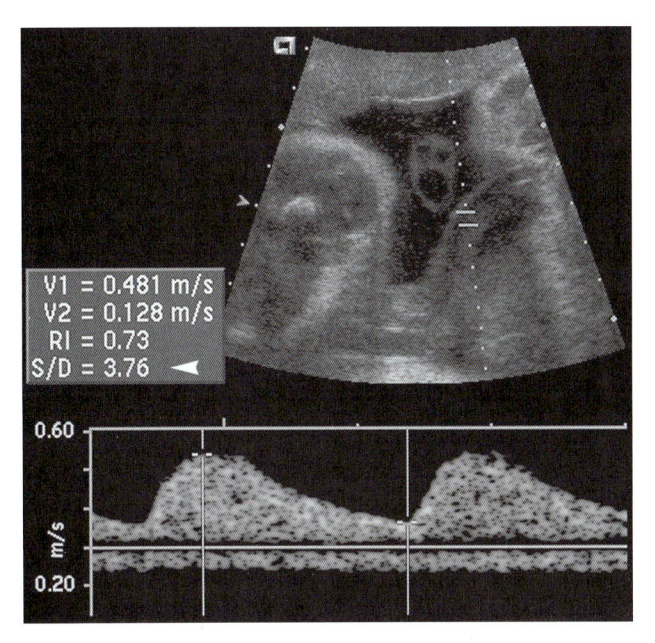

FIGURE 14.2. Doppler velocimetry. Umbilical artery Doppler of a 35-week fetus demonstrates an elevated S/D ratio of 3.76 (*arrowhead, calipers*) due to diminished diastolic flow. (From Doubilet PM, Benson CB. *Atlas of Ultrasound in Obstetrics and Gynecology*. Philadelphia, PA: Lippincott Williams & Wilkins; 2003:227.)

when umbilical artery Doppler velocimetry is combined with standard antepartum surveillance (non-stress test, biophysical profile) in the setting of IUGR. Fetal–placental circulation is evaluated in the umbilical artery and is measured by a systolic/diastolic (S/D) ratio. The S/D indirectly measures impedance or resistance downstream within the placental vessels. As placental resistance increases, diastolic flow decreases and the S/D ratio rises. A normal S/D ratio at term is 1.8 to 2.0. Fetuses with IUGR with absent or reversed end-diastolic flow have progressively worse perinatal outcomes (Figs. 14.2 and 14.3). Although other fetal vessels such as the middle cerebral artery and ductus venosus can be assessed, there is lack of current data to link use of these additional studies to improved outcome and they are not recommended as a standard component of monitoring.

Management

The goal of management of a growth-restricted fetus is to deliver the healthiest possible infant at the optimal time. Continued management of pregnancy with IUGR is based on the results of fetal testing. Serial evaluations of fetal biometry should be performed every 3 or 4 weeks to follow the extent of growth restriction. **Fetal surveillance** is important and may include fetal movement counting, nonstress testing, biophysical profiles, and umbilical artery Doppler studies. Antenatal surveillance should not begin before a gestational age when delivery would be considered for perinatal benefit. There are no specific therapies that have proven beneficial for pregnancies complicated by IUGR.

The fetus should be delivered if the risk of fetal death exceeds that of neonatal death, although in many cases these risks are difficult to assess. For example, a fetus with IUGR with normal anatomic survey, normal amniotic fluid volume, normal Doppler studies, and normal fetal testing may not benefit from early delivery. Conversely, the growth-restricted fetus with serial biometry measurements documenting decreasing growth rate and/or mildly abnormal Doppler studies may benefit from delivery. These decisions must be made while considering the gestational age of the fetus and the known risks associated with prematurity. Based on existing data and expert opinion, the following timing strategies have been recommended when IUGR has been diagnosed: (1) delivery at 38 0/7 to 39 6/7 weeks in cases of isolated IUGR and (2) delivery at 34 0/7 to 37 6/7 weeks in cases of IUGR with additional risk factors for adverse outcome (e.g., more severe IUGR, oligohydramnios, abnormal umbilical artery Doppler velocimetry, maternal co-morbidities).

Neonatal Management

Neonatal management of IUGR infants, which is partially dependent on gestational age, includes preparation for neonatal respiratory compromise, hypoglycemia, hypothermia, and hyperviscosity syndrome. Growth-restricted fetuses have less fat deposition in late pregnancy, so newborn euglycemia cannot be maintained by the normal mechanism of mobilization of glucose by fat metabolism. **Hyperviscosity syndrome** results from the fetus's attempt to compensate for poor placental oxygen transfer by increasing the hematocrit to more than 65%.

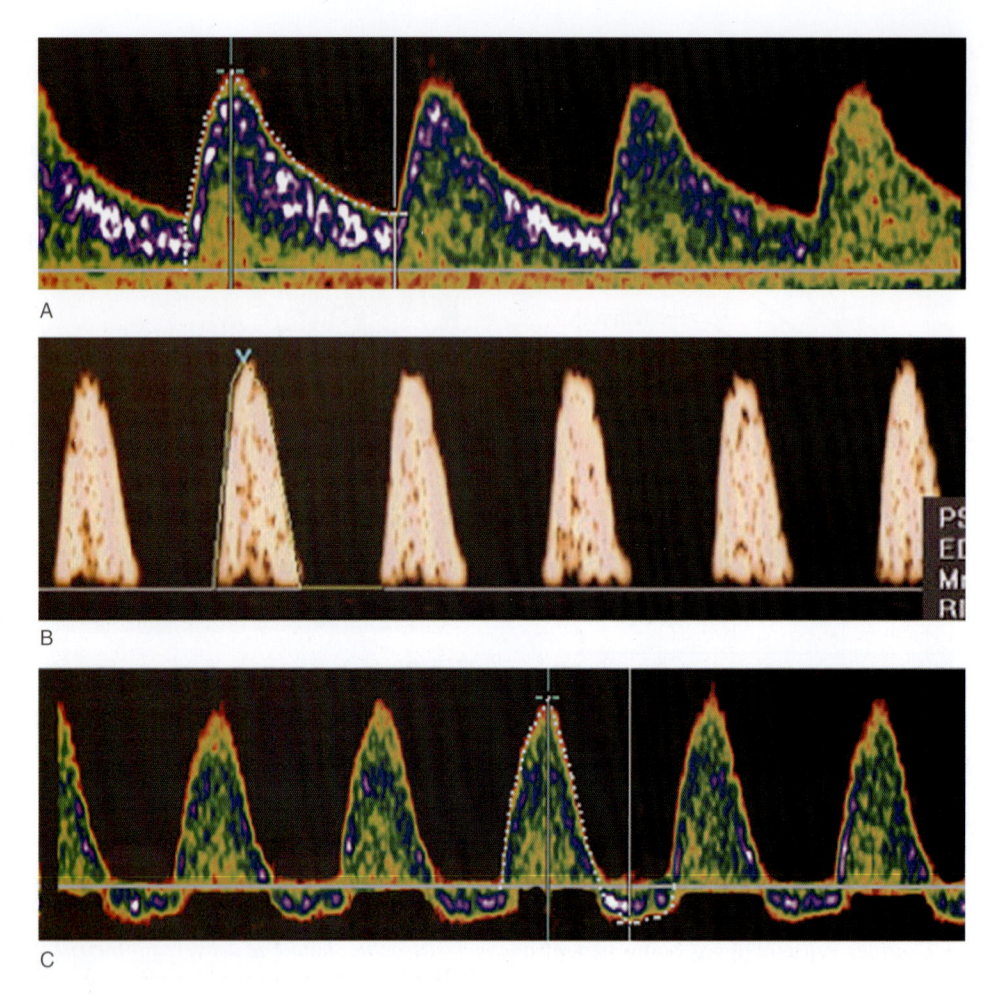

FIGURE 14.3. Umbilical artery Doppler velocimetry: (A) Normal, (B) absent, and (C) reversed end-diastolic flow.

After birth, this marked polycythemia can cause multiorgan thrombosis, heart failure, and hyperbilirubinemia. Overall, growth-restricted infants who survive the neonatal period have a generally good prognosis.

● MACROSOMIA

Two terms have been used to define excessive fetal growth. **Fetal macrosomia** is based on weight alone and refers to a very large fetus, typically with an estimated weight of greater than 4,000 to 4,500 g or more. There is no general agreement among obstetricians on the precise definition of macrosomia. However, morbidity increases sharply with birth weights ≥4,500 g when compared with the general population; thus, 4,500 g is often used as an estimate above which a fetus is considered macrosomic. **Large for gestational age (LGA)** generally implies a birth weight of >90% for a given gestational age and is dependent on both weight and gestational age with percentiles generated from population-specific norms (see Table 14.1). By definition, the prevalence of LGA is fixed, but not all neonates at the upper extreme of size are pathologically large. Growth potential, growth rate, and gestational age at onset may be important considerations.

Etiology

Macrosomia, like fetal growth restriction, has multiple potential causes, categorized into fetal or maternal factors (Box 14.2).

Maternal Factors

Maternal factors include a history of macrosomia, maternal prepregnancy weight, weight gain during pregnancy, multiparity, male fetus, gestational age greater than 40 weeks, ethnicity, maternal birth weight, maternal height, maternal age younger than 17 years, preexisting diabetes, and a positive 50-g glucose screen with a negative result on the 3-hour glucose tolerance test.

The magnitude of glucose intolerance during pregnancy and specific measures of control are correlated with fetal weight and fetal fat mass. Lipids are also associated with fetal size, with triglycerides and free fatty acids positively correlated to birth weight, and triglycerides independently associated with LGA infants. Maternal body composition and body mass index are major determinants of insulin sensitivity, independent of hypertension and pregestational or gestational diabetes. Also, maternal weight gain and pregravid weight contribute to the variance in fetal birth weight. Finally, increased parity is associated with larger babies.

Fetal Factors

Similar to fetal growth restriction, fetal factors include the genetic composition or inherent growth potential of the individual and genetic syndromes such as Beckwith-Wiedemann syndrome. Male fetuses are also more commonly affected than female fetuses.

Significance

Macrosomia is associated with both increased maternal and fetal/neonatal risks. Because of labor abnormalities, a patient with a macrosomic fetus has an increased risk of cesarean delivery. The risks of postpartum hemorrhage and vaginal lacerations are also elevated with macrosomia. Risks to the fetus are shoulder dystocia and fracture of the clavicle, although brachial plexus nerve injury is rare. Macrosomic infants also have an increased risk of lower Apgar scores.

Other neonatal risks are partially dependent on the underlying etiology of macrosomia, such as maternal obesity or diabetes, and may include an increased risk of hypothermia, hyperbilirubinemia, hypoglycemia, prematurity, and stillbirth. The relationship between gestational age and fetal size is important. Macrosomic preterm infants remain at risk for complications of prematurity. The fetal size and extent of maturity are independent. Long-term risks include overweight or obesity in later life, again illustrating that intrauterine growth may predict the foundation of many aspects of lifelong physiologic function.

Newborn mortality increases significantly with birth weights greater than 5,000 g. At this time, it seems reasonable to recognize a continuum of risk and to divide macrosomia into three categories:

1. Birth weight of 4,000 to 4,499 g with increased risk of labor abnormalities and newborn complications
2. Birth weight of 4,500 to 4,999 g with additional risk of maternal and newborn morbidity
3. Birth weight of 5,000 g or greater with additional risk of stillbirth and neonatal mortality

---

BOX 14.2 Risk Factors for Large for Gestational Age

Fetal
- Genetic potential
- Specific gene disorders
- Male sex

Maternal
- History of previous macrosomic pregnancy
- Metabolism (pre-existing diabetes)
- Body composition
- Pregnancy weight gain
- Parity

Diagnosis

The diagnosis of macrosomia is imprecise and can only be accurately diagnosed at delivery after weighing the infant. The diagnosis of suspected macrosomia is based on estimated fetal weight greater than 4500 g or LGA at greater than the 90th percentile for gestational age. Assessment of pregnancy duration becomes increasingly imprecise at later gestational ages, so careful dating of pregnancy as early as possible is important. The two primary methods for *clinical* estimation of fetal weight are Leopold maneuvers (abdominal palpation; see Fig. 9.7) and measurement of the height of the uterine fundus above the maternal symphysis pubis. Measurement of the symphysis–fundal height alone is a poor predictor of fetal macrosomia and should be combined with clinical palpation (Leopold maneuvers) to be useful.

Clinical findings may be combined with ultrasound to diagnose macrosomia. Ultrasound-derived estimates of fetal weight are obtained by entering the measurements of various fetal body parts, usually including the AC, into one of several popular regression equations. However, most of the regression formulas currently in use are associated with significant errors when the fetus is macrosomic. The superiority of ultrasound-derived estimates of fetal weight over clinical estimates has not been established.

The true value of ultrasound in management of macrosomia is its ability to rule out the diagnosis.

The differential diagnosis of an enlarged uterus includes a large fetus, more than one fetus (multiple gestation), extra amniotic fluid (polyhydramnios), large placenta (molar pregnancy), and large uterus (uterine leiomyomata, other gynecologic tumor, or uterine anomaly).

Management

For mothers without diabetes, no clinical interventions designed to treat or curb fetal growth when macrosomia is suspected have been reported. Current evidence does not support early delivery for macrosomia alone, because induction of labor does not decrease maternal and neonatal morbidity; however, it does increase the rate of cesarean deliveries. In addition, the data do not support a specific estimated fetal weight at which women should undergo elective cesarean delivery. Given the limitations of ultrasound estimations and the association with increasing injury with increasing infant weight, the American College of Obstetricians and Gynecologists recommends that a cesarean delivery should be offered for estimated fetal weights greater than 5,000 g in women without diabetes and greater than 4,500 g in women with diabetes.

Various techniques can be used to facilitate vaginal delivery in the case of shoulder dystocia, such as exaggerated flexion of the thighs (McRoberts maneuver; see Fig. 9.9A), suprapubic pressure, various rotations, episiotomy, delivery of the posterior arm, and intentional clavicular fracture. The Zavanelli maneuver, cephalic replacement with subsequent cesarean delivery, has yielded mixed results. A prolonged second stage of labor or arrest of descent in the second stage is an indication for cesarean delivery. Postpartum or neonatal management depends on gestational age and underlying etiology.

CLINICAL FOLLOW-UP

You should share your concerns about possible intrauterine growth restriction with your patient. Ultrasound evaluation is warranted. Once the diagnosis is established, careful, ongoing management of your patient throughout her pregnancy and delivery is important. Frequent counseling and addressing your patient's questions and concerns is also important. Caring for patients with fetal growth abnormalities, whether "too small" or "too big," can be challenging.

thePoint® Visit http://thePoint.lww.com/activate for an interactive USMLE-style question bank and more!

CHAPTER 15
Preterm Labor

This chapter deals primarily with APGO Educational Topic Area:

TOPIC 24   PRETERM LABOR

Students should be able to list risk factors, possible etiologies, and complications of preterm labor. They should be able to outline a basic approach to evaluation and management, including appropriate medications and their contraindications. They should be able to counsel a patient on risk reduction for preterm birth.

CLINICAL CASE

A 34-year-old patient was admitted to your antepartum service for advanced cervical dilation at 24 weeks of gestation. She had one other preterm delivery at 33 weeks of gestation. She was placed on progesterone for prevention of preterm delivery. She has intermittently had light vaginal bleeding. Today, at 27 weeks, the patient has another episode of bleeding and begins contracting regularly. She is very worried about her baby being delivered so early. What are the next steps in her evaluation and management? What can you do to prevent the sequelae of prematurity in the neonate?

INTRODUCTION

Preterm birth is delivery that occurs prior to the completion of 37 completed weeks (259 days) of gestation. Because it is the most common cause of perinatal morbidity and mortality in the United States, prevention and treatment of preterm birth is a major focus of obstetric care. The consequences of preterm birth occur with increasing severity and frequency the earlier the gestational age of the newborn. In addition to perinatal death in the very young fetus, common complications of preterm birth include respiratory distress syndrome, intraventricular hemorrhage, necrotizing enterocolitis, sepsis, neurologic impairment, and seizures. Long-term morbidity associated with preterm delivery includes bronchopulmonary dysplasia and developmental abnormalities, including cerebral palsy.

The 11% to 12% of babies born prematurely account for 70% of all perinatal mortality and 50% of long-term neurologic impairment in children in the United States.

Preterm births may be classified into two general presentations: **Spontaneous** and **indicated**. Approximately 40% to 50% of preterm births result from spontaneous preterm labor with intact membranes; 25% to 40% result from preterm premature rupture of membranes (PPROM; see Chapter 17). The remaining 20% to 30% occur following deliberate intervention for a variety of maternal or obstetric complications (e.g., eclampsia).

Preterm labor is defined as the presence of regular uterine contractions that occur before 37 completed weeks of gestation and are associated with cervical changes. It is often difficult to diagnose preterm labor because of the absence of definitive measurements. *The lack of diagnostic criteria presents a problem, because treatment appears to be more effective when initiated early in the course of preterm labor.*

CAUSE, PREDICTION, AND PREVENTION OF PRETERM LABOR

Causes

Preterm labor may represent a final common pathway for a number of pathogenic processes. The four main processes include (1) activation of the maternal or fetal hypothalamic–pituitary–adrenal axis due to maternal or fetal stress, (2) decidual–chorioamniotic or systemic inflammation caused by infection, (3) decidual hemorrhage, and (4) pathologic uterine distention (Fig. 15.1). Numerous risk factors have been associated with preterm labor (Box 15.1). The strongest risk factors are multifetal gestation and prior preterm birth. With a prior preterm birth, the risk in a subsequent pregnancy increases and continues to increase with each subsequent preterm pregnancy. Subclinical intra-amniotic infection has also been associated with preterm labor and PPROM, especially when it occurs at earlier gestational ages. *In most cases, however, no cause or risk factor for preterm labor can be identified.*

Factors Improving Outcomes

Despite the lack of effective strategies to predict and prevent preterm labor, infant morbidity and mortality following

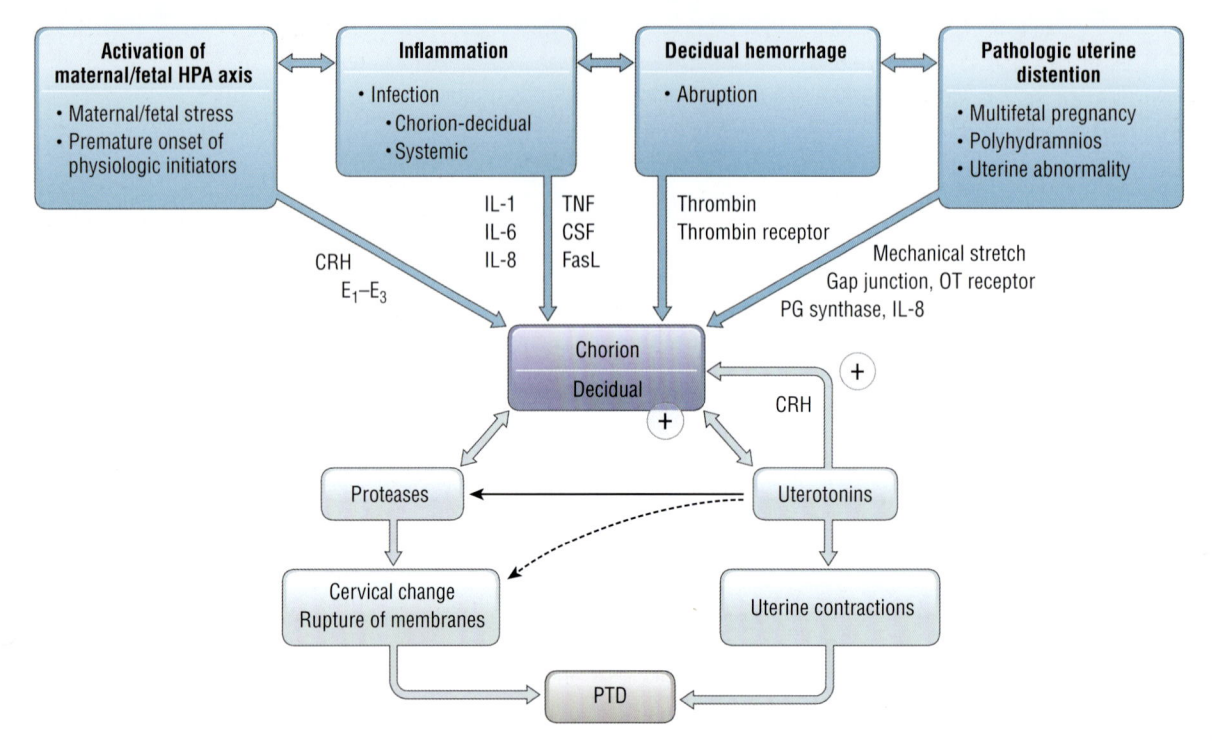

FIGURE 15.1. Preterm labor: final common pathway. The four main processes include activation of the maternal or fetal hypothalamic–pituitary–adrenal (HPA) axis, infection, decidual hemorrhage, and pathologic uterine distention. *CRH*, corticotropin-releasing hormone; *CSF*, colony-stimulating factor; E_1, estrone; E_3, estriol; *FasL*, FAS ligand; *IL*, interleukin; *OT*, oxytocin receptor; *PG*, prostaglandin; *PTD*, preterm delivery; *TNF*, tumor necrosis factor.

BOX 15.1 Factors Associated with Preterm Labor

- Prior history of preterm birth
- Preterm uterine contractions
- Premature rupture of membranes
- Behavioral risk factors:
  - Low maternal prepregnancy weight
  - Smoking
  - Substance abuse
  - Short interpregnancy interval
- Current pregnancy factors:
  - Short cervical length
  - Multifetal gestation
  - Vaginal bleeding
  - Urinary tract infections
  - Genital tract infection
  - Periodontal disease

BOX 15.2 Signs and Symptoms of Preterm Labor

- Menstrual-like cramps
- Low, dull backache
- Abdominal pressure
- Pelvic pressure
- Abdominal cramping (with or without diarrhea)
- Increase or change in vaginal discharge (mucous, watery, light bloody discharge)
- Uterine contractions, often painless

---

preterm birth have decreased over the past several decades as the result of several factors. First, neonatal intensive care management of preterm infants has greatly improved outcomes. Therefore, maternal transport to a regional tertiary care center is indicated for women in preterm labor presenting to hospitals without sophisticated neonatal intensive care. Second, the use of corticosteroids administered to a mother at immediate risk for preterm birth (such as a woman in preterm labor) has resulted in decreased incidence of respiratory distress syndrome, intraventricular hemorrhage, and associated infant morbidity and mortality. A major goal of therapy to stop contractions in a woman in preterm labor (**tocolytic therapy**) is to prolong pregnancy for up to 48 hours in order to allow time to administer corticosteroids. Third, magnesium sulfate administered prior to a preterm birth has been shown to decrease the rate of cerebral palsy in infants born preterm. Finally, prophylaxis against perinatal infection with group B streptococcus (GBS) in women with preterm labor or PPROM has also decreased infant morbidity and mortality rates in the United States.

Prediction of Preterm Labor

Patient and physician education has focused on recognition of the signs and symptoms that suggest preterm labor (Box 15.2). Patients with symptoms are counseled to seek prompt medical attention. Other screening modalities in asymptomatic women, such as fetal fibronectin, bacterial vaginosis screening, and home uterine contraction monitoring, have been advocated in the past; however, interventions based on results of these tests have not yielded improved perinatal outcome and are therefore not recommended as screening tests for preterm labor.

Cervical Changes

Cervical length can be used as a diagnostic factor. As cervical length decreases in mid-pregnancy, the risk of preterm birth has been shown to increase in a continuous fashion. **Transvaginal ultrasound** examination of the cervix is a reliable and reproducible method to assess cervical length. This test may be most helpful when evaluating women at high risk for recurrent preterm birth, those with uterine anomalies, and those who have had prior cervical cone biopsy or multiple dilation and curettage/evacuation procedures.

Early asymptomatic dilation and effacement of the cervix (**cervical insufficiency**) may be associated with an increased likelihood of preterm labor and delivery. Interventions such as prophylactic cervical cerclage on sonographic recognition of a shortened cervical length (often defined as less than 2.5 cm) in low-risk women have not improved outcomes; however, placement of a cerclage in high-risk women (e.g., history of prior preterm birth) with a shortened cervix may be beneficial.

Other screening modalities in asymptomatic women, such as fetal fibronectin, bacterial vaginosis screening, and home uterine contraction monitoring, have been advocated in the past; however, interventions based on results of these tests have not yielded improved perinatal outcomes and are, therefore, not recommended as screening tests for preterm labor.

Prevention

There are currently no uniformly effective interventions to prevent preterm labor, regardless of risk factors. Prophylactic therapy—including tocolytic drugs, bed rest, hydration, and sedation in asymptomatic women at high risk for preterm labor—has not been shown to be effective. However, in a select group of women at very high risk who have a documented history of preterm birth, the use of weekly intramuscular injections of progesterone (17-α-hydroxyprogesterone caproate) starting at 16 to 20 weeks of gestation and continuing until 36 weeks of gestation appears to reduce spontaneous preterm birth. Vaginal progesterone supplementation in women with a sonographically determined shortened cervical length has also shown some benefit.

● EVALUATION OF A PATIENT IN SUSPECTED PRETERM LABOR

Prompt evaluation is critical in the patient who describes symptoms and signs suggestive of preterm labor. Use of an external electronic fetal monitor (**tocodynamometer**) may help to quantify the frequency and duration of contractions. The status of the cervix should be determined, either by visualization with a speculum or by gentle digital examination. Because digital examination may increase the risk of infection in the setting of PPROM, speculum evaluation to assess cervical dilation and effacement should be performed first if there is a suspicion of rupture of fetal membranes. Changes in cervical effacement and dilation on subsequent examinations are important in the evaluation of both the diagnosis of preterm labor and the effectiveness of management. Subtle changes are often of great clinical importance, so serial examinations by the same examiner are optimal, when this is possible.

Laboratory Tests

Because urinary infections can predispose a patient to uterine contractions, a urinalysis and urine culture should be obtained. A vaginal/rectal culture should be obtained for GBS.

Women with GBS bacteriuria are candidates for intrapartum antibiotic prophylaxis. When indicated by history or physical examination findings, cultures for *Chlamydia trachomatis* and *Neisseria gonorrhoeae* should be obtained.

Ultrasound

Ultrasound examination is useful in assessing the gestational age of the fetus, estimation of the amniotic fluid volume (spontaneous rupture of membranes with fluid loss may precede preterm labor and may be unrecognized by the patient), fetal presentation, and placental location, as well as the existence of fetal congenital anomalies. Patients should also be monitored for bleeding, insofar as placental abruption and placenta previa may be associated with preterm labor (see Chapter 16).

Information concerning the length of the cervix can be obtained through ultrasound examination, although results are not particularly helpful unless the gestational age is less than 26 weeks.

Amniocentesis

Amniocentesis may be performed to assess for intra-amniotic infection. Either clinical or subclinical infection of the amniotic cavity (**chorioamnionitis, intra-amniotic infection**) is thought to be associated with preterm labor. Amniotic fluid can be evaluated for the presence of bacteria, white blood cells (WBCs), lactate dehydrogenase, and glucose. Evidence of WBCs in the amniotic fluid, decreased glucose, or elevated lactate dehydrogenase may indicate infection. The presence of bacteria in amniotic fluid is correlated not only with preterm labor but also with the subsequent development of infection. In a patient with preterm labor, a high suspicion of chorioamnionitis should prompt administration of antibiotics and delivery regardless of the gestational age. A high suspicion of intrauterine infection is an indication for intrapartum antibiotics. It may also warrant prompt delivery regardless of gestational age. Tocolysis is not appropriate in the setting of intrauterine infection. At the time of amniocentesis, additional amniotic fluid may be obtained for fetal pulmonary maturity studies, which could influence subsequent management.

MANAGEMENT OF PRETERM LABOR

The purpose in treating preterm labor is to delay delivery, if possible, until fetal maturity is attained. Management involves two broad goals: 1) the detection and treatment of disorders associated with preterm labor and 2) therapy for the preterm labor itself. Fortunately, more than 50% of patients with preterm contractions have spontaneous resolution of abnormal uterine activity. However, this complicates the evaluation of effectiveness of specific treatments, because it is unclear if the contractions would have resolved spontaneously or if their cessation was due to effective treatments.

Tocolytics

Various tocolytic therapies have been used in the management of preterm labor (Table 15.1). Different treatment regimens address specific mechanisms involved in the maintenance of uterine contractions, and each, therefore, may be best suited for certain patients.

Typically, patients with a diagnosis of preterm labor receive one form of tocolytic therapy, with the addition or substitution of other medications if the initial treatment is considered unsuccessful.

The use of nifedipine as a tocolytic is increasing. In the past, magnesium sulfate has been used as a tocolytic agent; however, accumulated data show that it is ineffective when used for this purpose. Evidence is building that magnesium sulfate, administered antenatally to women with preterm labor, has a neuroprotective effect on the fetus, appearing to lower the risk of developing cerebral palsy. Evidence as to the efficacy of tocolytics beyond several days is weak, but, often, intervention with medication allows enough time for administration of corticosteroid therapy to accelerate fetal lung maturation. Adverse side

TABLE 15.1 COMMON TOCOLYTIC AGENT

Agent or Class	Action	Maternal Side Effects	Fetal or Newborn Adverse Effects	Contraindications
Calcium-channel blockers (nifedipine)	Prevents calcium entry into muscle cells	Dizziness, flushing, and hypotension; suppression of heart rate, contractility, and left ventricular systolic pressure when used with magnesium sulfate; and elevation of hepatic transaminases	No known adverse effects	Hypotension and preload-dependent cardiac lesions, such as aortic insufficiency
Nonsteroidal anti-inflammatory drugs	Decreases PG production by blocking conversion of free arachidonic acid to PG	Nausea, esophageal reflux, gastritis, and emesis; platelet dysfunction is rarely of clinical significance in patients without underlying bleeding disorder	In utero constriction of ductus arteriosus[a], oligohydramnios[a], necrotizing enterocolitis in preterm newborns, and patent ductus arteriosus in newborn[b]	Platelet dysfunction or bleeding disorder, hepatic dysfunction, gastrointestinal ulcerative disease, renal dysfunction, and asthma (in women with hypersensitivity to aspirin)
β-Adrenergic receptor agonists	Increases cAMP concentration in cells, which decreases free calcium	Tachycardia, hypotension, tremor, palpitations, shortness of breath, chest discomfort, pulmonary edema, hypokalemia, and hyperglycemia	Fetal tachycardia	Tachycardia-sensitive maternal cardiac disease and poorly controlled diabetes mellitus
Magnesium sulfate	Competes with calcium for entry into cells	Causes flushing, diaphoresis, nausea, loss of deep tendon reflexes, respiratory depression, and cardiac arrest; suppresses heart rate, contractility and left ventricular systolic pressure when used with calcium channel blockers; and produces neuromuscular blockade when used with calcium-channel blockers	Neonatal depression[c]	Myasthenia gravis

[a] Greatest risk associated with use for longer than 48 hours.
[b] Data are conflicting regarding this association.
[c] The use of magnesium sulfate in doses and duration for fetal neuroprotection alone does not appear to be associated with an increased risk of neonatal depression when correlated with cord blood magnesium levels

Adapted from Johnson LH, Mapp DC, Rouse DJ, Spong CY, Mercer BM, Leveno KJ, et al. Association of cord blood magnesium concentration and neonatal resuscitation. Eunice Kennedy Shriver National Institute of Child Health and Human Development Maternal-Fetal Medicine Units Network. *J Pediatr*. 2011; DOI: 10.1016/j.jpeds.2011.09.016; American College of Obstetricians and Gynecologists. *Management of Preterm Labor, Practice Bulletin 171*. Washington, DC: American College of Obstetricians and Gynecologists; 2016. (based on Hearne AE, Nagey DA. Therapeutic agents in preterm labor: tocolytic agents. *Clin Obstet Gynecol*. 2000;43:787–801.)

effects, at times serious and even life threatening to the mother, can occur. The gestational age of the fetus is always a consideration in deciding how vigorously to pursue therapy. For example, maternal risks may be more acceptable when treating a 26-week fetus as compared with a 32-week fetus.

Contraindications

Contraindications to tocolysis include conditions in which the adverse effects of tocolysis may be significant, such as the following:

- Intrauterine fetal demise
- Lethal fetal anomaly
- Nonreassuring fetal status
- Severe preeclampsia or eclampsia
- Maternal bleeding with hemodynamic instability
- Intra-amniotic infection
- PPROM
- Maternal contraindications to tocolysis

In addition, a variety of obstetric complications, such as placental abruption, advanced cervical dilation, or evidence of fetal compromise or placental insufficiency, may contraindicate delay in delivery.

Corticosteroids

From 24 to 34 weeks of gestation, management generally includes administration of **corticosteroids** (betamethasone or dexamethasone) to enhance fetal pulmonary maturity.

A single course of corticosteroids should be given to pregnant women between 24 and 34 weeks of gestation who are at risk for preterm delivery within 7 days. Both the incidence and severity of fetal respiratory distress syndrome are reduced with such therapy. In addition, other sequelae of prematurity, such as intraventricular hemorrhage and necrotizing enterocolitis, occur less frequently in infants whose mothers received corticosteroid therapy. Maximal benefit to the fetus occurs if the therapy is administered within 7 days of delivery. Routine weekly courses of therapy are not recommended.

Antenatal steroids may be considered as early as 23 weeks for women with preterm labor who are at risk of delivering within 7 days, if the family's decision is to attempt resuscitation in this periviable period. A single rescue dose of steroids may be offered to a patient who previously received a full course of steroids (≥ two weeks previously) and is now deemed likely to deliver within a week. Current data only supports a rescue dose for those patients less than 34 weeks. Finally, recent data support offering a course of antenatal steroids for late preterm patients with preterm labor at 34 0/7 to 36 6/7 weeks who are at risk of delivering within a week, and who have not previously had antenatal steroids.

CLINICAL FOLLOW-UP

The patient's vital signs and hematocrit are stable. The fetal heart tone is reassuring. The bleeding has decreased; however, you are still concerned for possible abruption and decide not to tocolyse the patient. You do administer a course of antenatal steroids, antibiotic for group B streptococcus prophylaxis, and magnesium for neuroprotection of the fetus.

---

thePoint® Visit http://thePoint.lww.com/activate for an interactive USMLE-style question bank and more!

CHAPTER 16
Third-Trimester Bleeding

This chapter deals primarily with APGO Educational Topic Area:

TOPIC 23   THIRD-TRIMESTER BLEEDING

Students should be able to differentiate the causes and potential complications of third-trimester bleeding and describe the evaluation of a patient with this condition.

They should outline a basic approach for initial evaluation and management in a patient with acute blood loss including appropriate use of blood products.

CLINICAL CASE

A visitor to your community, a 26-year-old G1 P0 at 36 weeks of gestational age, presents to your labor and delivery urgent evaluation area. She indicated she has had "some" prenatal care and that everything seemed to be going well until 2 hours earlier when she experienced an episode of vaginal bleeding much like a light menstrual period, except that there was no pain as is usual with her menses. She had no history of bleeding disorders or sexually transmitted diseases and had not been sexually active since about the eighth week of her pregnancy. She had had a pelvic ultrasound at 7 weeks of gestational age because of a concern of ectopic pregnancy, which, obviously, proved unwarranted.

INTRODUCTION

Approximately 4% to 5% of pregnancies are complicated by vaginal bleeding in the third trimester. Bleeding ranges from spotting to life-threatening hemorrhage. Intercourse, trichomonas cervicitis, and recent pelvic examinations are common precipitants of spotting because the cervix is more vascular and friable in pregnancy. Bleeding from hemorrhoids may be mistaken for vaginal bleeding, but the difference is easily distinguished by examination. At term, a woman's total blood volume increases by about 40% and her cardiac output by about 30%. About 20% of this term cardiac output is shunted to the pregnant uterus, so significant bleeding can be quickly catastrophic. Severe hemorrhage is much less common than spotting but remains a leading cause of maternal and fetal morbidity and mortality.

The two most common causes of significant bleeding in the third trimester are **placenta previa** and **placental abruption**. In placenta previa, the placenta is located close to or over the cervical os. Placental abruption is premature separation of the placenta. The paradigm is that painful bleeding usually means placental abruption, whereas painless bleeding usually means placenta previa.

Other important causes of bleeding include preterm cervical change, preterm labor, and uterine rupture (see Chapters 15 and 17). In many cases, bleeding remains unexplained or is attributed to local lesions. Possible anatomic causes of third-trimester bleeding are listed in Box 16.1.

HISTORY AND PHYSICAL EXAMINATION

A timely, focused history and physical examination are crucial in assessing third-trimester bleeding once the patient is stable, and a reassuring fetal heart rate pattern is confirmed. Although diagnosis is rarely based solely on history, a differential diagnosis is usually possible after pertinent information has been gathered. It is always important to quantify bleeding and associated symptoms such as abdominal pain. A personal or family history of bleeding with procedures may lead to a diagnosis of a bleeding disorder such as **von Willebrand disease**, whereas a history of cervical dysplasia and no recent Pap tests would be worrisome for cervical cancer. It is also important to consider bleeding from other organs, such as hemorrhoids from the anus or gross hematuria from acute cystitis.

A physical examination should always begin with maternal vital signs, although significant changes are not seen until the blood loss exceeds 10% to 15% of the total blood volume. The fetal heart rate should be auscultated by either Doppler or electronic fetal monitor or assessed with bedside real-time ultrasound. A general review of respiratory and cardiovascular systems is warranted in all patients. Intravenous (IV) access should be established if the bleeding is heavy, estimated blood loss is significant, or the patient is unstable. A brief inspection for **petechiae**, or **bruising**, may be indicated if there is suspicion of a bleeding disorder including a coagulopathy. Abdominal examination should focus on whether the uterus is soft or firm and tender and if signs of hemoperitoneum are present. The presence or absence of bowel sounds can be misleading in this obstetric emergency situation. Bimanual pelvic

152

BOX 16.1 — Causes of Bleeding in the Second Half of Pregnancy

- Anal
  - Hemorrhoids
  - Trauma—tears and lacerations
- Vulvar
  - Varicose veins
  - Trauma—tears and lacerations
- Vaginal
  - Trauma—tears and lacerations
- Cervical
  - Labor
  - Cervicitis
  - Polyp
  - Ectropion
  - Friable glandular tissue
  - Trauma—tears and lacerations
  - Carcinoma
- Uterine
  - Uterine rupture
  - Placenta previa
  - Placental abruption
  - Vasa previa

examination should not be undertaken until placental position is confirmed by ultrasound, as it could cause hemorrhage by inadvertent detachment of the placenta. Instead, inspection of the vulva may be followed by a careful speculum examination of the vagina and cervix.

A common finding in pregnancy is a significant **ectropion** of the cervix, particularly among women with a history of using oral contraceptives. The ectropion is an area on the ectocervix where columnar epithelium has been exposed to vaginal acidity due to eversion of the endocervix. The ectropion may appear reddened and "raw looking," and mild bleeding can occur. These findings may raise concerns about cancer, but they are actually benign.

Bleeding

Significant bleeding is an obstetric emergency requiring immediate management, including ongoing monitoring of vital signs and placement of sufficient large-bore IV lines for the rapid administration of crystalloid fluid, blood, and blood products.

Baseline studies should be ordered when excessive blood loss is suspected and should be repeated periodically as clinical circumstances warrant. Clinicians should remember that the results of some studies may be misleading because equilibration may not have occurred. In addition, response to hemorrhage may be required before laboratory results are known. Baseline studies include a complete blood count with platelets, a prothrombin time, an activated partial thromboplastin time, fibrinogen, and a type and cross order. The blood bank should be notified that transfusion may be necessary. Patients who are Rh D-negative may require immunoglobulin to protect against the Rh D antigen, and a **Kleihauer-Betke test** to determine fetomaternal bleeding should be performed to determine the amount of immunoglobulin needed once the bleeding has been controlled (see Chapter 15).

Because stored blood has a higher concentration of potassium, hyperkalemia may occur, especially if a large number of units of blood is transfused. Staff should be ready for delivery, which is facilitated by having a rapid response system in place for such emergency situations. Most likely, this will require an emergency caesarean delivery and, possibly, a general anesthetic. If the bleeding is not sufficient to warrant emergency delivery and/or the fetus is preterm, then blood studies should be continued and IV access maintained. An ultrasound examination should be performed to assess placental location and condition of the fetus. The patient should be admitted to the hospital to allow for close monitoring.

Vaginal hemorrhage in the third trimester is one of the few true obstetric emergencies.

PLACENTA PREVIA

Placenta previa is a placental location close to or over the internal cervical os and is associated with an increase in preterm birth and perinatal mortality and morbidity. It can be classified as **complete**, in which the placenta completely covers the internal os, or **partial**, in which the placenta overlies part but not all of the internal os. A placental edge within 2 centimeters of the internal os without covering it is called a **marginal previa** while a placenta that extends into the lower uterine segment but is more than 2 centimeters from the os is called a **low-lying placenta** (Fig. 16.1).

Painless bleeding in the third trimester is classically associated with placenta previa. In many cases there may be small amounts of bleeding prior to a more significant episode of bleeding. About 75% of women with placenta previa will have at least one episode of bleeding. On average, this episode occurs at around 29 to 30 weeks of gestation. The number of bleeding episodes is unrelated to the degree of placenta previa or to fetal outcome. In general, placenta previa occurs in about 1 in 200 pregnancies. The incidence of placenta previa earlier in pregnancy (approximately 24 weeks) is 4% to 5% and decreases with increasing gestational age.

Complete placenta previa rarely resolves spontaneously, but partial and low-lying placenta previa will often resolve by 32 to 35 weeks of gestation. The mechanism of this resolution does not involve an upward "migration" of the placenta but, rather, a stretching and thinning of the lower uterine segment, which effectively moves the placenta away from the os.

Diagnosis, Etiology, and Risk Factors

Transvaginal ultrasonography is more accurate in diagnosing placenta previa than abdominal ultrasonography, which gives many false-positive results, particularly when the placenta is

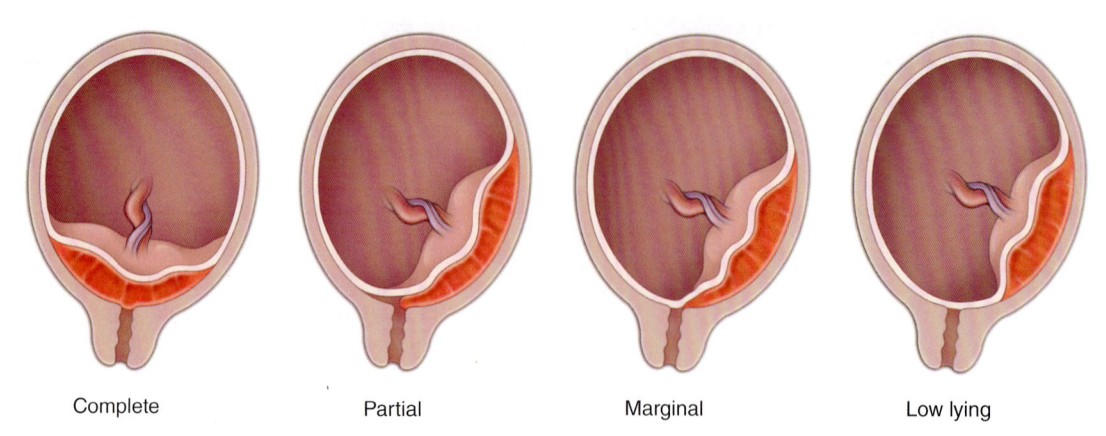

FIGURE 16.1. Placenta previa. (Adapted from Oyelese Y, Smulian JC. Placenta previa, accreta, and vasa previa. *Obstet Gynecol*. 2006;10(4):927.)

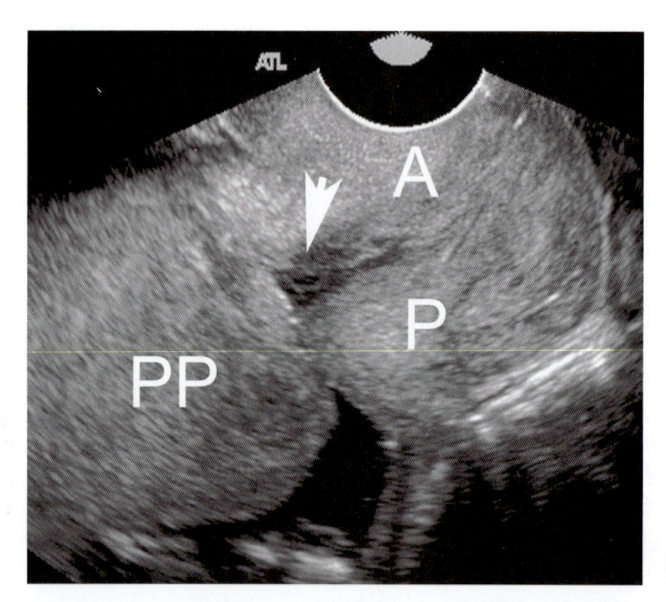

FIGURE 16.2. Transvaginal sonogram of a complete placenta previa (PP). Note that both the placenta and the internal cervical os *(arrow)* are clearly depicted. *A*, anterior lip of cervix; *P*, posterior lip of cervix. The placenta just overlaps the internal os. (From Oyelese Y, Smulian JC. Placenta previa, accreta, and vasa previa. *Obstet Gynecol*. 2006;107(4):927.)

located posteriorly (Fig. 16.2). The etiology of placenta previa is not known; however, it may be associated with abnormal vascularization. Risk factors for placenta previa include placenta previa in a prior pregnancy (4% to 8% recurrence), prior cesarean delivery or other uterine surgery, multiparty, advanced maternal age, cocaine use, and smoking. Placenta previa has been associated with a slight increase in fetal anomalies, although the precise mechanism is unclear. These anomalies include severe cardiovascular, central nervous system, gastrointestinal, and respiratory abnormalities.

Management

The first bleeding episode usually ceases in 1 to 2 hours if it was not severe enough to require delivery. Close observation, frequent blood pressure measurements, fluid administration, bed rest, and administration of steroids for fetal lung maturity may be appropriate if the fetus is premature and the bleeding is not heavy enough to warrant immediate delivery. The bleeding is usually painless, except when it is associated with labor or abruption (the premature separation of the placenta; see Table 16.1 for a comparison of placenta previa and placental abruption). For patients in a stable condition, cesarean delivery between 36 0/7 and 37 6/7 weeks is indicated. Delivery via caesarean birth is the rule unless it occurs earlier in pregnancy (i.e., at 20 weeks).

Complicating factors including abnormal fetal heart tracings, preeclampsia, or other conditions may be indications for immediate delivery at an earlier gestational age.

A single course of betamethasone is recommended for pregnant women between 34 0/7 and 36 6/7 weeks of gestation at risk of preterm birth within 7 days, and who have not received a previous course of antenatal corticosteroids.

Complications

Complications of placenta previa include increased bleeding from the lower uterine segment where the placenta was attached at the time of cesarean delivery. The placenta may also be abnormally adherent to the uterine wall. This is termed **placenta accreta** if the placental tissue extends into the superficial layer of the myometrium, **placenta increta** if it extends further into the myometrium, or **placenta percreta** if it extends completely through the myometrium to the serosa, and sometimes into adjacent organs such as the bladder (Fig. 16.3). The incidence of placenta accreta is about 1 in 533 deliveries but increases in patients with a history of cesarean delivery or previous uterine surgery. The risk of emergent hysterectomy (decision for the hysterectomy made intraoperatively or shortly postoperatively due to uncontrollable bleeding following a caesarean delivery) for patients with placenta previa is increased, which, in turn, increases the risk of maternal and perinatal morbidity and mortality. Generally, the recommended management of suspected placenta accreta is planned preterm cesarean hysterectomy with

TABLE 16.1 CHARACTERISTICS OF PLACENTA PREVIA AND PLACENTAL ABRUPTION

Characteristic	Placenta Previa	Placental Abruption
Magnitude of blood loss	Variable	Variable
Duration	Often ceases within 1–2 hours	Usually continuous
Abdominal pain	Absent	Present, often severe
Fetal heart rate pattern on electronic monitoring	Normal	Tachycardia, then bradycardia; loss of variability; decelerations frequently present; intrauterine demise not rare
Coagulation defects	Rare	Associated, but infrequent; disseminated intravascular coagulation often severe when present
Associated history	Placenta previa in a prior pregnancy (4%–8% recurrence); prior cesarean delivery or other uterine surgery; multiparty; advanced maternal age; cocaine use; smoking	Chronic hypertension, preeclampsia; multiple gestation; advanced maternal age; multiparty; smoking; cocaine use; and chorioamnionitis. Trauma is also a major risk factor, and patients involved in a vehicle accident (even if wearing a seat belt), fall, or other trauma should be evaluated for the possibility of abruption.

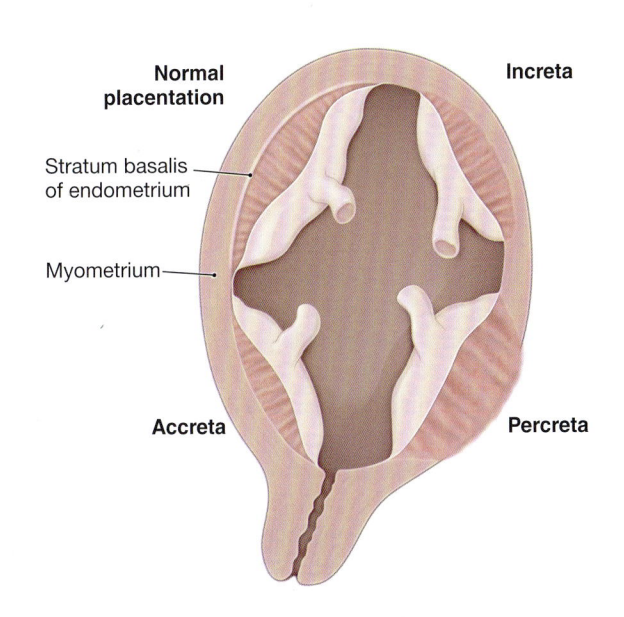

FIGURE 16.3. Placenta accreta, increta, and percreta.

the placenta left in situ because removal of the placenta is associated with significant hemorrhagic morbidity. Planned cesarean hysterectomy could actually decrease perinatal morbidity and mortality when compared to emergent rates.

PLACENTAL ABRUPTION

Placental abruption refers to an abnormal premature separation of an otherwise normally implanted placenta. There are various types of abruption depending upon the extent and region of separation. A **complete abruption** occurs when the entire placenta separates. A **partial abruption** exists when part of the placenta separates from the uterine wall. A **marginal abruption** occurs when the separation is limited to the edge of the placenta (Fig. 16.4). A significant abruption requiring delivery occurs in 1% of births.

Abruption occurs when bleeding in the decidua basalis causes separation of the placenta and further bleeding. The classic presentation of abruption is vaginal bleeding with abdominal pain. Smaller or marginal abruptions may present with bleeding only. **Concealed hemorrhage** occurs when blood is trapped behind the placenta and is unable to exit. Painful uterine contractions, significant fetal heart rate abnormalities, and fetal demise may occur in severe cases of concealed placental abruption.

Risk Factors

Risk factors for placental abruption include chronic hypertension, preeclampsia, multiple gestation, advanced maternal age, multiparty, smoking, cocaine use, and chorioamnionitis. Trauma is also a major risk factor, and patients involved in a vehicle accident (even if wearing a seat belt), fall, or other trauma should be evaluated for the possibility of abruption. Typically, fetal heart rate monitoring for a minimum of 4 hours is performed. Abruption in a prior pregnancy increases the risk of abruption in subsequent pregnancies by 15- to 20-fold. An elevated second-trimester maternal serum alpha-fetoprotein (AFP) level may be associated with up to a 10-fold increased risk of placental abruption due to possible entry of AFP into the maternal circulation through the placental uterine interface.

Diagnosis and Management

Abruption is often diagnosed by clinical examination, although an ultrasound examination may be useful in less severe cases not requiring immediate delivery. Abruption may occur in the absence of ultrasound findings.

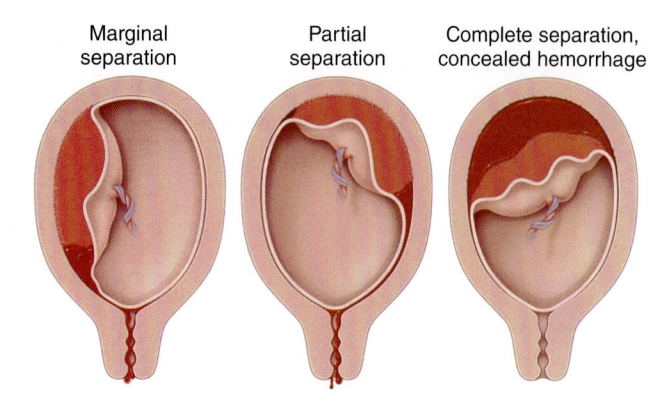

FIGURE 16.4. Types of placental abruption. Note that vaginal bleeding is absent when the hemorrhage is concealed.

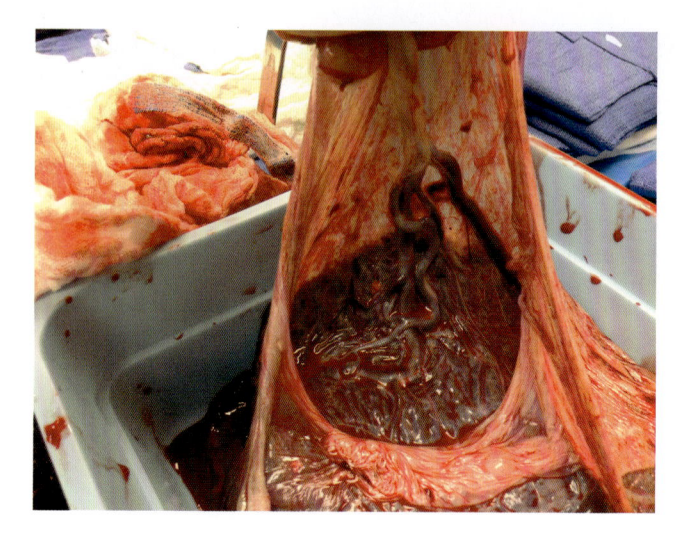

FIGURE 16.5. Velamentous insertion. Vessels are seen running unprotected through the membranes. *p*, placenta. From Robert Casanova Texas Tech University Health Sciences Center

Management of patients with placental abruption includes monitoring of vital signs, fluid administration, and delivery for severe hemorrhage. Expectant management may be appropriate for preterm patients with less severe abruptions and minimal bleeding. Decision for delivery is based on fetal status, the amount of bleeding, and gestational age. Delivery is often by cesarean birth, but vaginal delivery frequently is possible, and may even follow a rapid labor.

Complications

Rarely, blood penetrates the uterus to such an extent that the serosa becomes blue or purple in color. This condition is called **Couvelaire uterus**. A Kleihauer-Betke or similar test is essential to determine the amount of fetal–maternal hemorrhage. Results guide decisions regarding administration of Rh D immunoglobulin in women who are Rh D-negative and determine the need for blood transfusion in the potentially anemic neonate. Abruption is the most common cause of coagulopathy in pregnancy (see Table 16.1). Platelet counts may be low, and prothrombin time and partial thromboplastin time may be increased. Serum fibrinogen may also be depleted. Disseminated intravascular coagulation is a rare but extremely serious complication.

VASA PREVIA

Vasa previa describes the passage of fetal blood vessels over the internal os below the presenting part of the fetus. It can occur with a **velamentous insertion**, in which the fetal blood vessels insert into the membranes between the amnion and chorion instead of into the placenta and are not protected by Wharton jelly (Fig. 16.5), or when there is a succenturiate lobe across the os from the main placenta. Vasa previa occurs in 1 in 2000 to 5000 pregnancies. Rupture of a fetal vessel occurs rarely in pregnancy, but the risk is greatest with vasa previa. Rupture of a vessel can quickly lead to fetal death, as fetal blood volume is so small. Fetal mortality approaches 60% if rupture is not detected before delivery.

Tests

An **Apt test** can help distinguish fetal blood from maternal blood and may be useful if the test is rapidly available and bleeding is worrisome but not significant enough to warrant emergency delivery. This test mixes the blood specimen with water to achieve hemolysis. The centrifuged supernatant is mixed with sodium hydroxide (NaOH). Fetal blood remains pink, and maternal blood turns yellow-brown.

Rapidly performed transvaginal ultrasound examination with color Doppler may confirm a vasa previa engendering a rapid delivery—usually caesarean delivery. In actuality, though, complications from vasa previa usually remain unanticipated until unexpected bleeding occurs and is often iatrogenic. When performing artificial rupture of membranes, it is important to ensure that no pulsating vessels are present, which may represent a vasa previa.

UTERINE RUPTURE

Uterine rupture describes a spontaneous complete transection of the uterus from the endometrium to the serosa. If the peritoneum remains intact, it is referred to as a **partial rupture**, or **uterine dehiscence**. Most cases of uterine rupture occur at the site of a prior cesarean delivery. With complete rupture and fetal expulsion into the abdomen, fetal mortality ranges from 50% to 75%. Fetal survival depends in large part on whether a substantial portion of the placenta remains attached to the uterine wall until delivery is accomplished. Cesarean delivery is imperative to ensure neonatal survival and decrease maternal morbidity.

CLINICAL FOLLOW-UP

Her fundal height was consistent with her stated gestational age, and her uterus was not tender to palpation. The Leopold maneuvers are consistent with an unengaged cephalic presentation. There is no history of rupture of membranes. She was immediately placed on an electronic fetal monitor. No uterine contractions were noted, and the fetal heart rate was 140 beats per minute with good variability. Because her signs and symptoms were more consistent with third-trimester bleeding caused by placenta previa rather than placental abruption or other less common causes of third-trimester bleeding, pelvic examination was deferred, and an obstetric ultrasound was obtained. A complete placenta previa was discovered, and an appropriate obstetric management followed.

---

thePoint® Visit http://thePoint.lww.com/activate for an interactive USMLE-style question bank and more!

CHAPTER 17

Premature Rupture of Membranes

This chapter deals primarily with APGO Educational Topic Area:

TOPIC 25   PREMATURE RUPTURE OF MEMBRANES

Students should be able to list risk factors, possible etiologies, and complications of preterm rupture of membranes. They should be able to outline a basic approach to evaluation and management options, including a description of risks and benefits of expectant management versus immediate delivery. They should understand the role of gestational age in decision-making and describe appropriate maternal and fetal monitoring in the setting of premature rupture of membranes.

CLINICAL CASE

Your patient presents at 28 weeks of gestation complaining of a "gush" of fluid from her vagina while standing at work today. The triage nurse on Labor and Delivery obtains the patient's vital signs and places the fetal and uterine monitors, then calls you to evaluate the patient. What are your next steps in evaluation? What factors will affect how you manage this patient?

● INTRODUCTION

Amniotic fluid is normally produced continuously and, after approximately 16 weeks of gestation, is predominantly dependent on fetal urine production. However, passage of fluid across the fetal membranes, skin, and umbilical cord; fetal saliva production; and fetal pulmonary effluent also contribute. Amniotic fluid protects against infection, fetal trauma, and umbilical cord compression. It also allows for fetal movement and fetal breathing, which, in turn, permits fetal skeletal, chest, and lung development. Decreased or absent amniotic fluid can lead to compression of the umbilical cord and decreased placental blood flow. Disruption (rupture) of the fetal membranes is associated with loss of the protective effects and developmental roles of amniotic fluid.

● CLINICAL IMPACT

Premature rupture of membranes (PROM) is the rupture of the chorioamniotic membrane before the onset of labor. PROM is associated with about 8% of term pregnancies (37 weeks or more of gestational age) and is generally followed by the onset of labor. Preterm PROM (PPROM), defined as PROM that occurs before 37 weeks of gestation, is a leading cause of neonatal morbidity and mortality and is associated with approximately 30% of preterm deliveries. PROM leading to preterm delivery is associated with neonatal complications of prematurity such as respiratory distress syndrome, intraventricular hemorrhage, neonatal infection, necrotizing enterocolitis, neurologic and neuromuscular dysfunction, and sepsis. The most significant maternal risk of term PROM is intrauterine infection, a risk that increases with the duration of membrane rupture. The presence of lower genital tract infections with *Neisseria gonorrhoeae* and group B streptococcus (GBS), as well as bacterial vaginosis (BV) increases the risk of intrauterine infection associated with PROM. Other complications include prolapsed umbilical cord and abruptio placentae.

Consequences of PPROM depend on the gestational age at the time of occurrence. Rupture of the membranes before viability occurs in less than 1% of pregnancies. The probability of neonatal death and morbidity associated with PROM decreases with longer latency and advancing gestational age. PROM that occurs early in pregnancy following midtrimester genetic amniocentesis is very likely to seal with reaccumulation of amniotic fluid. Persistent oligohydramnios at <22 weeks of gestation is associated with incomplete alveolar development and the development of pulmonary hypoplasia. Survival is likely in the 24- to 26-week group, although the morbidities of extreme prematurity in this group of neonates are more substantial. Infants born with pulmonary hypoplasia cannot be adequately ventilated, regardless of the gestational age at birth, and soon succumb to hypoxia and barotrauma from high-pressure ventilation.

● ETIOLOGY

The cause of PROM is not clearly understood. Sexually transmitted infections (STIs) and other lower genital tract conditions, such as BV, may play a role, insofar as women with these infections are at higher risk for PROM than those without STI or BV. However, intact fetal membranes and normal amniotic fluid do not fully protect the fetus from infection, because it appears that subclinical intra-amniotic infection may contribute to PROM. Metabolites produced by bacteria and inflammatory mediators may either weaken the fetal membranes or initiate uterine contractions by stimulating prostaglandin synthesis.

Risk Factors

A history of PPROM is a major risk factor for preterm PROM or preterm labor in a subsequent pregnancy. Additional risk factors associated with PPROM are similar to those associated with spontaneous preterm birth and include short cervical length, second-trimester and third-trimester bleeding, low body mass index, low socioeconomic status, cigarette smoking, and illicit drug use. Although each of these risk factors is associated with PPROM, it often occurs in the absence of recognized risk factors or an obvious cause.

Chorioamnionitis

Chorioamnionitis (intra-amniotic infection), infection of the fetal membranes and amniotic fluid, poses a major threat to the mother and fetus. Fetal sepsis is associated with an increased risk of morbidity, particularly neurologic abnormalities, such as periventricular leukomalacia and cerebral palsy, secondary to increased inflammatory mediators in the fetal environment. Patients with intra-amniotic infection often experience significant fever (≥100.5°F), tachycardia (maternal and fetal), and uterine tenderness. Purulent cervical discharge is usually a very late finding. The maternal white blood cell (WBC) count is generally elevated, but this finding is nonspecific, and potentially misleading in pregnancy. It may also be the result of antenatal corticosteroid administration. Patients with chorioamnionitis frequently enter spontaneous and often dysfunctional labor. Once the diagnosis of chorioamnionitis is made, treatment consists of intravenous (IV) antibiotic therapy and delivery. Intra-amniotic infection alone is not an indication for urgent delivery, and the route of delivery in most situations should be based on standard obstetric indications. Intra-amniotic infection alone is rarely, if ever, an indication for cesarean delivery.

● DIAGNOSIS

Fluid passing through the vagina must be presumed to be amniotic fluid until proven otherwise. At times, patients describe a "gush" of fluid, whereas at other times they note a history of steady leakage of small amounts of fluid. Intermittent urinary leakage is common during pregnancy, especially near term, and this can be confused with PROM. Likewise, the normally increased vaginal secretions in pregnancy as well as perineal moisture (from perspiration) may be mistaken for amniotic fluid.

The differential diagnoses for PROM include urinary incontinence, increased vaginal secretions in pregnancy (physiologic), increased cervical discharge (pathologic, e.g., infection), and exogenous fluids (such as semen or douche). Most cases of PROM can be diagnosed on the basis of the patient's history and physical examination. Examination should be performed in a manner that minimizes the risk of introducing infection.

Nitrazine Test

The **nitrazine test** uses pH to distinguish amniotic fluid from urine and vaginal secretions. Amniotic fluid is alkaline, having a pH above 7.1; vaginal secretions have a pH of 4.5 to 6.0, and urine has a pH of ≤6.0. To perform the nitrazine test, a sample of fluid obtained from the vagina during a speculum examination is placed on a strip of paper or swab impregnated with nitrazine. If the pH is 7.1 to 7.3, reflecting that of amniotic fluid, the paper or swab turns dark blue. Cervical mucus, blood, and semen are possible causes of false-positive results (Box 17.1).

Fern Test

The **fern test** is also used to distinguish amniotic fluid from other fluids. It is named for the pattern of arborization that occurs when amniotic fluid is placed on a slide and is allowed to dry in room air. The resultant pattern, which resembles the leaves of a fern plant, is caused by the sodium chloride content of the amniotic fluid. The ferning pattern from amniotic fluid is fine, with multiple branches, as shown in Figure 17.1. Cervical mucus does not typically show ferning, or, if it does, the pattern is thick with much less branching. This test is considered more indicative of ruptured membranes than the nitrazine test, but as with any test, it is not 100% reliable.

Ultrasonography

Ultrasonography can be helpful in evaluating the possibility of rupture of membranes. If ample amniotic fluid around the fetus is visible on ultrasound examination, the diagnosis of PROM must be questioned. However, if the amount of amniotic fluid leakage is small, sufficient amniotic fluid will still be visible on scan. When there is less than the expected amount of fluid seen on ultrasound, the differential diagnosis of oligohydramnios, including PROM, must be considered. When the clinical history or physical examination is unclear, membrane rupture can be diagnosed unequivocally with ultrasonographically guided transabdominal instillation of indigo carmine dye, followed by observation for passage of blue fluid from the vagina. However, this procedure is performed very infrequently.

BOX 17.1 Causes of False-Positive and False-Negative Nitrazine Tests

False Positive
- Basic urine
- Semen
- Cervical mucus
- Blood contamination
- Some antiseptic solutions
- Vaginitis (especially trichomonas)

False Negative
- Remote PROM with no residual fluid
- Minimal amniotic fluid leakage

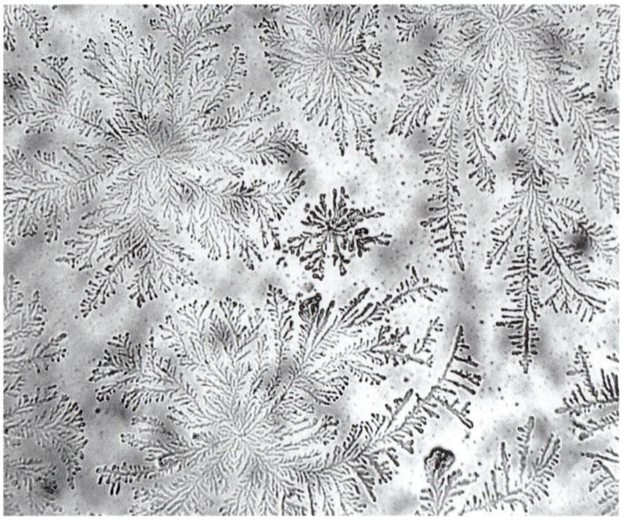

FIGURE 17.1. Ferning pattern from amniotic fluid. (Courtesy of Dr. Dwight Rouse. Gibbs RS, Karlan BY, Haney AF, Nygaard IE. *Danforth's Obstetrics and Gynecology.* 10th ed. Philadelphia, PA: Lippincott Williams & Wilkins; 2008, p. 27.)

● EVALUATION AND MANAGEMENT

Factors to be considered in the management of the patient with PROM include the gestational age at the time of rupture, assessment of fetal well-being, the presence of uterine contractions, the likelihood of chorioamnionitis, the amount of amniotic fluid around the fetus, and the degree of fetal maturity. These management factors, together with the patient's history, must be carefully evaluated for information relevant to the diagnosis and approach.

Physical Examination

Abdominal examination includes palpation of the uterus for tenderness and fundal height measurement for evaluation of gestational age and fetal lie.

A sterile speculum examination is performed to assess the likelihood of vaginal infection and to obtain cervical or vaginal cultures for *N. gonorrhoeae*, *Chlamydia trachomatis*, and Group B streptococcus. The cervix is visualized for its degree of dilation as well as for the presence of free-flowing amniotic fluid. Fluid is obtained from the vaginal vault for nitrazine and/or fern testing. Because of the risk of infection, **digital examination** should be kept to a minimum and is best avoided until the patient is in active labor or imminent delivery is planned.

Ultrasound examination can be helpful in determining gestational age, verifying the fetal presentation, and assessing the amount of amniotic fluid remaining within the uterine cavity. It has been shown that labor and infection are less likely to occur when an adequate volume of amniotic fluid remains within the uterus.

Term Premature Rupture of Membranes

If PROM occurs at term (≥37 weeks of gestation), spontaneous labor will ensue in 90% of women within about 24 hours. For women with PROM at term, labor should be induced at the time of presentation, generally with oxytocin infusion, to reduce the risk of chorioamnionitis.

However, with informed consent, induction of labor at any time after presentation of a PROM at term is also considered appropriate. The physician should discuss induction versus expectant management, taking into account, in addition to the risk of infection, that oxytocin administration is associated with a decreased risk of chorioamnionitis and endometritis. There appears to be a decrease in the incidence of cesarean delivery in patients managed expectantly. Serial evaluation for the development of intrauterine infection (fever, uterine tenderness, and maternal and/or fetal tachycardia) and other complications of PROM is requisite with expectant management, which, in most cases, should not extend beyond 24 hours in term pregnancy. When the decision to deliver is made, GBS prophylaxis should be given based on prior culture results or risk factors if cultures have not been previously performed.

Preterm Premature Rupture of Membranes

The time from PROM to labor is called the **latency period** and is inversely related to gestational age. Between 28 weeks and term, about 50% of patients go into labor within 24 hours and 80% within 1 week. Only 50% of patients whose gestational age is 24 to 28 weeks go into labor within 1 week of PROM. It also appears that the more severe the **oligohydramnios**, the greater the risk of infection and, consequently, the shorter the latency.

Amniocentesis can be helpful in assessing fetal lung maturity (FLM) but can be difficult in the setting of PROM and oligohydramnios. In addition to tests of FLM, evaluation for intra-amniotic infection (using the presence of bacteria on Gram stain, elevated WBC count, low glucose level, or a positive culture) can also be performed. If there is sufficient volume, FLM tests can also be performed on amniotic fluid obtained vaginally.

If there is strong clinical suspicion for the presence of uterine infection, delivery should be effected as soon as possible, regardless of gestational age. If the evaluation suggests intrauterine infection, IV antibiotic therapy and delivery are indicated, regardless of gestational age. The antibiotic prescribed should have a broad spectrum of coverage because of the polymicrobial nature of the infection. The effect of tocolysis to permit antibiotic and antenatal corticosteroid administration in the patient with PPROM who is having contractions has yet to be conclusively evaluated; therefore, specific recommendations for or against tocolysis administration cannot be made. Evidence does suggest neonatal benefit from administration of a single course of steroids (betamethasone or dexamethasone) regardless of membrane status in PPROM, and likely even for those in the late preterm period (34 0/7 to 36 6/7 weeks) who have not previously received a course of steroids. If the gestational age is thought to be in the transitional time of fetal maturity (i.e., from 34 to 36 weeks), the management is variable, depending on individual circumstances (Table 17.1).

TABLE 17.1 MANAGEMENT OF PREMATURE RUPTURE OF MEMBRANES CHRONOLOGICALLY

Gestational Age	Management
Term (37 weeks or more)	Proceed to delivery, usually by induction of labor, if spontaneous labor does not occur soon after ROM
	Group B streptococcal prophylaxis as indicated
Late Preterm (34 weeks to 36 completed weeks)	Same as for term
	Consider corticosteroids if not previously received
Preterm (32 weeks to 33 completed weeks)	Expectant management, unless fetal pulmonary maturity is documented
	Group B streptococcal prophylaxis as indicated
	Single-course of corticosteroids recommended
	Antibiotics recommended to prolong latency, if there are no contradictions
Preterm (24 weeks to 31 completed weeks)	Expectant management
	Group B streptococcal prophylaxis as indicated
	Single-course corticosteroids recommended
	Tocolytics—no proven benefit
	Magnesium sulfate for fetal neuroprotection, if delivery thought to be imminent
	Antibiotics recommended to prolong latency, if there are no contradictions
Less than 24 weeks[a]	Patient counseling
	Expectant management or induction of labor
	Group B streptococcal prophylaxis, tocolysis, magnesium sulfate for fetal neuroprotection, and corticosteroids are not recommended before viability
	Antibiotics may be considered as early as 20 0/7 weeks of gestation

[a] The combination of birth weight, gestational age, and sex provides the best estimates of changes of survival and should be considered in individual cases.
Adapted from the American College of Obstetricians and Gynecologists. Premature rupture of membranes. *ACOG Practice Bulletin No. 172.* Washington, DC: American College of Obstetricians and Gynecologists; 2016.

32 Weeks to 33 Completed Weeks

Because of the increased risk of chorioamnionitis, delivery is recommended when PROM occurs at or beyond 34 weeks of gestation. If PROM occurs at 32 to 33 completed weeks of gestation, the risk of severe complications of prematurity is low if FLM is evident by amniotic fluid samples collected vaginally or by amniocentesis.

24 Weeks to 31 Completed Weeks

If PROM occurs at 24 to 31 completed weeks of gestation, patients should be admitted to the hospital and cared for expectantly, if no maternal or fetal contraindications exist, until 33 completed weeks of gestation. Prophylaxis using antibiotics to prolong latency and a single course of antenatal corticosteroids can help reduce the risks of infection and gestational age–dependent neonatal morbidity. Patients are assessed carefully on a daily basis for uterine tenderness as well as maternal or fetal tachycardia. WBC counts may be obtained and compared with baseline, although the maternal WBC count is, again, nonspecific and can be affected by glucocorticoid administration. Intermittent ultrasound assessment helps to determine amniotic fluid volumes, because leaking of fluid from the vagina may cease and allow amniotic fluid to reaccumulate around the fetus. Periodic antepartum testing, such as nonstress tests, can also be helpful to assess fetal well-being. In the absence of sufficient amniotic fluid to buffer the umbilical cord from external pressure, compression of the cord can lead to fetal heart rate decelerations. If the decelerations are repetitive and the fetal heart tracing nonreassuring, there should be early and expeditious delivery to avoid fetal compromise or death. Unfortunately, umbilical cord accidents often are unrecognized for a significant period of time, regardless of the monitoring regimen instituted. Electronic fetal monitoring is used frequently during the initial evaluation period to search for any fetal heart rate decelerations, although the fetal cardiac control mechanisms are often insufficiently developed in preterm fetuses to allow meaningful evaluation for fetal heart rate variability and reactivity.

Midtrimester Preterm Premature Rupture of Membranes

PROM at very early gestational ages (i.e., prior to 24 weeks of gestation) presents additional problems. Along with the risks of prematurity and infection already discussed, the very premature fetus faces the further hazards of pulmonary hypoplasia, skeletal malformations, and other consequences of prolonged oligohydramnios. The relation of PROM with both of these entities is both interesting and important. The inability of the fetus to move freely within the amniotic sac can lead to skeletal contractures, which can become permanent deformities. For normal fetal lung development to occur, fetal breathing must occur. During intrauterine life, the fetus normally inhales and exhales amniotic fluid, with the net movement out into the amniotic fluid space. This adds substances generated in the respiratory tree to the amniotic fluid pool, including the phospholipids that form the basis for many of the fetal maturity tests. If rupture of fetal membranes occurs before 22 weeks of gestation, the lack of amniotic fluid interferes with respiratory efforts and, thus, with sufficient pulmonary development. The result is a failure of normal growth and differentiation of the respiratory tree and fetal chest. If severe, pulmonary hypoplasia may occur, which leads to an inability to maintain ventilation.

Women presenting with PROM before potential viability should be counseled regarding the impact of immediate delivery and the potential risks and benefits of expectant management. Counseling should include a realistic appraisal of neonatal outcomes, including the availability of obstetric monitoring and neonatal intensive care facilities. Because of advances in perinatal care, morbidity and mortality rates continue to decline. An attempt should be made to provide parents with the most up-to-date information possible. Women with previable PPROM are usually managed expectantly, either at home or in the hospital. Once the pregnancy has reached viability, administration of antenatal corticosteroids for fetal maturation is appropriate, given that early delivery remains likely.

CLINICAL FOLLOW-UP

The sterile speculum examination you performed on your patient was positive for PPROM. You further evaluate the mother and fetus to rule out any obvious signs of chorioamnionitis, abruption, or active labor prior to determining whether you will move toward delivery or attempt to prolong the latency period from rupture of membranes to delivery.

---

thePoint® Visit **http://thePoint.lww.com/activate** for an interactive USMLE-style question bank and more!

CHAPTER 18
Post-term Pregnancy

This chapter deals primarily with APGO Educational Topic Area:

TOPIC 30 POST-TERM PREGNANCY

Students should be able to define post-term pregnancy and list possible maternal and fetal complications associated with post-term pregnancy. They should be able to outline a basic approach to evaluation and management options for post-term pregnancy.

CLINICAL CASE

A 26-year-old patient with lifelong irregular and infrequent periods presents with increasing abdominal girth and fatigue. She does not think she is pregnant because she had been told by a previous physician that she would have a hard time conceiving. Her pregnancy test is positive, and ultrasound of the abdomen shows a 39-week intrauterine pregnancy with an estimated fetal weight of 7 lb. She is unsure when she would have conceived. In addition to having routine prenatal laboratory tests performed, she asks about plans for timing of delivery.

INTRODUCTION

Normal full-term pregnancy lasts from 37 to 42 weeks. The "due date" or **estimated date of delivery** (**EDD**) is calculated to be 40 weeks from the first day of the **last menstrual period** (**LMP**), presuming regular, 28-day cycles and without recent, prior use of oral contraceptives. *Post-term pregnancy is a pregnancy lasting 42 weeks of gestation or beyond.* This condition occurs in approximately 6% of pregnancies and carries with it an increased risk of adverse outcome. The increased morbidity and mortality in a small percentage of cases, however, warrant careful evaluation of all post-term pregnancies. In addition, post-term pregnancies can create significant stress for the patient, her family, and those caring for her. Therefore, the physician should understand the condition and the options for management.

"Postdates" is a commonly used, but misleading synonym and should be avoided.

CAUSE

The most common "cause" of post-term pregnancy is inaccurate estimation of gestational age (dating). Inaccurate dating is more likely in women with irregular menses and, thus, inconsistent ovulation; women who seek prenatal care later in pregnancy; women with delayed ovulation (e.g., women who have recently discontinued oral contraceptives); and women who inaccurately recall their LMP. Inaccurate dating that leads to the erroneous classification of a pregnancy as post-term has important sequelae. These pregnancies are erroneously labeled "high risk," resulting in the use of costly and unnecessary evaluations. This, in turn, increases the likelihood of intervention, specifically, induction of labor and cesarean delivery, both of which are potentially associated with increased maternal and fetal morbidity. Other less common causes of post-term pregnancy are listed in Table 18.1.

Whatever the cause, there is a tendency for recurrence of post-term pregnancy. Approximately 50% of the patients who have one post-term pregnancy will experience prolonged pregnancy with the next gestation. Other important risk factors include maternal obesity, nulliparity, and post-term delivery of the mother. Based on twin studies, there also appears to be a genetic influence.

EFFECTS

Compared with term pregnancies, the morbidity and mortality rates for both mother and fetus increase severalfold with post-term pregnancy.

Risks of maternal vaginal trauma, labor dysfunction, and cesarean delivery increase. Cesarean delivery carries increased risks of infection, bleeding, thromboembolic phenomenon, and visceral injury. Stillbirth and neonatal mortality rates increase steadily after 37 weeks, approaching 1 in 300 at 42 weeks and increasing severalfold as the 44th week approaches. Post-term gestations are associated with several conditions that present diagnostic and management challenges: Macrosomia, shoulder dystocia, meconium aspiration syndrome (MAS), dysmaturity syndrome, and oligohydramnios.

163

TABLE 18.1	FACTORS ASSOCIATED WITH POST-TERM PREGNANCY
Factor	Discussion
Inaccurate or unknown dates	Most common cause; more common with late or no prenatal care
Irregular ovulation; variation in length of follicular phase	Results in overestimation of gestational age
Anencephaly	Decreased production of 16α-hydroxydehydroepiandrosterone beta-sulfate, a precursor of estriol
Fetal adrenal hypoplasia	Decreased fetal production of estriol precursors
Placental sulfatase deficiency	X-linked disease prevents placenta conversion of sulfated estrogen precursors
Extrauterine pregnancy	Pregnancy not in uterus, no labor (see Chapter 19)

Macrosomia

Macrosomia is defined as an abnormally large infant size, specifically, an infant weighing 4,500 g or greater. It occurs in approximately 2.5% to 10% of postterm pregnancies. Maternal obesity, diabetes mellitus, or a previous macrosomic infant further raises the risk. Macrosomia is associated with an increased incidence of birth trauma, particularly if the infant is delivered vaginally. Such trauma includes shoulder dystocia; fracture of the clavicle; and associated brachial plexus injury, specifically, Erb–Duchenne palsy.

Shoulder dystocia is an obstetric emergency caused by impaction of the anterior fetal shoulder behind the symphysis pubis during the process of vaginal delivery. A series of particular maneuvers (see Chapter 9) can be accomplished to release this impaction. Brachial plexus injury is reported in approximately 0.85 to 1.89 per 1,000 term deliveries, but increases 18- to 21-fold in macrosomic infants delivered vaginally; it can also occur during cesarean deliveries. In **Erb–Duchenne palsy**, paralysis, stretch, or tear injury to the upper roots of the brachial plexus, at C5 and C6, results in paralysis of the deltoid and infraspinatus muscles and flexor muscles of the forearm, causing the limb to hang limply close to the side, with the forearm extended and internally rotated. Finger function is usually retained. Less frequently, damage is limited to the lower nerves of the brachial plexus, C8 and T1, causing **Klumpke paralysis**, or paralysis of the hand. Because most brachial injuries are mild, treatment is expectant with splints and physical therapy in anticipation of complete or nearly complete recovery in 3 to 6 months. Around 80% to 90% of brachial plexus injuries completely resolve by age 1 year.

Maternal risks with fetal macrosomia include perineal and vaginal lacerations and postpartum hemorrhage if the fetus is delivered vaginally and a twofold increase in the rate of cesarean delivery, with its associated operative risks and maternal trauma.

Meconium Aspiration Syndrome

Another special concern in post-term pregnancies is **meconium passage** and **MAS**. MAS can lead to severe respiratory distress from mechanical obstruction of both small and large airways, as well as to meconium chemical pneumonitis. Meconium passage is not limited to post-term pregnancies, although prolonged pregnancy, particularly in the setting of oligohydramnios, is a significant risk factor. Meconium passage occurs in 12% to 22% of women in labor, with aspiration occurring in up to 10% of these infants.

The incidence of meconium passage increases as pregnancy becomes prolonged, as does the incidence of MAS.

Dysmaturity Syndrome

Dysmaturity syndrome, which refers to infants with characteristics resembling chronic growth restriction, affects up to 20% of post-term pregnancies. This syndrome may be associated with an aging placenta that is unable to provide adequate nutrition and/or oxygen diffusion for the fetus. These pregnancies are at increased risk of meconium aspiration, umbilical cord compression due to oligohydramnios, as well as short-term neonatal complications such as hypoglycemia, seizures, and respiratory insufficiency.

In post-term pregnancies, there is an increased incidence of nonreassuring fetal testing, both antepartum and intrapartum.

Oligohydramnios

Oligohydramnios is defined as decreased amniotic fluid for gestational age and is generally quantified as an amniotic fluid index less than 5 cm. This is measured by dividing the gravid abdomen into quadrants and totaling the measurements of the largest vertical pockets of fluid in each of those quadrants. In some facilities, a maximum vertical pocket less than 2 cm is used to define oligohydramnios. Amniotic fluid is a reflection of fetal swallowing, fetal breathing, fluid transfer across the amniotic sac, and, especially, fetal urination. The amniotic fluid reaches its maximum volume at approximately 34 to 36 weeks and stays constant or slightly decreases from then through the remainder of the pregnancy. Any alterations in the above processes can cause changes in amniotic fluid volume.

Oligohydramnios is associated with poor outcomes due to umbilical cord compression, uteroplacental insufficiency, and meconium aspiration.

Because of these risks, after 40 weeks of gestation, close antepartum surveillance is warranted if the pregnancy is allowed to continue. After 36 0/7 to 37 6/7 weeks gestation, oligohydramnios is an indication for delivery.

DIAGNOSIS

The diagnosis of post-term pregnancy rests on establishment of the correct gestational age.

The first step in management of a patient with suspected post-term pregnancy is a careful review of the criteria used to establish the gestational age. The most common information used to determine gestational age includes the patient's reported LMP and the first-trimester ultrasound. Ultrasound is most accurate for determining dating for gestational age when it is performed from 8 to 13 6/7 weeks of gestation. If dating by ultrasonography performed between 14 0/7 weeks and 15 6/7 weeks of gestation (inclusive) varies from LMP dating by more than 7 days, or if ultrasonography dating between 16 0/7 weeks and 21 6/7 weeks of gestation varies by more than 10 days, the EDD should be changed to correspond with the ultrasonography dating. Once the EDD is determined, it should not be changed unless more accurate information is subsequently available.

With improved access to prenatal care and greater importance placed on accurate gestational age assessment, the percentage of patients in whom post-term pregnancy is suspected has diminished. Nonetheless, a substantial number of patients do not seek prenatal care early in pregnancy or do not have an accurate gestational age determination. The prevalence of post-term pregnancy varies regionally, depending on the use of first-trimester ultrasound for gestational dating and routine labor induction.

MANAGEMENT

Once the gestational age is believed to be firmly established and the patient approaches 41 weeks of gestation, the two management options are (1) induction of labor and (2) **antepartum fetal surveillance**, which continues either until spontaneous labor occurs or until approximately 42 weeks. In the United States, very few pregnancies are allowed to progress beyond 42 weeks and virtually none beyond 43 weeks.

Factors that influence management include the patient's concerns, the assessment of fetal well-being, and the status of the patient's cervix.

Induction of labor is appropriate if the cervix is favorable and if the patient prefers such management. The risk of failed induction is low with a favorable cervix, and most authorities believe it is low enough to recommend delivery in light of the risk of increased fetal morbidity in the post-term period.

The data on preventing post-term pregnancy are controversial. Some studies show that **sweeping the membranes** may decrease post-term pregnancy; other studies differ. Sweeping the membranes is a procedure by which the amniotic sac is gently detached from the uterine wall at the level of the cervix and/or lower uterine segment. This procedure is thought to release prostaglandins, which can increase cervical dilation, making the cervix more favorable and sometimes leading to the onset of labor. Sweeping the membranes should not be performed unless the gestational age is verified and the fetus is at least 39 weeks gestation.

If the gestational age is not well established and the menstrual history and early ultrasound findings are not available, there is little additional information that can be used to determine the best estimate of gestational age.

Fetal Assessment

If the cervix is not favorable for induction, fetal well-being is monitored intermittently until either spontaneous labor occurs or the cervix "ripens," thereby making induction more feasible. Fetal evaluation has not been definitively shown to decrease mortality in post-term pregnancy because studies are either underpowered or are not randomized controlled trials; however, it is also not associated with any negative outcomes. Although a variety of management schemes have been devised to monitor fetal well-being, none has been shown to be superior. Thus, it is common practice to assess fetal well-being using several methods. Weekly monitoring of **amniotic fluid volume** is commonly used, insofar as oligohydramnios at term is a sufficient indication for delivery. **Nonstress tests** (fetal heart rate monitoring), **biophysical profiles** (ultrasound evaluation of fetal fluid, movement, tone, and breathing), or oxytocin challenge tests are typically done once a week. Another option is the combination of amniotic fluid assessment and nonstress test, known as the **modified biophysical profile**. Doppler flow studies of the umbilical artery are not considered useful. **Daily fetal movement counting** is included in most management plans, with decreased perceived fetal movement being an indication for immediate evaluation of fetal well-being. Results of these tests are most useful when considered within the context of other conditions affecting the mother and the fetus. If fetal test results are nonreassuring, delivery is indicated.

Labor Induction

Induction of labor between 41 0/7 weeks and 42 0/7 weeks of gestation can be considered. Induction of labor after 42 0/7 weeks and by 42 6/7 weeks of gestation is recommended given evidence of an increase in perinatal morbidity and mortality. The patient with an unfavorable cervix should be counseled about risks of induction of labor and the risks of continuing pregnancy with fetal evaluation to assist in clinical decision making. Both management plans—inducing labor and continued fetal surveillance—are associated with low rates of maternal and fetal morbidity in the low-risk patient. Although there is no absolute time by which labor must be induced, most physicians believe that delivery should occur before 42 completed weeks. Compared with expectant management, several studies have demonstrated that routine induction at 41 weeks, using cervical ripening agents, is associated with lower cesarean delivery rates, lower perinatal mortality, decreased length of hospital stay, decreased hospital cost, and higher patient satisfaction.

Several different agents are now available for cervical ripening, including intracervical or intravaginal preparation of prostaglandin, intracervical Foley bulb placement, and misoprostol. Oxytocin should ideally be initiated after the cervix is ripened.

Induction at 41 weeks is becoming the preferred management of post-term pregnancy. Because of the risk of macrosomia-associated birth trauma, ultrasonographic estimation of fetal weight should be obtained before induction of labor in a post-term pregnancy when macrosomia is suspected. If the estimated fetal weight is more than 5,000 g in a woman who does not have diabetes or 4,500 g in a woman with diabetes, elective cesarean delivery may be considered.

It should be noted that there is no accurate way of estimating fetal weight at term; ultrasonographic estimates have a calculation error up to 500 g late in pregnancy. Clinically determined estimated fetal weights by palpation of the patient's abdomen and Leopold maneuvers are similarly inaccurate.

For patients who are post-term, special precautions are taken at the time of delivery to provide prompt evaluation of the infant in the event of meconium passage. In a depressed infant, aggressive suctioning of the fetus with a laryngoscope decreases, but does not eliminate, the likelihood of MAS. In a vigorous infant with meconium passage, laryngoscopy and aggressive suctioning have not been shown to decrease the risk of MAS and are no longer recommended. Similarly, routine amnioinfusion is not recommended during labor when meconium passage has been noted.

CLINICAL FOLLOW-UP

Without a firm due date, and with an advanced pregnancy at the time of presentation, the concern for this patient's pregnancy is not prematurity, but the risk of a post-term delivery. Weekly fetal evaluation with testing such as a biophysical profile can be reassuring that the fetus is not in jeopardy. If testing is no longer reassuring prior to the spontaneous onset of labor, induction of labor would be appropriate.

CHAPTER 19
Ectopic Pregnancy and Abortion

This chapter deals primarily with APGO Educational Topic Areas:

TOPIC 15 ECTOPIC AREA PREGNANCY
TOPIC 16 SPONTANEOUS ABORTION
TOPIC 34 INDUCED ABORTION

Students should be able to outline a basic approach to evaluation and management of first-trimester bleeding. They should be able to discuss the differential diagnosis, associated risk factors, etiologies, and complications. Finally, they should be able to counsel a patient about pregnancy options including medical and surgical terminations and associated complications. They should understand the public health impact of access to abortion.

CLINICAL CASE

A 25-year-old woman reports that she had a positive home pregnancy test last week and now has spotting and low abdominal pain of 2 days' duration. Her last menstrual period was 6 weeks ago. Her abdomen is minimally tender in the left lower quadrant with no rebound tenderness. The pelvic examination is normal except for tenderness and a 4 cm mass in the left adnexa. Pelvic ultrasound shows an intact pregnancy consistent with her last period and a simple left ovarian cyst.

● ECTOPIC PREGNANCY

An **ectopic** or **extrauterine pregnancy** is one in which the blastocyst implants anywhere other than the endometrial lining of the uterine cavity. Ectopic pregnancies account for approximately 1.5% of reported pregnancies in the United States. As shown in Figure 19.1, 98% of ectopic pregnancies implant in the fallopian tube, with 80% occurring in the ampullary segment. Other locations include, but are not limited to, the ovary, cervix, and abdomen.

In the past, ectopic pregnancy was life threatening. Currently, earlier diagnosis made possible by the ability to detect the β-subunit of human chorionic gonadotropin (hCG), combined with high-resolution transvaginal sonography (TVS), has reduced this threat. Nevertheless, ectopic pregnancies remain an important cause of morbidity and mortality in the United States.

Tubal Ectopic Pregnancy

Without intervention, the natural course of a tubal pregnancy will result in any of three outcomes: tubal abortion, tubal rupture, or spontaneous resolution. **Tubal abortion** is the expulsion of the pregnancy through the fimbriated end. This tissue can then either regress or reimplant in the abdominal cavity. **Tubal rupture** is associated with significant intra-abdominal hemorrhage, often necessitating surgical intervention.

Pathophysiology and Risk Factors

An appreciation of risk factors for ectopic pregnancy can lead to making a more timely diagnosis resulting in both improved maternal survival and future reproductive potential. Inflammation resulting in tubal damage can disrupt the normal migration of a fertilized ovum through the tube, thereby predisposing to an ectopic pregnancy. Specific examples of an inflammatory process include **salpingitis** and **salpingitis isthmica nodosa**. An acute **chlamydial infection** causes intraluminal inflammation and subsequent fibrin deposition with tubal scarring. Despite negative cultures, persistent chlamydial antigens can trigger a delayed hypersensitivity reaction with continued scarring. Whereas endotoxin-producing *Neisseria gonorrhoeae* causes virulent pelvic inflammation with a rapid clinical onset, chlamydial inflammatory response is indolent and peaks at 7 to 14 days. The incidence of ectopic pregnancy has increased consistently with the rise in chlamydial infections.

Pregnancy after tubal sterilization is rare, but, when it does occur, there is a substantial risk that the pregnancy will be ectopic due to the distorted tubal anatomy created by the tubal ligation. Previous concerns that intrauterine device use and pregnancy termination are predisposing risks for ectopic pregnancy have been dispelled. A history of infertility, independent of tubal disease, and ovulation induction also appear to be risk factors in ectopic pregnancy. Additional risk factors include prior ectopic pregnancy, smoking, prior tubal surgery, diethylstilbestrol exposure, and advanced age.

Symptoms

With the availability of early pregnancy testing, the ability to diagnose ectopic pregnancy before rupture—even before the onset of symptoms—is not unusual. The classic symptoms associated with ectopic pregnancy are amenorrhea followed by vaginal bleeding and abdominal pain on the affected side; however, there is no constellation of symptoms that are diagnostic.

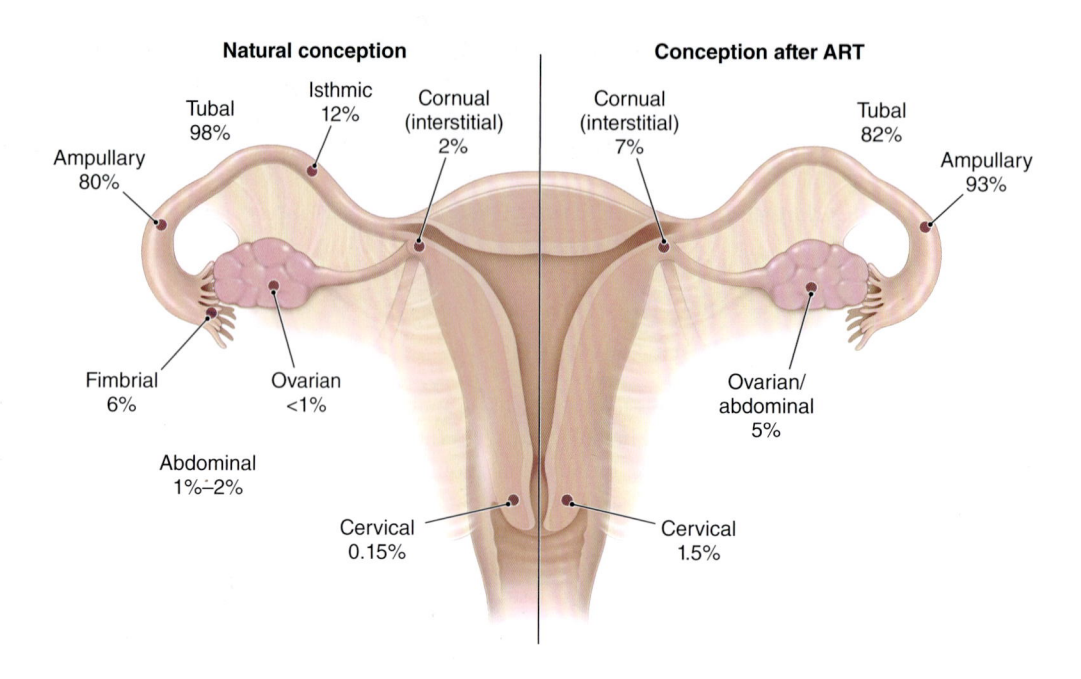

FIGURE 19.1. Incidence of types of ectopic pregnancy by location. ART, assisted reproductive technologies.

Normal pregnancy symptoms, such as breast tenderness, nausea, and urinary frequency, may accompany more ominous findings. These include shoulder pain worsened by inspiration and caused by phrenic nerve irritation from subdiaphragmatic blood as well as vasomotor disturbances, such as vertigo and syncope from hemorrhagic hypovolemia. As long as placental hormones are produced, there is usually no vaginal bleeding. Irregular vaginal bleeding results from the sloughing of the decidua from the endometrial lining. Vaginal bleeding in patients with an ectopic gestation may range from little or none to heavy, menstrual-like flow. In some patients, the entire "decidual cast" is passed intact, simulating a spontaneous abortion. Histologic evaluation of this tissue confirms whether placental villi are present. In any pregnant patient with no histopathologic confirmation of chorionic villi within the uterus, an ectopic implantation should be assumed to be present until proven otherwise.

Many women with a small unruptured ectopic pregnancy may have unremarkable clinical findings. Nevertheless, the diagnosis should be considered strongly when any of the above symptoms are reported by reproductive age women, especially those with risk factors for an extrauterine pregnancy.

Clinical Findings

Abdominal and pelvic findings are notoriously scant in many women before tubal rupture.

Prior to rupture, the diagnosis of an ectopic pregnancy is primarily based on laboratory and ultrasound findings. With rupture, however, nearly three-fourths of women will have marked tenderness on both abdominal and pelvic examination, and pain is aggravated with cervical manipulation. A pelvic mass, including fullness posterolateral to the uterus, can be palpated in about 20% of women. Initially, the ectopic pregnancy may feel soft and elastic, whereas extensive hemorrhage produces a firmer consistency. Many times, discomfort precludes palpation of the mass. Not performing a pelvic examination may actually help avert iatrogenic rupture.

Given the available technology and the natural course of an ectopic pregnancy, the role of physical examination in the diagnosis of this condition is minimal. Fever is not expected, although a mild elevation in temperature in response to intraperitoneal blood may occur. A temperature of 38°C may suggest an infectious cause of a patient's symptoms. Abdominal distention and tenderness, with or without rebound, rigidity, or decreased bowel sounds may be seen in cases of intra-abdominal bleeding. Abdominal tenderness is present in 50% to 90% of patients with ectopic pregnancies. Cervical motion tenderness caused by intraperitoneal irritation and adnexal tenderness are commonly found.

An adnexal mass is present in roughly one third of cases, but its absence does not rule out the possibility of an ectopic implantation. The uterus may enlarge and soften throughout the first trimester, thus simulating an intrauterine pregnancy. A slightly open cervix with blood or decidual tissue may be found and mistaken for a threatened and/or spontaneous abortion.

Differential Diagnosis

Symptoms of ectopic pregnancy can mimic multiple entities. Early pregnancy complications (threatened, incomplete, or missed abortion), placental polyp, and hemorrhagic corpus luteal cyst are difficult to differentiate from ectopic pregnancy. Since early bleeding occurs in up to 20% of women with normal, intact pregnancies, the physician must take care to avoid any action that might compromise a possible ongoing pregnancy. A number of nonpregnancy-related disorders, such as appendicitis and renal calculi, can also mimic ectopic pregnancy.

The rapid and accurate diagnosis of ectopic pregnancy is imperative to reduce the risk of serious complications or death. Up to half of the women who have died as a result of ectopic pregnancy had a lag in treatment because of delayed or inaccurate diagnoses. Any sexually active woman in the reproductive age group who presents with pain, irregular bleeding, and/or amenorrhea should have ectopic pregnancy as a part of the initial differential diagnosis.

Diagnostic Procedures

TVS and serial serum β-hCG measurements are the most valuable diagnostic aids to confirm a suspicion of ectopic pregnancy. The initial assessment in the otherwise hemodynamically stable patient must include a pregnancy test. A negative pregnancy test excludes the possibility of ectopic pregnancy. Urinary pregnancy tests, which detect hCG levels to 20 IU/L, are now commonly available. These tests detect hCG as early as 14 days after fertilization and are positive in more than 90% of cases of ectopic pregnancy. Serum assays can detect the presence of hCG as early as 5 days after fertilization, that is, before the missed menstrual cycle; however, because they require additional time and expertise to perform, they are often not utilized in a potentially emergent clinical setting.

Serum Human Chorionic Gonadotropin Levels

If a positive pregnancy test is found when ectopic pregnancy is suspected, the remainder of the workup should focus on evaluating the viability and location of the pregnancy. In normal pregnancies, serum β-hCG levels rise in a log-linear fashion until 60 or 80 days after the last menses, at which time levels plateau at about 100,000 IU/L. During this early phase of pregnancy, a 53% or greater increase in serum β-hCG levels should be observed every 48 hours. A rise of hCG levels less than this should raise suspicion for an abnormal gestation, either intrauterine or ectopic. Complicating this scenario is the recognition that approximately 15% of normal intrauterine pregnancies are associated with less than a 53% increase in hCG, and 17% of ectopic pregnancies have normal hCG doubling times. Although inappropriately rising serum β-hCG levels suggest (but do not diagnose) an abnormal pregnancy, they do not identify its location.

Transvaginal Ultrasonography

A key adjunct to serial quantitative levels of hCG is transvaginal pelvic ultrasonography (Fig. 19.2). Using TVS, a gestational sac is usually visible between 4½ and 5 weeks from the last menstrual period (LMP). The yolk sac appears between 5 and 6 weeks, and a fetal pole with cardiac activity is first detected at 5½ to 6 weeks. With transabdominal sonography, these structures are visualized slightly later. Each institution must define a β-hCG **discriminatory value** (i.e., the lower limit of serum hCG at which a TVS can reliably visualize pregnancy). It is not uncommon for TVS to demonstrate an intrauterine pregnancy by the time the hCG level is 1,000 to 2,000 IU/L. Transabdominal ultrasonography should be able to identify an intrauterine gestation by the time the hCG level reaches 5,000 to 6,000 IU/L. The absence of an intrauterine pregnancy with β-hCG levels above the discriminatory value signifies an abnormal pregnancy—ectopic, incomplete abortion, or resolving completed abortion. Care must be taken to differentiate between a uterine gestation and a **pseudogestational sac**. This one-layer sac is the result of an intracavitary fluid collection caused by sloughing of the decidua typically situated in the midline of the uterine cavity, whereas a normal gestational sac is eccentrically located (Fig. 19.3).

Serum Progesterone Level

Serum progesterone concentration is higher in a viable pregnancy than an ectopic pregnancy. There is minimal variation in serum progesterone concentration between 5 and 10 weeks of gestation; thus a single value is sufficient. A serum progesterone level of <5 ng/mL has been used to identify a nonviable

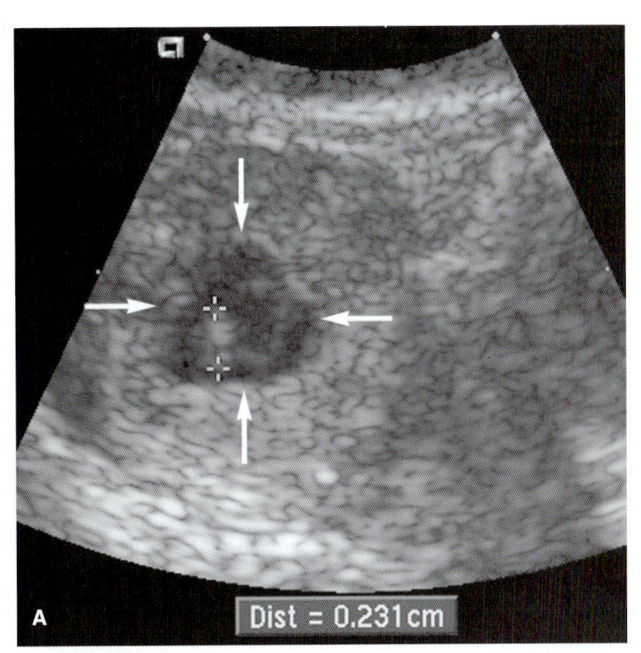

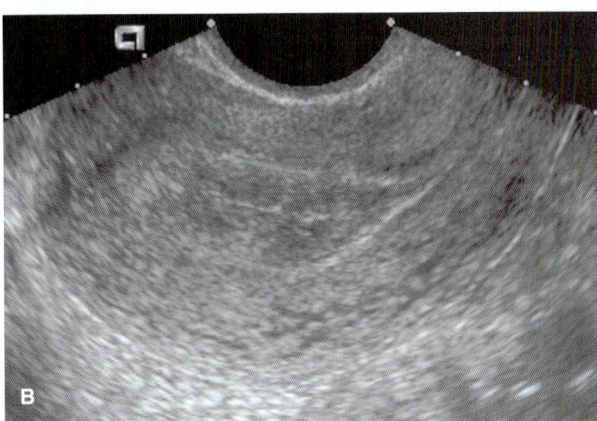

FIGURE 19.2. Ectopic pregnancy with an extrauterine gestational sac containing a live embryo. (A) Coronal transvaginal view of the right adnexa demonstrates an extrauterine sac (*arrows*) containing an embryo (calipers). (B) Sagittal transvaginal view of the uterus reveals no evidence of a gestational sac. (From Doubilet PM, Benson CB. *Atlas of Ultrasound in Obstetrics and Gynecology.* Philadelphia, PA: Lippincott Williams & Wilkins; 2003:319.)

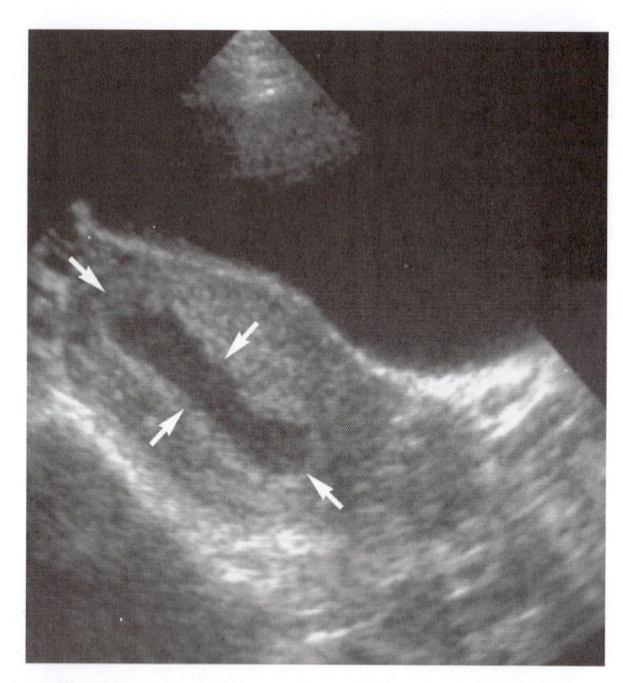

FIGURE 19.3. Pseudogestational sac. Sagittal transabdominal view of the uterus demonstrates a pseudogestational sac, a collection of fluid within the uterus. (From Doubilet PM, Benson CB. *Atlas of Ultrasound in Obstetrics and Gynecology*. Philadelphia, PA: Lippincott Williams & Wilkins; 2003:320.)

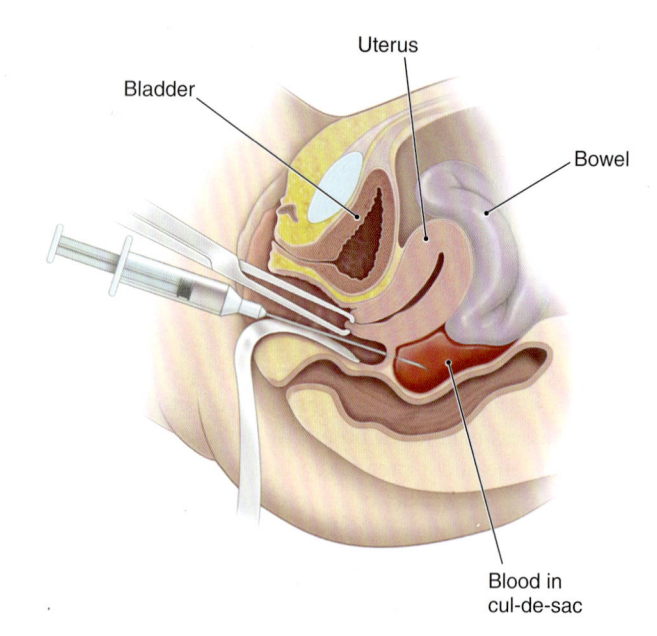

FIGURE 19.4. Culdocentesis.

pregnancy with 98% specificity and with a sensitivity of 75%. Conversely, a serum progesterone of >20 ng/mL has a sensitivity of 95%, with a specificity of approximately 40% to identify a healthy pregnancy. Serum progesterone values cannot differentiate between an ectopic and an intrauterine pregnancy.

Endometrial Curettage

Curettage of the uterine cavity can also help rule out ectopic pregnancy but should only be undertaken after the possibility of interrupting an intact pregnancy has been considered. Although intrauterine and ectopic pregnancies can exist simultaneously in rare cases (heterotopic pregnancy), identification of chorionic villi in tissue samples identifies an intrauterine location of the pregnancy and essentially rules out ectopic pregnancy. The presumptive diagnosis of ectopic pregnancy is reportedly inaccurate in nearly 40% of cases without histologic exclusion of a spontaneous pregnancy loss. The **Arias-Stella reaction**, a hypersecretory endometrium of pregnancy seen on histologic examination, occurs with both ectopic and intrauterine pregnancies and, therefore, is not useful in identifying an ectopic pregnancy.

Culdocentesis

Culdocentesis can identify **hemoperitoneum** (blood in the peritoneal cavity), which may indicate a ruptured ectopic pregnancy, although it is also consistent with other causes, such as a ruptured corpus luteum cyst. An 18G needle is inserted posterior to the cervix, between the uterosacral ligaments, and into the cul-de-sac of the peritoneal cavity (Fig. 19.4). Aspiration of clear peritoneal fluid (negative culdocentesis) indicates no hemorrhage into the abdominal cavity but does not rule out an unruptured ectopic pregnancy. Aspiration of blood that clots can indicate either penetration of a vessel or such rapid blood loss into the peritoneal cavity that the blood clot has not had time to undergo fibrinolysis. Aspiration of nonclotting blood is evidence of hemoperitoneum (positive culdocentesis), in which the blood clot has undergone fibrinolysis. If nothing is aspirated (equivocal or nondiagnostic culdocentesis), no information is obtained. Purulent fluid suggests a number of infection-related causes, such as salpingitis and appendicitis. Because none of the possible findings on culdocentesis can definitively confirm the presence or absence of ectopic pregnancy, its use in clinical practice is limited.

When used, the principal useful result is that a positive culdocentesis identifies blood in the peritoneal cavity and confirms the need for further evaluation to identify the source of the bleeding. With the availability of other diagnostic technology, particularly ultrasound, in many regions the use of culdocentesis has become almost obsolete.

Laparoscopy

The most accurate technique of identifying an ectopic pregnancy is by **direct visualization**, *which is done most commonly via* **laparoscopy**. Even laparoscopy, however, has a 2% to 5% misdiagnosis rate. For example, an extremely early tubal gestation may not be identified because it may not distend the fallopian tube sufficiently to be recognized as an abnormality (false negative). Conversely, a false-positive diagnosis may result from a **hematosalpinx** (blood in the fallopian tube) being misinterpreted as an unruptured ectopic pregnancy or tubal abortion.

Management

Management may be either surgical or medical, depending on a variety of factors. In any individual case, surgery can be a simple procedure, but it can also be far more extensive, depending on the location of the ectopic pregnancy, whether or not it is ruptured, the gestational age of the pregnancy, and the patient's desire for future fertility.

Due to the inherent risks of each, medical therapy is preferred over surgery in appropriate patients.

Medical Management

Methotrexate is the medical treatment usually used as an alternative to surgical therapy. Methotrexate is a folic acid antagonist that competitively inhibits the binding of dihydrofolic acid to dihydrofolate reductase, which, in turn, reduces the amount of the active intracellular metabolite, folinic acid. It stops the growth of rapidly dividing placental, embryonic, and fetal cells.

An appropriate candidate for medical therapy is the woman who is asymptomatic, motivated, and has resources to be compliant with follow-up. Relative and absolute contraindications for medical management are listed in Box 19.1.

Factors that can be assessed in predicting the success of medical therapy include the initial β-hCG level, the size of ectopic pregnancy as determined by TVS, and presence or absence of fetal cardiac activity. The initial serum β-hCG level is the best prognostic indicator of treatment success in women managed with a single-dose methotrexate protocol. An initial serum value <5,000 IU/L is associated with a success rate of 92%, whereas an initial concentration >15,000 IU/L has a success rate of 68%. Ectopic pregnancy size also appears to have an effect on methotrexate success rates. Success rates are reported as high as 93% in cases with ectopic masses <3.5 cm. A diameter >3.5 cm and the presence of cardiac activity are considered relative contraindications to medical management because these findings are associated with a lower success rate.

The most common side effects of methotrexate include nausea, vomiting, diarrhea, gastric distress, dizziness, and stomatitis. Intramuscular methotrexate given as part of a single-dose protocol has been the most widely used medical treatment of ectopic pregnancy. Close monitoring is imperative. A serum β-hCG level is determined before administering methotrexate and is repeated on days 4 and 7 following injection. Levels may continue to rise until day 4. Comparison is then made between the day 4 and the day 7 serum values. If there is a decline by 15% or more, serum β-hCG levels are measured weekly until they are undetectable. If the β-hCG level does not decline, the patient may require either surgery or a second dose of methotrexate if no contraindications exist. Surgical intervention may be required for patients who do not respond to medical therapy.

During the first few days following methotrexate administration, up to half of women experience abdominal pain that can be controlled with nonsteroidal anti-inflammatory drugs. This pain presumably results from tubal distention, tubal abortion, and/or hematoma formation.

Methotrexate given in a multidose protocol has also been used successfully, but the single-dose protocol described appears to reduce the amount of potential complications while achieving similar success rates. Other medical treatments that have been used include hyperosmolar glucose, potassium chloride, prostaglandins, and the progesterone receptor antagonist mifepristone (formerly referred to as *RU-486*). In some cases, an agent may be administered systemically, but sometimes it may be injected directly into the ectopic pregnancy.

Surgical Management

Women who are hemodynamically stable and in whom there is a small ectopic diameter, no fetal cardiac activity, and serum β-hCG concentrations <5,000 IU/L have similar outcomes with medical or surgical management. Conservative surgical techniques have been developed that maximize preservation of the fallopian tube. If removal is done through the laparoscope, definitive diagnosis as well as treatment can be accomplished at the same operation with minimal morbidity, cost, and hospitalization. In a **linear salpingostomy**, the surgeon makes an incision on the fallopian tube over the site of implantation, removes the pregnancy, and allows the incision to heal by secondary intention. A **segmental resection** is the removal of a portion of the affected tube (Fig. 19.5). **Salpingectomy** is removal of the entire tube, a procedure reserved for those cases in which little or no normal tube remains.

When conservative surgery or nonsurgical treatment is used, the patient must be followed post-therapy with serial quantitative β-hCG levels to monitor regression of the pregnancy. Subsequent surgery or methotrexate therapy is needed if trophoblastic function persists as evidenced by persistent or rising levels of hCG. Rh-negative mothers with ectopic pregnancy should receive **Rh immunoglobulin** to prevent Rh sensitization (see Chapter 23).

Non–Fallopian Tube Ectopic Pregnancy

Ovarian Pregnancy

Ectopic implantation of the fertilized egg in the ovary is rare. Improved imaging modalities have facilitated this diagnosis being made. Risk factors are similar to those for tubal

---

BOX 19.1 Contraindications to Medical Therapy for Ectopic Pregnancy

Absolute
- Breastfeeding
- Overt or laboratory evidence of immunodeficiency
- Known sensitivity to methotrexate
- Active pulmonary disease
- Peptic ulcer disease
- Hepatic, renal, pulmonary, or hematologic dysfunction
- Heterotopic pregnancy with viable intrauterine gestation
- Unable to comply with management protocol

Relative
- Gestational sac greater than 3.5 cm
- Embryonic cardiac motion
- Free peritoneal fluid (possible hemoperitoneum)

Modified from American Society of Reproductive Medicine. Medical Treatment of Ectopic Pregnancy: a committee opinion. Fertility and Sterility, Vol 100(3); September, 2013.

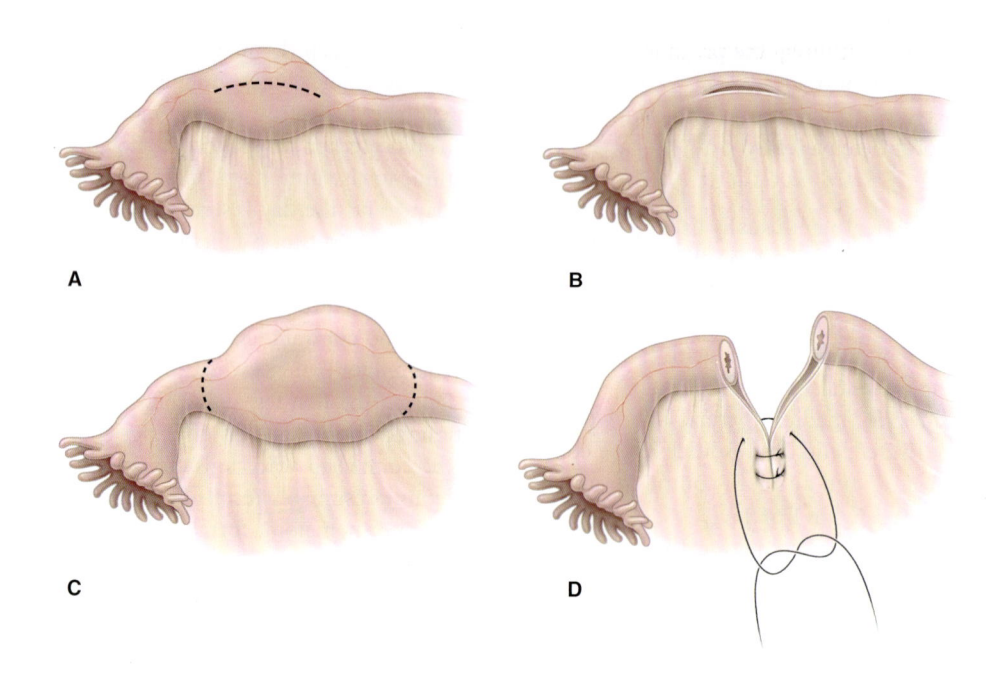

FIGURE 19.5. Surgical management of ectopic pregnancy. (A) Site of linear incision for linear salpingostomy. (B) Linear incision. (C) Segmental resection. (D) Tubal reanastomosis.

pregnancies, although ovarian pregnancies are not associated with a history of salpingitis. Diagnosis is based on the classic sonographic description of a cyst with a wide echogenic vascular outer ring located on or within the ovary.

Medical management as well as surgery can be used to conserve the ovary.

Interstitial Pregnancy
Also termed **cornual pregnancy**, interstitial pregnancies implant in the proximal tubal segment that lies within the muscular uterine wall. Swelling lateral to the insertion of the round ligament is the characteristic anatomic finding. A pregnancy that implants in the cornual segment of the tube tends to present several weeks later in pregnancy, because the muscular cornu of the uterus is better able to expand and accommodate an enlarging pregnancy. As a result, rupture of a cornual pregnancy typically occurs between the 8th and 16th gestational weeks and is often associated with massive hemorrhage, sometimes requiring hysterectomy.

Mortality rates are quoted as high as 2.5%. If detected prior to rupture, medical management is potentially successful. If surgery is needed, resection of the cornual region is performed.

Cervical Pregnancy
Cervical pregnancy occurs in 1 in 9,000 to 12,000 pregnancies, when the ovum implants in the cervical mucosa below the level of the histologic cervical internal os. Two diagnostic criteria are necessary for confirmation of cervical pregnancy: (1) the presence of cervical glands opposite to the placental attachment site and (2) a portion of or the entire placenta must be located below either the entrance of the uterine vessels or the peritoneal reflection on the anterior and posterior uterine surface. Both medical and surgical management have been used successfully to preserve the cervix in cases where future fertility is desired.

Heterotopic Pregnancy
Heterotopic pregnancy (coincident or combined pregnancy) is the coexistence of an ectopic and an intrauterine pregnancy. The incidence was previously estimated to be 1 in 30,000 pregnancies. As a result of assisted reproduction, however, the rate of heterotopic pregnancies has increased to as high as 1 in 100 pregnancies in some series. Mechanisms that have been proposed to explain this include (1) hydrostatic forces delivering the embryo into the cornual or tubal area, (2) the tip of the catheter directing transfer toward the tubal ostia, or (3) reflux of uterine secretions leading to retrograde tubal implantation. In addition to the option of surgical management of the ectopic pregnancy while attempting to preserve the intrauterine pregnancy, medical therapy in which potassium chloride can be injected into the pregnancy sac is another option. Methotrexate is contraindicated due to potential detrimental effects on the normal pregnancy.

Abdominal Pregnancy
The estimated incidence of **abdominal pregnancy** ranges from 1 in 10,000 to 1 in 25,000 live births. Abdominal pregnancies may result from primary implantation onto the peritoneal surface or secondary implantation via tubal rupture or tubal abortion. Physical findings and symptoms are widely variable, depending on gestational age and site of implantation. Diagnosis is confirmed primarily by ultrasonography. Abdominal pregnancy is usually discovered long before fetal viability, and removal of the pregnancy is the mainstay of therapy.

Survival of the fetus occurs in only 10% to 20% of cases; up to one half of those surviving have significant deformity. The patient is given the option of continuing the pregnancy to fetal viability with operative delivery or operative termination of the pregnancy at the time of diagnosis. In either case, removal of the placenta is usually not attempted because of the risk of uncontrollable hemorrhage. Allowing the placenta to spontaneously regress is often the management chosen. Alternative treatments include administration of methotrexate and embolization of placental vessels.

MISCARRIAGE

Abortion is a pregnancy loss that occurs at less than 20 weeks of gestation. **Miscarriage** (spontaneous abortion) occurs in the absence of any medical or surgical intervention. The incidence of recognized miscarriage is commonly cited as 15% to 25%, with 80% occurring during the first 12 weeks of pregnancy. This rate of miscarriage may be even higher because losses that occur at 4 to 6 weeks of gestation may be misinterpreted by the patient and her physician as a delayed menstrual cycle. Half of recognized early miscarriages are attributed to chromosomal abnormalities, most of which are trisomies.

Compared with first-trimester miscarriages, second-trimester miscarriages are less likely to be caused by chromosomal abnormalities and more likely to be caused by maternal systemic disease, abnormal placentation, or other anatomic considerations. This difference is clinically significant, because maternal systemic conditions often can be treated, and recurrent second-trimester abortions can, thereby, potentially be prevented.

Etiology

Infectious Factors

Infections are an uncommon cause of early spontaneous abortion. *Chlamydia trachomatis* and *Listeria monocytogenes* have been associated with spontaneous abortion. Serological evidence supports a role for *Mycoplasma hominis* and *Ureaplasma urealyticum* in some cases. In addition, miscarriage is independently associated with serological evidence of syphilis, human immunodeficiency virus 1 infection, and vaginal colonization with group B streptococci.

Endocrine Factors

Thyroid autoantibodies are associated with an increased incidence of spontaneous abortion, even in the absence of clinical hypothyroidism. In women with type 1 diabetes, the degree of metabolic control in early pregnancy has been found to be related to an increased risk of spontaneous abortion and major congenital malformation.

Environmental Factors

The miscarriage risk increases in a linear fashion with the number of cigarettes smoked per day. Both *miscarriage* and fetal anomalies may result from frequent, high doses of alcohol during the first 8 weeks of pregnancy. Radiation administered at therapeutic doses to treat cancer may be an abortifacient.

However, exposure to most diagnostic procedures that expose the patient to less than 5 rads does not increase the risk of miscarriage. The rates of spontaneous abortion and birth defects increase when the pregnancy is exposed to over 20 rads.

Immunologic Factors

There are a number of genetic disorders of blood coagulation that may increase the risk of both arterial and venous thrombosis. Among thrombophilias, only antiphospholipid antibody syndrome has consistently been significantly associated with increased risk of early spontaneous abortion.

Uterine Factors

Large and multiple **uterine leiomyomas** are common, and they may cause miscarriage.

In most instances, their location is more important than their size, with submucous leiomyomata playing a more significant role than others, presumably because of their effect on implantation.

In utero exposure to diethylstilbestrol has been associated with abnormally shaped uteri and cervical insufficiency, both of which can lead to spontaneous abortion, usually during the second trimester. **Intrauterine synechiae** (**Asherman syndrome**), a condition that is caused by uterine curettage with subsequent destruction and scarring of the endometrium, may also be a cause of spontaneous abortion. A uterine septum can similarly cause spontaneous abortion.

Classification and Differential Diagnosis of Spontaneous Abortions

Because the differential diagnosis of bleeding in the first trimester of pregnancy includes a wide range of possibilities, including ectopic pregnancy, hydatidiform mole, cervical polyps, cervicitis, and neoplasm, the patient should be examined whenever there is bleeding in early pregnancy.

Types of Spontaneous Abortion

Threatened abortion is characterized by bleeding in the first trimester without loss of fluid or tissue. About half of women with a threatened abortion proceed to spontaneous abortion. Those who carry a pregnancy complicated by threatened abortion to viability are at greater risk for preterm delivery and an infant of low birth weight. There does not, however, appear to be a higher incidence of congenital malformations in these newborns. Some patients describe bleeding at the time of their expected menses, sometimes referred to as **implantation bleeding**, which may be related to implantation of the pregnancy in the endometrium.

In cases of miscarriage, bleeding usually begins first, and cramping abdominal pain follows a few hours to several days later. The pain may present as anterior rhythmic cramps; as a persistent low backache, associated with a feeling of pelvic pressure; or as a dull, midline, suprapubic discomfort. The combination of persistent bleeding and pain usually indicates a poor prognosis for pregnancy continuation. *Ectopic pregnancy should* always be considered in the differential diagnosis of threatened abortion.

An **inevitable abortion** is vaginal bleeding and/or the gross rupture of the membranes in the presence of cervical dilation. Typically, uterine contractions begin promptly, resulting in expulsion of the pregnancy. It is unusual for the progress of an inevitable abortion to be halted and for a pregnancy to successfully reach viability in this circumstance. Conservative management (i.e., nonintervention in an attempt to prolong the pregnancy in these patients) significantly increases the risk of maternal infection.

In an **incomplete abortion**, the internal cervical os opens and allows passage of blood and some tissue. In some cases, retained placental tissue remains in the cervical canal, allowing easy extraction from an exposed external os with ring forceps. If needed, a suction curettage is used to remove remaining tissues from the uterine cavity.

Complete abortion refers to a documented pregnancy that spontaneously passes all of the contents of the uterus. Before 10 weeks of gestation, the fetus and placenta are commonly expelled together.

A **missed abortion** is the retention of a failed intrauterine pregnancy for an extended period, usually defined as more than two menstrual cycles. These patients have an absence of uterine growth and may have lost some of the early symptoms of pregnancy. Many women have no symptoms during this period except persistent amenorrhea. If the missed abortion terminates spontaneously, and most do, the process of expulsion is the same as in any spontaneous abortion.

Recurrent Pregnancy Loss

Recurrent pregnancy loss is a term that refers to two or more intrauterine pregnancy losses. Historically, the diagnosis required that the pregnancy losses be consecutive, but this is no longer the case. The timing of the pregnancy losses may provide a clue to their cause. Genetic and autoimmune factors most frequently result in early embryonic losses, whereas anatomic abnormalities are more likely to result in second-trimester losses.

First-Trimester Pregnancy Loss

Karyotyping is recommended for both parents when recurrent early pregnancy loss occurs, because there is a 3% chance that one parent is an asymptomatic carrier of a genetically balanced chromosomal translocation. The immune system also has a role in up to 20% of early recurrent pregnancy loss. **Antiphospholipid antibodies** are a family of autoantibodies that bind to negatively charged phospholipids. Lupus anticoagulant and anticardiolipin antibody have been linked with excessive pregnancy wastage. Treatment may include low-dose aspirin along with unfractionated heparin. This therapy, begun when pregnancy is diagnosed, may be continued until delivery. Intrauterine synechiae associated with **Asherman syndrome** may occur after a curettage procedure has denuded the endometrium past the layer of the basalis, which promotes the formation of webs of scar tissue to develop within the uterine cavity. Asherman syndrome and other anatomic abnormalities account for approximately 10% of early recurrent pregnancy losses. Asherman syndrome can be associated with not only early recurrent pregnancy loss but also amenorrhea, hypomenorrhea, cyclic pain, and infertility. The diagnosis is confirmed by a hysterogram that shows the characteristic webbed pattern or by hysteroscopy. Treatment involves lysis of the synechiae and postoperative treatment with high doses of estrogen to facilitate endometrial proliferation, leading to the reestablishment of a normal endometrial layer.

Second-Trimester Pregnancy Loss

Recurrent pregnancy losses that occur later than the first trimester are typically caused by anatomic abnormalities, such as septate uteri or fibroids. In these cases, management including hysterography, operative hysteroscopy, and/or laparoscopy may be required to correct the problem. If leiomyomata are felt to be the causative factor of recurrent second-trimester pregnancy loss, myomectomy is appropriate. Similarly, reconstructive surgery of the uterus may be necessary for congenital uterine malformations.

Recurrent pregnancy loss in the second trimester can also be caused by **cervical insufficiency**, a condition in which the increasing pressure within the uterus causes a weakened cervix to efface and dilate painlessly. Predisposing factors include uterine anomalies as well as previous trauma to the cervix including mechanical dilation or history of conization. **Cervical cerclage** is used to tie the cervix closed during the early second trimester if cervical insufficiency is deemed the etiology of recurrent second-trimester loss.

Treatment

No intervention is necessary for patients with threatened abortion even if the bleeding is accompanied by low abdominal pain and cramping. If there is no evidence of significant abnormality on ultrasound evaluation, and if the pregnancy is found to be intact, the patient can be reassured and allowed to continue normal activities. In cases of complete abortion, the uterus is small and firm, the cervix is closed, and ultrasound identifies an empty uterus. No further intervention is needed.

For incomplete, inevitable, or missed abortions, treatment may be expectant, medical, or surgical. Surgical treatment is definitive and predictable but is invasive and not necessary for all women. Expectant or medical management using prostaglandins may obviate curettage, but both approaches are associated with unpredictable bleeding, with some women still requiring surgery to empty the uterus.

In cases of significant pain, hemorrhage, or infection, prompt completion of abortion is warranted. In such cases, immediate considerations include control of bleeding, prevention of infection, pain relief, and emotional support. Bleeding is controlled by ensuring that the uterus is completely evacuated. The use of ultrasound to evaluate the uterus helps to determine whether surgical intervention is needed. If tissue remains in the uterus, curettage is typically used to remove the remaining tissue. Hemostasis is enhanced through uterine contraction stimulated by oral methylergonovine. Removal of the uterine contents and vaginal rest (no tampons, douches, or intercourse) decreases the risk of infection. A mild analgesic may be required and should be offered. Rh-negative mothers should receive Rh immunoglobulin (RhoGAM). Chromosomal evaluation of spontaneous abortions is not recommended, unless there is a history of recurrent abortion.

Emotional support is important for both the short- and long-term well-being of both the patient and her partner. No matter how well-prepared a couple is for the possibility of pregnancy loss, the event is a significant disappointment and cause of stress. When appropriate, the couple should be reassured that the loss was not precipitated by anything that they did or did not do and that there was nothing that they could have done to prevent the loss.

FOLLOW-UP

A follow-up office visit is generally scheduled for 2 to 6 weeks after the loss of a pregnancy. This is an appropriate time to evaluate uterine involution, assess the return of menses, and discuss reproductive plans. The causes (or lack of causes) of the pregnancy loss should also be reiterated. The impact of this loss on future childbearing should be discussed. A single pregnancy loss does not significantly increase the risk of future losses. Multiple pregnancy losses carry an increased risk of future pregnancies and warrant further evaluation for treatable etiologies.

• INDUCED ABORTION

Induced abortion has been legal in the United States since the 1973 Supreme Court decision of *Roe v. Wade*. Since that time, various local and state laws have been proposed to limit access to induced abortion based on physician and facility requirements, gestational age limits, state and private insurance restrictions, waiting periods, requirements for parental involvement, and mandatory patient information requirements.

The health care provider should maintain a nonjudgmental position in treating women who may be considering termination of pregnancy. **Induced abortion** is the medical or surgical termination of pregnancy before the time of fetal viability. In 2013, approximately 664,000 induced abortions were reported to the Centers for Disease Control and Prevention. The abortion rate was 12.5 abortions per 1,000 women ages 15 to 44 years, and the abortion ratio was 200 abortions per 1,000 live births. The number of abortions and the rate and ratio all represent a 5% decrease from the year before, reflecting a downward trend in induced abortions over the past decade. Induced abortion is a very safe procedure, with the fewest complications related to induced abortion in the first trimester.

Three medications for first-trimester **medical abortion** have been widely studied and used: the antiprogestin **mifepristone** (formerly known as **RU-486**), the antimetabolite **methotrexate**, and the prostaglandin **misoprostol**. A combined misoprostol–mifepristone regimen is the most commonly used. These agents cause abortion by increasing uterine contractility either by reversing the progesterone-induced inhibition of contractions—mifepristone and methotrexate, or by stimulating the myometrium directly—misoprostol. Abortion with this medical method is not always complete. As a result, the patient should be made aware that suction curettage may be required.

The most common form of suction curettage for first-trimester abortions, vacuum aspiration, requires a rigid cannula attached to an electric-powered vacuum source. Alternatively, manual vacuum aspiration uses a similar cannula that attaches to a handheld syringe for its vacuum source. Outpatient medical abortion is an acceptable alternative to surgical abortion in appropriately selected women with pregnancies up to 70 days of gestation (calculated from the first day of the LMP).

Second-trimester abortions are most commonly performed through the cervix, using suction and/or extraction forceps, but also can be induced with medication.

Complications

Overall, there is a very low rate of complications. *The most common complications associated with an induced abortion include uterine perforation, cervical laceration, hemorrhage, incomplete uterine evacuation, and infection.* In cases of postabortal infection, the patient usually presents with fever, pain, a tender uterus, and mild bleeding. Oral antibiotics and antipyretics are typically sufficient to manage these mild infections. If tissue remains in the uterus (incomplete abortion), a repeat suction curettage is necessary. The second most common complication following induced abortion is bleeding. Risk of death from abortion during the first 2 months of pregnancy is less than 1 per 100,000 procedures, with increasing rates as pregnancy progresses (vs. 7.7 maternal deaths per 100,000 live births).

Septic Abortion

An infected abortion, either complete or incomplete, is known as a **septic abortion**. Patients may present with sepsis, shock, hemorrhage, and, possibly, renal failure. Septic abortion rarely occurs as a complication of an induced abortion that is performed by a trained health care provider. *Broad-spectrum parenteral antibiotics, intravenous fluid therapy, and prompt evacuation of the uterus are indicated.* A careful evaluation for trauma, including perforation of the uterus, vagina, or intra-abdominal structures, should also be carried out.

Postabortal Syndrome

Postabortal syndrome (also called postabortal hematometra) develops when the uterus fails to remain contracted after miscarriage (with or without suction curettage) or induced abortion. The patient presents with cramping pain and/or bleeding and is found to have an open cervix, bleeding, and a large, "softer-than-expected" uterus, a result of the collection of blood in the uterus (**hematometra**). *The clinical presentation is often indistinguishable from incomplete abortion.* Suction curettage is the treatment for both conditions. Postevacuation treatment with an ergot derivative and an antibiotic reduces the risk of postabortal syndrome, further bleeding, and infection.

CLINICAL FOLLOW-UP

Bleeding can occur with both an ongoing pregnancy (threatened abortion) and a nonviable pregnancy (incomplete, complete, or missed abortion). Determining whether the pregnancy is intrauterine or extrauterine is of immediate concern because of the potential need for emergent treatment of an ectopic pregnancy. Ultrasound is useful to identify both the location of an early pregnancy and whether or not it is intact. The ovarian cyst is most likely a corpus luteum of pregnancy. No treatment for this patient is indicated at this time because both the intrauterine pregnancy and the corpus luteum cyst are normal at this time.

thePoint® Visit **http://thePoint.lww.com/activate** for an interactive USMLE-style question bank and more!

III Medical and Surgical Disorders in Pregnancy

CHAPTER **20**

Endocrine Disorders

This chapter deals primarily with APGO Educational Topic Area:

TOPIC 17   MEDICAL AND SURGICAL DISORDERS IN PREGNANCY

Students should be able to identify how pregnancy affects the natural history of various endocrine disorders and how a preexisting endocrine disorder affects maternal and fetal health. They should be able to outline a basic approach to evaluation and management of endocrine disorders in pregnancy.

CLINICAL CASE

A 22-year-old primigravida is in your office for her initial obstetric visit. Her menstrual history suggests that she is about 12 weeks' pregnant. In reviewing her history, you find that she was diagnosed with diabetes 6 years ago and has been taking insulin twice daily since then. She checks her blood glucose values "every now and then" and reports them to be in the 150 to 180 range. She has not had regular diabetic care. In looking over her laboratory reports from studies done 2 days ago, you note that her HgbA$_{1c}$ is elevated at 9.5. How do you counsel her about this HgbA$_{1c}$ result as well as overall obstetric care in a patient with diabetes?

INTRODUCTION

Maternal medical or surgical conditions can complicate the course of a pregnancy and can be affected by pregnancy. Physicians providing obstetric care must have a thorough understanding of the effect of pregnancy on the natural course of a disorder, the effect of the disorder on a pregnancy, and the change in management of the pregnancy and disorder caused by their coincidence.

DIABETES MELLITUS

Approximately 6% to 9% of pregnancies are complicated by diabetes that either develops during pregnancy (**gestational diabetes**) or was antecedent to pregnancy (**pregestational diabetes mellitus**). In either case, diabetes has significant implications for the mother and fetus during pregnancy, and conversely, pregnancy significantly affects diabetes. Whether diabetes is newly diagnosed or long standing, intense management may be stressful, and all those involved with obstetric care should be mindful of the extra emotional attention many of these patients need.

Classification of Diabetes in Pregnancy

The American Diabetes Association (ADA) identifies three forms of glucose intolerance:

- **Type 1 diabetes mellitus** refers to diabetes diagnosed in childhood. It is thought to be caused by immunologic destruction of cells of the pancreas, resulting in necessary insulin replacement. **Diabetic ketoacidosis (DKA)** is more common in patients with this type of diabetes.
- **Type 2 diabetes mellitus** is adult-onset glucose intolerance. Patients with type 2 diabetes mellitus are frequently overweight, and the disease can often be controlled with weight control and a carefully followed diet. This type of diabetes is thought to result from insulin resistance and exhaustion of the cells, rather than their destruction.
- **Gestational diabetes mellitus** (GDM) refers to glucose intolerance identified during pregnancy. In most patients, it subsides postpartum, although glucose intolerance in subsequent years occurs more frequently in this group of patients.

The White's Classification was developed in 1949 by Priscilla White and has been historically used as a descriptive classification system based on duration of diabetes, age of onset and presence of vasculopathy to predict risk of adverse perinatal outcome. The ADA classification system is recommended. However, some obstetricians still use White's Classification as an adjunct to the ADA system to help with assessment of pregnancy risk (Box 20.1).

BOX 20.1 White's Classification of Diabetes in Pregnancy

- A1 GDM, diet controlled
- A2 GDM, medical therapy (insulin or oral hypoglycemic)
- B   Onset at age ≥20 and/or duration < 10 years
- C   Onset at age 10-19 or duration 10 to 19 years
- D   Onset at age <10 or duration ≥20 years
- R   Proliferative retinopathy or vitreous hemorrhage
- F   Nephropathy, >500 mg/day of proteinuria
- H   Evidence of arteriosclerotic heart disease
- T   Prior transplant

Physiology of Glucose Metabolism in Pregnancy

Dietary habits frequently change during pregnancy. Food intake may decrease early in pregnancy because of nausea and vomiting, and food preferences may change later in pregnancy. Several pregnancy-associated hormones also have a major effect on glucose metabolism. Most notable of these is **human placental lactogen (hPL)**, which is produced in abundance by the enlarging placenta. hPL affects both fatty acid and glucose metabolism. It promotes lipolysis with increased levels of circulating free fatty acids and causes a decrease in glucose uptake. In this manner, hPL can be thought of as an anti-insulin. The increasing production of this hormone as pregnancy advances generally requires ongoing changes in insulin therapy to adjust for this effect.

Other hormones that have demonstrated lesser effects include **estrogen** and **progesterone**, which interfere with the insulin–glucose relationship, and **insulinase**, which is produced by the placenta and degrades insulin to a limited extent. These effects of pregnancy on glucose metabolism make the management of pregnancy-associated diabetes difficult. DKA, for example, is more common in pregnant patients.

With increased renal blood flow, the simple diffusion of glucose in the glomerulus increases beyond the ability of tubular reabsorption, resulting in the normal **glucosuria of pregnancy**, commonly of approximately 300 mg/day. In patients with diabetes, this glucosuria may be much greater, but, because of the poor correlation of pregnancy glucosuria values and simultaneous blood glucose concentrations, using urinary glucose levels is of little value in glucose management during pregnancy.

Fetal Morbidity and Mortality

Congenital Anomalies

Infants of mothers with diabetes are at a sixfold increased risk for congenital anomalies over the 1% to 2% baseline risk of all patients. The most commonly encountered anomalies are cardiac, central nervous system (CNS), renal, and limb deformities. Sacral agenesis is a unique but rare anomaly for this group (Fig. 20.1). The risk of congenital anomalies increases with increasing **glycosylated hemoglobin levels (HgbA$_{1c}$)** when entering pregnancy. The HgbA$_{1c}$ level is an indication of glycemic control over the prior 2 to 3 months. Levels of 5% to 6% are associated with a fetal malformation rate of 2% to 3%, which is close to the rate in normal pregnancies, whereas HgbA$_{1c}$ levels >9.5% are associated with a malformation rate of 22% or higher.

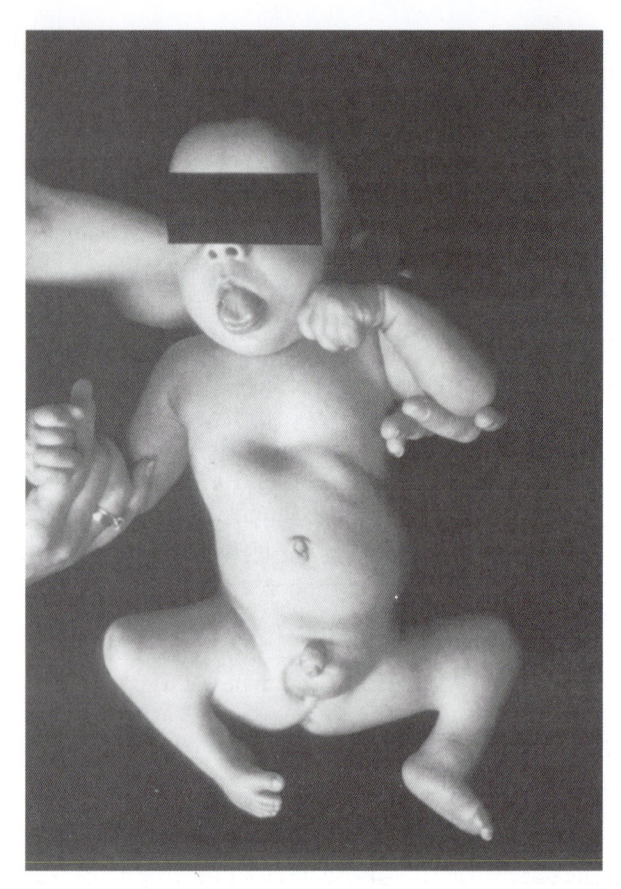

FIGURE 20.1. Infant born to a diabetic mother with poor glycemic control. Hypoplastic lower extremities and lack of lumbosacral spine are evident. (From Gabbe SG, Graves CR. Management of diabetes mellitus complicating pregnancy. *Obstet Gynecol.* 2003;102(4):857–868.)

Spontaneous Abortion and Stillbirth

The risk of spontaneous abortion is similar in patients with well-controlled diabetes and in patients without diabetes. However, the risk of spontaneous abortion is significantly increased for patients with diabetes if glucose control is poor when entering pregnancy. There is also an increased risk of intrauterine fetal demise and stillbirth, especially when diabetic control is inadequate. Because of this potentially devastating outcome, beginning at approximately 32 weeks of gestation, various antepartum fetal tests may be initiated to monitor fetal health (see Sections "Antepartum Fetal Monitoring").

Macrosomia

Excessive fetal growth, or **macrosomia** (usually defined as a fetal weight in excess of either 4,000 or 4,500 g), is more common in pregnant patients with diabetes because of the fetal metabolic effects of increased glucose transfer across the placenta. However, intrauterine growth restriction can also occur due to uteroplacental insufficiency. For these reasons, serial ultrasonography is often performed to follow fetal growth. When the estimated fetal weight by ultrasound late in pregnancy is greater than 4,500 g, cesarean delivery is often recommended to avoid the risk of fetopelvic disproportion, shoulder dystocia, and other birth trauma associated with large infants, insofar as these risks are increased even further in the setting of diabetes.

Polyhydramnios

Another complication of pregnancy in patients with diabetes is an increase in amniotic fluid volume greater than 2,000 mL, a condition known as **hydramnios** or **polyhydramnios**. Encountered in approximately 10% of mothers with diabetes, the increases in amniotic fluid volume and uterine size are associated with an increased risk of placental abruption and preterm labor as well as postpartum uterine atony. This condition is monitored while serial ultrasonography is performed for fetal growth, at which time the amount of amniotic fluid can be evaluated.

Other Complications

Neonatal hypoglycemia is often encountered in infants of women with diabetes. It results from the sudden change in the maternal–fetal glucose balance, in which an increased maternal glucose crossing the placenta is countered by an increase in fetal production of insulin. However, when the maternal supply of glucose is removed, this higher level of insulin can cause significant neonatal hypoglycemia. In addition, these newborns are subject to an increased incidence of neonatal hyperbilirubinemia, hypocalcemia, and polycythemia.

Infants of mothers with diabetes also tend to have an increased frequency of respiratory distress syndrome. The usual tests of lung maturity may be less predictive for these infants.

Pregestational Diabetes

Approximately 2% of all pregnant patients are diabetic before pregnancy. Type 2 pregestational diabetes mellitus is most common. Although 90% of diabetes cases encountered during pregnancy are GDM, up to 70% of these eventually develop type 2 pregestational diabetes mellitus later in life.

Antepartum Fetal Monitoring

Women with pregestational diabetes should receive an ultrasound examination early in pregnancy to check for fetal viability and accurately date the gestational age. At 18 to 20 weeks of gestation, a comprehensive ultrasound examination that focuses on identification of congenital anomalies, especially those of the CNS, genitourinary system, heart and great vessels, is indicated. Echocardiography may also be done if there are suspected cardiac defects or when the fetal heart and great vessels could not be visualized by ultrasonography.

Antepartum fetal monitoring, including fetal movement counting as well as the nonstress test, biophysical profile, and/or contraction stress test, performed at appropriate intervals, is a valuable approach and can be used to monitor fetal well-being in women with pregestational diabetes. This testing is usually initiated at 32 to 34 weeks of gestation but can be undertaken earlier if other high-risk conditions such as fetal growth restriction exist. The frequency is typically weekly, however, twice weekly or more may be recommended in the setting of poor glycemic control, maternal co-morbidities, or fetal growth disturbances.

Maternal Complications

Pregnant patients with pregestational diabetes, especially type 1 diabetes, are at higher risk for DKA, the management of which is not altered in pregnancy. Fetal death can accompany DKA, so electronic fetal monitoring is recommended until the maternal metabolic status is stabilized.

Hypoglycemia may also occur periodically, especially early in pregnancy, when nausea and vomiting interfere with caloric intake. Although hypoglycemia does not have adverse effects on the fetus, patients and their families should be taught how to respond quickly and appropriately to hypoglycemia for maternal benefit.

In addition to the added difficulties of glucose management and the increased risk of DKA during pregnancy, mothers with pregestational diabetes have a twofold increase in the incidence of pregnancy-induced hypertension, or **preeclampsia**, compared with patients without diabetes. Because of this increased risk of preeclampsia, 24-hour urine collections to determine the level of proteinuria and creatinine clearance are often used in pregestational diabetics. Additionally, if patients have preexisting **diabetic nephropathy**, manifested by prepregnancy creatinine >1.5 mg/dl or severe **proteinuria**, they are at an increased risk for progression to end-stage renal disease, and serial monitoring of renal function is warranted.

Diabetic retinopathy worsens in approximately 15% of pregnant patients with preexisting diabetes, some proceeding to proliferative retinopathy and loss of vision if the process remains untreated by laser coagulation. Therefore, women with pregestational type 1 or type 2 diabetes should have an ophthalmologic evaluation once in their first trimester if asymptomatic and as needed if symptoms arise.

Management

The patient with long-standing diabetes should realize that strict control of her glucose levels is advised during pregnancy, with greater attention to and more frequent monitoring of glucose values. For these patients, management ideally begins before conception, with the goal of optimal glucose control before and during pregnancy. Women with pregestational diabetes mellitus should be offered preconception counseling and care to reduce the risks of spontaneous abortion and congenital anomalies (see Section "Fetal Morbidity and Mortality" and Chapter 6). $HgbA_{1c}$ levels can be measured to reflect average glucose values over the preceding 12 weeks. These levels can then be used to monitor glucose control both before and during pregnancy and to predict the likelihood of congenital anomalies in the fetus (see Section "Fetal Morbidity and Mortality"). Multivitamins containing at least 400 µg of folic acid should be prescribed to all women contemplating pregnancy. This is particularly important in women with diabetes given their increased risk of neural tube defects. Higher doses of folic acid may be beneficial in some cases, especially in the presence of other risk factors for neural tube defects.

Excellent glucose control is achieved using a careful combination of diet, exercise, and insulin therapy. Insulin requirements will increase throughout pregnancy, most markedly in the period between 28 and 32 weeks of gestation.

The impact of pregnancy on diabetes, and vice versa, must also be emphasized to the pregnant patient with pregestational diabetes. Patients may need to be seen every 1 to 2 weeks during the first two trimesters and weekly after 28 to 30 weeks of gestation.

Gestational Diabetes

The prevalence of GDM is estimated to be about 7%, and this rate is increasing with higher rates of obesity. GDM is usually identified by prenatal screening of pregnant patients. It may be suspected, however, in patients with known risk factors for GDM, which include age, ethnicity, past obstetric history (gestational diabetes in a previous pregnancy, a history of an infant weighing more than 4,000 g at birth, repeated spontaneous abortions, or a history of unexplained stillbirth), a strong family history of diabetes, and obesity. However, 50% of patients identified as having gestational diabetes do not have such risk factors.

Laboratory Screening

The most commonly used screening test for glucose intolerance during pregnancy is given at 24 to 28 weeks of gestation and consists of a 50-g, 1-hour oral glucose challenge. Fasting is not necessary for this test. Patients whose glucose value exceeds a determined cut-off (typically 130, 135, or 140 mg/dL) require a standard 3-hour glucose tolerance test using 100 g of glucose. Two or more abnormal results of the 3-hour test establish the diagnosis of gestational diabetes.

In patients lacking any risk factors, the 1-hour glucose screening is usually performed between 24 and 28 weeks of gestation because glucose intolerance is generally evident by that time. Using this screening method, approximately 15% of patients have an abnormal screening test. Of those patients who then proceed to have the standard 3-hour oral glucose tolerance test, approximately 15% are diagnosed as having GDM. Treatment of women with GDM is associated with reduced rates of maternal and fetal complications including excessive weight gain, macrosomia, preeclampsia, shoulder dystocia, and cesarean delivery. Although many practitioners choose to screen high-risk patients early in pregnancy, the benefit of early treatment of women with GDM identified early in pregnancy has not been demonstrated but, rather, has been accepted on a theoretical basis.

Antepartum Fetal Monitoring

There is currently insufficient evidence to determine the optimal antepartum testing regimen for women with relatively normal glucose levels on diet therapy and no other risk factors. Despite the lack of evidence, it is reasonable to conclude that women whose GDM is not well controlled, who require insulin, or who have other risk factors such as hypertension should receive the same antepartum testing regimen as women with pregestational diabetes. Although ultrasonography can be used to assess congenital anomalies, the reliability of ultrasonography to estimate fetal weight and predict macrosomia prior to delivery has not been established.

Management

Often overlooked or underemphasized in the overall management of a patient whose pregnancy is complicated by diabetes mellitus is the importance of patient education. The patient with newly diagnosed diabetes should receive general diabetic counseling, along with information about the unique features of the combination of diabetes and pregnancy. Home glucose monitoring is the norm, and instruction in technique should be provided.

Diet and Glucose Monitoring

The overall goal of managing GDM is to control glucose values within circumscribed limits: fasting glucose levels of less than 95 mg/dL, 1-hour postprandial levels less than 140 mg/dL, or 2-hour postprandial values less than 120 mg/dL. The mainstay of GDM management is diet. The recommended diet is about 30 kcal/kg/day of ideal body weight, composed of approximately 33% to 40% complex carbohydrates, 40% fat, and 20% protein. With careful attention to diet, many mothers with GDM do not require insulin. Current available evidence does not support a recommendation for or against moderate caloric restriction in obese women with GDM. However, if caloric restriction is used, the diet should be restricted by no more than 33% of calories. In practice, three meals and two to three snacks are recommended to distribute carbohydrate intake and to reduce postprandial glucose fluctuations.

Patients are instructed to obtain a morning fasting glucose, along with pre- and/or postprandial glucose values throughout the day and evening. The precise goals for glucose control vary, but, in general, the fasting plasma glucose should be maintained at less than 95 mg/dl and the postprandial values obtained throughout the day at <120 to 140 mg/dl. For those patients who are able to control their gestational diabetes with diet alone, the perinatal outcome is good. Pregnancy is allowed to continue to term, with delivery planned no earlier than 39 to 40 weeks gestation.

Medical Therapy

For patients with GDM whose glucose levels cannot be controlled with diet, exogenous insulin is needed. Frequently, a combination of intermediate-acting **neutral protamine hagedorn** (**NPH**) and fast-acting insulin (such as regular or **lispro**) is used together near breakfast and dinner in order to suppress gluconeogenesis in the liver as well as to counter the rises in glucose that occur with meals. This necessitates only twice-daily injections. However, some advocate splitting the evening insulin dose, giving the short-acting insulin at dinner and then

NPH at bedtime, in order to decrease the risk of nocturnal hypoglycemia. Some groups use basal-bolus insulin regimens in pregnancy with a combination of long-acting insulin (insulin detemir or insulin glargine) with three times daily short-acting insulin (lispro or aspart) with meals. However, the longer-acting insulin analogs have not been as extensively studied in pregnancy. Insulin does not cross the placenta and, therefore, does not directly affect the fetus.

However, glucose does cross the placenta (by facilitated diffusion); the higher the maternal glucose level, the higher the fetal glucose level. In response, the fetus produces more insulin. This increased insulin production converts glucose to fat, resulting in the heavier infants (macrosomia) often noted in patients with diabetes. Following delivery, the high maternal glucose transfer ceases, but the continuing high fetal insulin concentration may lead to significant neonatal hypoglycemia temporarily.

Although insulin has always been the mainstay of medical treatment of GDM, therapy with oral hypoglycemic agents has been previously recommended for diabetic therapy in pregnancy by some groups. However, based on more recent studies with less optimal outcomes and concern for the unknown long-term effects of oral hypoglycemic exposure in utero, insulin remains the treatment of choice. **Glyburide**, which crosses the placenta in very low levels, and Metformin, which crosses the placenta, have been studied in comparison to insulin with inconsistent benefit. Metformin has been used in many patients with polycystic ovary syndrome (PCOS) to achieve pregnancy but is discontinued in the first trimester if utilized solely for PCOS. The use of oral hypoglycemic agents in pregnancy may be considered but should be individualized based on type of diabetes or limited resources or inability to administer insulin. Patients with more severe hyperglycemia despite a diabetic diet (fasting glucose levels >110–120 mg/100 mL or 2-hour postprandial glucose levels >140 mg/100 mL) may not be adequately controlled on oral hypoglycemic agents and need to be started directly on insulin.

Patients with diabetes are monitored closely throughout pregnancy, usually at 1- to 2-week intervals. Insulin adjustments are made on the basis of the glucose logs maintained by the patient. Also, as previously described, insulin requirements of a pregnant patient are expected to increase as pregnancy advances because of the rising production of hPL by the placenta, with its insulin-resistant effect.

Infection

Infections occur more frequently in mothers with diabetes. The glucose-rich urine is an excellent environment for bacterial growth; the risk of urinary tract infection and pyelonephritis is approximately double that of nondiabetic pregnant patients. Patients should be told to promptly report any symptoms that suggest infection so that identification and treatment can be initiated.

Labor and Delivery of the Patient with Diabetes

The goal is for the patient with diabetes to deliver a healthy child vaginally. The adequacy of glucose control, the well-being of the infant, estimated fetal weight by ultrasound, presence of hypertension or other complications of pregnancy, gestational age, presentation of the fetus, and status of the cervix are all factors involved in decisions regarding delivery. In the well-controlled patient with diabetes who has no complications, induction at term (39 weeks) is often undertaken. For women with GDM or pregestational diabetes and an estimated fetal weight of 4,500 g or more, cesarean delivery may be considered. Earlier delivery may be necessary for either fetal or maternal indications and may be accomplished without fetal lung maturity studies if medically indicated. If antepartum steroids for fetal lung maturity become necessary (e.g., for patients with preterm labor), frequent glucose monitoring and, at times, increased doses of insulin are necessary to counter the hyperglycemic effects of corticosteroids.

Whether the patient's labor begins spontaneously or is induced, the goal of intrapartum insulin therapy is strict glucose control. Once active labor begins or glucose levels decrease to 70 mg/dL, a constant glucose infusion of a 5% dextrose solution delivered at a rate of 100 to 150 mL/hour is administered to maintain a glucose level of 100 mg/dL. The plasma glucose level should be assessed every 1 to 2 hours. Short-acting insulin may be administered, usually by constant intravenous infusion, if glucose levels exceed 100 mg/dL. Maternal ketonuria is also monitored and can be managed during labor using the glucose-insulin infusion.

With delivery of the placenta, the source of the "anti-insulin" factors, most notably hPL, is removed. With its short half-life, the effect on plasma glucose is evident within hours. Many patients do not require any insulin for a few days postpartum. Routine management generally consists of frequent glucose assessments and a sliding-scale approach with minimal insulin injections. The goals for optimal glucose values are less stringent in the puerperium than during pregnancy. For patients with GDM, no further insulin is required postpartum. In patients with pregestational diabetes, insulin is generally resumed at 50% of the prepregnant dose once a patient is consuming a normal diet. Thereafter, insulin can be adjusted over the ensuing weeks, with requirements usually reaching the prepregnancy level.

More than 95% of mothers with gestational diabetes return to a completely normal glucose status immediately postpartum; however, up to 70% of these women go on to develop type 2 diabetes later in life and need to be educated about the importance of maintaining a healthy diet and regular exercise program. Glucose tolerance screening is advocated 4 to 12 weeks postpartum to detect the 3% to 5% who remain diabetic and require treatment. Typically, such screening involves a 75-g glucose load, followed by plasma glucose determination 2 hours later. A value above 140 mg/dL requires follow-up. The ADA and ACOG recommend repeat testing at least every 1 to 3 years for women who had a pregnancy affected by GDM and normal results of postpartum screening.

For contraception, barrier methods or intrauterine contraceptives are often chosen; patients who choose oral contraceptives should monitor their glucose values to identify an increase that is sometimes seen with this method (see Chapter 26).

THYROID DISEASE

As with diabetes mellitus, thyroid disease may predate pregnancy or may initially manifest during pregnancy. Obstetric conditions, such as gestational trophoblastic disease or hyperemesis gravidarum, may themselves affect thyroid function. All neonates of women with thyroid disease are at risk for neonatal thyroid dysfunction. For this reason, the neonate's pediatrician should be informed about the maternal diagnosis.

Pathophysiology

Thyrotoxicosis is the condition that results from excess production of and exposure to thyroid hormone from any cause. **Hyperthyroidism** is thyrotoxicosis caused by hyperfunctioning of the thyroid gland. **Graves' disease** is an autoimmune disease characterized by abnormal production of thyroid-specific immunoglobulins that either stimulate or inhibit thyroid function. Exacerbation of the signs and symptoms of hyperthyroidism is called a **thyroid storm**. **Hypothyroidism** is caused by inadequate thyroid hormone production. **Postpartum thyroiditis** is an autoimmune inflammation of the thyroid gland that presents as new-onset, painless hypothyroidism, transient thyrotoxicosis, or thyrotoxicosis followed by hypothyroidism within 1 year postpartum.

Levels of thyroid-binding globulin (TBG) normally increase in pregnancy. Test results that change significantly in pregnancy are those influenced by TBG concentration, including total thyroxine (TT4), total triiodothyronine (TTd), and resin triiodothyronine uptake (TR3U). A transient increase may also occur in free thyroxine (FT4) and free thyroxine index (FTI) levels in the first trimester (Fig. 20.2).

Plasma iodide levels decrease during pregnancy, and this change may cause a noticeable increase in thyroid gland size (up to 30% change) in 15% of women. However, in most women, the thyroid returns to normal size postpartum.

Laboratory Screening

There is insufficient evidence to warrant routine screening of asymptomatic pregnant women for hypothyroidism. Testing should be performed in women with a prior history of thyroid disease or symptoms of thyroid disease. Thyroid function is evaluated by measuring thyroid-stimulating hormone (TSH) levels. TSH does not cross the placenta, so this test is an accurate measure of hormone function during pregnancy. In pregnant women suspected of being hyperthyroid or hypothyroid, FT4 and FTI levels should be measured in addition to TSH.

Management of Existing Thyroid Disease in Pregnancy

Hyperthyroidism

Hyperthyroidism in pregnancy is treated with thionamides, specifically propylthiouracil (PTU) and methimazole. Both drugs cross the placenta but methimazole more so than PTU, theoretically causing greater fetal thyroid suppression. Methimazole has been associated with reports of fetal scalp defects (**aplasia cutis**) and **choanal atresia** and should be avoided in the first trimester. With more recent reports of hepatotoxicity with PTU, although rare, methimazole is recommended in pregnancy beyond the first trimester. Both drugs are considered compatible with breastfeeding.

The goal of treatment during pregnancy is to maintain the FT4 or FTI in the high normal range using the lowest possible dosage of thionamides to minimize fetal exposure. Thionamide treatment for Graves' disease in pregnancy may suppress fetal and neonatal thyroid function and has also been associated with fetal goiter. Neonatal hypothyroidism is usually transient and does not require treatment.

Thyroid Storm

Thyroid storm is a medical emergency characterized by an extreme hypermetabolic state. Although rare (it occurs in 1% to 2% of pregnant patients with hyperthyroidism), it carries a high risk of maternal heart failure. It is often precipitated by infection, surgery, labor, or delivery and is more common in women with poorly controlled hyperthyroidism. Thyroid storm must be diagnosed and treated quickly in order to prevent shock, stupor, and coma (Box 20.2). Treatment of thyroid storm consists of a standard series of drugs, each of which plays a role in suppressing thyroid function. The underlying precipitating event should also be treated. The fetus should be appropriately evaluated with ultrasonography, biophysical profile, or nonstress test, depending on the gestational age. It is also important to note that even if fetal status is not reassuring in the acute setting of thyroid storm, that status may improve as maternal status is stabilized. In general, it is prudent to avoid delivery in the presence of thyroid storm.

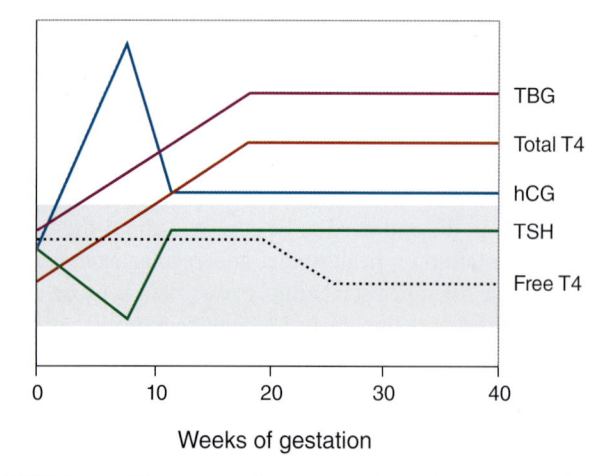

FIGURE 20.2. The pattern of changes in thyroid function and human chorionic gonadotropin (hCG) concentration according to gestational age. The shaded area represents the normal range of thyroid-binding globulin (TBG), total thyroxine (T4), thyroid-stimulating hormone (TSH), and free T4 in the nonpregnant woman. (Modified from Brent GA. Maternal thyroid function: interpretation of thyroid function tests in pregnancy. *Clin Obstet Gynecol.* 1997;40(1):3–15.)

BOX 20.2 Symptoms of Thyroid Storm

- Fever
- Tachycardia out of proportion to the fever
- Altered mental status (including restlessness, nervousness, confusion, and seizures)
- Vomiting
- Diarrhea
- Cardiac arrhythmia

Hypothyroidism

Treatment of hypothyroidism in pregnant women is the same as for nonpregnant women and involves administration of levothyroxine at sufficient dosages to normalize TSH levels. Maternal thyroxine requirements increase in women with hypothyroidism diagnosed before pregnancy. Levothyroxine levels should be adjusted at 4- to 6-week intervals by 25- to 50-µg increments until TSH levels normalize. Thereafter, levels should be checked once per trimester.

Management of Thyroid Disease Diagnosed during and after Pregnancy

Biochemical Hyperthyroidism

Severe nausea and vomiting of pregnancy (**hyperemesis gravidarum**) may cause biochemical hyperthyroidism, in which levels of TSH are undetectable, FTI levels are elevated, or both. This condition resolves spontaneously by 18 weeks of gestation. Routine measurements of thyroid function are not recommended in patients with hyperemesis gravidarum unless other overt signs of hyperthyroidism are evident.

Postpartum Thyroiditis

Postpartum thyroiditis occurs in 5% to 10% of women during the first year after childbirth who have no prior history of thyroid disease. Postpartum thyroiditis also may occur after pregnancy loss and has a 70% risk of recurrence. Almost half of women with postpartum thyroiditis have hypothyroidism, whereas the remaining women are evenly split between thyrotoxicosis and thyrotoxicosis followed by hypothyroidism. Postpartum thyrotoxicosis usually resolves on its own without treatment. Of those with hypothyroidism, approximately 40% of women require treatment for extremely high TSH levels or an increasing goiter size. Only 11% of women diagnosed with postpartum hypothyroidism develop permanent hypothyroidism.

CLINICAL FOLLOW-UP

With major changes on the way, your patient manages her diabetes with frequent visits and close monitoring of her glucose values and her fetus. She delivers a healthy child vaginally at 39 weeks. If she plans to have another pregnancy in the future, she knows that preconception care and strict control of her diabetes promote another healthy infant outcome.

thePoint® Visit http://thePoint.lww.com/activate for an interactive USMLE-style question bank and more!

CHAPTER 21

Gastrointestinal, Renal, and Surgical Complications

This chapter deals primarily with APGO Educational Topic Area:

TOPIC 17 MEDICAL AND SURGICAL COMPLICATIONS OF PREGNANCY

Students should be able to identify how pregnancy affects the natural history of various gastrointestinal, renal, and surgical disorders and how a preexisting gastrointestinal or renal disorder affects maternal and fetal health. They should be able to describe gastrointestinal disorders unique to pregnancy. They should be able to outline a basic approach to evaluation and management of gastrointestinal, renal, and surgical disorders in pregnancy.

CLINICAL CASE

You are seeing a new patient in your office who is complaining of frequent nausea and vomiting over the past few weeks. She recently found out she is pregnant. She has had to miss several days of work due to the vomiting and is worried that she is ill. She was seen by another physician who did some blood tests and told her she needed to be treated for hyperthyroidism. She is concerned about taking anything to help relieve her symptoms or to treat her thyroid disorder because she knows that many medications can cause birth defects.

● INTRODUCTION

Maternal medical or surgical conditions can complicate the course of a pregnancy and can be affected by pregnancy. Physicians providing obstetric care must have a thorough understanding of the effect of pregnancy on the natural course of a disorder, the effect of the disorder on a pregnancy, and the change in management of the pregnancy and disorder caused by their coincidence.

● GASTROINTESTINAL DISORDERS

The normal anatomical, physical, and functional changes that occur in the gastrointestinal (GI) tract in normal pregnancy can appreciably alter clinical findings or symptoms typically used for diagnosis of GI diseases (see Chapter 5). In addition, the implications of these signs and symptoms may change depending on the time of onset during the pregnancy (see Section "Nausea and Vomiting of Pregnancy"). Several disorders of the liver are unique to pregnancy including intrahepatic cholestasis of pregnancy (ICP), acute fatty liver of pregnancy, and preeclampsia/HELLP syndrome. Prompt diagnosis and appropriate management of these disorders are essential in preventing potentially serious adverse outcomes for the mother and fetus. Viral hepatitis is covered in Chapter 24. Management of cholelithiasis, cholecystitis, and appendicitis is covered later in this chapter in Section "Surgical Conditions."

Nausea and Vomiting of Pregnancy

Symptoms of nausea and vomiting are common in pregnancy (see Chapters 5 and 6), especially in the first trimester, and affect 70% to 85% of pregnant women. Because symptoms of **nausea and vomiting of pregnancy (NVP)** are so common, clinicians and pregnant women may minimize their importance and fail to offer or seek treatment. NVP may significantly impact the daily life of a pregnant woman, making it difficult for her to function at home or at work. Safe and effective treatment, in the form of dietary or lifestyle changes as well as pharmacological therapies, is available and should be offered.

Although the etiology of NVP is unknown, the timing is associated with the typical early pregnancy rise in human chorionic gonadotropin ([hCG] Fig. 21.1) as well as the higher estrogen and progesterone levels noted in pregnancy. Most women with NVP begin having symptoms before 9 weeks of gestation, with the peak in severity occurring between 7 and 12 weeks of gestation. The most severe form of NVP, **hyperemesis gravidarum**, occurs in 0.3% to 3% of pregnancies and is associated with ketonuria, dehydration, and significant weight loss (>5% prepregnancy weight). Hyperemesis gravidarum is the most common indication for hospital admission in the first half of pregnancy. Fortunately, 85% to 90% of women will stop experiencing symptoms of NVP by 16 weeks of gestation, with a very small proportion having persistent symptoms beyond 20 weeks. Women with multiple gestation, molar pregnancy, and family history or personal history of hyperemesis gravidarum in a prior pregnancy are at increased risk for NVP.

Symptoms

Symptoms of NVP can occur at any time of the day or night so the term "morning sickness" can be misleading. NVP can be

Peak symptoms of NVP and hCG levels

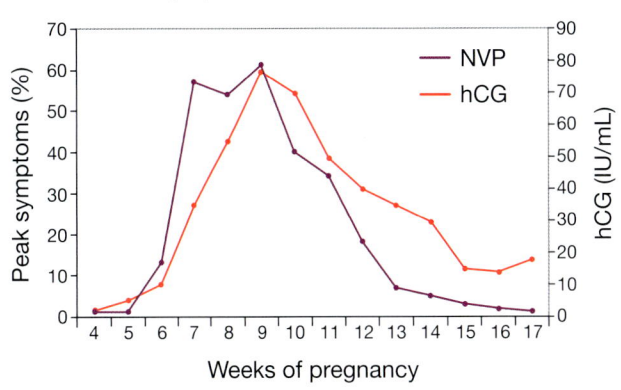

FIGURE 21.1. Nausea symptoms and human chorionic gonadotropin (hCG) levels by week of gestation. NVP, nausea and vomiting of pregnancy. (APGO Educational Series on Women's Health Issues, Nausea and Vomiting of Pregnancy, from www.apgo.org, by S.T. Phelan, MD, et al., 2017. Retrieved by https://www.apgo.org/ed-series-log-in. Copyright 2017 by the Association of Professors of Gynecology and Obstetrics (APOG). Reprinted with permission.)

classified as *mild* (nausea only), *moderate* (nausea with retching and/or vomiting), or *severe* (nausea and persistent vomiting leading to dehydration). However, even mild NVP may be perceived by some women as having a significant impact on their daily life. Therefore, NVP may be best classified according to the impact on a pregnant woman's daily family life or employment; this assessment of impact should guide the need for intervention. Other than quality of life and productivity, NVP has limited negative impact on outcomes of pregnancy; women with severe NVP or hyperemesis gravidarum and poor total weight gain during the pregnancy may be at increased risk for delivering an infant with lower birth weight compared with women with milder NVP or no symptoms. However, miscarriage rates are statistically lower in women with NVP compared with women without symptoms.

Diagnosis

NVP is essentially a diagnosis of exclusion, with the time of onset of symptoms in pregnancy being an important clue; onset of symptoms at >9 weeks of gestation and especially in the second half of pregnancy should prompt evaluation for diagnoses other than NVP. In addition, certain physical examination findings suggest a diagnosis other than NVP (Box 21.1). Conditions that should be considered in the differential diagnosis of NVP are listed in Box 21.2. A careful history will identify underlying medical disorders; this information combined with physical examination findings not consistent with NVP will direct the need for laboratory or other diagnostic evaluation. An ultrasonographic evaluation may be useful in cases of severe presumed nausea and vomiting of pregnancy. It may identify a predisposing factor such as multiple gestation or molar gestation. A "biochemical hyperthyroidism" has been associated with NVP due to the action of hCG on the thyroid-stimulating hormone receptor. Hyperthyroidism as a cause of NVP is very rare; if there are no overt signs of thyroid disease such as goiter, routine thyroid function tests are not indicated. NVP cannot be attributed to underlying psychological

---

BOX 21.1 Physical Examination Findings Not Characteristic of Nausea and Vomiting of Pregnancy

- Abdominal pain or tenderness (other than mild epigastric discomfort)
- Fever
- Headache
- Abnormal neurological examination
- Goiter

BOX 21.2 Selected Differential Diagnosis of Nausea and Vomiting of Pregnancy

Gastrointestinal Disorders
- Gastroenteritis
- Gastroparesis
- Gallbladder and biliary tract disease
- Hepatitis
- Bowel obstruction
- Peptic ulcer disease
- Pancreatitis
- Appendicitis

Genitourinary Tract Conditions
- Pyelonephritis
- Ovarian torsion
- Kidney stones

Metabolic Disease
- Diabetic ketoacidosis
- Porphyria
- Addison disease
- Hyperthyroidism

Neurologic Disorders
- Pseudotumor cerebri
- Migraines
- Tumors of the central nervous system

Miscellaneous
- Drug toxicity
- Psychologic and psychiatric disorders

Pregnancy-Related Conditions
- Acute fatty liver of pregnancy
- Preeclampsia

Modified from APGO monograph "Nausea and Vomiting of Pregnancy," 2011-2015 and Nausea and Vomiting of Pregnancy. Practice Bulletin No. 153. American College of Obstetricians and Gynecologists. *Obstet Gynecol*. 2015;126:e12–24.

or psychiatric disorders although the symptoms of NVP may exacerbate these problems.

Treatment

If symptoms of NVP are impacting the daily life and functioning of a pregnant woman, some form of intervention should be offered and instituted. The woman's perception of the severity of her symptoms and her desire for treatment are influential in clinical decision-making. Fear of teratogenicity may cause providers or pregnant women to avoid drug therapy for NVP; this is unwarranted insofar as safe and effective medical treatments are readily available. In addition, treatment of milder symptoms of NVP may prevent progression to more severe symptoms and hyperemesis gravidarum. Management of NVP includes dietary and lifestyle modifications (Box 21.3) as well as pharmacologic therapies (Fig. 21.2). First-line therapy should be vitamin B_6 with or without doxylamine. Effective and safe treatments for more serious cases include antihistamines other than doxylamine (H_1-receptor blockers) and dopamine antagonists (phenothiazines and benzamides).

● HEPATIC DISORDERS UNIQUE TO PREGNANCY

Intrahepatic Cholestasis of Pregnancy

ICP is characterized by generalized pruritus (but no definitive rash) with elevated serum bile acids that typically occurs in the second half of pregnancy and resolves after delivery. This disorder occurs in 0.2% to 1% of pregnancies in the United States and Western Europe but in much higher rates (4%) in other areas of the world (Bolivia and Chile). The cause of ICP is unknown but likely involves genetic and hormonal factors. Risk factors include multiple gestation and chronic hepatitis C. Recurrence is common in subsequent pregnancies. Maternal morbidity is low, with the main effect being discomfort from the intense itching, which is generalized but often involves the palms of the hands and soles of the feet. Fetal effects can be serious, with increased risk of stillbirth. Diagnosis is confirmed by the presence of elevated fasting levels of bile acids. Other laboratory abnormalities may include mild elevations in serum aminotransferases and total and direct bilirubin concentrations.

Treatment

Treatment consists of ursodeoxycholic acid, which decreases plasma bile acid concentrations and improves the symptoms of itching. Decreased levels of bile acids reduce the risk of adverse outcome, but there are no current studies documenting decreased perinatal morbidity and mortality with treatment. Once the diagnosis of ICP is made, antepartum fetal surveillance is initiated. It is not clear whether available methods of antepartum surveillance reliably predict fetal compromise in the setting of ICP. Therefore, delivery is generally recommended at 37 weeks of gestation.

Acute Fatty Liver of Pregnancy

The most common cause of acute liver failure in pregnancy is acute fatty liver. It is characterized by microvesicular fatty infiltration of hepatocytes most typically presenting in the third trimester. Fortunately, this serious disorder is uncommon, with rates of approximately 1 in 10,000 pregnancies. In some cases of acute fatty liver, there is a recessively inherited mitochondrial abnormality of fatty acid oxidation, similar to those in children with Reye-like syndromes. Recurrence in subsequent pregnancies is uncommon but has been described, especially if the woman is carrying a homozygous enzyme-deficient fetus. The most common symptoms of acute fatty liver of pregnancy are persistent nausea and vomiting. Other symptoms include malaise, anorexia, abdominal pain, edema, and progressive jaundice. In the most severe cases, women may present with hepatic encephalopathy. Common laboratory abnormalities include modestly elevated serum aminotransferase levels, elevated bilirubin, raised prothrombin time, leukocytosis, elevated serum creatinine, decreased fibrinogen, and thrombocytopenia. In more severe cases, hypoglycemia, elevated serum ammonia levels, lactic acidosis, and disseminated intravascular coagulation may be present. Imaging of the liver by ultrasound or other modalities may or may not be useful. Liver biopsy is rarely necessary to make the diagnosis but would show characteristic microvesicular steatosis and canalicular cholestasis. In about half of affected women, some combination of hypertension, proteinuria, and edema may be present, making it difficult to differentiate from severe preeclampsia. However, increased bilirubin, markedly decreased fibrinogen levels, and profound liver dysfunction are less common in preeclampsia. Viral serologies should be obtained to rule out viral hepatitis (see Chapter 24).

Management

Intensive supportive care and prompt delivery are key to optimal management. In the past, maternal mortality approached 75% and perinatal mortality 90%. More recent literature reports

---

> **BOX 21.3** Dietary and Lifestyles Measures for Managing Symptoms of Nausea and Vomiting of Pregnancy
>
> - Eating frequently in small amounts
> - Eating high-carbohydrate, low-fat foods
> - Adding protein to snacks and meals
> - Eating a bland, dry or salty diet
> - Drinking small amounts of cold, clear carbonated or sour liquids
> - Drinking between meals rather than with meals
> - Lying down as needed; getting plenty of rest
> - Changing position slowly, especially when rising
> - Going outside for fresh air as needed
> - Avoiding offensive foods and smells
> - Not brushing teeth after eating
>
> Modified from APGO monograph NVP 2011–2015.

Pharmacologic Therapy of NVP[a]

Monotherapy: Vitamin B6 10–50 mg orally 3–4 times daily
(for each option, if no improvement, proceed to the next step)

↓

Add: Doxylamine[b] 12.5 mg orally 3–4 times daily
Adjust dose and schedule according to severity of symptoms

↓

Add: Promethazine 12.5–25 mg every 4 hours orally or rectally
Or
Dimenhydrinate 50–100 mg every 4–6 hours orally or rectally
(not to exceed 400 mg/day; not to exceed 200 mg/day if also taking doxylamine)

IF NO EVIDENCE OF DEHYDRATION

Add any of the following (presented here in alphabetical order):
Chlorpromazine 10–25 mg every 4–6 hours orally or intramuscularly (IM)
Or
Metoclopramide 5–10 mg every 8 hours orally or IM
Or
Ondansetron 4–8 mg every 6–8 hours orally
Or
Prochlorperazine 5–10 mg every 6–8 hours orally or IM
Or
Promethazine 12.5–25 mg every 4 hours orally, rectally, or IM
Or
Trimethobenzamide 200 mg every 6–8 hours rectally

IF EVIDENCE OF DEHYDRATION

Intravenous fluid replacement
(No study has compared different intravenous [IV] fluid replacement for NVP but IV fluids should include dextrose for optimal clearance of ketosis/ketonuria)
Thiamine 100 mg IV daily for 2–3 days plus IV multivitamins should be administered with IV fluid replacement for any woman who has vomited for more than 3 weeks

↓

Add any of the following (presented here in alphabetical order):
Dimenhydrinate 50 mg every 4–6 hours IV
Or
Metoclopramide 5–10 mg every 8 hours IV
Or
Promethazine 12.5–25 mg every 4 hours IV

↓

Add one or both of the following:
Ondansetron 8 mg over 15 minutes every 12 hours IV
Or
Methylprednisolone 16 mg every 8 hours orally or IV for 3 days
(benefit should become apparent within 3 days; if no benefit noted then discontinue; if benefit noted, taper over 2 weeks to lowest effective dose; if beneficial, limit total duration of use to 6 weeks [Note: do not use during first 10 weeks of gestation due to increased risk of oral clefts])

[a] This algorithm assumes that other causes of nausea and vomiting have been ruled out. At any time, alternative therapies may be added depending on patient preference and clinician familiarity; consider ginger root powder, capsules, or extract up to 1,000 mg/day (ginger products are not standardized) or acupressure/acupuncture at acupoint P6. Enteral nutrition may be considered for those women with persistent nausea and vomiting and weight loss despite antiemetic therapy. Parenteral nutrition is associated with potentially life-threatening complications and should be reserved as a last resort for the rare patient who does not tolerate enteral tube feedings.

[b] In the United States, doxylamine is available as the active ingredient in some over-the-counter sleep aids; one half of a scored 25 mg tablet can be used to provide the 12.5 mg dose. Also, the combination of B6 and doxylamine is no longer commercially available in the United States. Individual compounding pharmacies in some communities will make the combination of B6 10 mg and doxylamine 10 mg on request.

FIGURE 21.2. Pharmacologic management of nausea and vomiting of pregnancy (NVP). (Modified from Nausea and Vomiting of Pregnancy. Practice Bulletin No. 153. American College of Obstetricians and Gynecologists; *Obstet Gynecol*. 2015;126:e12–24. Association of Professors of Gynecology and Obstetrics (APGO) Continuing Series on Women's Health Education, "Nausea and Vomiting of Pregnancy," 2011–2015.)

maternal mortality rates of 4% and perinatal mortality 12%. Delivery typically stops further decline in liver function, but recovery may be prolonged. Infants should be assessed for signs associated with defects in fatty acid oxidation.

Preeclampsia and HELLP Syndrome

Hypertensive disorders in pregnancy that affect the liver include severe preeclampsia–eclampsia syndromes and HELLP. These disorders and their effects on the liver are discussed extensively in Chapter 22.

URINARY TRACT DISORDERS

Urinary tract infections (**UTIs**) are common in pregnancy. Approximately 8% of all women (pregnant and nonpregnant) have >10^5 colonies of a single bacterial species on a midstream culture. Approximately 25% of the pregnant women in this group develop an acute, symptomatic UTI. Other urinary tract disorders that may complicate pregnancy include urinary calculi, nephrolithiasis, and preexisting renal disease.

Asymptomatic Bacteriuria and Uncomplicated Urinary Tract Infection

Compared with nonpregnant women with similar colony counts on urine culture, asymptomatic bacteriuria in pregnancy is more likely to lead to **cystitis** and **pyelonephritis**. The increased incidence of symptomatic infection during pregnancy is thought to be caused by **pregnancy-associated urinary stasis** and glucosuria. This relative urinary stasis in pregnancy is a result of progesterone-induced decreased ureteral tone and motility, mechanical compression of the ureters at the pelvic brim, and compression of the bladder and ureteral orifices. In addition, the pH of urine is increased because of increased bicarbonate excretion, which also enhances bacterial growth.

A urine culture is obtained at the onset of prenatal care, and patients with asymptomatic bacteriuria are treated with ampicillin, cephalexin or nitrofurantoin. Empiric treatment with a 3-day course of antibiotics is 90% effective. Alternatively, a standard 7- to 10-day course may be considered. The most common organism identified is Escherichia coli. Approximately 25% to 30% of patients not treated for asymptomatic bacteriuria proceed to symptomatic UTI; hence, this treatment should prevent a significant number of symptomatic UTIs in pregnancy. However, 1.5% of patients with initial negative cultures also develop symptomatic UTIs during pregnancy. Also, recurrence rates for asymptomatic bacteriuria approach 30% even with effective therapy. Suppressive antimicrobial therapy is indicated if there are repetitive UTIs during pregnancy or following pyelonephritis during pregnancy. Consideration should be given to postpartum radiographic evaluation of these patients to identify renal parenchymal and urinary-collecting duct abnormalities.

Acute cystitis occurs in approximately 1% of pregnancies and can manifest with dysuria, urinary frequency, and urgency. The treatment is the same as for asymptomatic bacteriuria.

Pyelonephritis

Patients with **pyelonephritis** (inflammation of the renal parenchyma, calices, and pelvis) are acutely ill, with fever; costovertebral tenderness; general malaise; and, often, dehydration. Approximately 20% of these ill patients demonstrate increased uterine activity and preterm labor, and approximately 10% have positive blood cultures if they are obtained in the acute febrile phase of the disease. Pyelonephritis occurs in 2% of all pregnant patients and is one of the most common medical complications of pregnancy requiring hospitalization, especially in its context as a major cause of maternal mortality (septic shock).

Treatment

After urinalysis and urine culture are obtained, patients are treated with intravenous hydration and antibiotics, commonly a cephalosporin or ampicillin and gentamicin. Uterine contractions may accompany these symptoms, and specific tocolytic therapy may be considered depending on the patient's status if preterm labor ensues. It is known that *E. coli* can produce phospholipase A, which, in turn, can promote prostaglandin synthesis, resulting in an increase in uterine activity. Fever is also known to induce contractions, so antipyretics are required for a temperature >100.4°F. Attention must be paid to the patient's response to therapy and her general condition; sepsis occurs in 2% to 3% of patients with pyelonephritis, and adult respiratory distress syndrome can occur. If improvement does not occur within 48 to 72 hours, urinary tract obstruction, urinary calculus, or renal abscess should be considered, along with a reevaluation of antibiotic coverage. Ultrasonography or other imaging study such as computed tomography will sometimes identify a calculus or abscess. The organisms most commonly cultured from the urine of symptomatic pregnant patients are *E. coli* and other gram-negative aerobes. Follow-up can be with either frequent urine cultures and/or empiric antibiotic suppression with an agent such as nitrofurantoin.

Recurrent symptoms or failure to respond to usual therapy suggests another cause for the findings. In these patients, a complete urologic evaluation 6 weeks after pregnancy may be warranted.

Nephrolithiasis and Urinary Calculi

Urinary calculi are identified in approximately 1 in 1,500 patients during pregnancy, although pregnancy per se does not promote stone development. Symptoms similar to those of pyelonephritis but without fever suggest urinary calculi. **Microhematuria** is more common with this condition than in uncomplicated UTI. Renal colic (pain) is a typical symptom in nonpregnant women but is seen less frequently in pregnant women because of the hormone-induced relaxation of ureteral tone. Usually, hydration and expectant management, along with straining of urine in search of stones, suffice as management. Occasionally, however, the presence of a stone can lead to infection or complete obstruction, which may require urology consultation and drainage by either ureteral stent or percutaneous nephrostomy.

Preexisting Renal Disease

During preconception counseling, patients who have preexisting renal disease (chronic renal failure or transplant) should be advised of the significant risks involved in a pregnancy. Pregnancy outcome is related to the degree of serum creatinine elevation and the presence of hypertension.

Overall, pregnancy does not seem to have a negative impact on mild chronic renal diseases. In general, patients with mild renal impairment (serum creatinine <1.5 mg/dL) have relatively uneventful pregnancies, provided other complications are absent. Patients with moderate renal impairment (serum creatinine 1.5–3.0 mg/dL) have a more guarded prognosis with an increased incidence of deterioration of renal function. Patients with severe renal impairment have the worst outcome. In approximately 50% of patients with renal disease, proteinuria is noted. An increase in proteinuria during pregnancy is not, by itself, a serious consequence. Many patients with renal disease also have preexisting or concurrent hypertension. These women are at increased risk for hypertensive complications of pregnancy.

In addition to hypertension, there is an increased incidence of intrauterine growth restriction in patients with chronic renal disease. Serial assessments of fetal well-being and growth are frequently performed. Pregnancy following renal transplantation is generally associated with a good prognosis if at least 2 years have elapsed since the transplant was performed and thorough renal assessment reveals no evidence of active disease or rejection. Drug therapy should be minimal.

● SURGICAL CONDITIONS

Patients who are pregnant can experience the same surgical conditions as those who are not pregnant, such as appendicitis, cholelithiasis, and bowel injury. In early gestation, ectopic pregnancy and torsion of the adnexa should be considered. Later in pregnancy, placental abruption and uterine rupture can cause acute abdominal signs and symptoms (see Section "Trauma in Pregnancy").

Considerations for Pregnant Patients

Surgical treatment of a pregnant woman should take into consideration both maternal and fetal health needs. Radiographic or other studies should not be avoided just because the patient is pregnant, though precautions should be used. For procedures such as radiographs of the chest, an abdominal shield may be used to avoid unnecessary exposure to the fetus. Exposure to low doses of radiation is safe for the fetus when considered against failure to treat or to diagnose a condition requiring surgery. In the perioperative period, fetal heart tones should be monitored to the extent possible, consistent with the stage of gestation and need for intervention, usually by electronic fetal monitoring.

The completely supine position should be avoided, if possible. Instead the patient should be placed in a decubitus lateral tilt to prevent supine hypotensive syndrome, in which pressure on the vena cava reduces venous return to the heart, causing a drop in blood pressure and uterine blood flow. Oxygen administration may be helpful. In general, clinicians caring for these patients should be constantly aware of both maternal and fetal considerations. For example, the residual lung volume is diminished in pregnancy, which provides less reserve for respiratory function. Delayed gastric emptying makes aspiration of stomach contents during a surgical procedure more likely.

Cholelithiasis in Pregnancy

Reproductive-aged women frequently have **gallstones**. **Cholelithiasis** can be exacerbated during pregnancy due to hormonal effects that slow gallbladder emptying and cause an increase in residual gallbladder volume. Asymptomatic cholelithiasis should be managed expectantly. If the patient develops biliary colic, attempts should be made to conservatively treat the patient with hydration, pain control, dietary restriction, and possible nasogastric tube. However, if **cholecystitis** occurs with common bile duct obstruction, ascending cholangitis, pancreatitis, or acute abdomen, immediate surgical management is required. Maternal and fetal outcomes tend to be excellent if surgical removal is undertaken before these serious consequences are allowed to worsen. As with appendicitis, traditional surgical management has been open cholecystectomy; however, in recent years, more evidence supports the safe use of laparoscopic cholecystectomy in pregnancy.

Appendicitis in Pregnancy

Appendicitis is a common surgical problem in reproductive-aged women, and, therefore, a common surgical problem in pregnancy. Similar symptoms of the disease occur in pregnancy; of note, leukocytosis associated with appendicitis may be masked with the normal **leukocytosis of pregnancy**. The appendix may be displaced upward as pregnancy advances and can cause a shift in the location of abdominal pain associated with appendicitis, though pain is still most commonly located in the right lower quadrant. When appendicitis is diagnosed and treated early (before appendiceal rupture and generalized peritonitis), fetal and maternal outcomes are good. Surgical management has traditionally been with open appendectomy; however, laparoscopy is increasingly being utilized for the management of appendicitis in pregnancy.

Adnexal Masses in Pregnancy

Abnormal **ovarian** or **adnexal masses** can occur in pregnancy. Often, they are discovered during routine ultrasound examination of the fetus. Most of these masses are benign and spontaneously resolve during pregnancy. For these reasons, expectant management is often advocated for adnexal masses in pregnancy. Approximately 1% to 7% of persistent complex masses are malignant. Serum biomarkers (CA 125) are not useful in pregnancy. With larger masses, there is an increased risk of ovarian torsion or cyst rupture. Surgical management is generally reserved for patients with symptoms or a high index of suspicion for malignancy. In general, surgical management is best performed in the second trimester and may be safely accomplished laparoscopically.

● TRAUMA IN PREGNANCY

Maternal trauma is one of the leading causes of morbidity and mortality in pregnancy. The most common cause of trauma in pregnancy is motor vehicle accidents. The second most common cause is physical violence against women, most frequently partner violence. Traumatic injury can result in maternal injury and death, as well as placental abruption, uterine rupture, fetal–maternal hemorrhage, premature rupture of membranes, or preterm labor. In addition to the above conditions, which can compromise fetal well-being, direct fetal injury is also possible.

Management

The primary goal for evaluation of a pregnant trauma patient is maternal stabilization. Management is essentially the same as for the nonpregnant patient. Vital signs should be assessed and the patient stabilized, followed by obstetric assessment. If the gestational age is 20 weeks or beyond, the patient should be placed in a decubitus lateral tilt position. If this is not feasible (e.g., due to cervical spine stabilization), tilting the backboard by placing a wedge underneath or manual displacement of the uterus off midline will promote adequate maternal venous return. Fetal assessment includes verification of fetal heart tones with Doppler, followed by electronic fetal monitoring once the secondary survey is complete. Fetal ultrasound is also helpful for identifying location of placenta, fetal well-being, amniotic fluid volume, and estimated gestational age.

After a minor trauma, electronic fetal monitoring (including tocometry) is recommended for at least 4 hours with a gestational age of 23 weeks or beyond (however, there are no large studies available to guide a consensus on the appropriate length of time for monitoring to occur). If, during that interval, there are any signs of uterine tenderness, irritability or contractions, vaginal bleeding, rupture of membranes, or nonreassuring fetal status, continued monitoring for at least 24 hours is advocated. Any major trauma necessitates at least 24 hours of continuous fetal monitoring.

Fetal–Maternal Hemorrhage

Fetal–maternal hemorrhage is another complication of maternal trauma, and determination of Rh status is an important part of the management. The extent of fetal–maternal hemorrhage can be determined using one of several tests (e.g., the **Kleihauer-Betke test**). Most often, a regular dose of Rh immunoglobulin is protective for all Rh-negative mothers.

If a pregnant woman undergoes cardiopulmonary arrest, attempts at resuscitation should begin immediately. Emergent cesarean delivery should be strongly considered after 4 minutes of failed resuscitation efforts if the patient is in the third trimester of pregnancy. Maternal resuscitation is made easier once the fetus has been delivered. Long-term outcomes for children are more likely to be favorable if the infant is delivered within 5 minutes of loss of maternal circulation. Fetal survival is not likely if maternal vital signs have been absent for more than 15 to 20 minutes.

CLINICAL FOLLOW-UP

You perform a careful history and physical examination; there are no symptoms other than the nausea and vomiting, no underlying medical disorders, and no abnormal physical findings (specifically, no goiter). An ultrasound shows a normal intrauterine pregnancy at 9 weeks of gestation. You draw some blood tests but reassure the patient that her nausea and vomiting are most likely related to the pregnancy and not hyperthyroidism. You recommend some dietary and lifestyle modifications as well as some medications for her symptoms. You reassure her that these medications will not harm her baby and may prevent her from missing work or having to come to the hospital with more severe vomiting. You plan to see her back to reassess her symptoms and review the blood tests.

CHAPTER 22

Cardiovascular and Respiratory Disorders

This chapter deals primarily with APGO Educational Topic Areas:

TOPIC 17   MEDICAL AND SURGICAL COMPLICATIONS OF PREGNANCY
TOPIC 18   PREECLAMPSIA-ECLAMPSIA

Students should be able to identify how pregnancy affects the natural history of various hematologic and immunologic disorders and how a preexisting hematologic and immunologic disorder affects maternal and fetal health. They should be able to outline a basic approach to evaluation and management of hematologic and immunologic disorders in pregnancy. Additionally, the student should understand the pathophysiology behind isoimmunization. They should be able to outline a basic approach to evaluation and prevention.

CLINICAL CASE

You are seeing a new patient in your office, and the nurse records her sitting blood pressure at 150/90 and on repeat, 154/98. The urine dip was negative except for 1+ protein. The patient complains of having a mild headache earlier that morning that resolved after eating breakfast. She also complains of increased swelling in her legs and feet and says that her blood pressure yesterday at the drug store was 150/100. She is 26 weeks' pregnant. Do you begin antihypertensive therapy? Do you need any further evaluation?

● INTRODUCTION

Maternal medical or surgical conditions can complicate the course of a pregnancy and can be affected by pregnancy. Physicians providing obstetric care must have a thorough understanding of the effect of pregnancy on the natural course of a disorder, the effect of the disorder on a pregnancy, and the change in management of the pregnancy and disorder caused by their coincidence.

● HYPERTENSIVE DISORDERS

Hypertensive disorders occur in up to 10% of pregnancies worldwide and cause substantial perinatal morbidity and mortality of both mother and fetus. Hypertensive disease is directly responsible for approximately 12.3% of maternal deaths in the United States. The incidence of preeclampsia has increased by 25% in the United States during the past two decades. The exact cause of hypertension associated with pregnancy remains unknown.

● CLASSIFICATION

Various classifications of hypertensive disorders in pregnancy have been proposed. Box 22.1 presents a commonly used classification. Because hypertensive disorders in pregnancy represent a spectrum of disease, classification systems should be used as a guide only.

Chronic Hypertension

Chronic hypertension is defined as hypertension present before pregnancy or before the 20th week of gestation or that persists longer than the postpartum period (i.e., 12 weeks after delivery). Criteria for chronic hypertension in pregnancy are as follows:

- **Mild-Moderate:** Systolic pressure of 140–159 mmHg or diastolic pressure of 90–109 mmHg
- **Severe:** Systolic pressure of 160 mmHg or greater or diastolic pressure of 110 mmHg or greater

A major risk with chronic hypertension is the development of preeclampsia or eclampsia later in the pregnancy, which is relatively common and difficult to diagnose. Up to 30% of women with chronic hypertension or gestational hypertension (see below) can develop preeclampsia. The acute onset of proteinuria and gestational hypertension in women with chronic hypertension is suggestive of superimposed preeclampsia.

Gestational Hypertension

Hypertension that develops for the first time after 20 weeks of gestation in the absence of proteinuria is termed gestational hypertension. Gestational hypertension develops in 5% to 10% of pregnancies, with a 30% incidence in multiple gestations, regardless of parity. Maternal morbidity is directly related to the severity and duration of hypertension.

Almost 50% of women with gestational hypertension go on to develop preeclampsia, and approximately 10% of eclamptic seizures occur before overt proteinuria develops. It is often difficult

> **BOX 22.1 Hypertensive Disorders in Pregnancy**
>
> - Gestational hypertension
> - Preeclampsia
>   - Without severe features
>   - With severe features
> - Eclampsia
> - Chronic hypertension preceding pregnancy (any cause)
> - Chronic hypertension (any cause) with:
>   - Superimposed gestational hypertension
>   - Superimposed preeclampsia
>   - Superimposed eclampsia

> **BOX 22.2 Risk Factors for Preeclampsia**
>
> - Nulliparity
> - Multifetal gestation
> - Maternal age 40 years or older
> - Preeclampsia in a previous pregnancy
> - Chronic hypertension
> - Pregestational diabetes
> - Vascular and connective tissue disorders
> - Nephropathy and other chronic renal disease
> - Antiphospholipid syndrome
> - Obesity
> - African American race
> - In vitro fertilization

to distinguish between chronic hypertension, preeclampsia, and gestational hypertension when a patient is seen in the second half of pregnancy with an elevated blood pressure level. In such cases, it is always wise to assume that the findings represent preeclampsia and evaluate accordingly. Gestational hypertension is considered transient hypertension if blood pressure returns to normal before 12 weeks postpartum or reclassified as chronic hypertension if it persists.

Preeclampsia

Preeclampsia is the development of hypertension with proteinuria after 20 weeks of gestation. Edema is typically present with the development of preeclampsia but is not useful as a diagnostic criterion insofar as some degree of edema is common in normal pregnancy. This condition can occur earlier in the presence of gestational trophoblastic disease (see chapter 45). Risk factors for preeclampsia are summarized in Box 22.2. The criteria for the diagnosis of preeclampsia are as follows:

- Blood pressure of ≥140 mmHg systolic or ≥90 mmHg diastolic that occurs after 20 weeks of gestation in a woman with previously normal blood pressure
- Proteinuria, defined as urinary excretion of 0.3 g protein or higher in a 24-hour urine specimen
- Severe preeclampsia is characterized by one or more of the following:
  - Blood pressure ≥160 mmHg systolic or ≥110 mmHg diastolic on two occasions at least 4 hours apart while the patient is on bed rest (severely elevated blood pressure that persists beyond 15 minutes should be treated, not waiting for 4 hours to make diagnosis)
  - Progressive renal insufficiency (serum creatinine >1.1 mg/dl or doubling of serum creatinine)
  - Cerebral or visual disturbances such as headache and scotomata ("spots" before the eyes)
  - Pulmonary edema
  - Epigastric or right-upper-quadrant (RUQ) pain (probably caused by subcapsular hepatic hemorrhage or stretching of Glisson capsule with hepatocellular edema)
  - Evidence of hepatic dysfunction (elevated serum transaminase levels more than two times normal)
  - Thrombocytopenia (platelet count <100,000/microliter)

These changes illustrate the multisystem involvement associated with preeclampsia. In most cases, severe preeclampsia is an indication for delivery, regardless of gestational age or maturity. In carefully selected pregnancies remote from term, expectant management of severe preeclampsia may be considered, predominantly to provide time for corticosteroid lung maturation benefit for the preterm infant (see preeclampsia with severe features below).

Eclampsia

Eclampsia is the additional presence of convulsions (grand mal or tonic–clonic seizures) in a woman with preeclampsia that is not explained by a neurologic disorder. Eclampsia occurs in 0.5% to 4% of patients with preeclampsia.

Most cases of eclampsia occur prior to or within 24 hours of delivery, but up to 10% of cases are diagnosed between 2 and 10 days postpartum.

HELLP Syndrome

HELLP syndrome is the presence of **h**emolysis, **e**levated **l**iver enzymes, and **l**ow **p**latelet count. HELLP syndrome is an indication for delivery to avoid jeopardizing the health of the woman. Women with HELLP syndrome who are less than 34 0/7 weeks gestational age should receive corticosteroids for fetal benefit. If maternal labs do not continue to worsen or the fetal status does not deteriorate, then an attempt to delay delivery for 24 to 48 hours to complete the corticosteroid course is reasonable. HELLP syndrome is now appreciated as a distinct clinical entity, occurring in 4% to 12% of patients with severe preeclampsia or eclampsia. Criteria for diagnosis are the following:

- Microangiopathic hemolysis
- Thrombocytopenia
- Hepatocellular dysfunction

PATHOPHYSIOLOGY

Hypertension in pregnancy affects the mother and newborn to varying degrees. Given the characteristic multisystem effects, it is clear that several pathophysiologic mechanisms are involved (Fig. 22.1). The predominant pathophysiologic finding in preeclampsia and gestational hypertension is maternal vasospasm.

Potential Causes of Maternal Vasospasm

Several potential causes for maternal vasospasm have been postulated:

- **Vascular changes:** Instead of noting the normal physiologic trophoblast-mediated vascular changes in the uterine vessels (decreased musculature in the spiral arterioles leads to the development of a low-resistance, low-pressure, high-flow system), inadequate maternal vascular remodeling is seen in cases of preeclampsia and IUGR. Endothelial damage is also noted within the vessels.
- **Hemostatic changes:** Increased platelet activation with increased consumption in the microvasculature is noted during the course of preeclampsia. Endothelial fibronectin levels are increased and antithrombin III and α_2-antiplasmin levels are decreased, reflecting endothelial damage. Low antithrombin III levels are permissive for microthrombi development. Endothelial damage is then thought to promote further vasospasm.
- **Changes in prostanoids:** Prostacyclin (PGI_2) and thromboxane (TXA_2) are increased during pregnancy, with the balance in favor of PGI_2. In patients who develop preeclampsia, the balance shifts to favor TXA_2. Again, PGI_2 functions to promote vasodilation and decrease platelet aggregation, and TXA_2 promotes vasoconstriction and platelet aggregation. Because of this imbalance, vessel constriction occurs.
- **Changes in endothelium-derived factors:** Nitric oxide, a potent vasodilator, is decreased in patients with preeclampsia and may explain the evolution of vasoconstriction in these patients.
- **Lipid peroxide, free radicals, and antioxidant release:** Lipid peroxides and free radicals have been implicated in vascular injury and are increased in pregnancies complicated by preeclampsia. Decreased antioxidant levels are also noted.

Effects on Organ Systems and Fetus

The above mechanisms, in any combination or permutation, are thought to contribute to the following common pathophysiologic changes seen in patients with preeclampsia:

- **Cardiovascular effects:** Elevated blood pressure is seen as the result of potential vasoconstriction as well as an increase in cardiac output.
- **Hematologic effects:** Plasma volume contraction or hemoconcentration may develop, with the risk of rapid-onset hypovolemic shock, if hemorrhage occurs. Plasma volume contraction is reflected in increased hematocrit values. Thrombocytopenia or disseminated intravascular coagulation may also develop from microangiopathic hemolytic anemia. Involvement of the liver may lead to hepatocellular dysfunction and further evolution of coagulopathy. Third spacing of fluid may be noted, because of increased blood pressure and decreased plasma oncotic pressure.

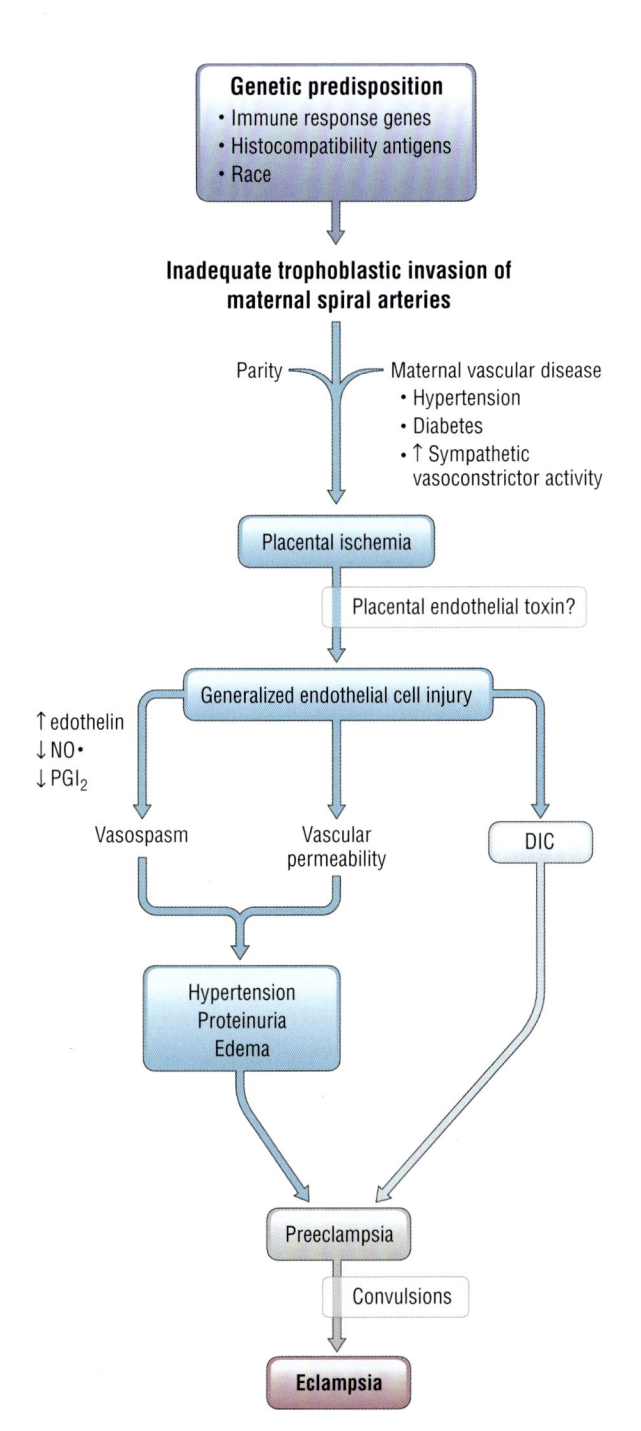

FIGURE 22.1. Proposed pathways and markers implicated in the development of preeclampsia and eclampsia. *DIC*, disseminated intravascular coagulation; *NO*, nitric acid; *PGI_2*, prostacyclin.

- **Renal effects:** Decreased glomerular filtration rate (increasing serum creatinine) and proteinuria (urine protein levels >300 mg per 24 hours) develop secondary to vasospasm and atherosclerotic-like changes in the renal vessels (glomerular endotheliosis). Uric acid filtration is decreased; therefore, elevated maternal serum uric acid levels may be an indication of evolving disease.
- **Neurologic effects:** Hyperreflexia/hypersensitivity may develop. Other neurologic manifestations include headache, blurred vision, and scotomata. In severe cases, grand mal (eclamptic) seizures may develop.
- **Pulmonary effects:** Pulmonary edema may occur and can be related to decreased colloid oncotic pressure, pulmonary capillary leak, left heart failure, iatrogenic fluid overload, or a combination of these factors.
- **Fetal effects:** Decreased intermittent placental perfusion secondary to vasospasm is thought to be responsible for the increased incidence of IUGR (<10% estimated fetal weight for gestational age) and oligohydramnios and increased perinatal mortality of infants born to mothers with preeclampsia. An increased incidence of placental abruption is also seen. With the stress of uterine contractions during labor, the placenta may be unable to adequately oxygenate the fetus. This may result in signs of intrapartum uteroplacental insufficiency. Specifically, a nonreassuring fetal heart rate pattern may necessitate cesarean delivery.

Presumably because of vasospastic changes, placental size and function are decreased. The results are progressive fetal hypoxia and malnutrition as well as an increase in the incidence of IUGR and oligohydramnios.

EVALUATION

The history and physical examination are directed toward detection of pregnancy-associated hypertensive disease and its signs and symptoms. A review of current obstetric records, if available, is especially helpful to ascertain changes or progression in findings. Visual disturbances, especially scotomata, or unusually severe or persistent headaches are indicative of vasospasm. RUQ pain may indicate liver involvement, presumably involving distension of the liver capsule. Any history of loss of consciousness or seizures, even in the patient with a known seizure disorder, may be significant.

Physical Examination

The position of the patient influences blood pressure. It is lowest with the patient lying in the lateral position, highest when the patient is standing, and at an intermediate level when she is sitting. The choice of the correct-size blood pressure cuff also influences blood pressure readings, with falsely high measurements noted when normal-sized cuffs are used on large patients. Also, during the course of pregnancy, blood pressure typically declines slightly in the second trimester, increasing to prepregnant levels as gestation nears term (Fig. 22.2). If a patient has not been seen previously, there is no baseline blood pressure against which to compare new blood pressure determinations, thereby making the diagnosis of pregnancy-related hypertension more difficult.

The patient's weight is compared with her pregravid weight and with previous weights during this pregnancy, with special attention to excessive or too rapid weight gain. Peripheral edema is common in pregnancy, especially in the lower extremities. However, persistent edema unresponsive to resting in the supine position is not normal, especially when it also involves the upper extremities, sacral region, and face. Indeed, the puffy-faced, edematous, hypertensive pregnant woman is the classic picture of preeclampsia. Careful blood pressure determination in the sitting and supine positions is necessary. Funduscopic examination may detect vasoconstriction of retinal blood vessels indicative of similar vasoconstriction of other small vessels. Tenderness over the liver, attributed partly to hepatic capsule distension, may be associated with complaints of RUQ pain. The patellar and Achilles' deep tendon reflexes should be carefully elicited and hyperreflexia noted. The demonstration of clonus at the ankle is especially worrisome.

Laboratory Tests

The maternal and fetal laboratory evaluations for pregnancy complicated by hypertension are presented in Table 22.1 and demonstrate, by the wide range of tests, the multisystem effects of hypertension in pregnancy. Maternal liver dysfunction, renal insufficiency, and coagulopathy are significant concerns and require serial evaluation. Evaluation of fetal well-being with

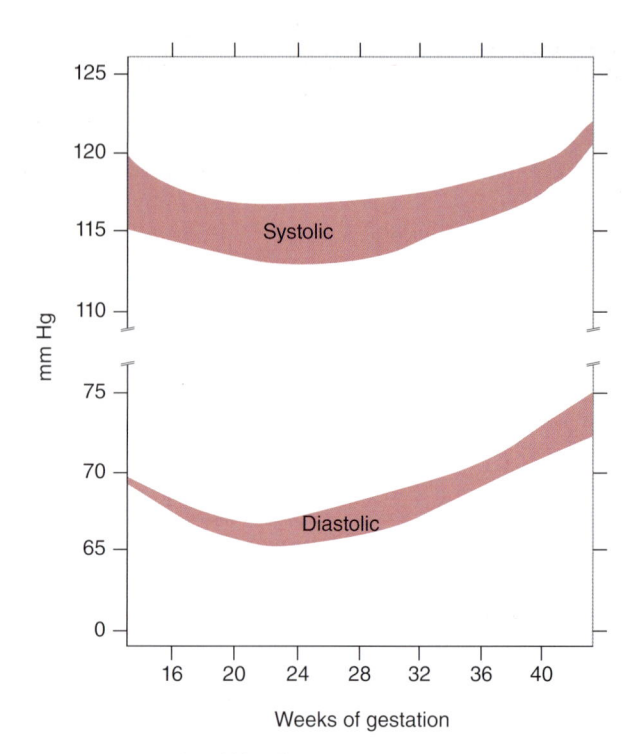

FIGURE 22.2. Range of blood pressures in normotensive pregnancy. Note the decrease in blood pressure in the second trimester.

TABLE 22.1 — LABORATORY ASSESSMENT OF PREGNANT HYPERTENSIVE PATIENTS

Test or Procedure	Rationale
Maternal studies	
Complete blood count	Increasing hematocrit may signify worsening vasoconstriction and decreased intravascular volume
	Decreasing hematocrit may signify hemolysis
Platelet count	Thrombocytopenia is associated with worsening disease
Coagulation profile (PT, PTT)	Coagulopathy is associated with worsening disease
Liver function studies	Hepatocellular dysfunction is associated with worsening disease
Serum creatinine	Decreased renal function is associated with worsening disease
Uric acid	
24-hour urine	
Creatinine clearance	
Total urinary protein	
Fetal studies (to assess for pregnancy-associated hypertension effects on the fetus)	
Ultrasound examination	
Fetal weight and growth	Intrauterine growth restriction
Amniotic fluid volume	Oligohydramnios
Nonstress test and/or biophysical profile	Uteroplacental insufficiency (indirect assessment)

PT, prothrombin time; PTT, partial thromboplastin time.

ultrasonography for fetal growth and amniotic fluid volume and a nonstress test (NST) and/or biophysical profile (BPP) are important.

● MANAGEMENT

The goal of management of hypertension in pregnancy is to balance the management of both fetus and mother and to optimize the outcome for each. Maternal blood pressure should be monitored and the mother should be observed for the sequelae of the hypertensive disease. Intervention for maternal indications should occur when the risk of permanent disability or death for the mother without intervention outweighs the risks to the fetus caused by intervention. For the fetus, there should be regular evaluation of fetal well-being and fetal growth, with intervention becoming necessary if the intrauterine environment provides more risks to the fetus than delivery with subsequent care in the newborn nursery.

Chronic Hypertension

The management of patients with chronic hypertension in pregnancy involves closely monitoring maternal blood pressure and watching for the superimposition of preeclampsia or eclampsia as well as following the fetus for appropriate growth and fetal well-being. Medical treatment of mild to moderate essential hypertension has been disappointing, in that no significant improvement in pregnancy outcome has been demonstrated with treatment. However, there are no consistent data to suggest harm in treatment of mild chronic hypertension in pregnancy.

Antihypertensive medication in women with chronic hypertension is generally recommended when the systolic blood pressure is ≥160 mmHg or the diastolic blood pressure ≥105 mmHg. The purpose of such medications is to reduce the likelihood of maternal stroke or major cardiac events. Labetalol (combined α- and β-blocker) is considered first-line antihypertensive therapy in pregnancy although calcium channel blockers (such as nifedipine or amlodipine) are also commonly used. Methyldopa was the most commonly used antihypertensive medication in pregnancy for many decades and still may be used although it is considered less effective than labetalol or calcium channel blockers. It was formerly taught that diuretics were contraindicated during pregnancy, but diuretic therapy is no longer discontinued and, indeed, is often continued in the patient who already has been on such therapy before becoming pregnant. Angiotensin-converting enzyme (ACE) inhibitors can cause fetal malformations when given in the first trimester and also in the second and third trimesters; they are not recommended in pregnancy or the preconception period. Angiotensin receptor blockers act in a similar manner to ACE inhibitors and are, therefore, presumed to have the same potential adverse fetal effects if used in pregnancy.

Preeclampsia

The severity of the preeclampsia and the maturity of the fetus are the primary considerations in the management of preeclampsia. Care must be individualized, but there are well-accepted general guidelines.

Preeclampsia diagnosed at term and beyond is generally an indication for delivery. The mainstay of management for patients with preeclampsia and no severe features who are being managed expectantly is rest and frequent monitoring of mother and fetus. Testing for suspected fetal growth restriction or oligohydramnios, weekly laboratory testing and twice-weekly NSTs, BPPs, or both is commonly employed and should be repeated more frequently as indicated, according to maternal condition. Ultrasound examination for fetal growth and amniotic fluid assessment is recommended every 3 weeks. Daily fetal movement assessment also may prove useful.

Hospitalization is often initially recommended for women with new-onset preeclampsia. After maternal and fetal conditions are serially assessed and there are no severe features, subsequent management for patients <37 weeks' gestation may be continued in the hospital, at a day-care unit, or at home on the basis of the initial assessment. Care must be individualized with attention to patient resources, other co-morbidities and reliability for consideration of outpatient management.

Preeclampsia with Severe Features

For the patient with worsening preterm preeclampsia or the patient who has preeclampsia with severe features, management is often best accomplished in a tertiary care setting. Daily laboratory tests and fetal surveillance may be indicated. Stabilization with magnesium sulfate, antihypertensive therapy (as indicated) and monitoring for maternal and fetal well-being are required. Administration of corticosteroids for fetal lung maturation is recommended if less than 37 weeks' gestation. Delivery by either induction or cesarean delivery should not be delayed, even if less than 34 weeks' gestation, if any of the following are noted: uncontrollable severe hypertension, eclampsia, pulmonary edema, abruptio placentae, disseminated intravascular coagulation, evidence of nonreassuring fetal status, intrapartum fetal demise, nonviable fetus. Otherwise, if less than 34 weeks' gestation and stabilized, expectant management in the hospital with frequent maternal and fetal assessment may be considered until maternal or fetal status worsens. Patients with the diagnosis of preeclampsia with severe features should be delivered if ≥34 weeks' gestation.

For almost a century, **magnesium sulfate** has been used to prevent and to treat eclamptic convulsions. Other anticonvulsants, such as diazepam and phenytoin, are rarely used because they are not as efficacious as magnesium and because they have potential adverse effects on the fetus. Magnesium sulfate is administered by intramuscular or intravenous (IV) routes, although the latter is far more common. In 98% of cases, convulsions will be prevented. Therapeutic levels are 4 to 6 mg/dL, with toxic concentrations having predictable consequences (Table 22.2). Frequent evaluations of the patient's patellar reflex and respirations are necessary to monitor for manifestations of rising serum magnesium concentrations. In addition, because magnesium sulfate is excreted solely from the kidney, careful attention for signs of magnesium toxicity is warranted in the setting of reduced urine output (<30 mL/hour) or diminished renal function (serum creatinine >1.0 mg/mL). In these situations, serum magnesium levels may be useful in adjusting the infusion rate and avoiding toxicity. Reversal of the effects of excessive magnesium concentrations is accomplished by the slow IV administration of 10% calcium gluconate, along with oxygen supplementation and cardiorespiratory support, if needed.

Antihypertensive therapy is initiated if, on repeated measurements, the systolic blood pressure is >160 mmHg or diastolic blood pressure exceeds 110 mmHg. Hydralazine is often the initial antihypertensive medication of choice, given in 5- to 10-mg increments IV until an acceptable blood pressure response is obtained. A 10- to 15-minute response time is usual. The goal of such therapy is to reduce the systolic and diastolic pressure to the 140- to 150-/90- to 100-mmHg range. Further reduction of the blood pressure may impair uterine blood flow to rates that are dangerous to the fetus. Labetalol is another agent used to manage severe hypertension (Table 22.3).

Once anticonvulsant and antihypertensive therapies are established in patients with preeclampsia and severe features or eclampsia, attention is directed toward delivery. As noted previously, patients with preeclampsia and severe features diagnosed at <34 weeks' gestation may be managed expectantly in the hospital with frequent assessment. Induction of labor is often attempted, although cesarean delivery may be needed either if induction is unsuccessful or not possible or if the maternal or fetal status is worsening. At delivery, blood loss must be closely monitored, because patients with preeclampsia or eclampsia have significantly reduced intravascular volumes and may not tolerate increased blood loss. After delivery, patients remain in the labor and delivery or antepartum high-risk area for 24 hours (longer if the clinical situation warrants) for close observation of their clinical progress and further administration of magnesium sulfate to prevent postpartum eclamptic seizures. Approximately 25% of eclamptic seizures occur before labor, 50% occur during labor, and 25% occur in the first 24 hours after delivery. Usually, the vasospastic process begins to reverse itself in the first 24 to 48 hours after delivery, as manifested by a brisk diuresis.

ECLAMPSIA

The eclamptic seizure is life-threatening for the mother and fetus. Maternal risks include musculoskeletal injury (including biting the tongue), hypoxia, and aspiration. Maternal therapy consists of inserting a padded tongue blade, restraining gently as needed, providing oxygen, assuring maintenance of an adequate airway, and gaining IV access. Eclamptic seizures are usually self-limited, so medical therapy should be directed at the initiation of magnesium therapy (4 to 6 g slowly, IV) to prevent further seizures. If a patient receiving magnesium sulfate experiences a seizure, additional magnesium sulfate (usually 2

TABLE 22.2 MAGNESIUM TOXICITY

Serum Concentration (mg/dL)	Manifestation
1.5–3	Normal concentration
4–6	Therapeutic levels
5–10	Electrocardiogram changes
8–12	Loss of patellar reflex
9–12	Feeling of warmth, flushing
10–12	Somnolence; slurred speech
15–17	Muscle paralysis; respiratory difficulty
30	Cardiac arrest

TABLE 22.3 TREATMENT OF CHRONIC HYPERTENSION IN PREGNANCY

Drug	Dosage	Maternal Side Effects
Oral antihypertensives used commonly in pregnancy		
Labetalol	200–2,400 mg per day in 2–3 divided doses	Dizziness, fatigue, orthostatic hypotension, nausea
Nifedipine	30–120 mg per day of a slow-release preparation	Headache, flushing, peripheral edema, orthostatic hypotension
Amlodipine	5-10 mg per day	Same as nifedipine
Methyldopa	0.5–3.0 g per day in 2–3 divided doses	Maternal sedation, elevated LFTs, depression
Adjunctive agents		
Hydralazine	50–300 mg per day in 2–4 divided doses	Use with methyldopa or labetalol to prevent reflextachycardia; risk of neonatal thrombocytopenia
Hydrochlorothiazide	12.5–50 mg per day	Can cause volume depletion and electrolyte disorders
Drugs for urgent control of severe acute hypertension in pregnancy		
Hydralazine	5 mg IV over 2 minutes or IM, then 5–20 mg every 20–40 minutes	Long experience of safety and efficacy Risk of delayed maternal hypotension, fetal bradycardia
Labetalol	20 mg IV, then 20–80 mg every 5–15 minutes, up to a maximum of 300 mg; or constant infusion of 1–2 mg per minute	Probably less risk of tachycardia and arrhythmia than with other vasodilators; increasingly preferred as first-line agent; switch to hydralazine if maternal heart rate <60 bpm
Nifedipine (immediate release)	10–30 mg PO, repeat in 45 minutes if needed	Theoretical higher risk for adverse effects if given with magnesium since both are calcium antagonists

Used with permission from American College of Obstetricians and Gynecologists. *Hypertension in Pregnancy.* Washinton, DC. American College of Obstetricians and Gynecologists; 2013.

g slowly) can be given and a blood level obtained. Other anticonvulsant therapy with diazepam or similar drugs is generally not warranted.

Transient uterine hyperactivity for up to 15 minutes is associated with fetal heart rate changes, including bradycardia or compensatory tachycardia, decreased variability, and late decelerations. These are self-limited and are not dangerous to the fetus unless they continue for 20 minutes or more. Delivery during this time of maternal stabilization imposes unnecessary risk for mother and should be avoided. Arterial blood gases are often obtained, any metabolic disturbance should be corrected, and a Foley catheter should be placed to monitor urinary output. If the maternal blood pressure is high, if maternal urinary output is low, or if there is evidence of cardiac disturbance, consideration of a central venous catheter and, perhaps, continuous electrocardiogram monitoring is appropriate. Delivery is indicated once the mother is stabilized.

HELLP Syndrome

Patients with HELLP syndrome are often multiparous and have blood pressure recordings lower than those of many preeclamptic patients. Liver dysfunction may manifest as RUQ pain and is all too commonly misdiagnosed as gallbladder disease or indigestion. Major morbidity and mortality with unrecognized HELLP make accurate diagnosis imperative. The first symptoms are often vague, including nausea and emesis and a nonspecific viral-like syndrome. Treatment of these gravely ill patients is best done in a high-risk obstetric center and consists of cardiovascular stabilization, correction of coagulation abnormalities, and delivery. Platelet transfusion before or after delivery is indicated if the platelet count is <20,000/mm^3, and it may be advisable to transfuse patients with a platelet count <50,000/mm^3 before proceeding with a cesarean birth. Management of cases of HELLP syndrome should be individualized based on gestational age at presentation, maternal symptoms, physical examination, laboratory findings, and fetal status. Delivery in these patients generally should not be delayed. In pregnancies less than 34 weeks' gestation, an attempt to administer 48 hours of corticosteroids for fetal benefit may be considered with frequent laboratory, maternal and fetal assessment. Worsening status should prompt delivery regardless of corticosteroid course and gestational age.

Cardiac Disease

With earlier diagnoses and more effective treatments, more women with congenital and acquired heart disease reach adulthood and may become pregnant. Patients with rheumatic heart disease (caused by untreated or delayed treatment of group A β-hemolytic streptococcal tonsillopharyngitis) and acquired infectious valvular heart disease (often associated with drug use) comprise only 50% of pregnant cardiac patients. The remainder consists of those with other cardiac conditions that traditionally have been less commonly seen in pregnancy. Because pregnancy is itself associated with an increase in cardiac output of 40%, the risks to mother and fetus are often profound for women with preexisting cardiac disease. Ideally, cardiac patients should have preconceptional care directed at maximizing cardiac function. They should also be counseled about the risks their particular heart disease poses in pregnancy.

Classification of Heart Diseases in Pregnancy

The classification of heart disease by the New York Heart Association is useful to evaluate all types of cardiac patients with respect to pregnancy (Table 22.4). It is a functional classification and is independent of the type of heart disease. Patients with septal defects, patent ductus arteriosus, and mild mitral and aortic valvular disorders often are in classes I or II and tend to do well throughout pregnancy. Primary pulmonary hypertension, uncorrected tetralogy of Fallot, Eisenmenger syndrome, Marfan syndrome with significant aortic root dilation, dilated cardiomyopathy, and certain other conditions are associated with a much worse prognosis (frequently death) through the course of pregnancy. For this reason, patients with such disorders are strongly advised not to become pregnant.

Management

General management of the pregnant cardiac patient consists of avoiding conditions that add additional stress to the workload of the heart beyond that already imposed by pregnancy, including prevention and/or correction of anemia, prompt recognition and treatment of any infections, a decrease in physical activity and strenuous work, and proper weight gain. Adequate rest is essential. For patients with class I or II heart disease, increased rest at home is advised; and in cases of higher class levels, hospitalization and treatment of cardiac failure may be required. Coordinated management between the obstetrician, cardiologist, and anesthesiologist is especially important for patients with significant cardiac dysfunction.

The fetuses of patients with functionally significant cardiac disease are at increased risk for low birth weight and prematurity. A patient with congenital heart disease is 1% to 5% more likely to have a fetus with congenital heart disease than is someone without this condition; antepartum fetal cardiac assessment using ultrasound is recommended.

The antepartum management of pregnant cardiac patients includes serial evaluation of maternal cardiac status as well as fetal well-being and growth. Anticoagulation, antibiotic prophylaxis for subacute bacterial endocarditis, invasive cardiac monitoring, and even surgical correction of certain cardiac lesions during pregnancy can all be accomplished if necessary. The intrapartum and postpartum management of pregnant cardiac patients includes consideration of the increased stress of delivery and postpartum physiologic adjustment. Labor in the lateral position to facilitate cardiac function is often desirable. Every attempt is made to facilitate vaginal delivery because of the increased cardiac stress of cesarean section. Because cardiac output increases by 40% to 50% during the second stage of labor, shortening this stage by the use of forceps or vacuum extractor is often advisable. Epidural anesthesia to reduce the stress of labor is also recommended, although fluid shifts induced by sympathetic nervous system blockade must be watched for. Even with patients who are stable at the time of delivery, cardiac output increases in the postpartum period because of the additional 500 mL added to the maternal blood volume as the uterus contracts. Indeed, most obstetric patients who die with cardiac disease do so following delivery.

Rheumatic Heart Disease
Rheumatic heart disease remains a common cardiac disease in pregnancy, particularly in non-Western countries. As the severity of the associated valvular lesion increases, the risk of thromboembolic disease, subacute bacterial endocarditis, cardiac failure, and pulmonary edema increases. A high rate of fetal loss also occurs in women with rheumatic heart disease. Approximately 90% of these patients have mitral stenosis, whose associated mechanical obstruction worsens as cardiac output increases during pregnancy. Women with mitral stenosis associated with atrial fibrillation have an especially high risk of developing congestive heart failure.

Cardiac Arrhythmias
Maternal cardiac arrhythmias are occasionally encountered during pregnancy. Paroxysmal atrial tachycardia is the most commonly encountered maternal arrhythmia and is usually associated with overly strenuous exercise. Underlying cardiac disease such as mitral stenosis should be suspected when atrial fibrillation and flutter are encountered.

Peripartum Cardiomyopathy
Peripartum cardiomyopathy is an unusual but especially severe cardiac condition identified in the last month of pregnancy or the first 6 months following delivery. It is difficult to distinguish from other cardiomyopathies (e.g., myocarditis) except

TABLE 22.4 NEW YORK HEART ASSOCIATION FUNCTIONAL CLASSIFICATION OF HEART DISEASE

Class	Description
I	No cardiac decompensation
II	No symptoms of cardiac decompensation at rest; minor limitations of physical activity
III	No symptoms of cardiac decompensation at rest; marked limitations of physical activity
IV	Symptoms of cardiac decompensation at rest; increased discomfort with any physical activity

for its association with pregnancy. In many cases, no apparent cause can be determined. Treatment is generally unchanged from cardiac failure unassociated with pregnancy, except that the use of ACE inhibitors is avoided if the patient is pregnant. Management includes bed rest, digoxin, diuretics, and, in some cases, anticoagulation. The mortality rate is high and is related to cardiac size and function 6 to 12 months later. If cardiac size and function returns to normal, prognosis is improved, although it remains guarded. Sterilization or long acting reversible contraception counseling is warranted for patients with persistent cardiomyopathy.

RESPIRATORY DISORDERS

Asthma

Asthma is a restrictive airway disease that is encountered in approximately 4% to 8% of pregnant patients. The effects of pregnancy on asthma are variable—in general, about one third of patients worsen, one third improve, and the remaining one third are unchanged. Women with mild or moderate asthma usually have excellent maternal and fetal outcomes (Table 22.5). However, suboptimal control of asthma during pregnancy may be associated with increased maternal or fetal risk. Decreased FEV_1 (forced expiratory volume in the first second of expiration) is associated with increased risk of low birth weight and prematurity.

Pregnant patients with asthma, even those with mild or well-controlled disease, should be monitored with peak expiratory flow rate or FEV1 testing as well as by close symptom observation. Routine evaluation of pulmonary function in pregnant women with persistent asthma is recommended. Serial ultrasound examinations and antenatal fetal testing should be considered for women who have moderate or severe asthma during pregnancy beginning at 32 weeks of gestation or for women recovering from a severe asthma exacerbation.

Management

The ultimate goal of asthma therapy in pregnancy is maintaining adequate oxygenation of the fetus by preventing hypoxic episodes in the mother. Inhaled corticosteroid therapy, particularly budesonide, is the first-line controller treatment for persistent asthma during pregnancy. Inhaled albuterol is the recommended rescue therapy. In the **step-care therapeutic approach**, the number and dosage of medications are increased with increasing asthma severity (see Box 22.3). Once control of symptoms is achieved, a "step-down" approach is usually implemented in the nonpregnant patient. In pregnant patients, it may be prudent to postpone a reduction in a therapy that is effectively controlling a patient's asthma until after the birth. Patients should be instructed to identify and control or avoid factors, such as allergens and irritants, particularly tobacco smoke.

Management of a severely asthmatic pregnant patient is similar to that of a nonpregnant patient. Evaluation consists of measurement of pulmonary function and arterial blood gases. Treatment may include administration of supplemental oxygen, treatment with nebulized β-agonists, corticosteroids (oral or IV), or intubation. Women who are currently receiving or recently have taken systemic corticosteroids should receive IV administration of corticosteroids during labor and for 24 hours after delivery to prevent adrenal crisis.

INFLUENZA

Respiratory infection caused by **influenza virus A** (including the H1N1 strain) or **B** in pregnancy can be serious, with increased susceptibility to pneumonia and higher rates of hospitalization for pregnant women compared with nonpregnant women. In addition, pregnancy has been associated with higher mortality rates with serious influenza respiratory illness, such as seen during the 2009 pandemic. Symptoms of influenza

TABLE 22.5 CLASSIFICATION OF ASTHMA SEVERITY AND CONTROL IN PREGNANT PATIENTS

Asthma Severity* (Control†)	Symptom Frequency	Nighttime Awakening	Interference with Normal Activity	FEV_1 or Peak Flow (Predicted Percentage of Personal Best)
Intermittent (well controlled)	2 days/week or less	Twice per month or less	None	More than 80%
Mild persistent (not well controlled)	More than 2 days/week, but not daily	More than twice per month	Minor limitation	More than 80%
Moderate persistent (not well controlled)	Daily symptoms	More than once per week	Some limitation	60%–80%
Severe persistent (very poorly controlled)	Throughout the day	Four times per week or more	Extremely limited	Less than 60%

* Assess severity for patients who are not taking long-term control medications.
† Assess control in patients taking long-term control medications to determine whether step-up therapy, step-down therapy, or no change in therapy is warranted.
American College of Obstetricians and Gynecologists. Asthma in pregnancy. *ACOG Practice Bulletin No. 90.* Washington, DC: American College of Obstetricians and Gynecologists; 2008;111(2):457–464. Used with permission.

infection include dry cough, fever, and systemic symptoms such as myalgias. Diagnosis can be confirmed using rapid flu assays. Treatment includes supportive care and antiviral therapy. There is no firm evidence that influenza virus causes congenital malformations; risk to the fetus is primarily that associated with maternal hypoxia and systemic inflammatory effects of maternal infection (preterm labor and exposure to hyperthermia with high maternal fever).

The influenza vaccine is safe during pregnancy, and women who will be pregnant during the influenza season (October through May in the United States) should be vaccinated with a current (based on predictions of prevalent strains for the season in the community) influenza vaccine at any time during the pregnancy. There are no contraindications to the inactivated influenza vaccine in pregnancy and vaccination prevents clinical illness in 70% to 90% of adults. Chemoprophylaxis with antiviral therapy should also be offered to pregnant women who are in close contact with an infected person.

CLINICAL FOLLOW-UP

This patient may have chronic hypertension or may be developing preeclampsia. Since she is a new patient, you obtain a careful history and perform a physical examination. She has no history of chronic hypertension and no other chronic medical disorders. Because of the risk of adverse outcome for mother and fetus if the diagnosis is preeclampsia, you plan to evaluate her further. You send her to Labor and Delivery for laboratory tests, maternal blood pressure monitoring, and fetal evaluation with ultrasonography and fetal heart rate monitoring.

BOX 22.3 Step Therapy Medical Management of Asthma during Pregnancy

Mild Intermittent Asthma
- No daily medications, albuterol as needed

Mild Persistent Asthma
- Preferred-low-dose inhaled corticosteroid
- Alternative-Cromolyn, leukotriene receptor antagonist or theophylline (serum level 5 to 12 mcg/mL)

Moderate Persistent Asthma
- Preferred-low-dose inhaled corticosteroid and salmeterol or medium-dose inhaled corticosteroid or (needed) medium-dose inhaled corticosteroid and salmeterol
- Alternative-low-dose or (if needed) medium-dose inhaled corticosteroid and either leukotriene receptor antagonist or theophylline (serum level 5 to 12 mcg/mL)

Severe Persistent Asthma
- Preferred-high-dose inhaled corticosteroid and salmeterol and (if needed) oral corticosteroid
- Alternative-high-dose inhaled corticosteroid and theophylline (serum level 5 to 12 mcg/mL) and oral corticosteroid if needed
- From Asthma in pregnancy. ACOG Practice Bulletin No. 90. American College of Obstetricians and Gynecologists. Obstet Gynecol. 2008;111:457–464.

From Asthma in pregnancy. ACOG Practice Bulletin No. 90. American College of Obstetricians and Gynecologists. Obstet Gynecol. 2008;111:457–464.

CHAPTER 23

Hematologic and Immunologic Complications

This chapter deals primarily with APGO Educational Topic Areas:

TOPIC 17 MEDICAL AND SURGICAL COMPLICATIONS OF PREGNANCY
TOPIC 19 ALLOIMMUNIZATION

Students should be able to identify how pregnancy affects the natural history of various hematologic and immunologic disorders and how a preexisting hematologic and immunologic disorder affects maternal and fetal health. They should be able to outline a basic approach to evaluation and management of hematologic and immunologic disorders in pregnancy. Additionally, the student should understand the pathophysiology behind isoimmunization. They should be able to outline a basic approach to evaluation and prevention.

CLINICAL CASE

A 24-year-old G3P1A1 patient is seen for her initial obstetric visit at about 12 weeks of gestation. She reports a history of a first-trimester loss with her first pregnancy. In her second pregnancy, she had "something in my blood that could make my baby anemic." She ruptured membranes and delivered at 36 weeks; her infant was anemic and was hospitalized for 6 days. What do you think is going on here? How would you approach the management of the current pregnancy?

● HEMATOLOGIC DISEASE

Anemia

The plasma and cellular composition of blood changes significantly during pregnancy, with the expansion of plasma volume proportionally greater than that of the red blood cell (RBC) mass. On average, there is a 1,000 mL increase in plasma volume and a 300 mL increase in RBC volume (a 3:1 ratio). Because the hematocrit (Hct) reflects the proportion of blood made up primarily of RBCs, it demonstrates a "physiologic" decrease during pregnancy; therefore, this decrease is often not actually an anemia but a dilutional effect.

The CDC defines anemia as a hemoglobin (Hb) or Hct value that is less than the fifth percentile for a healthy reference population based on the stage of pregnancy. Using these parameters, anemia in pregnancy should be diagnosed when the Hb (g/dl) and Hct (%) levels are below 11 g/dl and 33%, respectively, in the first trimester, 10.5 g/dl and 32% in the second trimester, and 11 g/dl and 33% in the third trimester. In practice, anemia in pregnancy is generally defined as an Hct less than 30% or a hemoglobin (Hb) of less than 10 g/dL.

The direct fetal consequences of anemia are minimal, although infants born to mothers with iron deficiency may have diminished iron stores as neonates. The maternal consequences of anemia are those associated with any adult anemia. If anemia is corrected, the woman with an adequate RBC mass enters labor and delivery better able to respond to acute peripartum blood loss and to avoid the risks of blood or blood product transfusion.

Iron-Deficiency Anemia

Iron-deficiency anemia is by far the most frequent type of anemia seen in pregnancy, accounting for more than 90% of cases. Because the iron content of the standard American diet and the endogenous iron stores of many American women are not sufficient to provide for the increased iron requirements of pregnancy, the National Academy of Sciences recommends 27 mg of iron supplementation (present in most prenatal vitamins) daily for pregnant women. Most prescription prenatal vitamin/mineral preparations contain 60 to 65 mg of elemental iron. It is not clear whether routine iron supplementation for pregnant women consuming a healthy diet actually improves perinatal outcome. All pregnant women should be screened for iron-deficiency anemia.

Severe iron-deficiency anemia is characterized by small, pale erythrocytes (Fig. 23.1) and RBC indices that indicate a low mean corpuscular volume and low mean corpuscular Hb concentration. Additional laboratory studies usually demonstrate decreased serum iron levels, an increased total iron-binding capacity, and a decrease in serum ferritin levels, but these studies are generally reserved for patients unresponsive to treatment of iron-deficiency anemia. This approach is warranted because the vast majority of anemia in pregnancy is of the iron-deficiency type. In evaluating the patient with anemia, a recent dietary history is obviously important, especially if **pica** (consumption of nonnutrient substances such as starch, ice, or dirt) exists. Such dietary compulsions may contribute to iron deficiency by decreasing the amount of nutritious food and iron consumed.

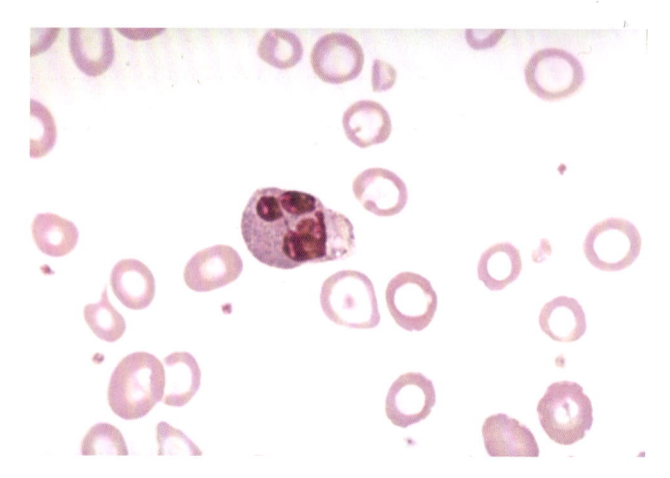

FIGURE 23.1. Peripheral blood smear of iron-deficiency anemia with microcytic, hypochromic erythrocytes. (From Rubin R, Strayer DS. *Rubin's Pathology: Clinicopathologic Foundations of Medicine*. 5th ed. Baltimore, MD: Williams & Wilkins; 2007:20–22.)

Treatment

Treatment of iron-deficiency anemia generally requires an additional 60 to 180 mg of elemental iron per day, along with folate to maximize RBC production, in addition to the iron in the prenatal vitamin/mineral preparation. Iron absorption is facilitated by or with vitamin C supplementation or ingestion between meals or at bedtime on an empty stomach. The response to therapy is first seen as an increase in the reticulocyte count approximately 1 week after starting iron therapy. Because of the plasma expansion associated with pregnancy, the Hct may not increase significantly but, rather, stabilizes or increases only slightly.

Folate Deficiency

Adequate intake of folic acid (folate) has been found to reduce the risk of neural tube defects (NTDs) in the fetus. The first occurrence of NTDs may be reduced by as much as 36% if women of reproductive age consume 0.4 mg of folate daily both before conception and during the first trimester of pregnancy. The Recommended Dietary Allowance for folate for pregnant women is 0.6 mg. Folate deficiency is especially likely in multiple gestations or when patients are taking anticonvulsive medications. Women with a history of a prior NTD-affected pregnancy or who are being treated with anticonvulsive drugs may reduce the risk of NTDs by more than 80% with daily intake of 4 mg of folate in the months in which conception is attempted and for the first trimester of pregnancy.

Folate is found in green, leafy vegetables and is now an added supplement in breakfast cereal, bread, and grain products in the United States. These supplements are designed to enable women to easily consume 0.4 mg of folate daily. Women who do not consume enough through food sources should take a supplement. Prescription prenatal vitamin/mineral preparations contain 1 mg of folic acid. Over-the-counter vitamin preparations generally contain less than 1 mg of folate.

Other Anemias

The **hemoglobinopathies** are a heterogeneous group of single-gene disorders that includes the structural Hb variants and the thalassemias. **Hereditary hemolytic anemias** are also rare causes of anemia in pregnancy. Some examples are hereditary spherocytosis, an autosomal dominant defect of the erythrocyte membrane; glucose 6-phosphate dehydrogenase deficiency; and pyruvate kinase deficiency.

The Hemoglobinopathies

More than 270 million people worldwide are heterozygous carriers of hereditary disorders of Hb, and at least 300,000 affected homozygotes or compound homozygotes are born each year. The hemoglobinopathies include the thalassemias (α-thalassemia and β-thalassemia) and the sickle cell spectrum: sickle cell trait (Hb AS), sickle cell disease (Hb SS), and sickle cell disorders (Hb SC and sickle cell β-thalassemia) (Table 23.1).

Hb consists of four interlocking polypeptide chains, each of which has an attached heme molecule. The polypeptide chains are called (α) alpha, (β) beta, (γ) gamma, (δ) delta, (ε) epsilon, and (ζ) zeta. Adult Hb consists of two alpha chains and either two beta chains (HbA), two gamma chains (HbF), or two delta chains (HbA$_2$). The beta chains are the oxygen-carrying subunits of the Hb molecule. HbF is the primary Hb of the fetus from 12 to 24 weeks of gestation. In the third trimester, production of HbF decreases as production of beta chains and HbA begins.

Thalassemias

α-Thalassemia is generally caused by missing copies of the α-globin gene; however, occasionally point mutations can cause functional abnormalities in the protein. Humans normally have four copies of the α-globin gene. Those with three copies are asymptomatic, those with two copies have mild anemia, and those with one copy have hemolytic anemia. Individuals in whom the gene is absent have **Hb Barts disease**, which results in **hydrops fetalis** and intrauterine death.

Phenotypic expressions of **β-thalassemia** vary because of the many possible mutations in the β-globin gene. Some mutations cause an absence of the protein, whereas others result in a defective globin protein. *β-Thalassemia major* occurs in homozygotes and is a severe disease, whereas a diagnosis of *β-thalassemia minor* (heterozygotes) may include asymptomatic to clinically anemic patients.

Sickle Cell Disorders

The **sickle cell disorders** are autosomal recessive disorders caused by point mutations that lead to functional abnormalities in the β-globin chains. Instead of normal HbA, individuals with this disorder have abnormal HbS. HbS is unstable, especially under conditions of low oxygen tension. The unstable HbS causes a structural change resulting in deformity of the normal spheroid shape of the RBC into the shape of a "sickle." These abnormally shaped cells lead to increased viscosity and hemolysis and a further decrease in oxygenation. Sickling that occurs in small blood vessels can cause a **vaso-occlusive crisis**, in which the blood supply to vital organs is compromised.

TABLE 23.1 THE HEMOGLOBINOPATHIES[a]

	Globin Abnormality	Genetics	Risk Groups
Sickle cell	**HbS** (valine substituted for glutamic acid at the sixth position)—classic sickle cell **HbC** (lysine substituted for glutamic acid at the sixth position)	Autosomal recessive **Sickle cell trait:** Hb AS heterozygous—one chain affected, <40% HbS 1/12 Black Americans **Sickle cell disease:** Hb SS or Hb SC homozygous—both chains affected 1/600 Black Americans	African, Mediterranean, Turkish, Arabian, East Indian heritage
α-Thalassemia	Normal hemoglobin; production of α-globin chains is decreased	Autosomal recessive severity of disease depends on amount of globin produced **Homozygous:** none = Hb Barts disease **Heterozygous:** 25%–75% of normal amount	Asian, African, East Indian, Mediterranean heritage
β-Thalassemia	Normal hemoglobin; point mutations cause decreased production of β-globin chains	Autosomal recessive **Homozygous:** β-thalassemia major (Cooley's anemia); no HbA is produced = severe disease **Heterozygous:** β-thalassemia minor; one normal and one abnormal β-globin allele = mild to moderate disease	Mediterranean, Middle Eastern, African, East Indian, and Asian heritage
Sickle cell/ β-thalassemia	One globin is HbS and one globin codes for β-thalassemia	Autosomal recessive in 1/1,700 pregnancies; severity of disease depends on the β-allele (no HbA production = severe disease; moderate production = milder disease)	Same as for sickle cell and β-thalassemia

[a] HbA is normal adult hemoglobin.

Heterozygotic individuals (Hb AS) have **sickle cell trait** and are asymptomatic. The most severe form of the disease, which occurs in homozygotic individuals (Hb SS), is called **sickle cell anemia**. Sickle cell disorders are found not only in patients who have Hb SS but also in those who have HbS and one other abnormality of β-globin structure. The most common are Hb SC disease and HbS/β-thalassemia. Women of Mediterranean, Southeast Asian, and African descent are at higher risk for being carriers of hemoglobinopathies and should be offered carrier screening. If both parents are deemed to be carriers of any hemoglobinopathy, genetic counseling is recommended. For individuals of non-African descent, initial testing may be done by complete blood count (CBC).

However, ethnicity is not always a good predictor of risk as individuals from at-risk groups may marry outside of their ethnic group. Because individuals of African descent, as well as those of other backgrounds (see Table 23.1) are at high risk for carrying a gene for sickle cell disease, these women should be offered Hb electrophoresis in addition to a CBC. Solubility testing, such as tests for the presence of HbS (Sickledex), isoelectronic focusing, and high-performance liquid chromatography are inadequate for screening and fail to identify important transmissible Hb gene abnormalities affecting fetal outcome. Although the course of pregnancy can vary according to the type of hemoglobinopathy, there is also individual variation among patients with the same type of disorder. Besides the genetic implications, patients with the sickle cell trait (Hb AS) have an increased risk of urinary infections but experience no other pregnancy complications. Pregnancies in patients with HbS/β-thalassemia are generally unaffected. Patients who are Hb SS or Hb SC, in contrast, may suffer vaso-occlusive episodes. Infections are also more common due to functional asplenia caused by repetitive end-organ damage to the spleen. Infection should be ruled out before attributing any pain to a vaso-occlusive crisis. Prophylactic maternal RBC transfusions for women with hemoglobinopathies were used in the past.

Now, however, transfusions are, for the most part, reserved for complications of hemoglobinopathies, such as congestive heart failure, sickle cell disease crises unresponsive to hydration and analgesics, and severely low levels of Hb.

Because fetal outcomes such as preterm labor, intrauterine growth restriction, and low birth weight are more common in women with hemoglobinopathies (except those with sickle cell trait), antenatal assessment of fetal well-being and growth is an important part of managing patients with hemoglobinopathies.

ALLOIMMUNIZATION

When any fetal blood group factor inherited from the father is not possessed by the mother, antepartum or intrapartum fetal–maternal bleeding may stimulate an immune reaction in the mother. Maternal immune reactions also can occur from blood product transfusion.

The formation of maternal antibodies is called **alloimmunization**. It can lead to various degrees of transplacental passage of these antibodies into the fetal circulation, causing an **antibody response** sufficient to destroy fetal RBCs. Although early exposures to maternal antigens during pregnancy may occur in the same pregnancy, alloimmunization more commonly occurs in a subsequent pregnancy. The binding of maternal antibodies to fetal RBC antigens leads to **hemolytic disease** in the fetus or newborn, characterized by **hemolysis**, **bilirubin release**, and **anemia**. The severity of the illness encountered by the fetus or newborn is determined by a number of factors, including the degree of immune response elicited (i.e., how much antibody is produced), how strongly the antibody binds the antigen, the gestational age at which the diagnosis is made, and the ability of the fetus to replenish the destroyed red cells to maintain an Hct sufficient for growth and development (Table 23.2).

Natural History

Any of the many blood group antigen systems can lead to alloimmunization, but the number of antigens involved in fetal and neonatal hemolytic disease is limited. The most common antigen involved is part of the **Rh** (**CDE**) **system**, specifically the **D antigen**. Rh alloimmunization is often called Rh-isoimmunization and was the first form of maternal alloimmunization described.

The Rh system is a complex of five antigens—including the **C**, **c**, **D**, **E**, and **e antigens**—each of which elicits a unique immune response. These antigens are inherited together in distinctive patterns, reflecting the underlying genotypic makeup of the parents. C and c are alternate forms of the same antigen, as are E and e, but there is no d antigen. The D antigen is either present or absent.

Patients with the D antigen are termed **Rh D-positive**, and those lacking this gene, and hence the antigen, are said to be Rh **D-negative**. Approximately 15% of whites, 5% to 8% of African Americans, and only 1% to 2% of Asians and Native Americans are Rh D-negative. A variant of the D antigen called the **weak D antigen** (formerly Du) also exists. If not appropriately diagnosed, patients can be mistakenly classified as Rh D-negative. For this reason, patients should not be considered Rh D-negative unless efforts have been made to look for the weak D antigen. Patients who are Rh weak D-positive should be managed the same as those who are Rh D-positive.

Alloimmunization can occur when an Rh D-negative woman is pregnant with a fetus who has inherited the Rh D antigen from its father and is, thus, Rh D-positive. Any event associated with fetal–maternal bleeding can potentially lead to maternal exposure to RBCs, which can trigger a maternal immune response. These events include the following:

- Childbirth
- Delivery of the placenta
- Threatened, spontaneous, elective, or therapeutic abortion
- Ectopic pregnancy
- Bleeding associated with placenta previa or abruption

TABLE 23.2 ATYPICAL ANTIBODIES AND THEIR RELATIONSHIP TO FETAL HEMOLYTIC DISEASE

Antigens Related to Hemolytic Disease	Hemolytic Disease	Severity	Proposed Management
Lewis		Not associated	Routine care
I		Not associated	Routine care
Kell	K	Mild to severe	Fetal assessment
	k	Mild	Routine care
Rh (non-D)	E	Mild to severe	Fetal assessment
	e	Mild to severe	Fetal assessment
	C	Mild to severe	Fetal assessment
	c	Mild to severe	Fetal assessment
Duffy	Fy^a	Mild to severe	Fetal assessment
	Fy^b	Not associated	Routine care
Kidd	Jk^a	Mild to severe	Fetal assessment
	Jk^b	Mild	Routine care
MNS	M	Mild to severe	Fetal assessment
	N	Mild	Routine care
	S	Mild to severe	Fetal assessment
Lutheran	Lu^a	Mild	Routine care
	Lu^b	Mild	Routine care
P	PP^{1pk}	Mild to severe	Fetal assessment

Adapted from Weinstein L. Irregular antibodies causing hemolytic disease of the newborn: a continuing problem. *Clin Obstet Gynecol*. 1982;25(2):321.

- Amniocentesis
- Abdominal trauma
- External cephalic version

The amount of Rh D-positive blood required to cause isoimmunization is small—<0.1 mL is sufficient.

Effects of Antibody Development on the Fetus and Newborn

One study indicates that 17% of Rh D-negative women who do not receive anti-D immune globulin prophylaxis during pregnancy will become isoimmunized. As with other antibody-mediated immune responses, the first immunoglobulin (Ig) type produced is of the **IgM** isoform, which does not cross the placenta to any extent. The chance of significant fetal or newborn disease in a woman's first at-risk pregnancy is, therefore, low. It is, however, important to consider prior pregnancy losses or terminations as potential exposures, because they could influence the risk of fetal or newborn disease. In a subsequent pregnancy, passage of minute amounts of fetal blood across the placenta into the maternal circulation, a relatively common occurrence, can lead to an **anamnestic response** of maternal antibody production, which is more robust and rapid than the initial response.

In the case of some antigens, the mother continues to produce predominantly IgM antibodies that fail to cross the placenta. In other cases, the secondary antibody response is characterized by the production of **IgG** antibodies that freely cross the placenta, enter the fetal circulation, and bind to antigenic sites on fetal red cells. RBCs that are highly bound with antibody are hemolyzed in the fetal reticuloendothelial system and are destroyed via complement-mediated pathways. Hemolysis releases bilirubin, and the fetus excretes the bilirubin and its breakdown products in urine. If the fetus is able to augment erythropoiesis to keep pace with the rate of hemolysis, serious anemia may not develop. However, if large amounts of antibody cross the placenta, resulting in destruction of large numbers of fetal RBCs, the fetus may be unable to sufficiently replenish the RBCs, and anemia may ensue.

Fetal Consequences

Typically, the first-affected pregnancy is characterized by mild anemia and elevated bilirubin at birth, often necessitating treatment for the newborn, such as ultraviolet light and exchange transfusion, because the newborn's liver may be unable to effectively metabolize and excrete the released bilirubin. Markedly elevated bilirubin levels can lead to **kernicterus** (bilirubin deposition in the basal ganglia), which can cause permanent neurologic symptoms or even death. This condition is rarely seen today in developed countries.

In some first-affected pregnancies, and in many, but not all, subsequent pregnancies with an antigen-positive fetus, antibody production increases as a result of the anamnestic response, leading to more significant hemolysis and anemia. Assessment of the amount of bilirubin excreted by the fetus into the amniotic fluid is one method used to monitor fetal status (see below). When fetal anemia is significant, fetal hematopoiesis increases, including the recruitment of alternative sites for RBC production. The fetal liver is an important site of extramedullary hematopoiesis. When the liver produces RBCs, the production of other proteins decreases, resulting in a lower oncotic pressure within the fetal vasculature. This consequence, in conjunction with the increase in intravascular resistance to flow caused by islands of hematopoietic cells in the liver, can lead to the development of ascites, subcutaneous edema, or pleural effusion.

Severe anemia affects fetal cardiac function in two ways. First, anemia can lead to a high-output cardiac failure. As the cardiac system attempts unsuccessfully to keep pace with the oxygen delivery demands, the myocardium becomes dysfunctional, resulting in effusions, edema, and ascites due to hydrostatic pressure increases. Second, the anemia itself can cause myocardial ischemia, thereby directly damaging and compromising myocardial function. This combination of fluid accumulation in at least two extravascular compartments (pericardial effusion, pleural effusion, ascites, or subcutaneous edema) is referred to as **hydrops fetalis**.

Alloimmunization usually progressively worsens in each subsequent pregnancy. Fetal anemia may occur at the same gestational age or earlier than in the prior affected pregnancies.

Significance of Paternal Antigen Status

Determination of the father's antigen status is important in assessing whether the fetus is at risk for developing anemia. Any individual can be either homozygous or heterozygous for a particular gene. If the father is heterozygous for the gene for the particular antigen of interest, there is a 50% chance that the fetus will not inherit the gene for that antigen. For many of the antigens, this information can be determined easily by looking at which antigens are expressed on the father's RBCs. For example, C and c are coded by the same gene but differ by a single base change. An individual can express C, c, or both. If he expresses both, he is *heterozygous*; if only one antigen is detected, then he must be *homozygous*. Unfortunately, the situation is not as straightforward with Rh D (because there is no **d** antigen). However, for antigens other than Rh D, direct **genotype testing** can be performed to determine if the father is homozygous or heterozygous.

In a pregnancy involving an alloimmunized patient, the first step in management is determination of the paternal erythrocyte antigen status. In pregnancies in which there is a heterozygous or unknown paternal genotype, the fetal antigen type may be assessed by genetic analysis of fetal cells obtained by **amniocentesis**. Newer noninvasive technologies utilizing cell-free fetal DNA testing from maternal plasma can assess for fetal D or Kell antigens and are becoming more widely available.

Regardless of the amount of maternal antibody present, if the subsequent fetus does not carry the antigen (because the father was a heterozygote or there is different paternity), then the fetus has a 98.5% probability of not being at risk.

Diagnosis

All pregnant women should be tested at the time of the first prenatal visit for ABO blood group and Rh D type and screened for the presence of erythrocyte antibodies. These laboratory assessments should be repeated in each subsequent pregnancy. Antibody screening is also recommended before administration of anti-D immunoglobulin at 28 weeks of gestation, postpartum, and the time of any event in pregnancy. Patients who are weak D-positive are not at risk for isoimmunization and should not receive anti-D immunoprophylaxis.

Any antibodies potentially associated with fetal hemolysis found during this routine screening are further evaluated based on the strength of the antibody response, which is reported in titer format (1:4, 1:8, 1:16, etc., or simply as 4, 8, 16, etc.), with higher numbers indicative of a more significant antibody response. Although often encountered during the process of antibody screening, **anti-Lewis** and **anti-I antibodies** are not associated with fetal hemolytic disease and, therefore, are not evaluated further.

Assessment

Although the antibody titer reflects the strength and the amount of the maternal antibody response, its utility in pregnancy management is limited. Titers provide little information about fetal status. In an initial sensitized pregnancy, serial antibody values can assist in determining when the maternal antibody response is strong enough to represent a risk of fetal anemia. A **critical titer** is that titer associated with a significant risk of severe fetal hemolytic disease and hydrops fetalis. In most centers, this is between 1:8 and 1:32. If the initial antibody titer is 1:8 or less, the Rh D-negative patient can be monitored with titer assessment every 4 weeks. In a first-sensitized pregnancy, titers are generally performed every 4 weeks. Once a critical titer is reached, further evaluation and surveillance of the fetus is warranted and serial titers are no longer necessary. With a history of an affected fetus or infant, titers are not helpful in predicting fetal hemolytic disease and further evaluation is warranted.

Amniotic Fluid Assessment

Evaluation for possible fetal anemia is usually undertaken in the second trimester, although management may be individualized depending on history and available expertise. Traditionally, amniotic fluid assessment of the level of bilirubin has been used as a measure of fetal status and an indirect means of estimating the potential for severe fetal anemia. In the second half of a normal pregnancy, the level of bilirubin in the amniotic fluid decreases progressively, whereas in an affected, isoimmunized patient, the amount of bilirubin detected can deviate significantly. The increase in the amniotic fluid bilirubin in affected pregnancies is thought to be a result of fetal urinary excretion of the increased amount of circulating bilirubin. Until recently, serial amniocenteses were performed to determine the level of bilirubin in the amniotic fluid, which in turn reflected the severity of fetal anemia.

Ultrasound Assessment

The current trend in management is the measurement of **peak velocity** of middle cerebral artery (MCA) flow using **Doppler ultrasound**. The velocity of flow through the MCA is related to the viscosity of the blood. In the setting of fetal anemia, the blood is less viscous due to fewer cells, and, therefore, the velocity of flow increases. Gestational age–specific peak velocity normal curves have been derived and correlated with the fetal Hct. The degree of peak velocity elevation above the median for that gestational age can be used to estimate the fetal Hct and, thus, the risk of fetal anemia. Using the peak systolic velocity of the MCA, almost all fetuses with moderate to severe anemia can be identified (Figs. 23.2 and 23.3).

Ultrasound assessment of the fetus is also helpful in detecting severe signs of hemolysis that have resulted in profound fetal anemia. Occasionally, the first presenting signs of fetal hemolysis may be hydropic changes in the fetus including subcutaneous edema, pericardial and pleural effusions, and ascites. When these findings are identified and hydrops fetalis is diagnosed, the fetal Hct is typically <15%.

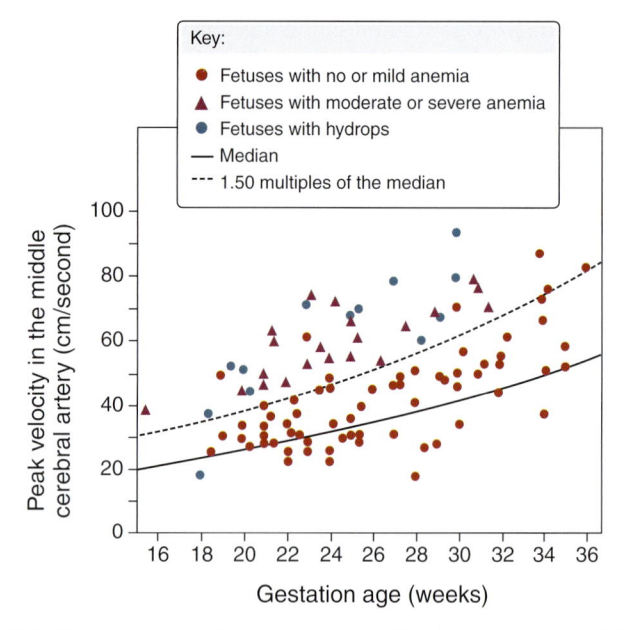

FIGURE 23.2. Peak velocity of systolic blood flow in the middle cerebral artery. Red circles indicate fetuses with no anemia or mild anemia; triangles indicate fetuses with moderate or severe anemia; and blue circles indicate fetuses with hydrops. (From Mari G, Deter RL, Carpenter RL, et al. Noninvasive diagnosis by Doppler ultrasonography of fetal anemia due to maternal red-cell alloimmunization. Collaborative Group for Doppler Assessment of the Blood Velocity in Anemic Fetuses. *N Engl J Med*. 2000;342(1):9–14.)

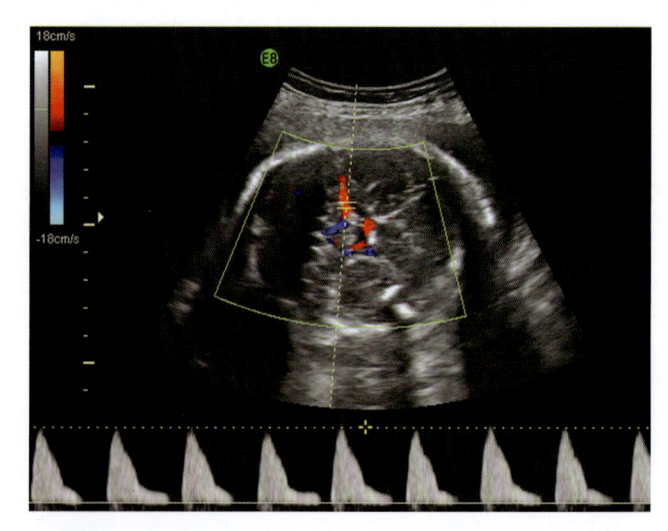

FIGURE 23.3. Image of fetal cerebral circulation demonstrating the middle cerebral artery and method of measuring peak flow.

Regardless of the methods used to monitor pregnancies at risk for fetal anemia, all techniques are designed to determine the fetal Hct using indirect measures. If the monitoring test indicates a risk of fetal anemia, or if hydrops is diagnosed, cordocentesis or **percutaneous umbilical blood sampling (PUBS)** is performed to directly measure the fetal Hct.

Under ultrasound guidance, a needle is advanced into the umbilical vein, a sample of fetal blood is removed, and the

Hct is measured. In general, the average fetal Hct is 36% to 44%, and with severe anemia, it is less than 30% (Box 23.1). In addition to procedures to monitor the fetus for anemia, general tests for fetal well-being are indicated in all isoimmunized women with titers above the critical threshold, because the ability of an affected fetus, even if only mildly anemic, to withstand the stresses of pregnancy and labor may be compromised.

Management

Previously, blood was transfused into the fetal abdominal cavity, where absorption of RBCs could take place over several days through the lymphatic channels. Currently, **transfusion of antigen-negative RBCs** (depending on the blood group involved) to the fetus is indicated when PUBS determines that the fetus has moderate or severe anemia with an Hct less than 30%.

Direct transfusion under ultrasound guidance into the umbilical vein has become the preferred technique. The procedure has a 1% to 3% risk of complications, including fetal death and preterm delivery, which must be weighed against the predicted course of the fetus if left untreated or delivered. The volume of RBCs to be transfused can be calculated based on the gestational age, estimated fetal weight, the Hct of the unit of blood, and the difference between the current fetal Hct and the desired Hct. Because the transfused cells are antigen negative, they are not subject to hemolysis by the maternal antibody and the predicted lifespan of the RBC is the only determinant of how long they persist in the fetal circulation. The timing and need for further transfusions can be based either on the predicted course given the severity of the disease or on MCA Doppler assessments. After two to three transfusions, most of the circulating RBCs in a fetus are transfused cells, because the hematopoietic system in the fetus has been suppressed.

> **BOX 23.1** Evaluation of a Pregnancy with a Positive Maternal Antibody Screen
>
> - Maternal antibody identification and antibody strength (titer)
> - Careful obstetric history for prior affected fetus
> - Paternal antigen testing, possible fetal DNA testing
> - Serial antibody titers, if first-sensitized pregnancy
> - Assessment of risk of fetal anemia if a critical titer is found or if there has been a prior affected child
> - Amniotic fluid bilirubin assessment (amniocentesis)
> - Middle cerebral artery Doppler (currently recommended since noninvasive)
> - Ultrasound, antenatal surveillance
> - Cordocentesis/percutaneous umbilical blood sampling if monitoring test is abnormal

Prevention

Maternal exposure and subsequent sensitization to fetal blood usually occurs at delivery, but it can occur at any time during pregnancy. In the late 1960s, it was discovered that an antibody to the D antigen of the Rh system could be prepared from donors previously sensitized to the antigen. Administration of the **anti-D immunoglobulin** soon after delivery prevents an active antibody response to the D antigen by the mother in most cases. Anti-D immunoglobulin is effective only for the D antigen of the Rh system. It is not effective in preventing sensitization to other Rh antigens or any other RBC antigens.

It is now standard for Rh D-negative women who deliver Rh D-positive infants to receive a dose of 300 μg of anti-D immunoglobulin within 72 hours of delivery. This practice reduces the risk of sensitization to the D antigen from around 16% to approximately 2%. The residual 2% risk is believed to result from sensitization occurring during the course of pregnancy, especially during the third trimester. For this reason, it is standard practice to administer a 300-μg dose of anti-D immunoglobulin to all Rh D-negative women at about 28 weeks of gestation, unless it is absolutely certain that the father is Rh D-negative. This prophylactic dose reduces the risk of sensitization from 2% to 0.2%. If there is any question regarding the need for prophylaxis, such as the certainty of paternity, anti-D immunoglobulin should be administered. Some authorities recommend that if delivery has not occurred within 12 weeks of the injection at 28 weeks of gestation, a second 300-μg dose of anti-D immunoglobulin should be given at 40 weeks in undelivered patients.

Because even a minute amount of fetal RBCs can result in sensitization to the Rh D antigen, in any circumstance when a fetal–maternal hemorrhage can occur, a prophylactic dose of 300 μg of anti-D immunoglobulin should be administered. Each dose of anti-D immunoglobulin provides protection against sensitization for up to 30 mL of fetal blood or 15 mL of fetal RBCs.

In cases of trauma or bleeding during pregnancy in which there is a potential for more than a 30-mL fetal–maternal transfusion, the extent of the fetal–maternal hemorrhage can be assessed using the **Kleihauer-Betke test**.

This test identifies fetal erythrocytes in the maternal circulation. The number of fetal cells as a proportion of the total cells can be determined, and the volume of fetal–maternal hemorrhage can be estimated. Based on this estimation, the appropriate dose of Rh immunoglobulin can be determined. An **indirect Coombs test** can also be used to determine if the patient has received sufficient antibody. A positive test indicates that she has received an adequate dose.

Management of Isoimmunization to Other Red Cell Antigens

Although the routine use of Rh immunoglobulin has decreased isoimmunization due to the D antigen, isoimmunization due to other blood group antigens has proportionally increased. The frequency of these antibodies varies depending on the frequency of the antigen in the general population and in various ethnic groups. In addition, the likelihood that these antibodies will result in significant fetal hemolytic disease depends on several factors, including the size of the sensitizing antigenic stimulus, the relative potency of the antigen, and the isoform (IgG or IgM) of antibody response.

Kell Antigen

Sensitization to any of these antigens can occur in any exposed woman lacking the particular antigen, regardless of her ABO or Rh type. An antibody screen will detect the presence of these antibodies. The most important cause of hemolytic disease of the fetus not associated with the D antigen is isoimmunization to the **Kell antigen** (see Table 23.2).

This sensitization commonly results from a prior blood transfusion. If a maternal antibody screen reveals the presence of an anti-Kell antibody, paternal blood typing for the Kell antigen should be performed. Because the direct phenotype of the erythrocyte for the Kell antigen and its complement—the Cellano antigen—can be performed, genotyping is not necessary. Ninety percent of individuals are Kell negative, so if paternity is certain, no further evaluation is required. Even among those who carry the Kell antigen, 98% are heterozygous, so consideration should be given to fetal genotype determination.

Anemia resulting from Kell isoimmunization is unique in that the predominant effect of the antibody is destruction and suppression of hematopoietic precursor cells; hemolysis is only a minimal component of the fetal problem. For this reason, amniotic fluid surveillance of bilirubin may not be as useful in monitoring these pregnancies, and MCA Doppler is the preferred surveillance method. Most providers use a critical titer measurement of 1:8 to initiate further evaluation in Kell-sensitized pregnancies.

ABO Hemolytic Disease

ABO hemolytic disease, due to maternal–fetal incompatibility for the major blood group antigens, can occur. It is usually associated with mild fetal and newborn hyperbilirubinemia. Typically, it is not associated with severe fetal disease, because there are fewer A and B antigenic sites on fetal RBCs than on adult blood cells. In addition, much of the anti-A and anti-B antibody produced is of the IgM isoform that does not cross the placenta to any extent.

CLINICAL FOLLOW-UP

In the case presented at the beginning of this chapter, the most likely diagnosis is isoimmunization. The initial sensitization could have occurred with her first-trimester loss. No mention of the patient having received prophylactic immunoglobulin is given. Inquiry into the father of each pregnancy is important in management, insofar as they each could possess different antigens. At this point in her current pregnancy, immediate management would consist of ultrasound to accurately assess her gestational age and blood type and screen for potentially dangerous antibodies. Paternal antigen testing is also important.

Subsequent management would depend on laboratory information. Close follow-up would likely be needed, to include periodic ultrasound examinations for fetal growth and to assess for evidence of fetal anemia. Intrauterine transfusions, steroid administration to promote fetal pulmonary maturity, and early delivery may be required.

---

thePoint® Visit http://thePoint.lww.com/activate for an interactive USMLE-style question bank and more!

CHAPTER 24

Infectious Diseases

This chapter deals primarily with APGO Educational Topic Area:

TOPIC 17   MEDICAL AND SURGICAL COMPLICATIONS OF PREGNANCY

Students should be able to identify how pregnancy affects the natural history of various infectious disorders and how a preexisting infectious disorder affects maternal and fetal health. They should be able to describe infectious disorders that are particularly concerning during pregnancy. They should be able to outline a basic approach to evaluation and management of infectious disorders in pregnancy.

CLINICAL CASE

You are seeing a patient with known human immunodeficiency virus (HIV) infection for her routine annual examination, and she tells you that she recently got married. She is interested in having children but has been told she should never get pregnant because she is infected with HIV. She wants to know whether pregnancy would cause her HIV infection to worsen and if there is anything she could do to prevent transmission of HIV to her baby.

INTRODUCTION

Screening for and preventing infectious disease is an integral part of routine prenatal care. Many of these agents can have devastating outcomes for mother, infant, or both. An understanding of the disease course in pregnancy; the maternal and fetal sequelae; and, most importantly, prevention and therapy are key to management of the pregnant patient. Screening recommendations for common sexually transmitted diseases (STDs) in pregnancy are listed in Table 24.1. Infections involving specific organ systems and not associated with significant risk of fetal infection (i.e., urinary tract infections) are covered elsewhere (see Chapters 11, 21, and 22).

GROUP B STREPTOCOCCUS

Group B streptococcus (**GBS**) (or *Streptococcus agalactiae*) is an important cause of perinatal infections. Asymptomatic lower genital tract colonization occurs in up to 30% of pregnant women, but cultures may be positive only intermittently, even in the same patient. Approximately 50% of infants exposed to the organism in the lower genital tract will become colonized. For most of these infants, such colonization is of no consequence, but without preventive treatment, GBS sepsis occurs in approximately 1.7 infants per 1,000 live births.

There are two manifestations of clinical infection of the newborn, termed *early onset* and *late onset*, occurring at roughly equal frequency. **Early-onset** infection manifests as septicemia and septic shock, pneumonia, or meningitis and occurs during the first week of life. Early-onset infection is much more common in preterm infants than in term infants. **Late-onset** infection occurs later, by definition, in infants older than 6 days (but has been reported beyond 3 months). GBS disease in newborns may occur as a result of vertical transmission or nosocomial or community-acquired infection.

With prevention strategies, current rates of early-onset GBS disease of the newborn have decreased to approximately 0.24 per 1,000 live births. Currently, the Centers for Disease Control and Prevention (CDC) and the American College of Obstetricians and Gynecologists (College) recommend universal screening for GBS between 35 and 37 weeks of gestation. All women who are GBS positive by rectovaginal culture should receive antibiotic prophylaxis in labor or with rupture of membranes.

If a patient's culture status is unknown, then prophylaxis should be given if any of the following conditions exists:

- Preterm labor (less than 37 weeks of gestation)
- Preterm premature rupture of membranes (less than 37 weeks of gestation)
- Rupture of membranes 18 hours or longer
- Maternal fever during labor (at or above 38°C [100.4°F])

Women with GBS bacteriuria during their current pregnancy or women who have previously given birth to an infant with early-onset GBS disease also are candidates for intrapartum antibiotic prophylaxis. When culture results are not available, intrapartum prophylaxis should be offered only on the basis of the presence of intrapartum risk factors for early-onset GBS disease. CDC and the College Guidelines include recommended medication regimens.

In the mother, significant postpartum fever may indicate postpartum endometritis; sepsis; and, rarely, meningitis, which may be caused by infection with GBS. With endometritis, the onset is often sudden and within 24 hours of delivery. Significant fever and tachycardia are typically present; sepsis may follow.

TABLE 24.1 SCREENING RECOMMENDATIONS FOR SEXUALLY TRANSMITTED DISEASES IN PREGNANCY

STI	Population to Be Screened
First Prenatal Visit	
HIV	All women (CDC/College)
Syphilis	All women (CDC/College)
Hepatitis B	All women (CDC/College)
Hepatitis C	High risk (CDC/College)
HSV	Inquire about history, no routine screening (CDC/College)
Chlamydia	All women (CDC/College)
Gonorrhea	High risk (CDC/College)
Third Trimester	
HIV	High risk or if previously undocumented (CDC/College)
Syphilis	High risk (CDC/College)
Chlamydia	Women aged 25 years or younger and high risk (CDC/College)
Gonorrhea	High risk (CDC/College)
Group B Streptococcus	All women at 35–37 weeks of gestation (CDC/College)
Delivery/Postpartum Stay	
HIV	High risk or if previously undocumented (CDC/College)
Syphilis	High risk or if previously undocumented (CDC)
	All women (College)
Hepatitis B	High risk or if previously undocumented (CDC/College)
HSV	With prior history of genital HSV or new diagnosis in pregnancy, inquire about symptoms and perform careful inspection of lower genital tract and perineum before delivery (College)

Note: State or local laws may supersede these recommendations. College, American College of Obstetricians and Gynecologists; CDC, Centers for Disease Control and Prevention; HIV, human immunodeficiency virus; HSV, herpes simplex virus.

HERPES

Herpes simplex virus (HSV) is a double-stranded DNA virus that can be differentiated into HSV type 1 (HSV-1) and HSV type 2 (HSV-2). HSV-1 is the primary etiologic agent of herpes labialis (fever blisters), gingivostomatitis, and keratoconjunctivitis.

Most genital infections with HSV are caused by HSV-2, but genital HSV-1 infections are becoming increasingly common, particularly among adolescent and young women. Up to 80% of new genital infections among women may be due to HSV-1, with the highest rates occurring in adolescents and young adults. Herpes infections are categorized as follows:

- **Primary** occurs in a woman with no evidence of prior HSV infection (seronegative to both HSV-1 and HSV-2).
- **Nonprimary first episode** occurs in a woman with a history of heterologous infection (e.g., first HSV-2 infection with a prior HSV-1 infection).
- **Recurrent** disease occurs in a woman with clinical or serologic evidence of prior genital herpes (of the same serotype).

The primary form poses the greatest risk to the fetus. The fetus/neonate is infected either from ascending infection following spontaneous rupture of membranes or from passage through an infected lower genital tract at delivery. With a primary infection at the time of delivery, the risk of neonatal infection approaches 50%; it is far lower (less than 1%) with recurrent infection, because the size of the inoculum is much decreased.

In utero fetal infection can occur, although this is much less common. Most infants with localized herpes infection ultimately do well; as a rule, infants with disseminated infection do very poorly.

Diagnosis

The diagnosis of HSV infection is suspected when clinical examination shows the characteristic tender vesicles with ulceration followed by crusting (Fig. 24.1). Confirmation is by identification of the virus in cell culture, with most positive results reported within 72 hours. Polymerase chain reaction (PCR) testing is commercially available and is more sensitive than culture. Serologic testing for HSV-1 and HSV-2 immunoglobulin (Ig) is also available and is a helpful ancillary test because cultures of crusted or healing lesions can often be negative. Type-specific serologic testing that accurately distinguishes between anti-HSV-1 and -2 Ig is recommended.

Treatment

All pregnant women should be asked about a history of HSV infection at their initial prenatal visit. If infection with herpes virus is suspected during the course of pregnancy in a woman with undocumented history of HSV, a culture or PCR from a lesion should be obtained to confirm the diagnosis. In such patients, or any patient with a history of herpes virus infection, careful inspection of the lower genital tract is important at the onset of labor or when rupture of membranes occurs. If no lesions are identified, vaginal delivery is deemed safe.

Cesarean delivery is recommended if herpes (or suspected herpes) lesions are identified on the cervix, in the vagina, or on the vulva at the time of labor or if spontaneous rupture of membranes occurs. This is true whether or not the lesions are

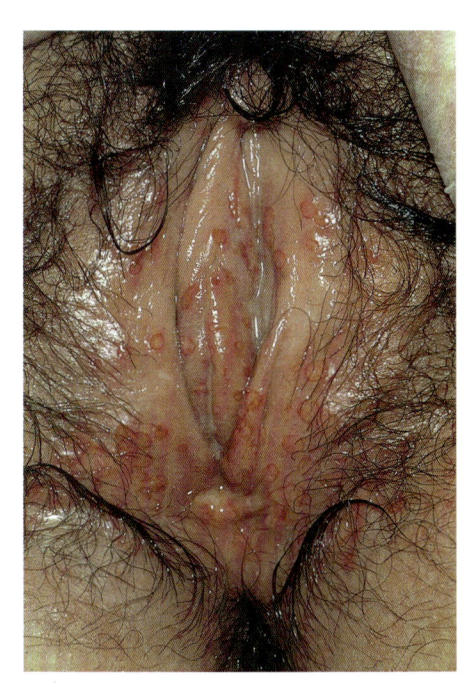

FIGURE 24.1. Herpes virus infection. Although herpes virus infection is primarily a blistering disease, on thin, moist skin, blisters quickly shear off to produce round, coalescing erosions. (Edwards L. *Genital Dermatology Atlas.* Philadelphia, PA: Lippincott Williams & Wilkins; 2004:90.)

associated with primary or recurrent infection due to the severity of neonatal disease.

Acyclovir and related compounds are safe in pregnancy and can be used if symptoms are severe. Additionally, in patients with recurrent HSV, these medications should be offered for suppression of outbreaks starting at 36 weeks of gestation to reduce the risk of viral shedding and cesarean delivery due to active lesions. Routine antepartum genital HSV cultures in asymptomatic women are not recommended, insofar as these tests do not predict viral shedding at delivery.

Routine type-specific serologic screening for HSV in pregnancy is not currently recommended. However, serologic screening may be considered in certain populations to identify women who may benefit from suppressive therapy or preventive measures.

● RUBELLA

Rubella (German, or 3-day, measles) is an RNA virus with important perinatal impact if infection occurs during pregnancy. Widespread immunization programs in the United States over the last 30 years have prevented large epidemics of rubella, but some women of reproductive age lack immunity to this virus and are, therefore, susceptible to infection. Foreign-born women may lack immunity and be susceptible to infection if their country of origin does not have a comprehensive vaccination program. Once infection occurs, immunity is lifelong. A history of prior infection is an unreliable indicator of immunity.

Symptoms

Up to 50% of adult women have had subclinical or asymptomatic infection; symptoms include fever, rash involving the face and spreading to the trunk and extremities, arthralgias, head and neck lymphadenopathy, and conjunctivitis. However, fetal effects are substantial. If a woman develops rubella infection in the first trimester of pregnancy, there is an increased risk of both spontaneous abortion and congenital rubella syndrome. Although most infants with congenital rubella appear normal at birth, many subsequently develop signs of infection. Common defects associated with the syndrome include congenital heart disease (e.g., patent ductus arteriosus), intellectual disability, deafness, and cataracts. The risk of congenital rubella is related to the gestational age at the time of infection; it is highest in the first 12 weeks of pregnancy (80% vertical transmission) and decreases with increasing gestational age (25% transmission in the second and third trimesters). Primary infection can be diagnosed by serologic testing for maternal IgM and IgG antibodies during the acute and convalescent stages of infection.

Screening

Because of the serious fetal implications, prenatal screening for IgG rubella antibody is routine. All pregnant women should be screened, unless they are known to be immune based on previous serologic testing.

Previously unvaccinated and susceptible women should be vaccinated when they are not pregnant. The vaccine induces antibodies in virtually all rubella nonimmune women. Because the vaccine itself is of the live, attenuated type, pregnant women should not be vaccinated. It is recommended that pregnancy be delayed 1 month following immunization, although congenital rubella syndrome following vaccination during an undiagnosed pregnancy has not been reported. In women whose prenatal screen identifies a lack of rubella antibody, vaccination postpartum at the time of hospital discharge is recommended. Such management poses no risk to the newborn or other children; breastfeeding is not contraindicated.

If rubella is diagnosed in a pregnant woman, the patient should be advised of the risk of fetal infection and counseled regarding options for continuing the pregnancy. Because there is no effective treatment for a pregnant patient infected with rubella, patients who do not have immunity are advised to avoid potential exposure. Although Ig may be given to an infected woman, it does not prevent fetal infection. The absence of clinical signs in a woman who has received Ig does not guarantee that infection of the fetus has been prevented.

Hepatitis

Viral hepatitis is one of the most common and potentially serious infections that can occur in pregnant women. Six forms of viral hepatitis have now been identified, two of which, hepatitis A and hepatitis B, can be prevented effectively through vaccination.

Hepatitis A

Hepatitis A virus (HAV) is transmitted from person to person primarily through fecal–oral contamination. Good hygiene and proper sanitation are important to prevent infection. However, vaccination is the most effective means of preventing transmission. The hepatitis A vaccine is available as both a single-antigen vaccine and a combination vaccine (containing both HAV and hepatitis B virus [HBV] antigens). Prior to vaccine availability, HAV accounted for one third of cases of acute hepatitis in the United States.

HAV infection does not progress to chronic infection. Diagnosis is confirmed by demonstration of anti-HAV IgM antibodies. HAV infection has no specific effects on pregnancy or the fetus. Breastfeeding is not contraindicated in HAV-infected women if appropriate hygienic precautions are followed. Vaccination safety during pregnancy has not been established, but the risk to the developing fetus is minimal because the vaccine contains inactivated purified viral proteins.

Vaccination is recommended for individuals who are intravenous (IV) drug users, who have certain medical disorders (e.g., chronic liver disease or receiving clotting factor concentrates), who are employed in specific occupations (e.g., working in primate laboratories or research laboratories), and who travel to countries with endemic HAV infection. HAV Ig is effective for both pre- and post-exposure prophylaxis and can be used during pregnancy.

Hepatitis B

Hepatitis B virus (HBV) infection is more serious than HAV infection regardless of pregnancy status. HBV is transmitted by the parenteral route and through sexual contact. Ten to fifteen percent of infected adults develop chronic infection, and, of those, some will become carriers.

Testing for hepatitis B surface antigen (HBsAg) during pregnancy is routine, as about half of pregnant women infected lack traditional high-risk factors. Vertical transmission of hepatitis occurs to a significant but variable extent and is related to the presence or absence of maternal hepatitis B e antigen (HBeAg): If the patient is positive for the "e" antigen, indicating a high viral load and active viral replication, her fetus has a 70% to 90% risk of becoming infected, and most of such infants will become chronic carriers with a 25% to 30% lifetime risk of serious or fatal liver disease. The risk of fetal infection is higher if maternal infection occurs in the third trimester. Neonatal infection can also occur via breast milk.

Women who are HBsAg negative with risk factors for HBV infection should be offered vaccination during pregnancy. Patients who have been exposed to HBV should be treated as soon as possible with hepatitis B immunoglobulin (HBIg) and begin the vaccination series. All infants now receive vaccination against hepatitis B, with the initial injection given between 2 days and 2 months of delivery. Infants of mothers who are HBsAg positive should receive the vaccine and HBIg within 12 hours of birth.

More recently, HBV viral load has been used as a predictor of disease progression and treatment response in chronically infected adults. Treatment with antiviral agents has demonstrated sustained viral suppression and lower rates of long-term disease risk. Although current neonatal immunoprophylaxis with HBIg and HBV vaccine has been highly successful, there are still 5% to 15% of newborns who are infected in the setting of chronic maternal HBV infection. High maternal HBV-DNA levels appear to be the strongest predicator of in utero maternal-to-child transmission and neonatal immunoprophylaxis failure. Based on limited but promising initial studies, the Society for Maternal-Fetal Medicine recommends targeted maternal antiviral therapy with tenofovir in women with chronic HBV infection and a high viral load (>6 to 8 log 10 copies/mL) to decrease the risk of intrauterine fetal infection.

Breastfeeding is not contraindicated in women who are chronic carriers if their infants have received both the vaccination and HBIg within 12 hours of delivery.

Hepatitis C

Hepatitis C virus (HCV) infection is a growing problem in the United States and has obstetric implications. Worldwide, HCV seroprevalence rates of 0.6% to 6.6% among pregnant women have been reported. Similar to HBV in transmission (i.e., sexual, parenteral, and vertical), HCV infection is often asymptomatic. Diagnosis is made by serologic evidence of anti-HCV IgG. However, antibodies may not be detectable until up to 10 weeks after onset of clinical illness. PCR identification of HCV RNA may be a useful adjunct to diagnosis in early and chronic infection. The presence of anti-HCV antibody does not confer immunity or prevent transmission of infection. Fifty percent of infected individuals go on to have chronic infection.

Risk Factors

Screening for evidence of HCV infection is not routine. However, the CDC recommends routine screening for certain groups (Box 24.1). Vertical transmission occurs in 2%

BOX 24.1 Risk Factors for Routine Screening

The following risk factors warrant routine screening:
- History of injection or intravenous drug abuse
- Human immunodeficiency virus infection
- History of blood transfusion or solid organ transplant before July 1992
- History of receiving clotting factor concentrates produced before 1987
- Long-term dialysis
- Signs and symptoms of liver disease
- Current evaluation or care for a sexually transmitted infection, including HIV

Adapted from Centers for Disease Control and Prevention, Workowski KA, Bolan GA. Sexually transmitted diseases treatment guidelines, 2015. *MMWR Recomm Rep*. 2015;64(RR-3):1–137.

to 8% of cases, with the risk of fetal infection directly related to the quantity of hepatitis C RNA virus in maternal blood. Vertical transmission is rare with an undetectable hepatitis C RNA viral load. Maternal co-infection with HIV is also associated with a higher risk (up to 44%) of vertical transmission of HCV. Other risk factors for fetal infection include prolonged rupture of membranes in labor and use of invasive fetal monitoring.

Currently, there are no preventive measures known to reduce the risk of mother-to-child transmission; cesarean delivery has not been consistently associated with a decreased rate of vertical transmission and should be performed for usual obstetric indications in HCV-infected women.

Breastfeeding is not contraindicated in women with HCV unless the mother has cracked or bleeding nipples. Newer therapies for HCV infection that clear detectable virus in the blood and normalize transaminase levels are promising in nonpregnant adults. Ig does not contain antibodies to HCV and has no role in post-exposure prophylaxis.

Hepatitis D

Hepatitis D virus (**HDV**) is an incomplete viral particle that can only cause infection in the presence of HBV. Transmission of HDV is through the parenteral route; chronic infection can occur, resulting in severe disease in 70% to 80% of chronically infected individuals and mortality rates as high as 25%. Vertical transmission has been documented but is uncommon. Diagnosis is made by identification of HDV antigen and anti-HDV IgM in acute disease; IgG antibodies develop but are not protective. No vaccine is currently available. Measures to prevent HBV infection are effective in the prevention of HDV transmission.

Hepatitis E

Hepatitis E virus (**HEV**) infection is a waterborne disease and is uncommon in the United States. The disease is typically self-limited, but it has been associated with higher rates of fulminant hepatitis E and mortality in pregnant women, which can be as high as 20% after infection in the third trimester. Co-infection with HIV results in severe disease and high mortality in pregnancy. Diagnosis is made by serologic testing for HEV-specific antibodies in women with travel exposure. The risk of vertical transmission is very low, but cases have been reported. No vaccine is currently available.

● ACQUIRED IMMUNE DEFICIENCY SYNDROME

Worldwide, women account for nearly 50% of those infected with HIV. The CDC estimates that 24% of those living with **acquired immune deficiency syndrome** (**AIDS**) in the United States are women. Of all Americans living with the diagnosis of HIV, 23% are women. Of these women, 86% were exposed through heterosexual contact and 13% through injection drug use. However, among white women, 32% of HIV diagnoses are attributed to injection drug use. Among women diagnosed with HIV, 61% are African American, 19% are White, and 15% are Hispanic/Latina. Less than one percent of those living with AIDS are children younger 13 years, most of whom acquired the infection perinatally.

The usual estimated latency period from untreated HIV to AIDS is about 11 years. HIV infection becomes AIDS as the helper (CD4+) lymphocyte count decreases, and the host becomes more susceptible to other types of infections. With the availability of increasingly effective antiretroviral drugs, lifespan and quality of life have improved dramatically.

Pathophysiology

HIV is a single-stranded, RNA, enveloped human retrovirus that has the ability to become incorporated into the cellular DNA of CD4+ cells such as lymphocytes, monocytes, and some neural cells. Once infected, seroconversion usually occurs within 2 to 8 weeks, but it may take up to 3 months and, in rare cases, 6 months. HIV infection appears to have no direct effect on pregnancy course or outcome. Likewise, pregnancy does not seem to affect the course of HIV.

Both HIV and pregnancy may affect the natural history, presentation, treatment, or significance of certain infections, and these, in turn, may be associated with pregnancy complications or perinatal infection. These infections include vulvovaginal candidiasis, bacterial vaginosis, genital herpes simplex, **human papillomavirus** (**HPV**), syphilis, cytomegalovirus (CMV), toxoplasmosis, and hepatitis B and C. All women demonstrate a decline in absolute CD4+ cell counts in pregnancy, which is thought to be secondary to hemodilution. On the other hand, the percentage of CD4+ cells remains relatively stable. Therefore, percentage, rather than absolute number, of CD4+ cells may be a more accurate measure of immune function for HIV-infected women. The baseline rate of perinatal HIV transmission without prophylactic therapy is approximately 25% and is generally related to higher viral loads and lower CD4+ counts.

With zidovudine monotherapy, perinatal transmission is reduced to ~8%. Currently, with combination antiretroviral therapy and an undetectable viral load, perinatal transmission is reduced to 1% from 2%. There is evidence that transmission can occur antepartum, intrapartum, or postpartum through breastfeeding; however, 66% to 75% of transmission appears to occur during or close to the intrapartum period, particularly in nonbreastfeeding populations.

Screening and Testing

Initial screening consists of **enzyme-linked immunosorbent assay** (**ELISA**), which is based on an antigen–antibody reaction. In 99% of cases, antibodies to HIV become detectable by 3 months after infection. If results of ELISA are positive, a **Western blot** test, which identifies antibodies to specific portions of the virus, is performed to confirm the diagnosis. A serologic test is reported as positive only if both the ELISA and the Western blot analyses are positive; this testing has a sensitivity and specificity of more than 99%. In the early stages of HIV infection, the ELISA may be reactive but the supplemental test may not yet be positive. Therefore, HIV RNA viral load should be performed in the setting of discordant results.

Universal, voluntary HIV screening for pregnant women is standard and should be part of the standard prenatal laboratory tests, unless a patient states that she does not want HIV testing. This "opt-out" approach is recommended by both the College and the CDC; however, state and local laws to the contrary may supersede these recommendations. Refusal of testing should be documented.

Additionally, third-trimester repeat screening is recommended for at-risk populations (including women with an STD or women who use illicit drugs, exchange sex for money or drugs, have multiple sexual partners in pregnancy, or have signs or symptoms suggesting acute HIV during pregnancy) as well as for women who declined testing in the first trimester or have undocumented HIV status at the time of labor and delivery.

Rapid HIV testing is a valuable alternative to the conventional testing previously discussed. Results can be available *within hours* after the blood sample is obtained and, thus, is especially useful when a patient of unknown HIV status presents in labor. A positive rapid HIV test must be confirmed by Western blot analysis or immunofluorescence assay before the woman is deemed HIV positive; however, immediate antiretroviral treatment should be started as soon as a rapid HIV-positive result is noted in a laboring patient, pending further confirmation.

Management

Management involves antiretroviral therapy and taking precautions during delivery to avoid transmission. Antiretroviral therapy in pregnancy is a key component to reduction of perinatal transmission to as low as 1% to 2%.

Effective combination antiretroviral therapy should be offered to all HIV-infected pregnant women and is administered in the antepartum and intrapartum period as well as to the neonate. Other than maternal disease status and viral load, risk factors for increased vertical transmission of HIV include chorioamnionitis, prolonged rupture of membranes, invasive fetal monitoring, and mode of delivery.

Awareness of maternal HIV status can help guide management of pregnancy and labor and delivery to minimize risk of transmission to the fetus. During pregnancy, amniocentesis and chorionic villus sampling should be avoided.

During labor, the likelihood of transmission increases linearly with increasing duration of rupture of membranes. The use of fetal scalp electrodes or fetal scalp sampling increases exposure of the fetus to maternal blood and genital secretions and may increase the risk of vertical transmission, depending on the serum and genital HIV viral load. These techniques should be avoided. Use of episiotomy or vacuum extraction or forceps may potentially increase risk of transmission by increasing exposure to maternal blood and genital secretions. However, these techniques may help shorten duration of labor or rupture of membranes with vaginal delivery and, thus, may decrease the likelihood of transmission.

Finally, cesarean delivery performed before the onset of labor and rupture of membranes significantly reduces the risk of perinatal HIV transmission. Planned cesarean delivery at 38 weeks of gestation to decrease the risk of perinatal transmission of HIV is recommended for women who have a viral load >1,000 copies/mL.

Breastfeeding plays a significant role in perinatal HIV transmission. It is estimated to have accounted for up to 50% of newly infected children globally. Breastfeeding in the setting of established maternal infection has a significant additional risk of transmission. When safe alternatives are available, breastfeeding should be avoided in HIV infection.

The field of HIV care and management is rapidly advancing, and care of HIV-infected pregnant women should be coordinated with a health care provider who regularly cares for HIV-infected women. Comprehensive information is also provided and regularly updated on the U.S. Department of Health and Human Resources Web site AIDS*info*, at www.aidsinfo.nih.gov, under "perinatal guidelines."

● HUMAN PAPILLOMAVIRUS

HPV is the most common sexually transmitted infection in the United States. There are over 100 types of HPV and at least 40 types can infect the genital area. Most sexually active women have been exposed to at least one type of HPV during their lifetime. Genital wart lesions (**condyloma acuminata**) are typically caused by nononcogenic HPV types 6 and 11 and often increase in size and area during pregnancy due to relative immune suppression. If extensive, cesarean delivery may be necessary to avoid excessive trauma to the lower genital tract. In pregnancy, cryotherapy, laser therapy, and trichloroacetic acid may be used to treat genital HPV lesions. Podophyllin, 5-fluorouracil, and interferon are not recommended, because they may be toxic to the fetus.

Because there are limited data regarding imiquimod use in pregnancy, it is generally avoided. Treatment of genital HPV lesions is often delayed until after pregnancy, insofar as spontaneous resolution may occur. Transmission of HPV from mother to infant is very rare but manifests as **laryngeal papillomatosis**. Cesarean delivery does not prevent perinatal transmission of HPV.

Certain oncogenic HPV types (16, 18, 31, 33, 45, 52, 58) cause abnormal Pap test results, cervical dysplasia, and cervical cancer. Management of abnormal Pap test results in pregnancy is similar to that in nonpregnant women; however, biopsies and other excisional procedures are often deferred until the postpartum period.

Close follow-up, which may include a repeat Pap test and/or colposcopy in pregnancy is often performed instead. HPV infection and abnormal Pap tests as well as recommendations regarding the **HPV vaccine** are discussed elsewhere in the text (see Chapters 29 and 47).

SYPHILIS

Syphilis is a systemic disease caused by the motile spirochete *Treponema pallidum*. The spirochete is transmitted by direct contact, invading intact mucous membranes or areas of abraded skin. A painless ulcer at the site of inoculation follows, usually within 6 weeks following exposure. The ulcer is firm, with elevated edges; it lasts for several weeks. One to three months later, a skin rash occurs or, in some patients, raised lesions (**condyloma lata**) appear on the genitalia. T. pallidum is generally considered to cross the placenta to the fetus after 16 weeks of gestation. Transmission can occur at any stage of maternal infection and has been documented at as early as 6 weeks of gestation.

Spontaneous abortion, stillbirth, and neonatal death are more frequent in any untreated patient, whereas neonatal infection is more likely in primary or secondary rather than latent syphilis. Newborns with congenital syphilis may be asymptomatic or have the classic signs of the syndrome, although most infants do not develop evidence of disease for 10 to 14 days after delivery. Early evidence of the disease includes a maculopapular rash, "snuffles," mucous patches on the oropharynx, hepatosplenomegaly, jaundice, lymphadenopathy, and chorioretinitis (Fig. 24.2). Later signs include Hutchinson teeth, mulberry molars, saddle nose, and saber shins.

Screening

Congenital syphilis is readily preventable with prompt and appropriate maternal treatment. Therefore, all pregnant women should be screened serologically as early as possible and again at delivery (and if exposed to an infected partner). Serologic testing is the mainstay of diagnosis. **Nontreponemal screening tests** (Venereal Disease Research Laboratory [VDRL] and rapid plasma reagin [RPR]) are sometimes falsely positive; **treponemal-specific tests** (fluorescent treponemal antibody absorbed and *T. pallidum* particle agglutination) are used to confirm infection and identify antibodies specific for *T. pallidum*. A positive treponemal-specific test result indicates either active disease or previous exposure; regardless of treatment, the test remains positive for life in most individuals.

Treatment

Therapy differs by stage of disease and is generally the same as that recommended for nonpregnant adults. There are no proven alternative therapies to penicillin for treating syphilis in pregnancy. Therefore, patients with penicillin sensitivity require skin testing, followed by desensitization for those with a true penicillin allergy. The **Jarisch-Herxheimer reaction** occurs most often among patients with early syphilis and is an acute febrile reaction that typically occurs in the first 24 hours after treatment. In pregnancy, this reaction may precipitate preterm labor or cause fetal distress and may warrant close observation of mothers after treatment.

Post-treatment titers (RPR or VDRL) should be followed serially for at least 1 year. A fourfold increase in serologic titer, or persistent or recurrent signs or symptoms, may indicate inadequate treatment or re-infection. Retreatment is indicated in either case. Response to therapy is again evaluated by following serologic titers.

Gonorrhea

Antepartum screening for Neisseria should be performed early in pregnancy for women with risk factors or symptoms and repeated in the third trimester for women at high risk (see Table 24.1). Rates in pregnancy range from 1% to 7%, depending on the population. Diagnosis is made by nucleic acid amplification testing (NAAT), which can be performed on a variety of specimen types including endocervical or vaginal swabs and urine. All cases of gonorrhea must be reported to health care officials.

Treatment is with an extended spectrum or third-generation cephalosporin (ceftriaxone) plus azithromycin. Tetracyclines and fluoroquinolones are contraindicated in pregnancy, although fluoroquinolones are no longer recommended as treatment for gonorrhea in nonpregnant women due to increased resistance.

Infection above the cervix (i.e., of the uterus, including the fetus, and the fallopian tubes) is rare after the first weeks of pregnancy. At delivery, however, infected mothers may transmit the organism, causing **gonococcal ophthalmia** in the neonate. All neonates receive routine prophylactic treatment with sterile ophthalmic ointment containing erythromycin, which is generally effective in preventing neonatal gonorrhea.

Chlamydia

Antepartum screening for *Chlamydia trachomatis* should be performed early in pregnancy and repeated in the third trimester

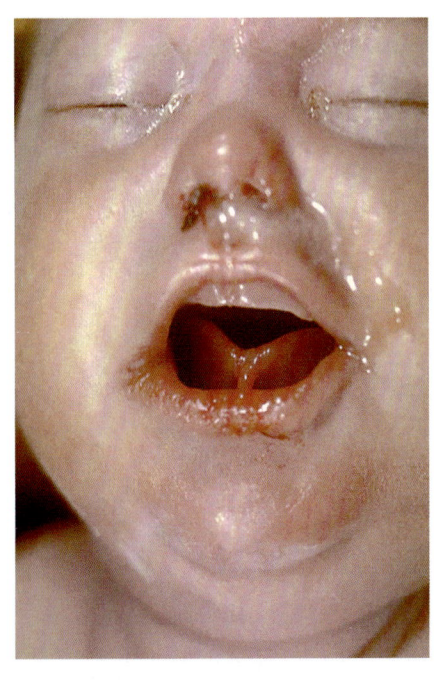

FIGURE 24.2. Congenital syphilis. Note the mucous patches on the oropharynx and the characteristic "snuffles." CDC/Dr. Norman Cole.

based on risk factors (see Table 24.1). It has been detected in 2% to 13% of pregnant women, depending on the population, and is generally found in 5% of all populations. In pregnant women, infection is often asymptomatic but may cause urethritis or mucopurulent cervicitis. Like gonorrhea, infection of the upper genital tract is uncommon during pregnancy, although *Chlamydia* infection has been associated with postpartum endometritis and infertility. Diagnosis is made by culture, direct fluorescent antibody staining, ELISA, DNA probe, or PCR. Maternal *Chlamydia* infection at the time of delivery results in colonization of the neonate in 50% of cases. Neonates colonized at birth may go on to develop purulent conjunctivitis soon after birth or pneumonia at 1 to 3 months of age. Routine prophylaxis against neonatal gonococcal ophthalmia is not generally effective against chlamydial conjunctivitis; systemic treatment of the infant is necessary. Fortunately, neonatal chlamydial ophthalmia and pneumonia are becoming less common with the institution of universal prenatal screening and treatment. Recommended treatment of genital infection with *C. trachomatis* in pregnancy includes azithromycin or amoxicillin. Doxycycline and ofloxacin are contraindicated during pregnancy.

Repeat testing to confirm successful treatment, preferably by culture or NAAT performed 3 to 4 weeks after completion of therapy, is recommended in pregnancy.

Cytomegalovirus

Approximately 1% of all neonates are infected with CMV in utero and excrete CMV at birth. Although the majority of CMV infections are asymptomatic, 12% and 18% of neonates infected in utero show symptoms at birth and up to 25% of these will develop sequelae.

A DNA herpesvirus, CMV may be transmitted in saliva, semen, cervical secretions, breast milk, blood, or urine. CMV infection is often asymptomatic, although it can cause a short febrile illness. Similar to HSV, CMV may have dormant periods, only to reactivate at a later time. There are multiple serotypes, and the presence of anti-CMV IgG does not confer immunity; recurrent infection may occur with a new strain of virus.

The prevalence of antibodies to CMV is inversely proportional to age and socioeconomic status. The risk of neonatal infection is significantly higher with primary maternal infection 30% to 40% risk of vertical transmission) than with recurrent infection; with recurrent infection the risk of neonatal infection is much lower, at 2% or less. Most infants are asymptomatic at birth; when signs occur, they include petechiae, hepatosplenomegaly, jaundice, thrombocytopenia, microcephaly, chorioretinitis, or nonimmune hydrops fetalis. Long-term sequelae include severe neurologic impairment and hearing loss. There is no effective vaccine or treatment for maternal or fetal infection. Therefore, routine serologic screening for CMV in pregnancy is not recommended. Congenital CMV may be suspected during the prenatal period when ultrasound findings suggesting fetal infection are noted; these include abdominal or intracranial calcifications, hepatosplenomegaly, echogenic bowel, ventriculomegaly, ascites, and intrauterine growth restriction. However, none of these findings are specific for CMV infection and are often found with other fetal abnormalities. Amniocentesis for CMV DNA PCR may be performed to confirm fetal infection.

Congenital CMV may also be suspected after a documented maternal primary infection. Anti-CMV IgG in maternal serum samples collected 3 to 4 weeks apart can confirm primary infection. Seroconversion from negative to positive or a fourfold increase in anti-CMV IgG titers are evidence of infection. Anti-CMV IgM is less useful in differentiating primary from recurrent CMV infection. IgG avidity assays measure the maturity of the IgG antibody and may be combined with IgM titers to improve diagnosis of primary infection. The presence of IgM and low-avidity IgG suggests primary infection within the preceding 2 to 4 months, high-avidity IgG suggests more remote primary infection.

Antiviral agents have been used to treat neonatal infection but remain experimental for prenatal treatment. The use of CMV-specific hyperimmune globulin has been investigated for prevention of congenital CMV infection in the setting of primary maternal CMV infection. Although initially promising, a subsequent randomized, placebo-controlled, double-blind trial did not demonstrate benefit and this treatment is not currently recommended in pregnancy.

Toxoplasmosis

Infection with the intracellular parasite **Toxoplasma gondii** occurs primarily through ingestion of the infectious tissue cysts in raw or poorly cooked meat or through contact with feces from infected cats, which contain infectious sporulated oocytes. The latter may remain infectious in moist soil for more than 1 year. Only cats that hunt and kill their prey are reservoirs for infection; those that eat prepared cat food are not.

In immunocompetent adult humans, infection is most commonly asymptomatic, and disease is self-limited. Prior infection confers immunity, unless the individual is immunosuppressed. Approximately 15% of reproductive-age women have antibodies to toxoplasmosis. Although congenital infection is more common following maternal infection in the third trimester, the sequelae following first-trimester fetal infection are more severe. More than half of infants whose mothers are infected during the last trimester of pregnancy have serologic evidence of infection, but three fourths of these show no gross evidence of infection at birth.

Signs of congenital infection include severe neurodevelopmental delay, chorioretinitis, blindness, epilepsy, intracranial calcifications, and hydrocephalus. Amniocentesis with PCR of the amniotic fluid to confirm the diagnosis should be offered in the setting of suspected congenital infection based on ultrasound findings (ventriculomegaly, intracranial calcifications, microcephaly, IUGR).

Screening

In some regions with high prevalence of disease (e.g., France and Central America), screening is routine in pregnancy. In the United States, routine screening in pregnancy is not recommended except in the presence of maternal HIV infection. Because identification of the organism in tissue or blood is complex and infection is usually asymptomatic, diagnosis depends on demonstration of seroconversion. A positive IgG titer indicates infection at some time. A negative IgM effectively rules out recent infection; however, IgM may persist for long periods and a positive test is not reliable in assessing duration of disease. In addition, false-positive IgM results are common with commercially available assays. Confirmatory testing in pregnancy should be performed in a *Toxoplasma* reference laboratory prior to initiating any therapy. IgG avidity testing can also be performed in a *Toxoplasma* reference laboratory; low-avidity indicates infection within the past 5 months and high-avidity indicates more remote infection.

Treatment and Prevention

Treatment of acutely infected pregnant women with spiramycin may reduce the risk of fetal transmission but does not prevent sequelae in the fetus if infection has occurred. This medication is only available through the Food and Drug Administration. If fetal infection has already been noted (through ultrasound findings or confirmed with testing of amniotic fluid), pyrimethamine and sulfadiazine therapy may reduce the severity of manifestations.

Prevention of infection should be an important part of prenatal care, including counseling regarding thoroughly cooking all meats, careful handwashing after handling raw meats, washing of fruits and raw vegetables before ingestion, wearing gloves when working with soil, and keeping cats indoors and feeding them only processed foods. If a cat is kept outside, someone other than a pregnant woman should feed and care for the cat and dispose of its waste.

Varicella

Congenital varicella (chicken pox) infection can be serious, but it is very uncommon due to high rates of immunity in women of reproductive age. Risk of **congenital varicella syndrome** (i.e., skin scarring, limb hypoplasia, chorioretinitis, and microcephaly) is limited to maternal infection occurring in the first half of pregnancy. Most patients are immune, even if they or their families do not recall the patient having been infected. A pregnant patient exposed to varicella can have serologic testing (IgM and IgG) and can be given varicella zoster immune globulin within 96 hours of exposure to reduce the severity of maternal infection.

A pregnant patient who develops the characteristic varicella rash can be given oral acyclovir within 24 hours of the rash to decrease symptoms and duration of disease (Fig. 24.3). However, maternal acyclovir has not been shown to decrease the rate or severity of fetal infection.

If clinical infection occurs in a patient from 5 days prior to delivery to 2 days after delivery, neonatal infection can be severe, even deadly. Varicella zoster Ig is given to infants in such situations, though protection is not complete.

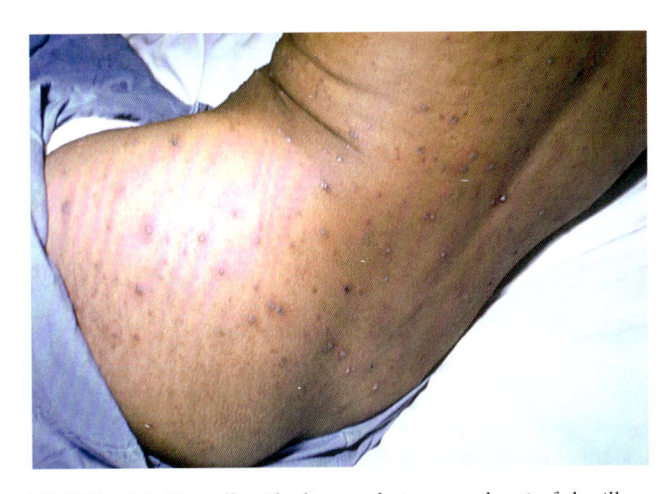

FIGURE 24.3. Varicella. Chickenpox lesions on day 6 of the illness. CDC/J. D. Millar.

Severe complications of varicella including pneumonia and encephalitis are much more common in adults than in children. Varicella pneumonia seems to occur more frequently with varicella infection during pregnancy and is associated with maternal mortality.

Treatment is with IV acyclovir. Effective vaccination against varicella has been available since 1995 and should be offered to susceptible nonpregnant women. Pregnant women with no history of varicella infection or immunization should have serologic testing for evidence of immunity; if non-immune, the first dose of the varicella vaccine should be administered in the postpartum period. The vaccine is a live attenuated virus and should be avoided in pregnancy and within 1 month of conception; however, no adverse outcomes have been reported if given in pregnancy. Vaccination of susceptible household contacts of pregnant women is safe.

Parvovirus

Maternal parvovirus **B19 infection** can cause devastating fetal outcomes such as spontaneous abortion, fetal nonimmune hydrops fetalis, and even death. Seroprevalence increases with age and is >60% in adolescents and adults. For susceptible pregnant women, the risk of seroconversion ranges from 20% to 50%, depending on closeness to the infectious contact (higher risk for closer contacts such as family members); however, the risk of transplacental infection is low.

Maternal immune status can be determined by serologic testing; IgM reflects recent infection and IgG indicates infection in the past and immunity. Routine serologic screening in pregnancy is not recommended. Exposed pregnant women should be offered B19-specific IgM and IgG serologic testing. If IgM is positive or seroconversion is confirmed, ultrasound testing every 1 to 2 weeks for 8 to 12 weeks to look for evidence of fetal hydrops (ascites and edema), placentomegaly, and growth disturbances is performed. Doppler assessment of the peak systolic velocity of the fetal middle cerebral artery (MCA) should also be performed to more accurately predict fetal anemia. Intrauterine transfusions may be necessary if hydrops develops more severe fetal anemia is suspected based on MCA Doppler assessment. There is no specific treatment for parvovirus infection. If hydrops does not develop in the fetus, long-term outcomes are overall good. Long-term neurodevelopmental outcomes are uncertain; previous studies suggested no long-term effects if the fetus survives but a more recent study suggests increased risk of neurodevelopmental impairment with survival after hydrops and fetal transfusion.

Zika Virus

Zika virus is transmitted to humans by infected mosquitoes (Aedes species) or through sexual contact. Zika virus can also be transmitted from mother to fetus at any time during pregnancy and is associated with severe abnormalities including microcephaly, IUGR, and stillbirth (see Figure 24.4).

The virus was first discovered in 1947 but a recent epidemic in South America in 2015 first highlighted the severe fetal effects of infection during pregnancy. Most adults infected with Zika virus are asymptomatic but symptoms include fever, rash, arthralgias, headache, and conjunctivitis. There is currently no available treatment for the infection. Prevention largely involves avoiding travel to high risk areas and implementing measures to avoid mosquito bites.

Since the reports in 2015, Zika virus infection and transmission have spread to many parts of the world, including some areas of the United States. There are specific travel advisories and recommendations for testing of pregnant women with suspected exposure or infection. Testing includes serology and NAT. Women with confirmed infection should have ultrasound screening and surveillance.

Zika virus infection in pregnancy continues to be an area of evolving care and recommendations. Regular updates and practice advisories are available on the ACOG website at www.acog.org and the CDC web site www.cdc.gov and should be accessed to guide counseling, screening, and management.

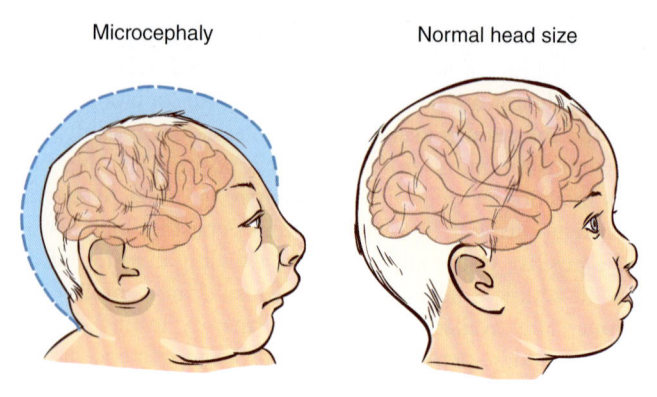

FIGURE 24.4. Zika virus transmitted from mother to fetus is associated with microcephaly.

CLINICAL FOLLOW-UP

You set up an appointment for preconception counseling with your patient and discuss the implications of HIV infection in pregnancy for the mother and fetus. You explain that, fortunately, pregnancy does not appear to worsen disease for the mother. However, there is a substantial risk of transmission of HIV from mother to infant if the mother is not on combination antiretroviral therapy during pregnancy and labor and delivery and if her HIV infection is not well controlled. There are also measures that can reduce the risk of transmission during labor and delivery. Fortunately, most antiretroviral agents have not been associated with fetal harm. With careful planning, effective therapy, good prenatal and intrapartum care, and avoiding breastfeeding if safe alternatives are available, she can reduce the risk of transmission of HIV to her baby from 25% or higher to less than 1% to 2%.

thePoint Visit http://thePoint.lww.com/activate for an interactive USMLE-style question bank and more!

CHAPTER 25
Neurologic and Psychiatric Disorders

This chapter deals primarily with APGO Educational Topic Areas:

TOPIC 17 MEDICAL AND SURGICAL COMPLICATIONS OF PREGNANCY
TOPIC 29 ANXIETY AND DEPRESSION

Students should be able to identify how pregnancy affects the natural history of various neurologic and mood disorders and how a preexisting neurologic and mood disorder affects maternal and fetal health. They should be able to outline a basic approach to evaluation and management of neurologic and mood disorders in pregnancy.

CLINICAL CASE

You are seeing a new patient who is at 14 weeks of gestation with her first pregnancy. She informs you that she has had significant depression for some years. When she has tried stopping her antidepressant medications, her symptoms became severe and on two occasions required hospital admission. Her psychiatrist discussed continued use of a selective serotonin reuptake inhibitor in pregnancy, and together they decided she should remain on such medications. In discussing general obstetric care, you counsel her on depression and management during pregnancy.

INTRODUCTION

Headaches are common in reproductive aged women and are therefore encountered during pregnancy, particularly in the first trimester. Depression and anxiety are seen quite frequently in the pregnant population, as they are in the general population. Postpartum depression (PPD) is an important entity that must be appreciated by anyone caring for patients during and after delivery. Other specific neurologic and psychiatric disorders are also seen, albeit less frequently, but they pose challenges for those providing obstetric care to patients with these conditions.

NEUROLOGIC DISORDERS

Headaches

Hormonal changes are thought to influence headaches in women in pregnancy, the postpartum period, and at other reproductive system changes throughout life. Headaches are especially common in pregnancy, particularly in the first trimester. In pregnant women presenting with headaches after 20 weeks gestation, the possibility of preeclampsia must always be considered and ruled out (see Chapter 22 for more details on the workup and management of preeclampsia). Although much less common, preeclampsia can develop during the postpartum period and should be considered in the evaluation of headache.

Patients who report the new onset of significant headaches in pregnancy, or describe acute worsening of symptoms, should undergo evaluation, including imaging. Computed tomography (CT) and magnetic resonance imaging (MRI) scans, and lumbar puncture, are considered safe. In general, contrast is avoided during CT (iodinated contrast agents) and MRI (Gadolinium-based contrast agents) in pregnancy due to potential risks to the fetus unless absolutely necessary to significantly improve diagnostic performance and maternal outcome.

Tension Headaches

Tension headaches are the most common type of headache experienced; symptoms include painful pressure or "tightness" all around the head, originating over the forehead or frontalis muscle, radiating over the crown of the head down to the posterior neck; the severity varies. Initial treatment is usually with acetaminophen, being careful not to exceed the manufacturer's recommendation for total consumption per day; nonsteroidal anti-inflammatory drugs are best avoided in pregnancy. Combination medications, some including narcotics, may be necessary short term. Alternative therapies for short-term use include combinations of acetaminophen, butalbital, and caffeine.

Migraine Headaches

Migraine headaches occur more often in women than in men, and they are thought to be related to hormonal fluctuations more than are tension headaches. The prevalence is highest during the childbearing years. Overall, the majority of patients experience an improvement in the frequency and severity of migraines during pregnancy, with the most improvement described in the third trimester. Return to the pre-pregnant pattern of migraines often occurs during the puerperium. Again, initial treatment is generally with

219

acetaminophen, alone or in combination with codeine, metoclopramide, or butalbital-caffeine. Prolonged use of narcotics is to be avoided, if at all possible, due to risk for medication overuse headaches, addiction, and neonatal abstinence syndrome. Triptans selectively vasoconstrict the blood vessels in the brain but are generally avoided in pregnancy due to the theoretical risk of vasoconstriction with decreased uterine blood flow or increased uterotonic activity. However, for patients with severe symptoms who do not respond to other medications, sumatriptan may be considered as the experience in human pregnancy has been generally favorable. Ergotamines should be avoided. Treatment for symptoms of nausea and vomiting associated with migraine headaches is individualized. Ondansetron and metoclopramide are sometimes used for severe gastrointestinal symptoms. Prophylaxis with β-blockers, oral magnesium, and other agents may be needed. Collaboration with a neurologist is appropriate and encouraged in patients with ongoing symptoms despite standard therapies.

Postdural Puncture Headaches

Women who have neuraxial anesthesia or analgesia for pain management in labor and delivery may develop a postdural puncture headache (PDPH). These headaches generally develop within 48 hours of the procedure and are typically positional; the headache is worse with standing or sitting and improves in the supine position. A neurologist or anesthesiologist should assist in the evaluation and management. PDPH typically resolve spontaneously in 24 to 48 hours; those that do not respond to conservative management or are severe may be treated with an epidural blood patch.

Epilepsy

Despite the fact that most women with **epilepsy** have successful pregnancies, optimal management may prove challenging. Pharmaceutical agents used to treat epilepsy appear to increase the risk of both major and minor congenital anomalies. However, the risk of obstetric complications appears to be less than previously thought. Adequate data concerning pregnancy loss rates are lacking.

Management

Preconception counseling is strongly recommended for patients contemplating pregnancy. At that time, drug choices and adjustments in doses can be reviewed, along with a discussion of risks and overall pregnant management. Folate supplementation (usually at a dose of 4 mg/day) to reduce the risk of neural tube defects should begin several months before conception is attempted and continued at least through the first trimester of pregnancy. High doses of folate may alter some antiepileptic drug levels and dosing may need to be altered. The frequency of seizure activity does not change during pregnancy for most patients.

Besides the risks noted below, fetal injury (e.g., placental abruption) or oxygen deprivation from a prolonged maternal seizure is possible. Offspring of patients with epilepsy are at increased risk for being diagnosed with epilepsy in later life.

All of the commonly used anti-epileptic drugs appear to increase the risk of congenital abnormalities by a factor of roughly two—from 2% to 3% to 4% to 6%. Valproate carries the highest risk of malformations, specifically with neural tube defects, and it should be avoided unless absolutely necessary for seizure control. The other agents commonly used in pregnancy (e.g., phenytoin, carbamazepine, topiramate, and phenobarbital) appear to have similar risk profiles, so there are no specific recommendations as to choice of drug. Some newer agents such as gabapentin, lamotrigine and levetiracetam appear to have a lower risk profile for major fetal malformations when used as monotherapy. The lowest dose that prevents seizure activity is preferred, of course. Monotherapy is also preferred if possible. If patients have been seizure free for several years, some neurologists recommend discontinuation of antiepileptic medications prior to conception, to see if ongoing medications are indeed necessary.

In addition to antiseizure medications, pregnancy management for patients with epilepsy include frequent visits, with folate supplementation, monitoring of free folate levels, and dose adjustments of antiseizure medicines as needed secondary to changes in maternal weight and plasma volume; screening for fetal congenital anomalies; possibly, maternal vitamin K supplementation in the third trimester; and preparation for treatment of an epileptic seizure during labor, delivery, or in the first-day postpartum.

Postpartum, medication dose adjustments to prepregnancy dosing should be coordinated with the patient's neurologist. Unless epileptic treatment includes sedatives, breastfeeding may be recommended, but data remain limited.

Multiple Sclerosis

Multiple sclerosis (MS) is also more common in women, with diagnosis most commonly around age 30 years. In general, pregnant patients report fewer, and less severe, relapses during pregnancy, though postpartum relapse occurs. Lower infant birth weights and a higher cesarean delivery rate have been noted in patients with MS. Medical management during pregnancy and the puerperium (if breastfeeding) must take into account the perinatal effects of the agents used. Many experts suggest stopping disease-modifying medications for MS prior to and during pregnancy and restarting in the postpartum period to avoid potential risks to the fetus. Anesthesia for delivery should be based on obstetric circumstances.

Carpal Tunnel Syndrome

Carpal tunnel syndrome is quite common in pregnancy. Although it can occur anytime during pregnancy, it is more common as pregnancy advances. Fluid retention is thought to be causative; compression of the median nerve within the carpal tunnel causes symptoms of pain, tingling, and numbness. Wrist splints widely available may offer significant relief. Symptoms subside postpartum but not immediately.

Bell's Palsy

For reasons that are unknown, paralysis of the facial nerve (**Bell's palsy**) more commonly occurs during pregnancy, especially in the third trimester or in the first week postpartum. Overall, the outcome with complete facial nerve paralysis during pregnancy is somewhat worse than when the palsy occurs in the nonpregnant state. Steroids remain the mainstay of therapy, preferably started within 3 days of onset of symptoms. The addition of antiviral medications (valacyclovir) in combination with steroids may be considered in severe cases although the evidence to support this is inconsistent.

● PSYCHIATRIC DISORDERS

Depression and Anxiety

Pregnancy and the puerperium are periods of life that can be very emotional. Although excitement and joy often exist, depression and anxiety may arise or recur, especially in the postpartum period. Pregnancy can present many stresses for patients and their families. Hormonal influences are thought to play a role but are not the only responsible factor.

Perinatal depression is defined as a major or minor depressive episode that occurs during pregnancy or during the first 12 months after delivery. Perinatal depression affects one in seven women and is one of the most common medical complications encountered in the perinatal period. Depression, in general, is twice as common in women than in men. Both genetic and environmental factors are thought to be involved.

Untreated perinatal mood disorders can have devastating effects on women, infants, and families. Therefore, awareness of the possibility of these disorders, and the screening and recognition of them, is important. The negative consequences of unrecognized and untreated perinatal depression, other mood disorders, and other maternal psychiatric illnesses are well documented; lack of treatment or inadequate treatment may result in poor compliance with prenatal care, inadequate nutrition, increased alcohol, tobacco and other substance use and abuse, poor maternal–infant bonding, and disruptive family environments.

Because of these concerns, ACOG recommends that clinicians screen all women at least once during the perinatal period for symptoms of depression and anxiety using a standardized, validated tool. All pregnant women should be asked about any individual or family history of mental health disorders including any past or current medication use during the intake history.

There are several screening instruments that have been validated for use in the perinatal period (Box 25.1). The Edinburgh Postnatal Depression Scale (see Appendix C) is short (10 questions), available in multiple languages, and includes anxiety symptoms, which are prominent in perinatal mood disorders. The Edinburgh Scale also excludes constitutional symptoms, such as sleep disturbances, which are common in the perinatal period. All of the instruments listed in Box 25.1 are available in Spanish, except the Zung Self-rating Depression Scale.

Risk Factors

A history of mental illness is important for optimizing care during pregnancy and beyond. The association of depression during and after previous pregnancies is also helpful in formulating care. Risk factors for perinatal depression are listed in Box 25.2. Maternal suicide now exceeds hemorrhage and hypertensive disorders as a cause of maternal mortality in the United States. Although, the risk factors listed in Box 25.2 are important to note, clinicians and patients should recognize that perinatal depression can affect any woman of any socioeconomic status.

BOX 25.1 Validated Screening Tools for Perinatal Depression

- Edinburgh Postnatal Depression Scale (may be used during pregnancy as well; see Appendix C)
- Postpartum Depression Screening Scale
- Patient Health Questionnaire 9
- Beck Depression Inventory
- Beck Depression Inventory-II
- Center for Epidemiologic Studies Depression Scale
- Zung Self-rating Depression Scale

Modified from Screening for Perinatal Depression. Committee Opinion No. 630. American College of Obstetricians and Gynecologists. *Obstet Gynecol.* 2015;125:1268–1271.

BOX 25.2 Risk Factors for Perinatal Depression

During Pregnancy
- Anxiety disorders
- Life stress
- History of depression
- Lack of social or family support
- Unintended pregnancy
- Lower socioeconomic status
- Lower educational level
- Smoking and other substance use/abuse
- Poor relationship quality

Postpartum
- Depression during pregnancy
- Anxiety during pregnancy
- Stressful life events during pregnancy or postpartum
- Traumatic or difficult birth experience
- Infant admission to neonatal intensive care unit
- Lack of social or family support
- Previous history of depression
- Problems with breastfeeding

Modified from Screening for Perinatal Depression. Committee Opinion No. 630. American College of Obstetricians and Gynecologists. *Obstet Gynecol.* 2015;125:1268–1271.

Management

Patients with inadequate treatment of depression and anxiety often will fail to care for themselves (and consequently their fetuses) during pregnancy. With depression, poor diet and nutrition, substance abuse, and other suboptimal care may be involved in the increased prevalence of low-birth-weight infants seen in women with depression. Anxiety alone does not seem to alter perinatal outcome.

Screening for perinatal depression alone is not sufficient to improve outcomes and must be coupled with appropriate follow-up as indicated. Management of depression and anxiety involves counseling and, at times, medications. Multidisciplinary care involving the obstetrician, mental health care provider, and pediatrician is recommended. Clinical staff in obstetrics and gynecology should be prepared to initiate medical therapy and refer patients for mental health counseling and therapy as appropriate to the situation. Prompt referral for psychiatric care is sometimes needed. Involvement of a patient's partner and/or other family members can be beneficial.

A variety of antidepressant medications are available, including selective serotonin reuptake inhibitors (SSRIs), which are more commonly used; tricyclic antidepressants; and others (e.g., bupropion). All appear to cross the placenta. Teratogenicity and fetal/neonatal effects are concerns, although the absolute risk of major congenital abnormalities appears to be quite low. Available studies offer varying levels of risk. The only SSRI that currently should be avoided in the first trimester pregnancy is paroxetine due to potential increased risk for fetal cardiac defects. For the fetus exposed to psychotropic medications in the third trimester, neonatal behavior may be altered, with a range of sequelae, such as tremors, to, rarely, persistent pulmonary hypertension.

When medications are to be considered part of the management of pregnant patients with depression and anxiety, a current search for new reports is wise, insofar as new data are commonly added to our information regarding the perinatal effects of such drugs. There are multiple electronic resources available to clinicians for information related to fetal and neonatal effects of medications considered for use in pregnancy and lactation including, but not limited to, Reprotox (https://reprotox.org), TERIS (http://depts.washington.edu/terisdb), and LactMed (https://toxnet.nlm.nih.gov/newtoxnet/lactmed.htm). Reprotox and TERIS require a subscription but LactMed is free. Reprotox and LactMed also have mobile app versions available. Careful counseling regarding benefits, risks, and alternatives should be thoroughly discussed with the patient prior to prescribing them.

Women with a history of mania or bipolar disorder should be referred for psychiatric evaluation prior to starting any medical therapy as antidepressant monotherapy in these women may trigger mania or psychosis. Prior to starting antidepressant medication, all women, regardless of history, should have a short screen for behavior or symptoms suggesting mania or bipolar disorder. If concern for bipolar disorder, referral to psychiatry is indicated to initiate appropriate therapy.

Postpartum Depression

Depression in varying degrees is common both during pregnancy and in the postpartum period. There is a wide spectrum of response to pregnancy and delivery, ranging from mild postpartum blues to severe **postpartum depression** (PPD) (see Table 25.1). Approximately 70% to 80% of women report feeling sad, anxious, or angry beginning 2 to 4 days after birth. These **postpartum blues** may come and go throughout the day, are usually mild, and abate within 1 to 2 weeks. Supportive care and reassurance are helpful in ensuring that symptoms are self-limited. Approximately 10% to 15% of new mothers experience PPD, which is a more serious disorder and usually requires medication and counseling. PPD differs from postpartum blues in the severity and duration of symptoms.

Women with PPD have pronounced feelings of sadness, anxiety, and despair that interfere with activities of daily living, including infant care. These symptoms do not abate but, instead, worsen over several weeks. Counseling and medical treatment are indicated. Although the exact cause of PPD is unknown, several associated factors have been identified. The normal hormonal fluctuations that occur following birth may trigger

TABLE 25.1 THREE CATEGORIES OF POSTPARTUM MOOD DISORDERS

	Postpartum Blues	Postpartum Depression	Postpartum Psychosis
Incidence (%)	70–80	≥10	0.1–0.2
Average time	2–4 days postpartum	2 weeks to 12 months postpartum	2–3 days postpartum
Average duration	2–3 days, resolution within 10 days	3–14 months	Variable
Symptoms	Mild insomnia, tearfulness, fatigue, irritability, poor concentration, depressed affect	Irritability, labile mood, difficulty falling asleep, phobias, anxiety; symptoms worsen in the evening	Similar to organic brain syndrome: confusion, attention deficit, distractibility, clouded sensorium
Treatment	None; self-limited	Antidepressant pharmacotherapy; psychotherapy	Antipsychotic pharmacotherapy; antidepressant pharmacotherapy (50% of patients also meet depression criteria)

depression in some women. Women who have a personal or family history of depression or anxiety may be more likely to develop PPD. Acute stressors, including those specific to motherhood (childcare), or other stressors (e.g., death of a family member) may contribute to the development of PPD. Having a child with a difficult temperament or health issues may lead the mother to doubt her ability to care for her newborn, which can lead to depression. The age of the mother may influence susceptibility to PPD, with younger women more likely to experience depression than older women. Toxins, poor diet, crowded living conditions, low socioeconomic status, and low social support may also play a role.

A strong predictor of PPD is depression during pregnancy. It is estimated that half of all cases of PPD may begin during pregnancy. PPD may also be a continuation of a depressive disorder that existed prior to pregnancy, rather than a new disorder.

Treatment

Treatment must be tailored to the patient's individual situation. Postpartum blues do not require treatment other than support and reassurance. Women with PPD should receive mental health counseling and medication, if warranted. Effective therapies for the treatment of PPD include cognitive–behavioral and interpersonal therapies.

Anxiety Disorders

Phobias, obsessive–compulsive disorders, and generalized anxiety disorders are among a number of anxiety disorders. Counseling and medications are sometimes necessary. Little is known about the effects of anxiety disorders on pregnancy, but potential risks seem to be small. Patients with anxiety disorders during pregnancy are prone to PPD.

Bipolar Disorders

Approximately 1% of the population is affected with bipolar disorder. Because its onset often occurs in early adulthood, pregnancy can be an important consideration in therapy. Preconceptional treatment planning is wise. There is a strong genetic component to bipolar illness. Manifestations include depression, mania, and psychosis. Teratogenic concerns exist for medications such as sodium valproate and carbamazepine; previous concern for lithium may have been exaggerated. Careful collaboration with mental health professionals is important in optimizing outcome.

Postpartum Psychosis

Postpartum psychosis is the most severe form of mental derangement and is most common in women with preexisting disorders, such as bipolar illness or schizophrenia. This condition should be considered a medical emergency, and the patient should be referred for immediate, often inpatient, treatment.

Schizophrenia

Schizophrenia is a serious condition that also affects approximately 1% of the population and manifests symptoms in young adulthood. It, too, has a strong genetic component. The offspring of a couple, one of whom has schizophrenia, has a 5% to 10% risk of having the disorder. Outcome with treatment is variable.

CLINICAL FOLLOW-UP

In your initial discussion with your G1 at 14 weeks of gestation, you review the potential adverse effects of antidepressants in pregnancy. Given her history of severe relapses when off medications, you concur with her decision to remain on a SSRI. You also discuss PPD, which is quite common in patients without a history of depression. She continues through pregnancy, delivers uneventfully at term, and continues her SSRI therapy through and after delivery.

IV Gynecology

CHAPTER 26
Contraception

This chapter deals primarily with APGO Educational Topic Area:

TOPIC 33 FAMILY PLANNING

Students should be able to compare and contrast common contraceptive methods in terms of benefits, risks, mechanism of action, and effectiveness. They should be able to counsel a patient on options and identify barriers to effective contraception.

CLINICAL CASE

A young couple returns to your obstetric office for a routine postpartum visit after normal vaginal delivery of a healthy boy. Because of your explanation of the benefits of breastfeeding for mother and baby, the mother had elected to breastfeed despite discouragement from other professional friends. With their confidence in you bolstered, the couple returns with a new, serious problem. They had planned to use condoms for contraception during breastfeeding, but now realize that the mother may breastfeed for a year or more and that they are not satisfied with the use of condoms, which distracts substantially from their sexual experience. They have never used a diaphragm, but feel it would present the same problems. As they plan to have more children, probably within the next 2 years, tubal ligation and vasectomy are inappropriate considerations. They did an Internet search for the issues of hormonal contraception during breastfeeding and found themselves bewildered by the conflicting information they found. They seek your advice.

● INTRODUCTION

Over 50% of all pregnancies in the United States are unplanned, the highest rate in the developed world. Yet every year new contraceptive options are introduced touting various "improvements." Although no method is effective if it is not used correctly, many methods are very reliable. We will take a look at the various contraceptive options from the most reliable to the least and compare their risks, benefits, and reliability (their efficacy rate).

Although there are many kinds of contraceptives, all work either by inhibiting the development or release of ova or blocking the meeting of ova and sperm. This goal is accomplished by two general mechanisms, each with many variations: (1) inhibiting the development and release of the egg (via oral contraceptive pills [OCPs], long-acting progesterone injection, or contraceptive patch and ring) and (2) imposing a mechanical, chemical, or temporal barrier between the sperm and egg (via condom, diaphragm, spermicide, intrauterine contraception, and fertility awareness). As a secondary mechanism, intrauterine devices (IUDs) placed as emergency contraception (EC) alter the ability of the fertilized egg to implant and grow. It is important to understand that the mechanism of action of the IUD not placed for EC is via changes in the amount and viscosity of cervical mucus, endometrial suppression, inhibition of sperm migration and viability, changes in transport speed of the ovum, and damage to or destruction of the ovum. Each approach may be used individually or in combination and has its own advantages, disadvantages, risks, and benefits.

Before helping any woman or couple choose among the many contraceptive options, the physician must consider two things. First, the physician must understand and be able to explain (in language the woman and partner can understand) the physiologic or pharmacologic mechanism of action of all of the available contraceptive methods, along with their effectiveness rates, indications, contraindications, complications, advantages, and disadvantages. Second, the physician must know the woman and her partner well enough to recognize personal, physical, religious, or cultural values affecting the use of each contraceptive method under consideration and be able to help them deal with those issues using empathic evidence-based discussions, regardless of any personal bias. When done correctly, these discussions allow the couple to understand the contraceptive options and the physician to freely provide evidence-based recommendations. In this manner, an appropriate individualized contraceptive method can be chosen whose correct, regular use is highly likely.

Seen from another perspective, contraception allows the woman or couple to formulate a reproductive health plan, allowing conception to be a planned rather than an unexpected event. This takes into account their desire for children and allows for planning the timing, spacing, and, ultimately, the optimal number of children.

When comparing all contraceptive methods, both the **typical use failure rate** (the failure rate seen when the method is actually used by patients, that is, factoring in the mistakes in usage everyone will make from time to time and actual noncompliance) and **method or perfect use failure rate** (the failure rate inherent in the method if the patient uses it correctly 100% of the time) should be considered, as described in Table 26.1. Throughout the chapter, failure rates will be included in parenthesis (as typical/perfect use) referring to the percentage of unintended pregnancies within the first year of typical versus perfect use. By helping a woman and her partner choose a personally acceptable and biologically appropriate contraceptive method, the gap between the typical failure rate and method failure rate is minimized.

FACTORS AFFECTING THE CHOICE OF CONTRACEPTIVE METHOD

Although efficacy is important in the choice of contraceptive methods, other factors to be considered include safety, availability, cost, acceptability, and, in some cases, the patient's physical ability to appropriately use the method. Although we tend to think of safety in terms of significant health risks, for many patients, this also includes the possibility of side effects. Women may obtain good information from reliable sites on the Internet, but there is also a huge amount of incorrect or biased information that can complicate the discussion between the physician and patient. Because good information empowers good decision making, and the converse is also true, physicians must take the time to explain the information brought in by patients. The Centers for Disease Control and Prevention's Medical Eligibility Criteria for Contraceptive Use (http://www.cdc.gov/reproductivehealth/contraception/usmec.htm) is a useful resource for patient counseling. How and when the method is used can also determine the acceptability. Options vary from methods that are coitus dependent (barriers) to methods that are placed by a health-care provider and last for up to 10 years (intrauterine contraception). Some women prefer methods they control. They can choose an oral daily preparation, whereas others consider the weekly transdermal (contraceptive patch) or the monthly transvaginal (contraceptive ring) forms easier to use successfully. Other women elect to use a method administered

Adapted from the American College of Obstetricians and Gynecologists. Guidelines for Women's Health Care. 3rd ed. Washington, DC: American College of Obstetricians and Gynecologists; 2007:184–185.

TABLE 26.1 CONTRACEPTIVE TECHNIQUE PREGNANCY RATES IN THE FIRST YEAR OF USE IN THE UNITED STATES

Method	Percentage of Women Experiencing an Unintended Pregnancy Within the First Year of Use	
	Typical Use[a]	Perfect Use[b]
No method of contraception	85.0	85.0
Withdrawal	22	4
Hormonal contraceptives		
Combination pill	9	0.3
Progestin-only pill	9	0.3
Contraceptive patch	9	0.3
Contraceptive ring	9	0.3
DMPA	6	0.2
Implantable contraceptive rods	0.05	0.05
Barrier contraceptives		
Spermicides	28	18
Male condom (without spermicide)	18	2
Female condom	21	5
Diaphragm and spermicide	12	6
Sponge (parous women)	24	20
Sponge (nulliparous women)	12	9
IUDs		
Progesterone IUD	0.2	0.2
Copper T-380A	0.8	0.6
Natural family planning		
Standard days method		5
Two-day method		4
Ovulation method		3
Symptothermal		0.4
Permanent—sterilization		
Male	0.15	0.10
Female	0.5	0.5

DMPA, depot medroxyprogesterone acetate; IUD, intrauterine device.
[a] Among typical couples who initiate the use of a method (not necessarily for the first time), the percentage who experience an accidental pregnancy during the first year if they do not stop use for any other reason.
[b] Among couples who initiate the use of a method (not necessarily for the first time) and who use it perfectly (both consistently and correctly), the percentage who experience an accidental pregnancy during the first year if they do not stop use for any other reason.

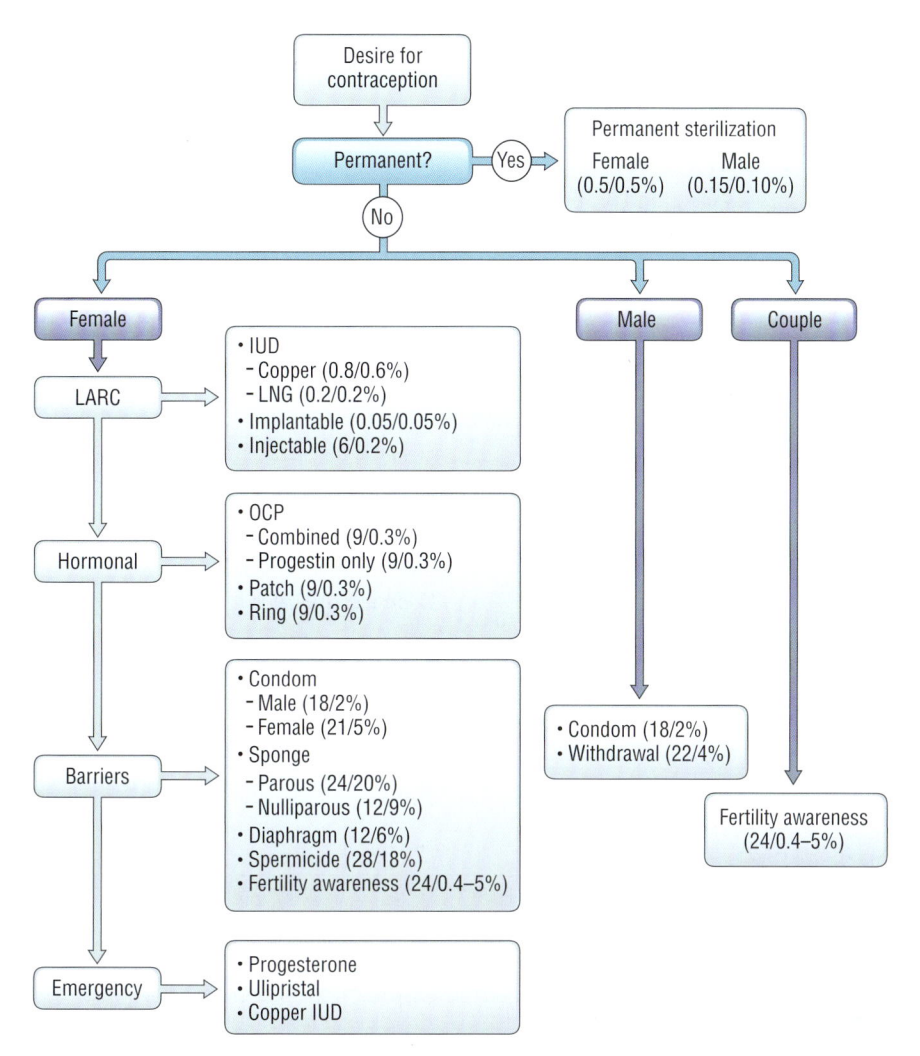

FIGURE 26.1. Decision tree for choosing a contraceptive method. IUD, intrauterine device; LARC, long- acting reversible contraception; LNG, levonorgestrel; OCP, oral contraceptive pill.

by their physician such as injections, implants, and intrauterine contraception. Methods that are not user or coitus dependent tend to be more effective. Sterilization (permanent contraception) is discussed in Chapter 27. Career or other life choices, as well as plans for future fertility, may influence the type and duration of the method chosen. Additionally, the couple's feelings about which partner should take responsibility for contraception may be important.

Finally, the ability of a contraceptive method to provide some protection against sexually transmitted diseases (STDs) may also be relevant, but the physician must explain that such protection is not the main intended use of most contraceptives. Helping patients understand that, aside from condoms, contraceptive methods do not provide protection from STD is one of the most important preventive care tasks.

The physician must be sensitive to all factors that might influence the decision and provide factual information that fits the needs of the woman and her partner. All practitioners should guard against imposing their own cultural or religious bias into the discussion. A decision tree based on this concept is presented in Figure 26.1. Table 26.2 offers a view of the multiple options.

LONG-ACTING REVERSIBLE CONTRACEPTION

Long-acting reversible contraception (LARC) can offer contraceptive efficacy equal to or better than permanent sterilization with the advantage of reversibility. In that respect, they are ideal for timing and spacing pregnancies. Additionally, they have few contraindications and the risks and side effects are low.

Implantable Hormonal Contraceptives (0.05/0.05%)

The **implantable contraceptive system** is a 4-cm by 2-mm rod containing a progestin (etonogestrel) that provides 3 years of contraception. With a typical and perfect use failure rate of 0.05%, it is the most effective form of contraception available, including female sterilization (0.5/0.5%). The implant works primarily by thickening the cervical mucus and inhibiting ovulation.

Insertion and Removal

Insertion is a simple office procedure under local anesthesia. A special applicator is used to place the rod "just underneath

TABLE 26.2 TYPES OF CONTRACEPTIVES

FDA-Approved Methods	Number of pregnancies expected (per 100 Women)*	Use	Some Risks or Side Effects*
Sterilization Surgery for Women	Less than 1	Onetime procedure. Permanent.	Pain Bleeding Infection or other complications after surgery
Sterilization Implant for Women	Less than 1	Onetime procedure. Permanent.	Pain/cramping Pelvic or back discomfort Vaginal bleeding
Sterilization Surgery for Men	Less than 1	Onetime procedure. Permanent.	Pain Bleeding Infection
IUD Copper	Less than 1	Inserted by a healthcare provider. Lasts up to 10 years.	Cramps Heavier, longer periods Spotting between periods
IUD with Progestin	Less than 1	Inserted by a healthcare provider. Lasts up to 3-5 years, depending on the type.	Irregular bleeding No periods (amenorrhea) Abdominal/pelvic pain
Implantable Rod	Less than 1	Inserted by a healthcare provider. Lasts up to 3 years.	Menstrual changes, Mood swings or depressed mood Weight gain, Headache Acne
Shot/Injection	6	Need a shot every 3 months.	Loss of bone density Irregular bleeding/bleeding between periods Headaches, Weight gain Nervousness, Dizziness Abdominal discomfort
Oral Contraceptives "The Pill" (Combined Pill)	9	Must swallow a pill every day.	Spotting/bleeding between periods Nausea Breast tenderness Headache
Oral Contraceptives "The Pill" (Extended/Continuous Use Combined Pill)	9	Must swallow a pill every day.	Spotting/bleeding between periods Nausea Breast tenderness Headache
Oral Contraceptives "The Mini Pill" (Progestin Only)	9	Must swallow a pill at the same time every day.	Spotting/bleeding between periods Nausea Breast tenderness Headache
Patch	9	Put on a new patch each week for 3 weeks (21 total days). Don't put on a patch during the fourth week.	Spotting or bleeding between menstrual periods Nausea, Stomach pain Breast tenderness, Headache Skin irritation
Vaginal Contraceptive Ring	9	Put the ring into the vagina yourself. Keep the ring in your vagina for 3 weeks and then take it out for one week.	Vagina discharge, discomfort in the vagina, and mild irritation. Headache, Mood changes Nausea, Breast tenderness
Diaphragm with Spermicide	12	Must use every time you have sex.	Irritation Allergic reactions Urinary tract infection
Sponge with Spermicide	12-24	Must use every time you have sex.	Irritation
Cervical Cap with Spermicide	17-23	Must use every time you have sex.	Irritation Allergic reactions Abnormal Pap test
Male Condom	18	Must use every time you have sex. Provides protection against some STDs.	Irritation Allergic reactions
Female Condom	21	Must use every time you have sex. Provides protection against some STDs.	Discomfort or pain during insertion or sex. Burning sensation, rash or itching
Spermicide Alone	28	Must use every time you have sex.	Irritation Allergic reactions Urinary tract infection

*This chart does not list all of the risks and side effects for each product.

From U.S. Food & Drug Administration. *Birth Control Guide.* Retrieved from https://www.fda.gov/downloads/ForConsumers/ByAudience/ForWomen/FreePublications/UCM517406.pdf

FIGURE 26.2. Subcutaneous contraceptive implant using etonogestrel (Nexplanon).

the skin." The procedure takes less than a minute with minimal discomfort (Figure 26.2). Postpartum insertion may be performed while the patient is still in hospital and decrease the risk of pregnancy that is accompanied by missed postpartum visits.

Removal of the device is also performed in the office under local anesthesia. Although it requires a small (2 mm) incision, it is also well tolerated. In addition, a new implant may be placed at the same time for 3 more years of highly effective contraception.

Side Effects
The most common side effect is irregular, unpredictable vaginal bleeding that may continue even after several months of use.

Intrauterine Contraception (0.2–0.8/0.2–0.6%)

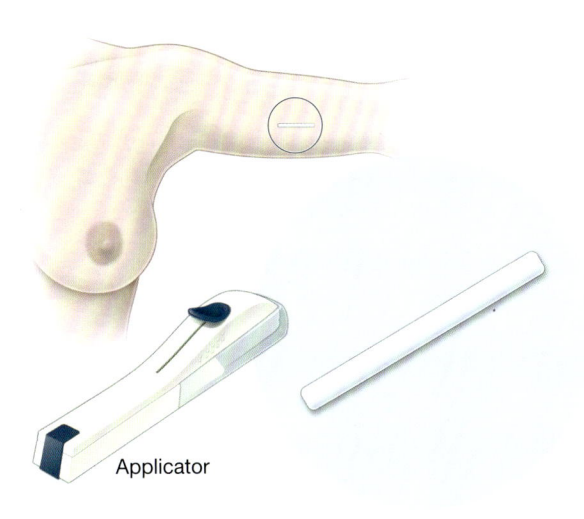

Intrauterine contraceptives, also known as **IUDs** or **intrauterine contraception devices**, are recommended for adolescent, nulliparous, and parous women and are among the most commonly used and safe methods of interval contraception worldwide. However, in the United States oral contraceptives and sterilization are more common despite lower efficacy. This continued disinterest in IUDs stems from early kinds of IUDs that were associated with an increased incidence of pelvic inflammatory disease (PID) and infertility. These devices were removed from use and the current IUDs are not associated with PID. Nonetheless, the fear continues to dissuade some women, and practitioners, from IUD use despite the proven safety profile of the current models.

There are four IUDs available in the United States—three hormonal and one nonhormonal. All are T shaped. The hormonal IUDs release a small amount of levonorgestrel (LNG-IUD) into the uterus (0.2/0.2%), and the nonhormonal IUD releases a small amount of copper (Cu-IUD) into the uterus (0.8/0.6%).

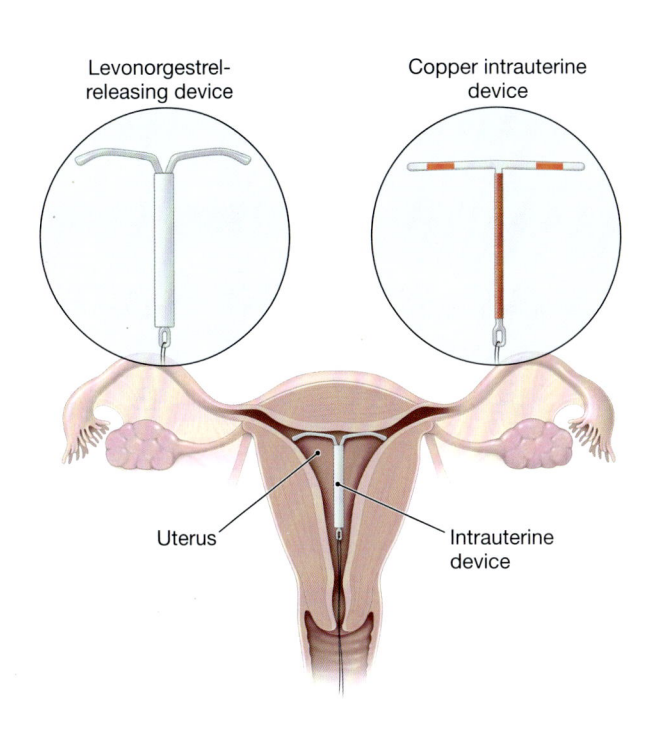

FIGURE 26.3. Intrauterine devices using levonorgestrel or copper.

Insertion
IUD insertion is best accomplished when the patient is menstruating. This timing is beneficial because it confirms the patient is not pregnant and her cervix is usually slightly open. If that timing cannot be achieved, it can be done at other times in the cycle as the patient is switching from another reliable method of contraception. The devices may also be inserted in breastfeeding women, who, in fact, demonstrate a lower incidence of postinsertional discomfort and bleeding.

All IUD insertion techniques share the same basic rules: careful bimanual examination before insertion to determine the likely direction of insertion into the endometrial cavity, proper loading of the device into the inserter, careful placement to the fundal margin of the endometrial cavity, and proper inserter removal while leaving the IUD in place (Figure 26.3). Sterile technique and a vaginal prep with povidone-iodine should be used prior to insertion of an IUD.

The overall expulsion rate for IUDs is 1% to 5%, with the greatest likelihood in the first few months of use. Expulsion is often preceded by cramping, vaginal discharge, or bleeding, although it may be asymptomatic, with the only evidence being the observed lengthening of the IUD string or the partner feeling the device during intercourse. Patients should be counseled to see their clinician if expulsion is suspected.

Insertion may be performed immediately postpartum (within 10 minutes of placental delivery) or intraoperatively during a cesarean before closure of the hysterotomy incision. Although the expulsion rate is higher, the success rate decreases the pregnancy rate from missed postpartum visits and lengthens the interval between pregnancies.

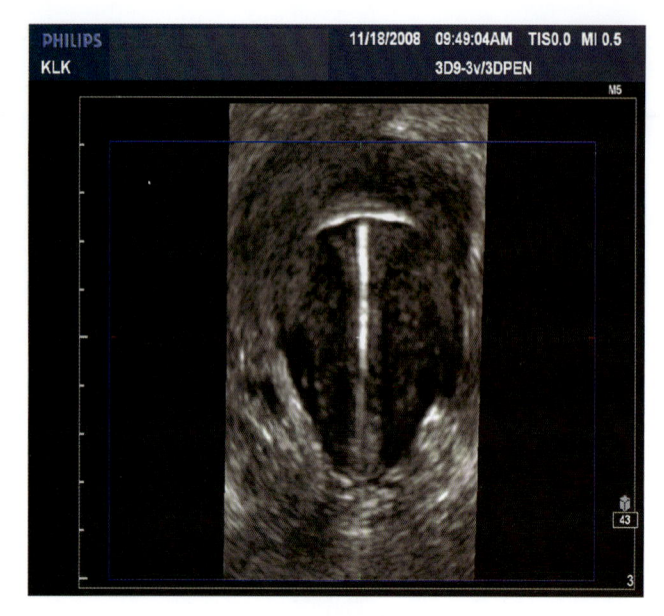

FIGURE 26.4. Reconstructed coronal view of uterus with appropriately placed progesterone-containing intrauterine device in endometrial cavity.

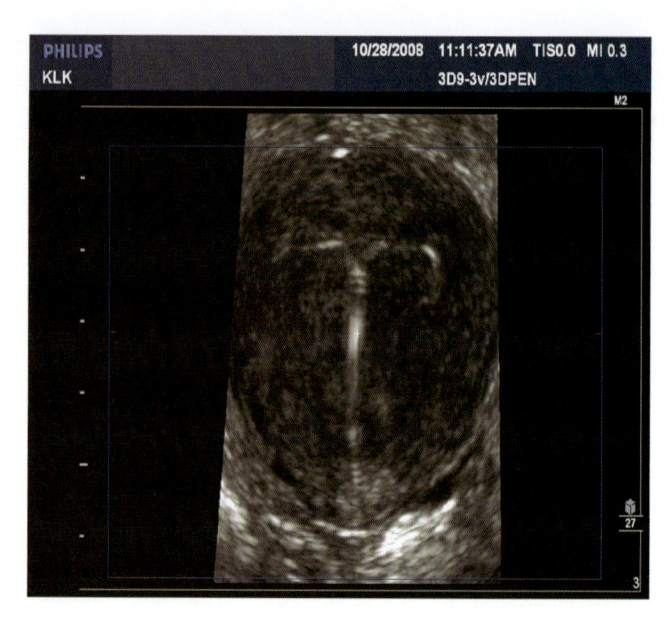

FIGURE 26.5. Reconstructed coronal view of uterus with appropriately placed copper-containing intrauterine device in endometrial cavity.

Mechanisms of Action

There are three hormonal IUDs (LNG-IUD's) that work by preventing the sperm and egg from meeting by thickening the cervical mucus, thus decreasing the number of sperms that enter the uterine cavity and creating an unfavorable uterine environment by thinning the uterine lining (Figure 26.4).

The copper ions from the copper IUD (Cu-IUD) act as a spermicide, inhibiting sperm motility and the acrosomal reaction necessary for fertilization (Figure 26.5). It rarely works by inhibiting implantation and does not function as an abortifacient in normal use. The Cu-IUD may also be used postcoitally as an EC. When used in this way, it may interfere with implantation.

Side Effects

A clinically important side effect of LNG-IUDs is a decrease in menstrual blood loss (up to 50%) and severity of dysmenorrhea.

Although the LGN-IUDs are associated with menstrual irregularities, typically lighter periods, or amenorrhea, serum progesterone levels are not affected. The local progesterone effect is used to relieve pain related to endometriosis and adenomyosis as well as for endometrial protection for women taking hormone replacement therapy who cannot take oral progestins.

The Cu-IUD is associated with heavier periods and dysmenorrhea that often result in discontinuation. The LGN-IUDs have a lesser incidence of this problem because of the progestin effect on the endometrium. Thus, increased menstrual flow and pain may be encountered in women choosing Cu-IUDs compared with LGN-IUDs.

Efficacy

The IUDs currently available in the United States are highly effective. The Cu-IUD has a recommended life span of 10 years and demonstrates a pregnancy rate of 0.8/0.6%. There are currently three LNG-IUDs in the market. The 5-year LNG-IUD was approved for parous women but is available for nulliparous women as well (0.2/0.2%). Two smaller LNG-IUDs are marketed for nulliparous women and are effective for 3 years.

Risks

There is a slight increased risk of infection the first 20 days after IUD insertion. Pelvic infection occurring 3 months or more after IUD insertion may be presumed to be an acquired STD and treated accordingly. Women at high risk for STDs may benefit from screening prior to insertion. Asymptomatic IUD users with positive cervical cultures for gonorrhea or chlamydia, or with bacterial vaginosis, should be treated promptly. The IUD may remain in place unless there is evidence of spread of the infection to the endometrium or fallopian tubes and/or failure of treatment with appropriate antibiotics.

IUDs do not increase the overall risk of ectopic pregnancy. However, because the IUD offers greater protection against intrauterine than extrauterine pregnancy, the relative ratio of extrauterine pregnancy is greater in a woman who uses an IUD than in a woman not using contraception. Therefore, in the rare instance that a woman with an IUD in place becomes pregnant, that pregnancy would have a high risk of being extrauterine. About 40% to 50% of patients who become pregnant with an IUD in place will spontaneously abort in the first trimester.

Because of this risk, patients should be offered IUD removal if the string is visible; this is associated with a decreased spontaneous abortion rate of about 30%. If the IUD string is not visible, instrumental removal may be performed, but the risk of pregnancy disruption is increased. If the IUD is left in place, pregnancy may proceed uneventfully. There is no evidence of an increased risk of congenital anomalies with LNG-IUD or Cu-IUD. There is, however, an approximate two- to four-fold increase in the incidence of preterm labor and delivery.

Patient counseling and skillful insertion are crucial to the successful use of the IUD as a method of contraception.

Removal

The IUD is removed by placement of a speculum and simply pulling on the string. If the string is not visible, rotating two cotton-tip applicators in the endocervical canal will often retrieve the strings. If this is not possible, a fine probe may be inserted, the IUD felt, and then removed with an "IUD hook" or small forceps. If needed, ultrasound guidance can assist in this process. Infrequently, IUDs become embedded in the uterine wall and require hysteroscopic removal. Even less frequently, an IUD perforates the uterus and requires laparoscopic removal.

Injectable Hormonal Contraceptives

Depot medroxyprogesterone acetate (DMPA) (6/0.2%) is an injectable progestin given as intramuscular or subcutaneous injections every 13 weeks. It can be given up to 15 weeks after the last injection without requiring additional contraceptive protection, providing a useful "safety margin." The injection should be given within the first 5 days of the current menstrual period, and, if not, a back-up method of contraception is necessary for 2 weeks. DMPA is not a sustained-release preparation, relying instead on higher peaks and sustained levels of progestin. In addition to thickening of the cervical mucus and decidualization of the endometrium, DMPA also acts by maintaining a circulating level of progestin high enough to block the LH surge and, thus, ovulation. FSH suppression does not occur with DMPA as it does with combination OCPs (cOCPs); therefore, ovulation suppression may not be as effective as with cOCPs.

Side Effects

DMPA suppresses production of estradiol and is associated with loss of bone mineral density (BMD). Special concern has been raised about this effect during adolescence, a critical period of bone accretion, although the decrease in BMD appears to be substantially reversible after discontinuation of this injectable contraceptive. Nonetheless, the U.S. Food and Drug Administration has added a warning to this formulation that use beyond 2 years should be carefully considered and alternate contraceptive methods be evaluated. Because the effects of DMPA on BMD are intermediate and reversible, the American College of Obstetricians and Gynecologists does not recommend that practitioners routinely limit use of DMPA to 2 years.

Concern about the use of DMPA in adolescents should be weighed against the advantages of compliance and effective contraception, and bone density monitoring is not warranted based on DMPA use alone. However, women at special risk for osteoporosis should be especially careful when considering the use of DMPA.

Noncontraceptive benefits of DMPA include decreased risk of endometrial carcinoma and iron deficiency anemia. It may also improve management of pain associated with endometriosis, endometrial hyperplasia, and dysmenorrhea. As with all contraceptive options, the balance of overall risk to benefit for DMPA should be weighed on an individual patient basis.

Efficacy

The typical versus perfect use efficacy of DMPA is 6% and 0.2%, respectively (see Table 26.1) and is not affected by weight or altered by patients taking medications that alter hepatic function. Contraindications of DMPA are outlined in Box 26.1. Note that they differ from contraindications to cOCPs (birth control pills that contain a combination of both estrogen and progesterone). The lack of contraindications to hypertension, smokers over age 35 years, and other conditions make DMPA an attractive and viable option for women who may not be cOCP candidates. DMPA injections may cause irregular bleeding, which decreases with each injection so that 80% of women are amenorrheic

---

BOX 26.1 Indications and Contraindications for DMPA Contraception

Indications

Desire for effective contraception
Women for whom compliance with other methods has been problematic
Breastfeeding
Women for whom estrogen-containing preparations are contraindicated
Women with seizure disorders
Sickle cell anemia
Anemia secondary to menorrhagia

Contraindications

- Known or suspected pregnancy
- Unevaluated vaginal bleeding
- Known or suspected malignancy of the breast
- Liver dysfunction or disease
- Known sensitivity to DMPA or any of its other ingredients

Discussion

One injection every 3 months, 2-week "safety" interval (i.e., can be delayed up to 2 weeks without loss of efficacy)
No effect on quality of breast milk or on baby; increases quantity of breast milk; can be administered immediately postpartum
See above for absolute contraindications
Antiseizure medications unaffected, and sedative effects of progestins may aid in seizure control
Not contraindicated for active thrombophlebitis or current or past history of thromboembolic disorders per U.S. Medical Eligibility Criteria (http://www.cdc.gov/reproductivehealth/contraception/usmec.htm)
Decreased menstrual flow

DMPA, depot medroxyprogesterone acetate.

after 5 years. Because 25% of users discontinue DMPA within the first year of use owing to this problem, extensive preinitiation counseling is very important. If needed, treatment with 7 to 10 days of conjugated estrogen (1.25 mg/day) may be useful in managing irregular bleeding patterns. When DMPA is discontinued, about 50% of patients resume normal menses within 6 months; 25% do not resume menses for more than 1 year. These patients should be evaluated to detect other possible causes. Patients should be counseled about the slower return to fertility compared to implants and IUDs. DMPA is associated with measurable weight gain in many, but not all women. Early weight gain may be indicative of future weight gain. The relatively large number of risk and benefit issues associated with the use of DMPA are often confusing to patients and require especially careful patient education to allow the best selection of this highly effective contraceptive method.

HORMONAL CONTRACEPTIVES

For many women, "birth control" is synonymous with pills. However, hormones are also used in many other contraceptive methods, including injectable hormonal preparations, implantable hormonal rod, hormone-containing intrauterine systems (as discussed earlier), and contraceptive patches and rings.

About one-third of all sexually active women in the United States use OCPs, including half of young women aged 20 to 24 years. Hormonal contraceptives have many health benefits, including decreasing a woman's risk of ovarian and uterine cancer and providing protection against menses-associated anemia. Although hormonal contraceptive methods are associated with risks, the use of one of these agents is safer than pregnancy for most women.

Method (perfect use) failure rates for oral, transdermal, and transvaginal contraceptives are in the range of ≤1%. Longer-acting hormonal methods (injections, implants, and intrauterine contraception) have effectiveness rates that equal or even surpass those of sterilization. Because OCP failures (typical use failure rate of 9%) are usually related to missed pills, injectable long-acting agents, patches, implants, intrauterine contraception, and rings share the additional advantage of lack of a need for daily use, which invites error.

Hormonal contraceptives do not protect against STDs. Women who use these techniques should be counseled about high-risk behaviors, safe sexual behaviors, and the need to use condoms for additional protection.

Mechanisms of Action

Most of the OCPs are combinations of an **estrogen** and a **progestin**, although there are also progestin-only products.

Combination Oral Contraceptives (9/0.3%)
Almost all cOCP preparations contain **ethinyl estradiol** as the estrogen component (although some now contain estradiol valerate) and one of the **19-nortestosterones** or a **spironolactone derivative** (**drospirenone**) as the progestin product. The most prominent effect is suppression of hypothalamic gonadotropin-releasing factors with subsequent suppression of pituitary production of follicle-stimulating hormone (FSH) and luteinizing hormone (LH). The progestational component provides the major contraceptive effect, acting primarily by suppressing secretion of LH and, in turn, ovulation. It also provides the added effects of thickening the cervical mucus, inhibiting sperm migration, and creating an unfavorable atrophic endometrium for implantation. The estrogenic component acts by suppressing secretion of FSH, preventing maturation of a follicle, as well as potentiation of the action of the progestational agent. The estrogen provides an additional modest contraceptive effect, thus increasing the efficacy of this method. Importantly, estrogen also improves cycle control by stabilizing the endometrium and resulting in more regular cycles, allows for less **breakthrough bleeding** (bleeding not related to the menstrual period in a woman using OCPs), and is associated with greater patient satisfaction and compliance. Common progestin compounds used in hormonal contraceptives include, in descending order of biologic progestin activity, norgestrel, ethynodiol diacetate, norethindrone acetate, norethynodrel, and norethindrone. cOCPs using the less androgenic agents, desogestrel, norgestimate, and drospirenone, are also available if less androgenic activity is desired. Although the progestin and estrogen components of cOCPs act in a synergistic manner, the progestin provides more of the contraceptive effect, whereas the estrogen regularizes menstrual cycles. Knowing the difference may help in the selection of the most appropriate and acceptable formulation for a patient.

Most cOCPs contain a fixed ratio of estrogen and progestin, although "**phasic**" formulations have been introduced that vary this ratio during the course of the month with the intent of lowering the total dose of hormones.

The classic regimen for hormonal contraception has been 21 days of active hormone (pill, patch, and ring) and 7 days of placebo or no hormones. Continuous hormone regimens are also available that produce shorter or less frequent menstrual periods, either every 3 or even every 12 months. Some women may prefer this usage pattern, although they should be aware that there is a higher incidence of breakthrough bleeding in the first 12-week cycle, compared with the 4-week cycle preparations. New preparations continue to be developed with the ultimate goal of maximizing the benefits and minimizing the side effects.

Progestin-Only Oral Contraceptives (9/0.3%)
Progestin-only oral contraceptives (progestin-only "minipill") act primarily by making the cervical mucus thick and relatively impermeable. Ovulation continues normally in about 40% of patients using the progestin-only formulation. Progestin-only OCPs are especially useful in lactating women and women over age 40 years. In the former group, the progestin effect coincides with the prolactin-induced suppression of ovulation; in the latter group, the inherent reduced fecundity adds to the progestin effect. There is no effect on the quality or quantity of breast milk or any evidence of short- or long-term adverse effects on

infants, and the progestin-only pill may be started immediately after delivery in the breastfeeding mother. The progestin-only pill is also an option for women in whom estrogen-containing formulations are contraindicated. Because of the low dosages of progestin, the minipill must be taken at approximately the same time each day, starting on the first day of menses. If a woman is more than 3 hours late in taking the minipill, a back-up contraceptive method should be used for 48 hours. The minipill, being progestin only, offers poor cycle control.

Progestin-only OCPs are good choices for breastfeeding women and women with contraindications to estrogen, but their use must be tempered with a clear understanding that they must be used in a very consistent manner because of their limited mode of action.

Effects of Hormonal Contraceptives

Hormonal contraception affects more than just the reproductive system. Estrogens affect lipid metabolism, potentiate sodium and water retention, increase renin substrate, stimulate the cytochrome P450 system, increase sex hormone–binding globulin, and can reduce antithrombin III. Progestins increase sebum, stimulate the growth of facial and body hair, induce smooth muscle relaxation, and increase the risk of cholestatic jaundice. The newer progestational agents—desogestrel, norgestimate, and drospirenone—have less metabolic impact.

Benefits

OCPs also have many beneficial effects. Menstrual periods are predictable (for cOCP users), shorter, and less painful, and, as a result, the risk of iron-deficiency anemia is reduced. OCP users have a lower incidence of endometrial and ovarian cancers, benign breast and ovarian disease, and pelvic infection. By decreasing conception, the risk of ectopic pregnancy is reduced, along with the complications of undesired intrauterine pregnancies.

Side Effects

Breakthrough bleeding occurs in 10% to 30% of women taking low-dose cOCPs during the first 3 months of use. Although it is an especially worrisome symptom, it is not associated with decreased efficacy as long as the pill-taking regimen is maintained. The abnormal bleeding pattern is the most common reason for discontinuation of contraception, and women should be counseled to expect irregularities before hormones are initiated. If breakthrough bleeding does occur, it is best managed by encouragement and reassurance, because it usually resolves spontaneously. Breakthrough bleeding after approximately 3 months is associated with progestin-induced decidualization, with the shallow and fragile endometrium prone to asynchronous breakdown and bleeding. A short course of exogenous estrogen (1.25 mg conjugated estrogen for 7 days) given while the patient continues cOCP use usually stabilizes the endometrium and stops the bleeding. Taking two or three of the pills each day is not an effective therapy for breakthrough bleeding, because the progestin component will predominate, often worsening the problem by causing further decidualization of the endometrium. Careful counseling about the possibility of irregular menses in the first 3 months of use is important to prevent user discontinuation based on fear that the bleeding change may be a sign that "something is wrong."

Amenorrhea occurs in approximately 1% of users of low-dose cOCPs in the first year of use, reaching perhaps 5% of users after several years of use. Contraceptive efficacy is maintained if the pill regimen is followed. Changing to a higher estrogen–containing pill or use of exogenous estrogen may be employed to induce bleeding, if the patient wishes. A pregnancy test should precede therapy for amenorrhea. No treatment is indicated if the amenorrhea is acceptable to the patient.

Serious complications (such as venous thrombosis, pulmonary embolism, cholestasis and gallbladder disease, stroke, and myocardial infarction) are more likely for women using high-dose formulations and in smokers over age 35 years. However, these complications also can occur occasionally in patients taking low-dose formulations. Hepatic tumors have also been associated with the use of high-dose cOCPs. Although all of these complications are 2 to 10 times more likely in pill users, they are still uncommon.

Less serious but more common side effects also depend on the dosage and type of hormones used. Estrogens may cause a feeling of bloating and weight gain, breast tenderness, nausea, fatigue, or headache. Studies have demonstrated no overall weight gain in pill users despite the patient's perception of weight gain. Altering the dose or composition of the progestational agent used may relieve some of these minor side effects.

The therapeutic principle of contraception is to select the method providing effective contraception with the greatest margin of safety, and then to use it as long as the patient wishes contraception or beneficial menstrual-related changes. If the patient experiences new signs or symptoms while using hormonal contraception, further evaluation is necessary to choose another contraceptive method of contraception. In some cases, cessation of the chosen hormonal method or hormonal methods in general may be required (Box 26.2).

Patient Evaluation for Combined Hormonal Contraceptive Use

Before considering estrogen- and progestin-containing contraceptives for a patient, a careful evaluation is required. Not only are hormones relatively or absolutely contraindicated in some patients but also factors such as previous menstrual history may have an impact on the choice of these agents. cOCP use is generally contraindicated in women over age 35 years who smoke or who have had a thromboembolism and in women with a history of coronary artery disease, congestive heart failure, cerebral vascular disease, or migraine with aura due to the estrogen component.

Approximately 3% of patients may experience problems with resumption of their periods after prolonged contraceptive use (**postpill amenorrhea**). Younger women and those who had irregular periods before the use of OCPs are more likely to experience this problem after discontinuing their use. These patients should be counseled about this potential complication.

> **BOX 26.2** Management of New Symptoms in Patients Using Oral Contraceptives
>
> **Discontinue OCP; Start Nonhormonal Methods, Immediate Evaluation**
> | | |
> |---|---|
> | Loss of vision, diplopia | (Possible retinal artery thrombosis) |
> | Unilateral numbness, weakness | (Possible stroke) |
> | Severe chest/neck pain | (Possible myocardial infarction) |
> | Slurring of speech | (Possible stroke) |
> | Severe leg pain, tenderness | (Possible thrombophlebitis) |
> | Hemoptysis, acute shortness of breath | (Possible pulmonary embolism) |
> | Hepatic mass, tenderness | (Possible hepatic neoplasm, adenoma) |
>
> **Continue OCP; Immediate Evaluation**
> | | |
> |---|---|
> | Amenorrhea | (Possible pregnancy) |
> | Breast mass | (Possible breast cancer) |
> | Right upper quadrant pain | (Possible cholecystitis, cholelithiasis) |
> | Severe headache | (Possible stroke, migraine headache) |
> | Galactorrhea | (Possible pituitary adenoma) |
>
> OCP, oral contraceptive pill.

Hormonal contraceptives may interact with other medications that the patient is taking. This interaction may reduce the efficacy of either the contraceptive or the other medications. Examples of drugs that decrease the effectiveness of contraceptives include barbiturates, benzodiazepines, phenytoin, carbamazepine, rifampin, and sulfonamides. Drugs that may show retarded biotransformation when contraceptives are also used include anticoagulants, methyldopa, phenothiazines, reserpine, and tricyclic antidepressants. Antibiotics may alter the intestinal flora and are thought to interfere with hormone absorption, but efficacy is not reduced.

Before prescribing medications to women using contraceptives, the clinician should consider possible drug interactions and discuss them with the patient.

Ring and Patch (9/0.3%)

The **transdermal contraceptive patch** contains synthetic estrogen and progestin and remains effective for an entire week (Fig. 26.6). The patient should start the patch during the first 5 days of her menstrual period and replace it weekly for 3 weeks. The fourth week is patch-free to allow a **withdrawal bleed**. Placement on clean, dry skin located on the buttocks, upper outer arm, or lower abdomen is recommended. Caution should be used when prescribing the patch for women weighing more than 90 kg (198 lb) because of its decreased efficacy with obesity. Side effects and contraindications are similar to those of the cOCPs, although recent research has identified an increased risk of thrombosis. A complaint specific to the patch, however, includes skin irritation from adhesive residue at the application site.

The **contraceptive vaginal ring** releases a sustained amount of synthetic estrogen and progestin daily (Fig. 26.7). Comparable with cOCPs in efficacy, the ring is associated with greater compliance because of its once-a-month usage. Placed into the vagina by the patient at the beginning of her menses, it is left in place for 3 weeks. Removal of the device results in a withdrawal bleed. The ring can be taken out of the vagina for up to 3 hours, if desired, without altering its efficacy. Because it is colorless and odorless, with a 2-in. diameter, most patients and their partners are unaware of the presence of the ring. An advantage of the ring over cOCPs is a decreased incidence of breakthrough bleeding.

Because the hormones in the vaginal ring and the transdermal patch are not absorbed through the gastrointestinal tract, some of the medication interactions that occur with cOCPs may not apply. However, metabolism still occurs in the liver; therefore, caution must be used.

BARRIER CONTRACEPTIVES

Among the oldest and most widely used contraceptive methods are those that provide a barrier between the sperm and egg. These barriers include condoms, diaphragms, and cervical caps. Some methods, such as fertility awareness, may be thought of as providing a "time" barrier between coitus and conception. Each of these methods depends on the proper use before or at the time of intercourse and, as such, is subject to a higher failure rate than noncoitus-dependent methods. This is the result of inconsistent or incorrect use as well as actual damage to the barrier material itself. For example, the latex in condoms, diaphragm, and cervical cap can be damaged by the application of oil-based lubricants. Despite this, these methods provide relatively good contraception and are inexpensive, and most require little or no medical consultation. In addition, condoms provide some protection against the transmission of STDs, including gonorrhea, herpes, chlamydia, human immunodeficiency virus (HIV), and human papillomavirus infection.

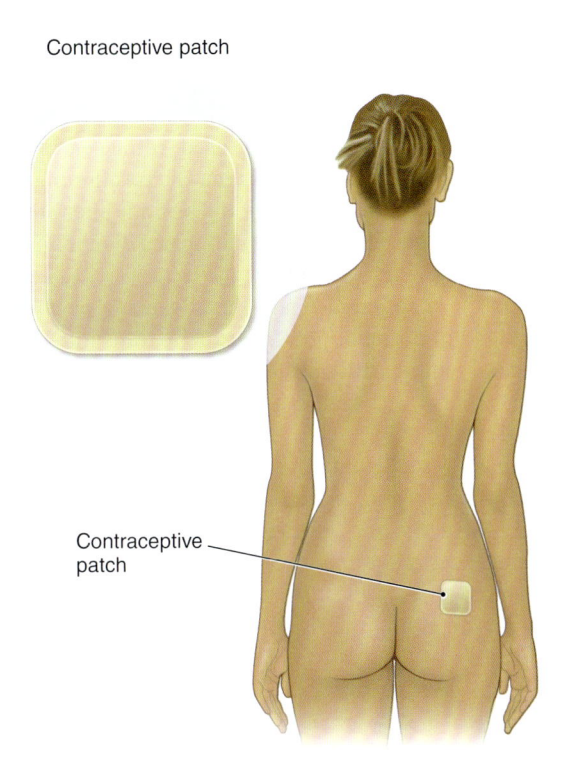

FIGURE 26.6. Contraceptive patch.

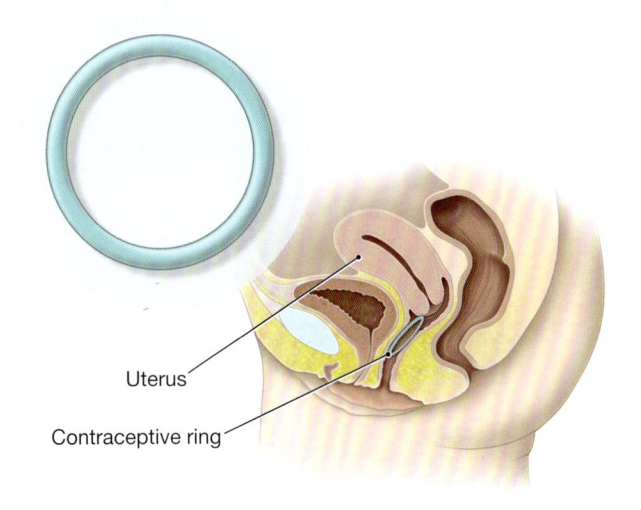

FIGURE 26.7. Contraceptive ring.

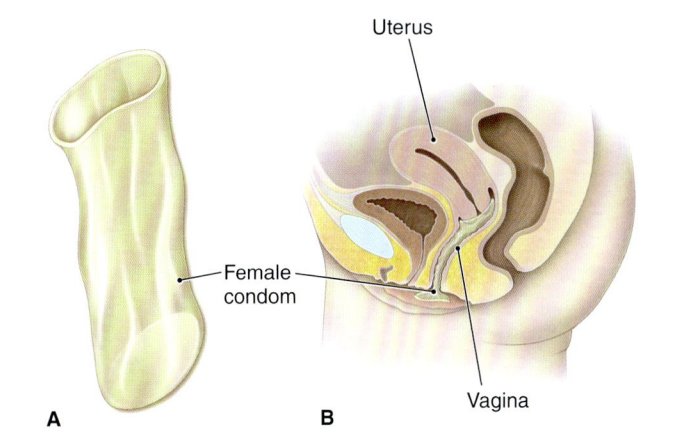

FIGURE 26.8. The female condom. (A) Preparation for insertion. (B) Condom in proper position.

condoms protect against HIV. A reservoir tip reduces the likelihood of breakage. ==Recommending reservoir tip condoms may decrease condom breakage, a common cause of contraceptive failure with the use of this contraceptive method.==

Condoms are well tolerated, with only rare reports of skin irritation or allergic reaction. Some men complain of reduced sensation with the use of condoms, but this may actually be an advantage for those with rapid or premature ejaculation. The slippage and breakage rate in normal use is estimated at 5% to 8%. In these cases, couples should be counseled to seek medical care within 120 hours so that emergency contraceptive methods may be used.

Sponge: Nulliparous (21/9%); Parous (24/20%)

The **contraceptive sponge** is a small, pillow-shaped sponge containing spermicide. The sponge has a dimple that is designed to fit over the cervix and remain in place during intercourse. The opposite side has a loop to facilitate removal. All have slippage and breakage rates of about 3%, and, as in the case of diaphragms, it is recommended that they be left in place 6 to 8 hours after coitus. ==The sponge is available only in one size, which may explain why it is more effective in a nulliparous woman than in one who has had children.== The sponge is moistened prior to insertion and can be used for repeated acts of intercourse in a 24-hour period. The sponge should be left in place for at least 6 hours after intercourse, but wearing it for more than 30 hours is not recommended because of the risk of toxic shock syndrome.

Diaphragm (12/6%)

The **diaphragm** is a small, latex-covered, dome-shaped device. Proper use of a diaphragm includes applying a contraceptive jelly or cream containing spermicide into the center and along the rim of the device, which is then inserted into the vagina, over the cervix, and behind the pubic symphysis. In this position, the diaphragm covers the anterior vaginal wall and cervix.

Condoms: Male (18/2%), Female (21/5%)

Condoms are sheaths worn over the erect penis (male condom) or inside the vagina (female condom) to prevent sperm from reaching the cervix and upper genital tract (Fig. 26.8). Although almost one half of all condoms are sold to women, the condom is the only reliable, nonpermanent method of contraception available to men. Condoms are widely available and inexpensive. They may be made of latex; nonlatex; or, less commonly, animal membrane (usually sheep cecum), but only latex it may buckle, causing discomfort, irritation, and leakage. The patient must be initially instructed in the proper positioning of the diaphragm, with the correct position subsequently verified by the patient each time it is used. If the cervix can be felt through the dome of the diaphragm, the positioning is correct. In postpartum women, fitting should be done after uterine involution is complete. Correct positioning of a diaphragm is shown in Figure 26.9.

Thus the diaphragm offers the advantage of being female controlled but does not prevent sexually transmitted infections (STIs) and requires fitting by a health care provider.

Side Effects

Women who use diaphragms are approximately twice as likely to have urinary tract infections (UTIs) as women using hormonal contraception. The increased risk of UTI may be caused by a combination of pressure against the urethra, causing urinary stasis, and an effect of spermicides on the normal vaginal flora, increasing the risk of *Escherichia coli* bacteriuria and infection.

Spermicides (28/18%)

Spermicides are preparations that contain an active chemical that kills sperm as well as some type of carrier or base (e.g., gel, foam, cream, film, suppository, and tablet). In the United States, the active ingredient is nonoxynol-9. Foams and tablets should be inserted high into the vagina against the cervix, 10 to 30 minutes before each act of intercourse. The duration of maximal spermicidal effectiveness is usually no more than 1 hour. Douching should be avoided for at least 8 hours after use. There is no known association between spermicide use and congenital malformation.

Spermicides are economical, well tolerated, and effective in protection against pregnancy. Spermicides used in combination with condoms have failure rates that approach those of hormonal methods. Spermicides provide little, if any, protection against STIs when used alone. For women who cannot or do not want to use hormonal contraceptives, the high effectiveness of the combined use of condoms and spermicides may be a good option.

FERTILITY AWARENESS METHODS (24/0.4–5%)

"Fertility awareness methods" refer to techniques that seek to identify the days when pregnancy is most likely to occur by tracking the menstrual cycle or other signs of fertility like cervical mucus or basal body temperature. Couples avoid unprotected intercourse during these days. In essence they provide "time" as a barrier to conception. Fertility awareness methods may be acceptable for women who prefer a more natural contraceptive option or who have a religious objection to other contraceptive methods.

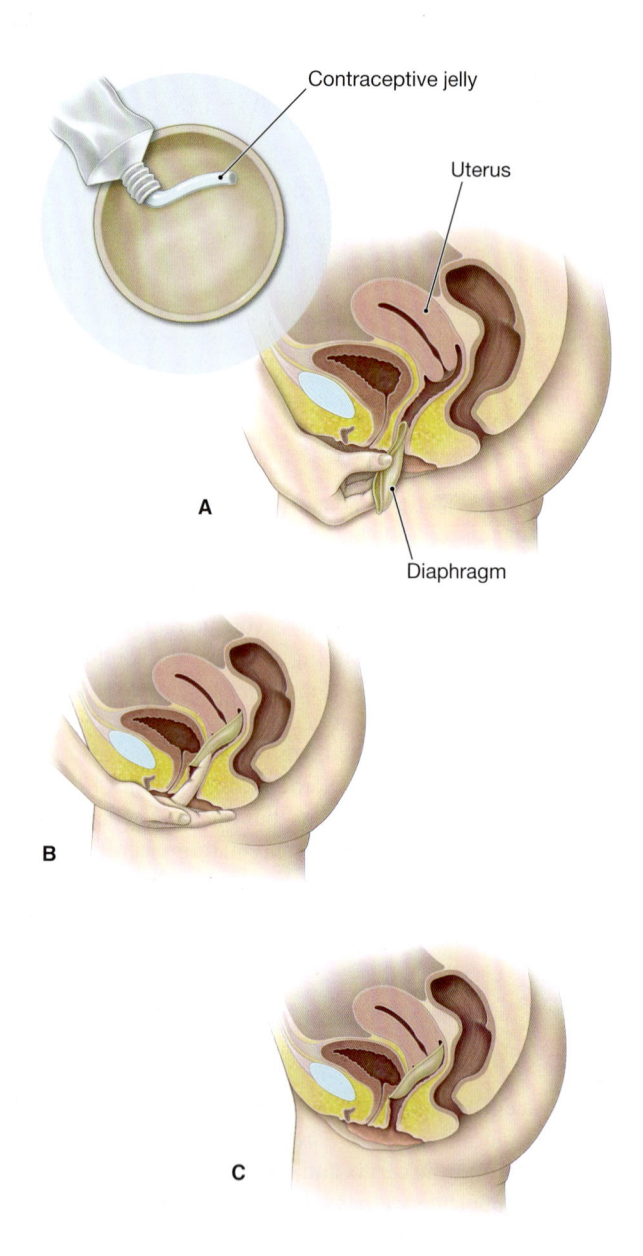

FIGURE 26.9. Diaphragm. (A) Insertion of the diaphragm. (B) Checking to ensure the diaphragm covers the cervix. (C) Diaphragm in place.

The diaphragm can be inserted up to 6 hours before intercourse and must be left in place for 6 to 8 hours afterward, but not more than 24 hours. It may then be removed, washed, and stored. Users should be cautioned not to use talc to dry the diaphragm. If additional intercourse is desired during the 6- to 8-hour waiting time, additional spermicide should be applied without removing the diaphragm, and the waiting time should be restarted.

There are several sizes of diaphragm available and one must be fitted to the individual patient. Fit may change with significant weight change, vaginal birth, or pelvic surgery. The diaphragm should be the largest that can be comfortably inserted, worn, and removed. If the diaphragm is too small, it may slip out during coitus because of vaginal elongation; if it is too large,

Calendar Methods

The **calendar methods** (which include the standard days method) are based on calculation of a woman's fertile period. She charts her periods for 6 months to calculate this fertile period. The first day of the fertile period is determined by subtracting 18 days from the total length of her shortest menstrual cycle. The last day of the fertile period is calculated by subtracting 11 days from the total length of her longest cycle. For a woman with regular 28-day cycles, the fertile period is from Day 10 (28 – 18) to Day 17 (28 – 11). Sex is avoided during this span. If the cycle varies from 25 to 35 days, however, the fertile period is from Day 7 (25 – 18) to Day 24 (35 – 11).

Basal Body Temperature Method

The **basal body temperature method** is based on temperature variations that occur around the time of ovulation. The temperature is checked daily upon awakening, but before getting out of bed, using a special thermometer and recorded on a graph. A biphasic pattern with a rise in basal body temperature of 0.5°F to 1°F is indicative of ovulation. The couple must abstain from intercourse from the end of the menstrual period until 3 days after the temperature increase.

Cervical Mucus Methods

The **cervical mucus methods** (which include the 2-day method) depend on the woman daily assessing her cervical mucus and noting the changes surrounding ovulation. The vagina is usually dry just after menstruation. Subsequently, a thick, sticky mucus appears. The mucus then changes to thin, "stretchy," clear cervical mucus, called **spinnbarkeit**. The last day of wetness, called the "peak" day, often coincides with ovulation. The fertile period occurs with the first signs of mucus and continues until 4 days after the peak day.

Symptothermal Method

The **symptothermal method** combines the assessment of cervical mucus and basal body temperature methods. In addition to checking her temperature and cervical mucus, the woman also checks for other signs of ovulation, such as abdominal cramping, spotting, breast tenderness, and changes in the position or firmness of her cervix. The fertile period is from the first sign of ovulation until 3 days after temperature rise or 4 days after peak mucus.

Lactational Amenorrhea

The contraceptive effect of lactational amenorrhea is based on the concept that the intensity and frequency of suckling in breastfeeding is associated with elevated prolactin levels, amenorrhea, and anovulation (see Chapter 11). This method is excellent for up to 6 months as long as menses has not resumed and there is exclusive or near exclusive (85%) breastfeeding. Pumping does not have the same effect as suckling.

EMERGENCY CONTRACEPTION

EC may be used to prevent pregnancy within 5 days of unprotected intercourse but is more effective if taken within the first 24 hours after intercourse. Making EC widely and easily available is one of the most important steps that can be taken to reduce the high rates of unintended pregnancy and abortion. It is estimated that the regular use of EC would prevent more than 1.5 million unintended pregnancies in the United States each year.

cOCP regimens used for EC, known collectively as the **Yuzpe method**, were first reported by Albert Yuzpe in 1974. They require a regimen of tablets within the first 72 hours of unprotected sexual intercourse. Modern-day progestin-only EC is better tolerated and more effective than cOCP regimen. The use of a progestin-only pill was approved for behind-the-counter dispensing to women over age 17 years without a prescription. Women younger than age 17 years require a physician's prescription to obtain the medication. The prescription consists of single-dose regimen or a two-dose regimen of levonorgestrel taken 12 hours apart and can be used up to 120 hours after unprotected intercourse.

A prescription-only formulation using ulipristal acetate 30 mg is just as effective as the progestin formulation up to 72 hours postintercourse but is more effective between 72 and 120 hours. EC should not be confused with the so-called "abortion pills" that are used to induce abortion but are not approved or appropriate for use as an EC. All approved EC methods act by preventing ovulation and fertilization rather than by preventing implantation and will not terminate an existing pregnancy.

The failure rate for the progestin method is 1.1%. Multiple unprotected coital events or an interval greater than 72 hours may be associated with an increasing failure rate, although some evidence of success is seen up to 120 hours after unprotected intercourse. If the woman is already pregnant, these medications have no ill effect on the fetus. The amount of hormone in these regimens is not associated with alterations in clotting factors or teratogenic risk. Body weight influences the effectiveness of oral EC; however, it should not be withheld from women who are overweight or obese as no research to date has established the weight threshold at which it would be less effective. There is no medical contraindication to the use of EC. Therefore, EC should be made available to women who may have contraindications to other contraceptive agents.

Cu-IUD is another recommended option for EC (except in patients with Wilson disease) and, in limited studies, has a failure rate of approximately 0.1%. An additional advantage of IUD insertion is the contraceptive effect that is provided for up to 10 years. Before using this method, a pregnancy test is required because of the risk to an implanted pregnancy.

POSTPARTUM CONTRACEPTION

In the past, postpartum contraception generally included lactational amenorrhea, barriers and progestin-only preparations like the progestin-only pill, and injectable progesterone. Lately there has been great interest in the use of immediate postpartum LARC to reduce unintended and short-interval pregnancy by bypassing barriers to interval placement (6-week postpartum visit) of LARC. The contraceptive rod may be inserted any time before hospital discharge including in the delivery room. It requires no additional didactic training.

Immediate postpartum IUD placement (LNG or copper) does require additional didactic training and is accomplished shortly after delivery of the placenta in vaginal or cesarean deliveries. Contraindications include intrauterine infection, postpartum hemorrhage, or sepsis. The patient should be counseled that expulsion rates are higher (up to 27%) and should be counseled on signs of expulsion, but the continuation rate in the immediate postpartum IUD group was significantly higher than in the 6-week postpartum group.

INEFFECTIVE METHODS

The clinician must be prepared to use empathic communication skills to counsel against the routine use of folklore-based, ineffective techniques such as postcoital douching, makeshift barriers (such as food wrap), and various "contraceptive coital positions."

Coitus interruptus, or withdrawal before ejaculation (24/4%), although not as effective as other methods, is somewhat effective if used regularly and certainly may be encouraged if it is the only method with which the couple is comfortable.

CLINICAL FOLLOW-UP

Using empathic communication skills, you first reassure them of the "correctness" of their concern and your comfort with the issue. You then explain the various hormonal methods of contraception but quickly move to the progestin-only oral contraceptive formulations, providing an explanation of how they work, and, especially, that they are the recommended hormonal contraceptive method during breastfeeding. They are reassured and elect a progestin formulation. You subsequently explain that, unlike estrogen–progestin combination hormonal preparations, the exact timing of the use of the progestin formulation is crucial to assure effectiveness.

---

thePoint®   Visit http://thePoint.lww.com/activate for an interactive USMLE-style question bank and more!

CHAPTER 27
Sterilization

This chapter deals primarily with APGO Educational Topic Areas:

TOPIC 32   OBSTETRIC PROCEDURES
TOPIC 33   FAMILY PLANNING
TOPIC 41   GYNECOLOGIC PROCEDURES

Students should be able to compare and contrast common methods of permanent sterilization. They should be able to describe the risks and benefits.

CLINICAL CASE

A couple in their mid-30s comes to you for contraceptive counseling. With their third of three planned pregnancies ending with the birth of twin sons, they are "quite certain that their family is complete" and wish to consider long-term contraception and sterilization procedures. Despite the high efficacy, they rapidly discard ideas of long-acting reversible contraception because the mother is only 34 years old and, thus, would need repeat insertion of implants or intrauterine devices until menopause. You then review the risks and benefits of laparoscopic tubal ligation and hysteroscopic tubal blockage for her versus vasectomy for him.

STERILIZATION AS A METHOD OF CONTRACEPTION

Sterilization offers highly effective birth control without continuing expense, effort, or motivation. It is the most frequently used method of controlling fertility in the United States. Approximately 47% of married couples have chosen surgical sterilization as their method of contraception. Sterilization is the leading contraceptive method for couples in whom the wife is older than 30 years and who have been married more than 10 years.

All available surgical methods of sterilization prevent the union of sperm and egg, either by preventing the passage of sperm into the ejaculate (*male sterilization*: vasectomy) or by permanently occluding the fallopian tube (*female sterilization*: tubal ligation and hysteroscopic sterilization).

Although it is possible to reverse some forms of surgical sterilization, the difficulty of doing so combined with the generally poor rates of success and the financial expense demands that women or couples consider the decision for surgical sterilization to be permanent.

The physician should counsel couples who are considering surgical sterilization using empathic communication skills combined with the latest evidence-based information about the methods under consideration and assist them with counseling specific to their circumstances in determining the best method.

Changes in operative techniques; anesthesia methods; and attitudes of the public, insurance providers, and physicians have contributed to the rapid increase in the number of sterilization procedures performed each year. Modern methods of surgical sterilization are less invasive, less expensive, safer, and as effective—if not more effective—as those used in the past (Table 27.1).

STERILIZATION OF MEN

About one third of all surgical sterilization procedures are performed on men. The technique for **vasectomy** varies and includes excision and ligation, electrocautery, and mechanical or chemical occlusion of the vas deferens. Because vasectomy is performed outside the abdominal cavity, the procedure is safer, more easily performed in most cases, less expensive, and generally more effective than procedures done on women. Vasectomy is also more easily reversed than most female sterilization procedures (Fig. 27.1), although its reversal is still uncertain in outcome. The main benefit of tubal ligation (but not hysteroscopic sterilization) over vasectomy is immediate sterility.

Minor postoperative complications occur in 5% to 10% of cases and include bleeding, hematomas, acute and chronic pain, and local skin infections. Some authors report a greater incidence of depression and change in body image after vasectomy than after female sterilization. This risk may be minimized with preoperative counseling and education. Concern has been raised about the formation of sperm antibodies in approximately 50% of patients, but no adverse long-term effects of vasectomy have been identified. Likewise, concerns about an increased risk of

239

TABLE 27.1 FAILURE RATES (10-YEAR) PER 1,000 PROCEDURES AND COMPLICATIONS FOR STERILIZATION METHODS

Tubal Ligation	10-Year Failure Rates per 1,000 Procedures	Complications
Bipolar coagulation	24.8	Injury to gastrointestinal and urinary systems, anesthesia-associated complications, hemorrhage, infection, and ectopic pregnancy
Silicone band methods	17.7	
Spring clip	36.5	
Ligation methods		
Postpartum	7.5	
Interval	20.1	
Hysteroscopy	1.6 for Essure in 5 years	Uterine perforation, bleeding, and infection
Vasectomy	11.3	Infection, bleeding, hematoma formation, and granuloma formation

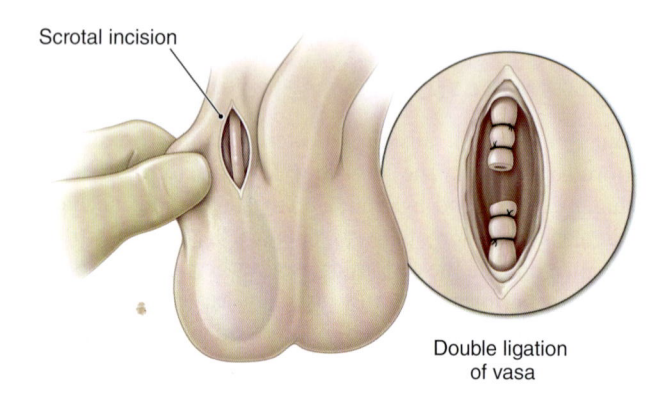

FIGURE 27.1. Vasectomy.

prostate cancer following vasectomy are not supported in the literature; indeed, in countries with the highest rates of vasectomy, there is no increase in the incidence of prostate cancer. Pregnancy after vasectomy occurs in about 1% of cases. Many of these pregnancies result from intercourse too soon after the procedure, rather than from recanalization. *Vasectomy is not immediately effective.* Multiple ejaculations are required before the proximal collecting system is emptied of sperm. Couples should use another method of contraception until male sterility is reasonably assured or postoperative azoospermia is confirmed by semen analysis (98 to 99% at 6 months). Unlike occlusion of the fallopian tubes by tubal ligation, occlusion of the vas deferens is not immediately effective. Complete azoospermia is usually not obtained until 10 weeks after vasectomy.

STERILIZATION OF WOMEN

Surgical sterilization techniques for women can be performed by laparoscopy, minilaparotomy, or hysteroscopy. Sterilization can be performed as an interval procedure, after a spontaneous or elective abortion, or as a postpartum procedure at the time of cesarean delivery or following vaginal delivery. Some nonsurgical methods based on principles of immunization as well as sclerosing agents are under investigation, but remain experimental although promising. Regardless of the method chosen, patients should be counseled about the various components of the procedure, effectiveness rates, and possible complications. Because of the relative safety, low cost, and ease of most sterilization procedures, care must be taken to be certain that the patient understands that the procedure should be considered as a permanent decision.

Patients should understand that reversal is sometimes possible, but at a high cost and usually with low success rates. Failure rates of tubal sterilization are roughly comparable with those of the intrauterine contraceptive. Pregnancy should also be ruled out prior to performing any sterilization procedure.

Laparoscopy

Performed as an outpatient interval procedure, laparoscopic techniques may be carried out under local, regional, or general anesthesia (see Chapter 34). Small incisions, a relatively low rate of complications, and a degree of flexibility in the procedures have led to high physician and patient acceptability.

Occlusion of the fallopian tubes may be accomplished through the use of electrocautery (unipolar or bipolar) or the application of a plastic and spring clip (Filshie clip) or silastic band (Yoon or Falope ring). The choice among laparoscopic methods and cautery or occlusive device is often based more on operator experience, training, and personal preference than on outcome data. It can also be based on patient characteristics, such as body habitus or condition of the fallopian tube. Total salpingectomy can also be done through laparoscopy and is being revisited as an ovarian cancer reduction procedure.

Electrocautery-Based Methods
Electrocautery-based methods are fast, but carry a risk of inadvertent electrical damage to other structures, poorer reversibility, and greater incidence of ectopic pregnancies when failure does occur. Most operators coagulate at the isthmus, taking care that the coagulation forceps is placed over the entire fallopian tube and onto the mesosalpinx so that the entire tube and its lumen are coagulated >3 cm in length. Bipolar cautery is safer than unipolar one; it has less risk of spark injury to adjacent tissue, because the current passes directly between the blades of the coagulation forceps (Fig. 27.2). Unipolar cautery, however,

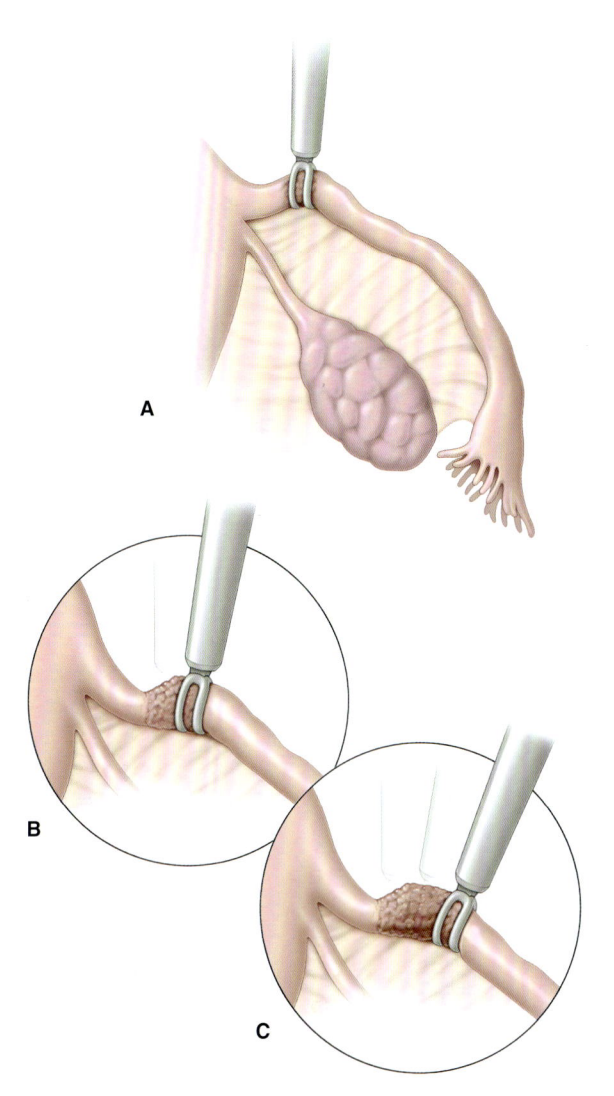

FIGURE 27.2. Electrocautery. (A) Placement of electrocautery forceps. (B) Cauterization of the fallopian tube. (C) Tube coagulated to >3 cm in length.

has a lower failure rate than bipolar. The surgeon, therefore, needs to carefully weigh the risk of the individual procedure with its respective effectiveness.

Hulka Clip

The **Hulka clip** is the most readily reversible method because of its minimal tissue damage, but also carries the greatest failure rate (>1%) for the same reason. As in coagulation, care must be taken to place the jaws of the Hulka clip over the entire breadth of the fallopian tube at a 90° angle. This can be especially difficult when performed immediately postpartum, due to the natural edematous dilation of the tubes.

Falope Ring

The **Falope ring** has intermediate reversibility and failure rates. Patients may, however, have a higher incidence of postoperative pain, requiring strong analgesics. Care must be taken to draw a sufficiently long segment of fallopian tube (the so-called

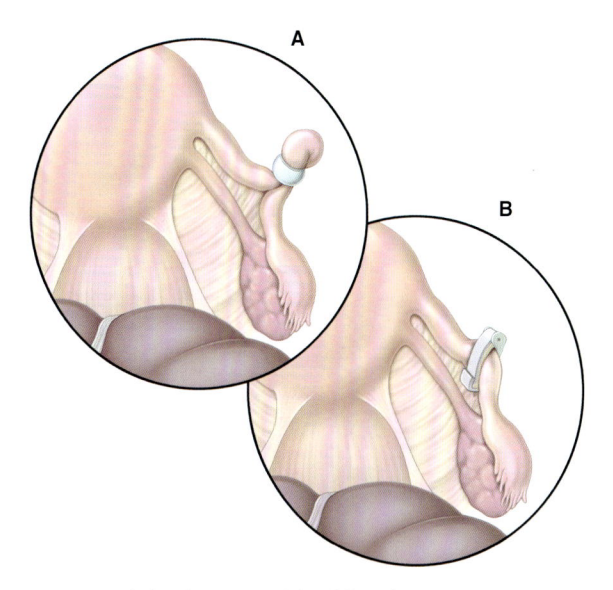

FIGURE 27.3. (A) Falope ring. (B) Filshie clip.

"knuckle" of fallopian tube) into the Falope ring applicator so that the band is placed below the outer and inner borders of the fallopian tube, thus occluding the lumen completely (Fig. 27.3A). Bleeding is a potential complication if too much pressure is placed on the mesosalpinx during the application of the ring.

Filshie Clip

The **Filshie clip** has a lower failure rate than the Hulka clip because of its larger diameter, ease of application, and atraumatic locking device (see Fig. 27.3B). To maximize effectiveness, this clip should be placed at the isthmic portion of the fallopian tube.

Minilaparotomy

Minilaparotomy is the most common surgical approach for tubal ligation throughout the world. Minilaparotomy can be accomplished with a small infraumbilical incision made in the postpartum period or a small lower abdominal suprapubic incision used as an interval procedure, both of which provide ready access to the fallopian tubes. The infraumbilical approach is preferred postpartum, but the suprapubic approach is rarely used in the United States, with laparoscopy being the preferred method for interval tubal ligation. Occlusion of the fallopian tubes may then be accomplished by excision of all or part of the fallopian tube or the use of clips, rings, or cautery. Again, total salpingectomy is currently being revisited as an ovarian cancer reduction procedure.

A common method of tubal interruption utilized in minilaparotomy is Pomeroy tubal ligation (Fig. 27.4). In this procedure, a segment of tube from the midportion is elevated, and an absorbable ligature is placed across the base, forming a loop, or knuckle, of tube. This knuckle is then excised. Because of the similarity in appearance between the fallopian tube and the round ligament, this tissue is sent for histologic

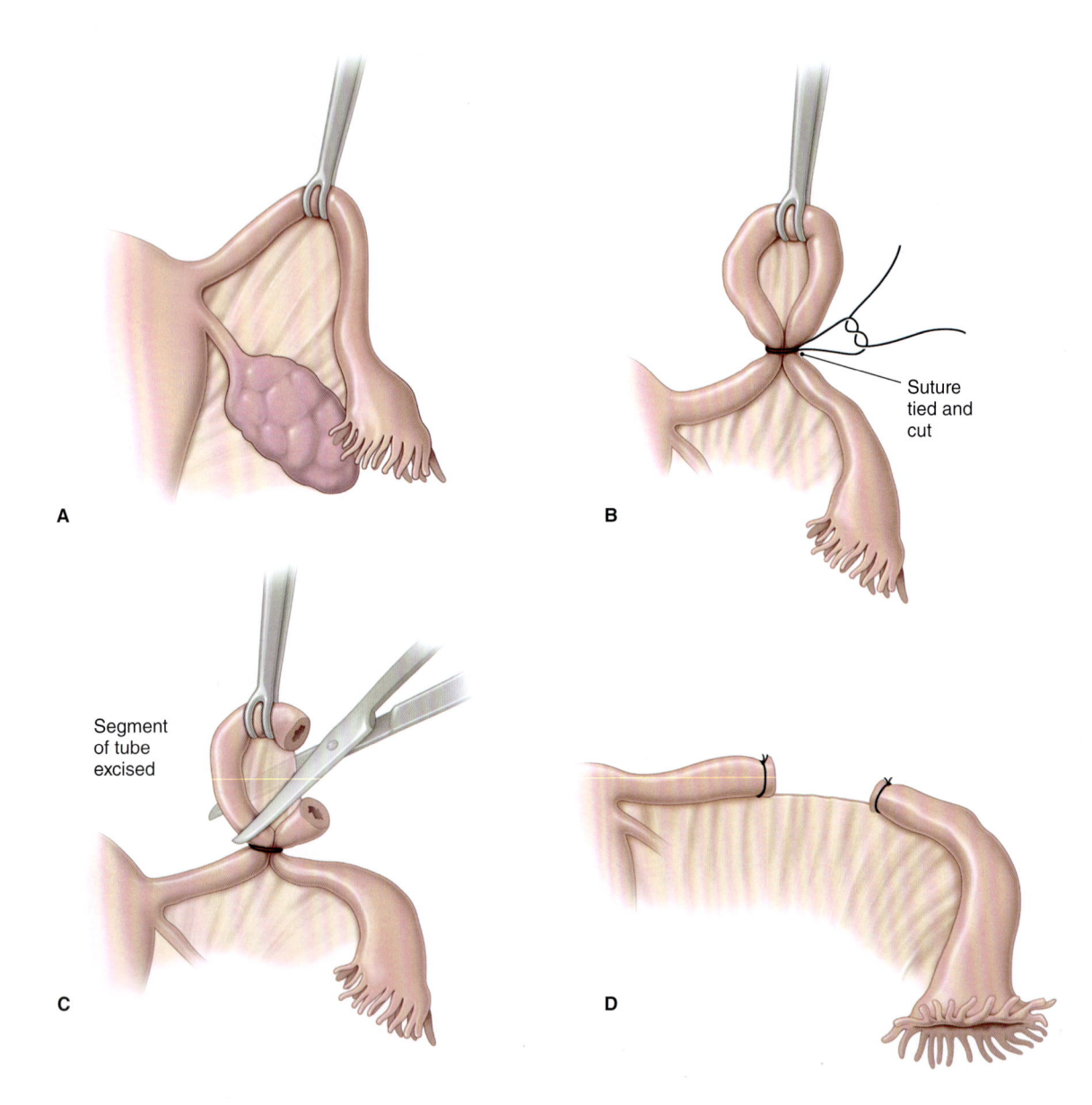

FIGURE 27.4. Pomeroy technique. (A) A segment of the tube is elevated. (B) A suture is tied, forming a loop in the tube. (C) The loop is excised. (D) A 1- to 2-cm gap forms between the ends of the cut tube when healing is complete.

confirmation. When healing is complete, the ends of the tube will have sealed closed, with a 1- to 2-cm gap between the ends. Electrocoagulation or the application of clips or bands may also be accomplished through a minilaparotomy incision, although these are more widely used with laparoscopy.

Hysteroscopy

Transcervical approaches to sterilization include **hysteroscopy** and involve gaining access to the fallopian tubes through the cervix. The Essure system involves the introduction of a 3.6-cm stainless steel inner coil and a nickel titanium outer coil into each fallopian tube (Fig. 27.5). Patients are instructed to use an additional form of contraception for 3 months after the procedure, until the efficacy of the device can be proven with **hysterosalpingography**. Contraindications include contrast allergies, active pelvic infection, and suspected pregnancy. Patients with nickel sensitivity should be counseled about the presence of minute amounts of nickel in the microinserts, but that they are likely of no clinical significance. These procedures can be used for obese patients who may otherwise not be suitable candidates for laparoscopic tubal ligation due to their body habitus. The efficacy of this procedure has been reported to be as high as 99.8%.

Side Effects and Complications

No surgically based technology is free of the possibility of complications or side effects. Infection, bleeding, injury to surrounding structures, or anesthetic complications may occur with any of the

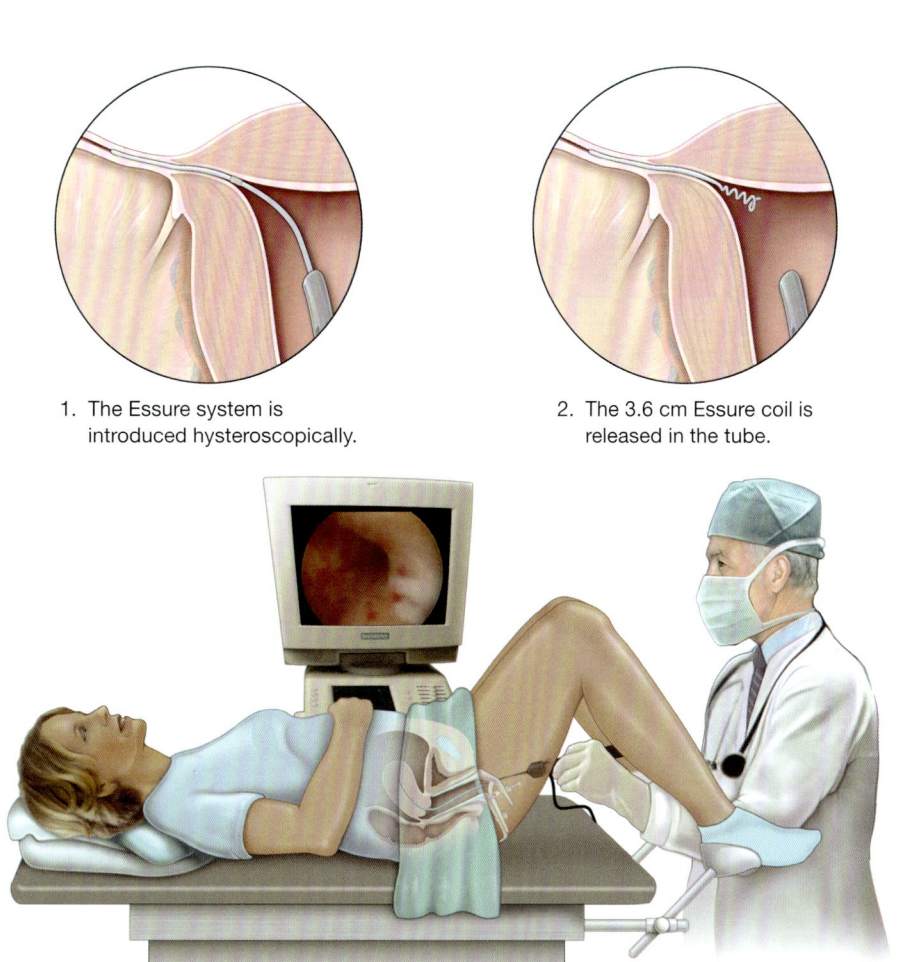

FIGURE 27.5. Hysteroscopic sterilization.

1. The Essure system is introduced hysteroscopically.
2. The 3.6 cm Essure coil is released in the tube.

techniques discussed in this chapter. Complications of laparoscopic and minilaparotomy procedures occur in approximately 1 of every 1,000 procedures. The most common complications include unplanned major surgery, reoperation, infection, injury to other organs, internal bleeding, and problems related to anesthesia. The complication rate with hysteroscopic sterilization is approximately 0.02 per 1,000 procedures. The most common complication is perforation of the uterus (when an instrument creates a small tear through the uterine wall). This usually does not require treatment and rarely has any long-term consequences. The overall fatality rate attributed to sterilization is about 1–4 per 100,000 procedures, significantly lower than that for childbearing in the United States, estimated at about 10 per 100,000 births. Although pregnancy after sterilization is uncommon, there is substantial risk that any poststerilization pregnancy will be ectopic. The risk varies with the type of procedure and the age of the patient. Ectopic pregnancy occurs after tubal ligation, more commonly after cautery than after mechanical tubal occlusion, probably because of microscopic fistulae in the coagulated segment connecting to the peritoneal cavity. Overall, the 10-year cumulative probability of ectopic pregnancy after tubal ligation is 7.3 per 1,000 procedures.

Noncontraceptive Benefits

Patients who undergo tubal ligation not only gain effective contraception but also benefit from a decreased lifetime risk of ovarian cancer. The mechanism for this risk reduction may be related to the newly established link between the fallopian tubes and some ovarian cancers. In fact, tubal ligation has been associated with a significant reduction in ovarian cancer in both the general population and high-risk women. Although tubal sterilization has not been shown to protect against sexually transmitted diseases, it may offer some protection against pelvic inflammatory disease.

REVERSAL OF TUBAL LIGATION

Reversal of tubal ligation by microsurgical techniques is most successful when minimal damage is done to the smallest length of the fallopian tube (e.g., Hulka clip, Filshie clip, and Falope ring). In some series, success rate approaches 50% to 75%. In most cases, however, rates of 25% to 50% are more reasonable expectations; therefore, many specialists in infertility recommend the use of assisted reproductive technology (e.g., in vitro fertilization) rather than attempts at tubal ligation reversal with its attendant low success rates and increased risk of tubal ectopic pregnancy. A patient who has undergone tubal reversal and becomes pregnant is presumed to have an ectopic pregnancy until intrauterine pregnancy is established.

THE DECISION FOR STERILIZATION

The decision for sterilization is an important one, and the patient should be fully informed about the procedure and its risks, effectiveness, and long-term implications. Despite careful counseling, up to 20% of women aged 30 years or younger who undergo sterilization subsequently report regret, although only 1% of all women actually request reversal of the procedure.

CLINICAL FOLLOW-UP

The idea of having to get a confirmation hysterosalpingogram 3 months after hysteroscopic tubal procedures makes them unattractive to the couple. They feel that from their perspective, the risks of both surgical procedures are similar enough to be inconsequential. However, learning that the 10-year failure rate per 1,000 procedures is 2.5 times greater for tubal ligation when compared with vasectomy, they choose vasectomy and a urology appointment is arranged. After learning about the 10-week "waiting period" after vasectomy they choose an estrogen–progestin combined hormonal formulation for interval contraception until the procedure.

---

thePoint®   Visit **http://thePoint.lww.com/activate** for an interactive USMLE-style question bank and more!

CHAPTER 28
Vulvovaginitis

This chapter deals primarily with APGO Educational Topic Area:

TOPIC 35 VULVAR AND VAGINAL DISEASE

Students should be able to outline a basic approach to evaluation and management of vulvar and vaginal complaints, including defining the role of the wet mount preparation.

CLINICAL CASE

A 20-year-old virginal woman presents to the office with a 2-day history of thick white discharge, redness of her "bottom," and intense vaginal itching. She had a course of oral antibiotics the prior week for sinusitis. She denies ever having anything like this in the past. Her symptoms are confirmed on physical examination.

INTRODUCTION

Vulvovaginitis is the spectrum of conditions that cause vaginal or vulvar symptoms such as itching, burning, irritation, and abnormal discharge. Vaginal and vulvar symptoms are among the most common reasons for patient visits to obstetrician–gynecologists. Symptoms may be acute, subacute, or chronic and may range in intensity from mild to severe. Vulvovaginitis may have important consequences in terms of discomfort and pain, days lost from school or work, sexual functioning, and self-image. Depending on the etiology, vulvovaginitis may also be associated with adverse reproductive outcomes in pregnant and nonpregnant women.

VULVOVAGINITIS

Vulvovaginitis has a broad differential diagnosis, and successful treatment typically depends on accurately identifying its cause. The most common causes of vaginitis are **bacterial vaginosis** (**[BV]** 22%–50% of symptomatic women), vulvovaginal **candidiasis** (17%–39%), and **trichomoniasis** (4%–35%). These common vaginal infections often present with characteristic patterns (Table 28.1). The vulva and vagina are also sites of symptoms and lesions of several sexually transmitted infections, such as herpes genitalis, human papillomavirus, syphilis, chancroid, granuloma inguinale, lymphogranuloma venereum, and molluscum contagiosum (see Chapter 29). It is estimated that up to 70% of women with vaginitis remain undiagnosed. In this undiagnosed group, symptoms may be caused by a broad array of conditions, including atrophic vaginitis, various vulvar dermatologic conditions, and vulvodynia.

Although sexually transmitted and other infections are common etiologies of vulvovaginitis, the patient's history and symptoms may point to chemical, allergic, or other noninfectious causes. Evaluation of women with vulvovaginitis should include a focused history about the entire spectrum of vaginal symptoms, including change in discharge, vaginal malodor, itching, irritation, burning, swelling, dyspareunia, and dysuria. Questions about the location of symptoms (vulva, vagina, and anus), duration, the relation to the menstrual cycle, the response to prior treatment including self-treatment and douching, and a sexual history can yield important insights into the likely etiology. In patients with vulvar symptoms, the physical examination should begin with a thorough evaluation of the vulva; however, evaluation may be compromised by patient self-treatment with nonprescription medications.

Easily performed office tests available to aid in diagnosing the cause of vulvovaginitis include vaginal pH testing, the **amine ("whiff") test**, as well as microscopic examination of discharge mixed in normal saline or 10% potassium hydroxide (KOH). Laboratory tests such as rapid tests for enzyme activity from BV-associated organisms, *Trichomonas vaginalis* antigen, and point-of-care testing for DNA of *Gardnerella vaginalis*, *T. vaginalis*, and *Candida* species are also available, although the role of these tests in the proper management of patients with vulvovaginitis is unclear. Depending on the risk factors, DNA amplification tests can be obtained for *Neisseria gonorrhoeae* and *Chlamydia trachomatis*.

NORMAL VULVOVAGINAL ECOSYSTEM

The vulva and vagina are covered by stratified squamous epithelium. The vulva contains hair follicles and sebaceous, sweat, and apocrine glands, whereas the epithelium of the vagina

245

TABLE 28.1	DIAGNOSIS AND TREATMENT OF PHYSIOLOGIC VAGINAL SECRETIONS AND COMMON VAGINAL INFECTIONS			
Characteristic	Normal	Bacterial Vaginosis	Candidiasis	Trichomoniasis
Common symptoms	None	Discharge odor that gets worse after intercourse; may be asymptomatic	Itching Burning Irritation Thick, white discharge	Frothy discharge Bad odor Dysuria Dyspareunia Vulvar itching and burning
Amount of discharge	Small	Often increased	Sometimes increased	Increased
Appearance of discharge	White Clear Flocculent	Thin, homogeneous White Adherent	White Curdy "Cottage cheese-like"	Yellow-green Frothy Adherent
Vaginal pH	3.8–4.2	>4.5	Normal	>4.5
KOH "whiff test" (amine odor)	Absent	Present (fishy)	Absent	Possibly present (fishy)
Microscopic appearance	Normal squamous epithelial cells Numerous lactobacilli	Increased white blood cells Decreased lactobacilli Many clue cells	Hyphae and buds	Normal epithelial cells Increased white blood cells Trichomonads
Treatment	N/A	Metronidazole (oral or intravaginal) Clindamycin (oral or intravaginal)	Intravaginal synthetic imidazoles or oral fluconazole	Oral metronidazole or tinidazole

is nonkeratinized and lacks these specialized elements. At puberty, with maturation of the epithelial cells that occurs with estrogen stimulation, increased levels of glycogen in the vaginal tissues favor the growth of lactobacilli in the genital tract. These bacteria break down glycogen to lactic acid, lowering the pH from the 6 to 8 range, which is common before puberty and after menopause, to the normal vaginal pH range of 3.5 to 4.7 in reproductive-age woman. In addition to lactobacilli, a wide range of other aerobic and anaerobic bacteria are normally found in the vagina at concentrations of 10^8 to 10^9 colonies per mL of vaginal fluid. Because the vagina is a potential space, not an open tube, a ratio of 5:1 anaerobic to aerobic bacteria is normal.

Discharge from the vagina is normal; therefore, not all discharges from the vagina indicate infection. This distinction is important to the diagnostic process. Vaginal secretions arise from several sources. The majority of the liquid portion consists of mucus from the cervix. A small amount of moisture is contributed by endometrial fluid; exudates from accessory glands, such as the Skene and Bartholin glands; and from vaginal transudate. Exfoliated squamous cells from the vaginal wall give the secretions a white to off-white color and provide some increase in consistency. The action of the indigenous vaginal flora also can contribute to the secretion. These components form vaginal secretions that provide physiologic moisture, which prevents symptoms of dryness and irritation. The amount and character of this normal wetness may vary under the influence of factors such as hormonal and fluid status, pregnancy, immunosuppression, douching, and coital activity. Asymptomatic women produce approximately 1.5 g of odorless vaginal fluid each day.

BACTERIAL VAGINOSIS

BV is a polymicrobial infection characterized by a lack of normal hydrogen peroxide–producing lactobacilli and an overgrowth of facultative anaerobic organisms including *G. vaginalis*, *Mycoplasma hominis*, *Bacteroides* species, *Peptostreptococcus* species, *Fusobacterium* species, *Prevotella* species, and *Atopobium vaginae*. Women with BV generally complain of a "musty" or "fishy" odor with an increased thin gray-white to yellow discharge. The discharge may cause mild vulvar irritation in approximately 25% of the cases. The vaginal discharge is mildly adherent to the vaginal wall and has a pH greater than 4.5. Adding a few drops of KOH to the vaginal discharge produces an "amine" or "fishy" odor, commonly referred to as a "positive whiff test."

Microscopic examination made under saline wet mount shows a slight increase in white blood cells (WBCs), clumps of bacteria, loss of normal lactobacilli, and characteristic "clue cells" (Fig. 28.1). These are epithelial cells with numerous coccoid bacteria attached to their surface, which makes their borders appear indistinct and their cytoplasm resemble "ground glass." Because the bacteria that cause BV are part of the normal vaginal flora, the mere presence of these organisms is not diagnostic.

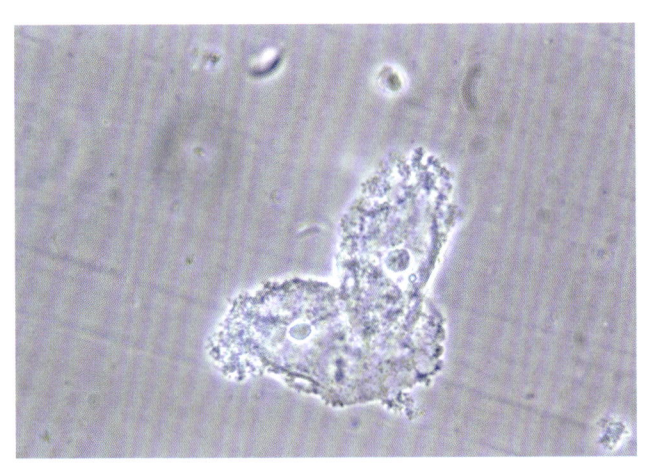

FIGURE 28.1. Clue cells. Clue cells are epithelial cells with clumps of bacteria clustered on their surfaces. Clue cells indicate the presence of a vaginal bacterial infection. CDC/M. Rein.

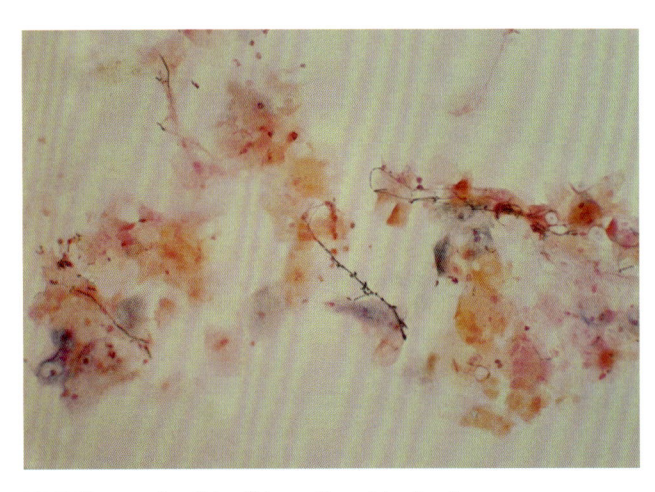

FIGURE 28.2. *Candida albicans.* Branching hyphae are present among epithelial cells in this Gram stain of a vaginal smear. CDC/ Dr. Stuart Brown.

In symptomatic women with BV on a Pap smear, a vaginal pH, amine test, and wet mount should be performed; asymptomatic women do not need evaluation or treatment given that the diagnosis on Pap smear is uncertain and it is unclear that asymptomatic nonpregnant women with BV benefit from treatment. The "gold standard" for laboratory diagnosis of BV is the Gram stain, but, more commonly, the diagnosis is made clinically and is defined by any three of the following four criteria: (1) abnormal gray discharge, (2) pH greater than 4.5, (3) positive whiff test, and (4) the presence of clue cells.

Treatment

BV may be treated with oral or topical metronidazole as well as topical clindamycin. Treatment with oral tinidazole, oral clindamycin, or clindamycin intravaginal ovules is an effective alternative. Symptomatic pregnant women can be treated with either metronidazole or clindamycin, insofar as neither drug has been shown to have teratogenic effects. There are data suggesting that treatment of BV in women with high-risk pregnancies may reduce the incidence of premature rupture of membranes (PROM) and preterm delivery; however, there is no apparent benefit to either universal BV screening or treatment of asymptomatic pregnant women. In nonpregnant women, BV has been associated with both pelvic inflammatory disease (PID) and postoperative infections. It has also been associated with an increased risk of acquisition of HIV and herpes simplex virus (HSV). Although preoperative BV treatment may help prevent postoperative infections, treatment for BV has not been shown to decrease the risk of HIV or HSV infection. Treatment of partners of patients with BV does not help prevent recurrence.

● VULVOVAGINAL CANDIDIASIS

Vulvovaginal candidiasis is caused by ubiquitous airborne fungi. Approximately 90% of these infections are caused by *Candida albicans* (Fig. 28.2). The remaining cases are caused by *Candida glabrata*, *Candida tropicalis*, or *Torulopsis glabrata*. *Candida* infections generally do not coexist with other infections and are not considered to be sexually transmitted, although 10% of male partners have concomitant penile infections. Candidiasis is more likely to occur in women who are pregnant, diabetic, obese, immunosuppressed, on oral contraceptives or corticosteroids, or have had broad-spectrum antibiotic therapy. Practices that keep the vaginal area warm and moist, such as wearing tight clothing or the habitual use of panty liners, may also increase the risk of *Candida* infections. Because **Candida** species typically require estrogenized tissue, vulvovaginal candidiasis is more common during reproductive years and less so before menarche or after menopause.

Signs and Symptoms

The most common presenting complaint for women with candidiasis is itching, although up to 20% of women may be asymptomatic. Burning, external dysuria, and dyspareunia are also common. The vulva and vaginal tissues are often bright red in color, and excoriation is not uncommon in severe cases. A thick, odorless, adherent "cottage cheese" discharge with a pH of 4 to 5 is generally found.

Diagnosis

A reliable diagnosis cannot be made on the basis of history and physical examination alone. Over-the-counter (OTC) treatments are safe and effective, but any woman who does not respond to OTC treatment or who has a recurrence soon after treatment should be seen by a physician for a definitive diagnosis. Patients who have self-administered OTC medications should be advised to stop treatment 3 days before their office visit. Diagnosis requires visualization of either blastospores or pseudohyphae on saline or 10% KOH microscopy or a positive culture in a symptomatic woman. The diagnosis can be further classified as *uncomplicated* or *complicated* vulvovaginal candidiasis (Box 28.1). Latex agglutination tests may be of particular use for non–*C. albicans* strains, because they do not demonstrate the pseudohyphae on wet prep.

Treatment

Treatment of uncomplicated *Candida* infections is primarily with the vaginal application of one of the synthetic imidazoles, such as miconazole, clotrimazole, butoconazole, tioconazole, and terconazole in cream or suppository form. Single-dose oral therapy with fluconazole 150 mg has become widely used. This same low dose is safe for pregnant women despite findings that there is an increased risk of birth defects associated with high daily doses (400–800 mg) of fluconazole. The antifungal nystatin is also used in pregnant women. It is recommended that treatment for vulvovaginal candidiasis begin with topical imidazoles for 7 days.

Although these agents are associated with high cure rates, approximately 20% to 30% of patients experience recurrences 1 month after treatment. Weekly therapy with oral fluconazole for 6 months has been shown to be effective in preventing recurrent candidiasis in 50% of nonpregnant women. Weekly or twice-weekly topical therapy can also be used for prevention. *T. glabrata* is resistant to all azoles and may respond to therapy with intravaginal boric acid capsules or gentian violet.

Patients with frequent recurrences should be carefully evaluated for possible risk factors such as diabetes and autoimmune disease. Prophylactic local therapy with an antifungal agent should be considered when systemic antibiotics are prescribed. Because it is not considered a sexually transmitted disease (STD), the Centers for Disease Control and Prevention does not recommend routine treatment of sexual partners.

BOX 28.1 Classification of Vulvovaginal Candidiasis

Uncomplicated
- Sporadic or infrequent episodes or
- Mild to moderate symptoms or findings or
- Likely instead of suspected *C. albicans* infection or
- Nonimmunocompromised women

Complicated
- Recurrent episodes (four or more per year) or
- Severe symptoms or findings or
- Suspected or proven non–*C. albicans* infection or
- Women with diabetes, severe medical illness, or immunosuppression

Modified from Centers for Disease Control and Prevention. Sexually Transmitted Diseases Treatment Guidelines, 2010. MMWR Recomm Rep. 2002;51(RR-6):1–78.

Trichomonal Vulvovaginitis

T. vaginalis is a flagellate protozoan that lives only in the vagina, Skene ducts, and male or female urethra. The infection can be transmitted by sexual contact, but can also occur via fomites, and the organism has been known to survive in swimming pools and hot tubs.

Trichomoniasis is associated with PID, endometritis, infertility, ectopic pregnancy, and preterm birth. It often coexists with other STDs as well as BV and has also been shown to facilitate HIV transmission.

Symptoms

Symptoms of *Trichomonas* infection vary from mild to severe and may include vulvar itching or burning, copious discharge with rancid odor, dysuria, dyspareunia, and postcoital bleeding. Although not present in all women, the discharge associated with *Trichomonas* infections is generally "frothy," thin, and yellow-green to gray in color, with a pH above 4.5. Examination may reveal edema or erythema of the vulva.

Petechiae, or strawberry patches, are classically described as present in the upper vagina or on the cervix but are actually found in only about 10% of affected patients. A significant number of women with trichomoniasis are asymptomatic.

Diagnosis

The diagnosis is confirmed by microscopic examination of vaginal secretions suspended in normal saline. This wet smear will show large numbers of mature epithelial cells, WBCs, and the *Trichomonas* organism (Fig. 28.3). Point-of-care tests include the OSOM Trichomonas Rapid Test, which uses an immunochromatographic capillary flow dipstick technology, and the Affirm VP III, a nucleic acid probe test that can identify *T. vaginalis*, *G. vaginalis*, and *C. albicans*. Other options include culture and amplification testing such as polymerase chain reaction testing. Women diagnosed with trichomoniasis should also undergo screening for other STDs, especially gonorrhea and chlamydia.

Treatment

Treatment of uncomplicated *Trichomonas* infections is with oral metronidazole or tinidazole. Treating sexual partners of women with trichomoniasis is recommended. An individual undergoing treatment should avoid intercourse until she and her partner have completed the prescribed medication and are asymptomatic. Abstinence from alcohol use when taking metronidazole is necessary to avoid a possible disulfiram-like reaction.

Trichomoniasis has been associated with preterm delivery, PROM, and low birth weight.

Pregnant patients should be treated, and metronidazole is considered safe for use during pregnancy; however, treatment may not prevent these pregnancy complications. Although follow-up examination of patients with trichomoniasis for test of cure is often advocated, it is usually not cost-effective, except in

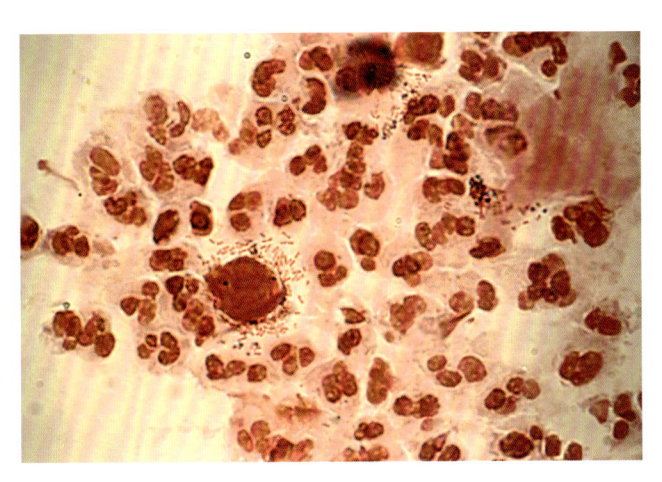

FIGURE 28.3. Trichomonads. The flagella of this parasite can be clearly seen in this image. CDC.

the rare patient with a history of frequent recurrences. In these patients, reinfection or poor compliance must be considered as well as the possibility of infection with more than one agent or other underlying disease. Infections with metronidazole-resistant *T. vaginalis* have been reported. Although absolute resistance is rare, relative resistance may be as high as 5%. These infections are treated with high doses of tinidazole.

OTHER CAUSES

Atrophic Vaginitis

Atrophic vaginitis is defined as atrophy of the vaginal epithelium due to diminished estrogen levels. Although more common in postmenopausal women, atrophic vaginitis can be observed in younger premenopausal women.

Estrogen status plays a crucial role in determining the normal state of the vagina. When estrogen levels decrease, there is loss of cellular glycogen with resulting loss of lactic acid. In the prepubertal and postmenopausal states, the vaginal epithelium is thinned, and the pH of the vagina is usually elevated (4.7 or greater). Loss of elasticity in the connective tissue may also occur, resulting in shortening and narrowing of the vagina. The urinary tract may also be affected and may demonstrate atrophic changes. Patients with atrophic vaginitis may have an abnormal (decreased) vaginal discharge, dryness, itching, burning, or dyspareunia. Diagnosis can be made on the basis of an elevated vaginal pH and the presence of parabasal or intermediate cells on microscopy. An amine test result will be negative. Typical urinary symptoms include urgency, frequency, recurrent urinary tract infections, and incontinence. Atrophic vaginitis is treated with local water-based moisturizing preparations or topical or oral estrogen therapy. **Desquamative inflammatory vaginitis** is generally seen in perimenopausal and postmenopausal women and is characterized by purulent discharge, exfoliation of epithelial cells with vulvovaginal burning and erythema, relatively little lactobacilli, and overgrowth of Gram-positive cocci; usually streptococci are seen. This condition is easily mistaken for trichomoniasis; however, in cases of desquamative inflammatory vaginitis, no motile trichomonads are present and cultures for *T. vaginalis* are negative. Vaginal pH is greater than 4.5. Initial therapy is clindamycin cream 2%, applied daily for 14 days.

CLINICAL FOLLOW-UP

The patient's presentation strongly suggests candidal vulvovaginitis. The course of broad-spectrum antibiotics is a likely predisposing factor. The KOH prep confirms the diagnosis, and the normal saline prep is negative for BV and trichomoniasis. A culture is not necessary in relatively straightforward cases, as this one appears to be, and surveillance for STD is not needed because she denies sexual activity. A single dose of oral fluconazole successfully treats this patient's symptoms.

thePoint Visit http://thePoint.lww.com/activate for an interactive USMLE-style question bank and more!

CHAPTER 29
Sexually Transmitted Infections

This chapter deals primarily with APGO Educational Topic Area:

TOPIC 36 SEXUALLY TRANSMITTED INFECTIONS AND URINARY TRACT INFECTIONS

Students should be able to describe preventive measures and screening protocols for sexually transmitted infections (STIs). They should be able to outline a basic approach to evaluation and management for common STIs. Further, they should be able to discuss the pathophysiology of pelvic inflammatory disease (PID), describe initial evaluation and management, and identify long-term consequences.

CLINICAL CASE

A 24-year-old patient complains of a vaginal discharge and burning with urination for 2 weeks. The symptoms persist despite having taken a course of over-the-counter yeast medication and drinking cranberry juice to treat what she suspects is a bladder infection. She was contacted yesterday by her new boyfriend because he had been told by his doctor that he tested positive for chlamydia. She uses oral contraceptives and does not use condoms. Her urinalysis and wet prep of vaginal secretions in the office are normal. There is a moderate amount of gray discharge at the cervical os and in the vagina.

INTRODUCTION

STIs are one of the most common gynecologic problems in sexually active women, both those who have sex with men and those who have sex with women. STIs can be transmitted by oral, vaginal, or anal sex. The transmission of an STI may have varied consequences, including infertility, cancer, and even death. STIs are the most common cause of preventable infertility and are strongly associated with ectopic pregnancy. The risk of acquiring HIV may be associated with some STIs, making effective STI prevention, screening, and treatment an even greater public health priority. STIs can also take an individual toll, resulting in pain, discomfort, and strain on personal relationships. Most STIs require skin-to-skin contact or exchange of body fluids for transmission.

Anal sex poses a particularly high risk, because tissues in the rectum break easily, and organisms can be transmitted through these breaks. Several STIs can be transmitted through oral–genital contact. Some patients have the misconceptions that this type of sexual contact is not at-risk behavior, or that they are not sexually active when engaging in this behavior. It is important to counsel patients, especially adolescents, about the health risks of noncoital sexual activity. Assessment for STIs should be a routine part of women's health care.

GENERAL DIAGNOSTIC PRINCIPLES

Many STIs are asymptomatic in women or are asymptomatic during the initial stages. As a result, a thorough sexual history and physical examination are both essential in detecting the presence of an STI. About 20% to 50% of patients with one STI have a coexisting infection; as a result, when one infection is confirmed, other infections must be suspected.

On physical examination, the inguinal region should be evaluated for rashes, lesions, and adenopathy. The vulva, perineum, and perianal areas should be inspected for lesions or ulcerations, and palpated for thickening or swelling. The Bartholin glands, Skene ducts, and urethra should be evaluated because these are frequent sites of gonorrheal infection. In patients with urinary symptoms, the urethra should be gently milked to express any discharge. The vagina and cervix should be inspected for lesions and abnormal discharge.

The signs of many STIs may be characterized by genital ulcers or infection of the cervix (cervicitis), urethra (urethritis), or both (Table 29.1). If a patient engages in anal intercourse, the rectum should be considered a potential site for infection. For completeness, the oral cavity as well as the cervical and other lymph nodes should be evaluated, if appropriate, based upon the patient's modes of sexual expression. The Centers for Disease Control and Prevention (CDC) has a guide for taking a sexual history. It can be found at https://www.cdc.gov/std/treatment/sexualhistory.pdf.

SCREENING

STI screening for nonpregnant women depends on the age of the patient and assessment of risk factors (Box 29.1).

TABLE 29.1 DISEASES CHARACTERIZED BY GENITAL ULCERS

	Herpes	Syphilis	Chancroid	Granuloma Inguinale	Lymphogranuloma Venereum
Prevalence	• At least 50 million persons in the United States have HSV infection	• Decreasing; more prevalent in metropolitan areas	• Usually in discrete outbreaks—high rates of HIV coinfection • Declining in the United States and worldwide	• Occurs rarely in the United States; endemic in India, Papua New Guinea, central Australia, Caribbean, southern Africa	• Unknown in the United States
Presentation	• Classic presentation of painful vesicles/ulcers absent in many cases • Recurrences much less common with HSV-1; important fact for counseling	• Primary: ulcer or chancre • Secondary: skin rash, lymphadenopathy, mucocutaneous lesions • Neurologic: ophthalmic and auditory abnormalities • Tertiary: cardiac or ophthalmic manifestations, auditory abnormalities, gummatous lesions • Latent: no symptoms, diagnosed by serology	• Combination of a painful genital ulcer and tender suppurative inguinal adenopathy	• Painless, raised, red lesions that bleed easily	• Self-limited vesicle or ulcer at the site of infection (sometimes) • Inguinal or femoral lymphadenopathy
Diagnosis	• Clinical diagnosis should be confirmed by laboratory testing • Isolation of HSV in cell culture and PCR is the preferred virologic test • Viral culture isolates should be typed to determine if HSV-1 or HSV-2 is the cause of the infection • The serologic type-specific glycoprotein G–based assays should be specifically requested when serology is performed	• Dark-field examinations and direct fluorescent antibody tests of lesion exudate or tissue are the definitive methods for diagnosing early syphilis • Presumptive diagnosis is possible with nontreponemal tests (VDRL and RPR) and treponemal tests (e.g., FTA-ABS and TP-PA). • The use of only one type of serologic test is insufficient; false-positive nontreponemal test results are sometimes associated with medical conditions unrelated to syphilis	• Culture media and PCR testing not readily available • Probable diagnosis: patient with painful ulcers, no evidence of syphilis, typical chancroid presentation, and diagnostic tests negative for herpes	• Clinical suspicion • Wright or Giemsa-stained smears or biopsies of granulation tissue; presence of dark-staining Donovan bodies is diagnostic	• Clinical suspicion • Exclusion of other causes • Positive test for causative agent (*Chlamydia trachomatis*)

FTA-ABS, fluorescent treponemal antibody absorbed; HSV, herpes simplex virus; PCR, polymerase chain reaction; RPR, rapid plasma reagin; TP-PA, *Treponema pallidum* particle agglutination; VDRL, Venereal Disease Research Laboratory. All patients should be tested for syphilis and herpes.
Centers for Disease Control and Prevention. Sexually Transmitted Diseases Treatment Guidelines 2015. https://www.cdc.gov/STI/tg2015/default.htm Accessed February, 2017.

BOX 29.1 Sexually Transmitted Disease Screening Recommendations from the American College of Obstetricians and Gynecologists

Routine Screening
- Sexually active women ages 24 years and younger should be routinely screened for chlamydial and gonorrheal infection.
- Women with developmental disabilities should be screened for STIs.
  - HIV screening is recommended for females aged 13 to 64 years at least once in their lifetime and annually thereafter based on factors related to risk. (Physicians should be aware of and follow their states' HIV screening requirements.)

Screening Based on Risk Factors
- Women with a history of multiple sexual partners or a sexual partner with multiple contacts, sexual contact with culture-proved STIs, a history of repeated episodes of STIs, or attendance at clinics for STIs should be regularly screened for STIs.
- Asymptomatic women aged 25 years and older who are at high risk for infection should be routinely screened for chlamydial infection and gonorrhea.

Used with permission from American College of Obstetricians and Gynecologists. *Guidelines for Women's Health Care*, 4th ed. Washington, DC: American College of Obstetricians and Gynecologists; 2014:404–405.

When a patient is diagnosed with cervicitis, she should also be screened for **PID**, chlamydial infection, gonorrhea, bacterial vaginosis, and trichomoniasis and treated, if necessary. A woman diagnosed with PID should be tested for chlamydial infection, gonorrhea, trichomoniasis, and HIV. Hepatitis B and C screening should also be considered for at-risk populations.

PREVENTION

Prevention of STIs includes educating patients about delaying sexual activity, limiting the number of sexual partners, and using male and female condoms. For some STIs, including **human papillomavirus** (**HPV**) and hepatitis B, immunizations are available to reduce or prevent transmission.

Patient notification is an important part of prevention. When an STI is diagnosed, the patient's sexual partner(s) should also be evaluated. In the United States, cases of gonorrhea, chlamydial infection, and syphilis must be reported to local health departments. Treatment of male sexual partners is important in the prevention of reinfection.

In **expedited partner therapy**, a patient's sexual partner receives drug therapy for an STI without undergoing physical evaluation or testing. The American College of Obstetricians and Gynecologists supports the use of expedited partner therapy in accordance with the CDC guidelines as a method for preventing reinfection of patients with gonorrhea and chlamydia when their partners are unable or unwilling to otherwise seek medical care. Although this approach to therapy typically does not result in adverse reactions, potential risk does exist. Sexual partners should always be encouraged to seek medical evaluation on their own. In some states, expedited partner therapy is prohibited or restricted; therefore, it is important for providers to be familiar with local laws and regulations.

SPECIFIC INFECTIONS

Tables 29.1 and 29.2 summarize the prevalence, signs and symptoms, evaluation, and special considerations of the most common STIs according to whether they present as cervicitis or genital ulcers. Treatment protocols change frequently, and the most current guidelines can be found on the CDC web site (www.cdc.gov).

Chlamydia trachomatis (Chlamydia)

C. trachomatis is a Gram-negative obligate intracellular bacterium that lacks the metabolic and biochemical ability to produce adenosine triphosphate and preferentially infects columnar epithelial cells. Chlamydial infection is the most frequently reported infectious disease in the United States. In 2015, over 1.5 million cases were reported to the CDC. Despite the high number of reported cases, most cases of chlamydial infection are unreported. It is estimated that over a million cases of chlamydial infections remain undiagnosed each year.

If untreated, up to 40% of women with chlamydia will develop PID, which can result in significant complications, including ectopic pregnancy, chronic pelvic pain, and infertility. Chlamydial infections are also responsible for nongonococcal urethritis and inclusion conjunctivitis. Because of the serious consequences of untreated infection, it is recommended that all sexually active women age 24 years and younger should be screened annually. Older women with risk factors, such as multiple sexual partners, a new partner, a sex partner with concurrent partners, or a sex partner who has an STI, should also receive annual screening.

Diagnosis

Chlamydial infection may be asymptomatic, or the clinical presentation can be subtle and nonspecific. Symptoms may include abnormal vaginal discharge and vaginal bleeding. **Cervicitis**, characterized by a mucopurulent discharge from the cervix and eversion or ectropion of the cervix that results in intermittent cervical bleeding, may also suggest the diagnosis (Fig. 29.1). Ascending infection causes mild **salpingitis** (infection of the fallopian tubes) with insidious symptoms. Once salpingitis is established, it may remain active for many months, with increasing risk of tubal damage. Because chlamydia is frequently found in conjunction with Neisseria gonorrhoeae infection, any patient with known or suspected gonorrhea infection should also be evaluated for chlamydia.

TABLE 29.2 DISEASES CHARACTERIZED BY CERVICITIS OR URETHRITIS

	Chlamydial Infection	Gonorrhea
Prevalence	• Most frequently reported infectious disease in the United States • Highest prevalence in persons aged 25 years and younger	• Estimated 600,000 new infections in the United States each year • Prevalence varies widely among communities and populations • Women younger than 25 years are at highest risk
Presentation	• Asymptomatic infection common • Other presentations: mucopurulent cervicitis, abnormal vaginal discharge, irregular intermenstrual vaginal bleeding	• Frequently asymptomatic
Evaluation	• All sexually active women aged 24 years and younger should be screened annually • Urogenital infection in women can be diagnosed by testing urine or swab specimens collected from the endocervix or vagina • Culture, direct immunofluorescence, EIA, nucleic acid hybridization tests, and NAATs are available for the detection of *Chlamydia trachomatis* on endocervical swab specimens • NAATs are the most sensitive tests for endocervical swab specimens and are FDA cleared for use with urine, and some tests are cleared for use with vaginal swab specimens • The College recommends consideration of urine screening or vaginal swab specimen for adolescents reluctant to have pelvic examination or seen where pelvic examination is not feasible	• Testing appropriate in patients at high risk for STIs • The College recommends annual screening if female is 24 years and younger and sexually active. Pharyngeal and anorectal infections should be considered based on sexual practices elicited during the sexual history • Consider urine screening or vaginal swab specimen when adolescents are reluctant to have pelvic examination or are seen where pelvic examination is not feasible
Special considerations	• Persons treated for chlamydial infection should be instructed to abstain from sexual intercourse for 7 days after single-dose therapy or until completion of a 7-day regimen and be instructed to abstain from sexual intercourse until all of their sex partners are treated • Test of cure (repeated testing 3 to 4 weeks after completing therapy) is not recommended for persons treated with the recommended or alternative regimens, unless therapeutic compliance is in question, symptoms persist, or reinfection is suspected • Because of high rates of reinfection, consider advising all women with chlamydial infection to be retested approximately 3 months after treatment and encourage retesting for all women treated for chlamydial infection whenever they next seek medical care within the following 3 to 12 months	• Patients with gonorrhea should be treated routinely for chlamydial infection unless it has been excluded by NAAT • Consider advising all patients with gonorrhea to be retested 3 months after treatment; if patients do not seek retesting in 3 months, encourage retesting whenever these patients seek medical care within the following 12 months

CDC, Centers for Disease Control and Prevention; EIA, enzyme immunoassay; FDA, Food and Drug Administration; NAAT, nucleic acid amplification test; STI, sexually transmitted infection.
Centers for Disease Control and Prevention. *Sexually Transmitted Diseases Treatment Guidelines* 2015. https://www.cdc.gov/STI/tg2015/default.htm Accessed February, 2017.

Laboratory testing for chlamydial infection is accomplished by culture, direct immunofluorescence, enzyme immunoassay, nucleic acid hybridization tests, and nucleic acid amplification tests (NAATs) of endocervical swab specimens. NAATs are the most sensitive tests for endocervical swab specimens and are Food and Drug Administration (FDA) approved for use with vaginal swab specimens. Self-collected vaginal swab specimens are equivalent in sensitivity and specificity to those collected by a clinician using NAATs and women find this screening strategy highly acceptable. Adolescents who are reluctant to undergo a pelvic examination or who receive care where pelvic examination is not possible can be tested with urine screening.

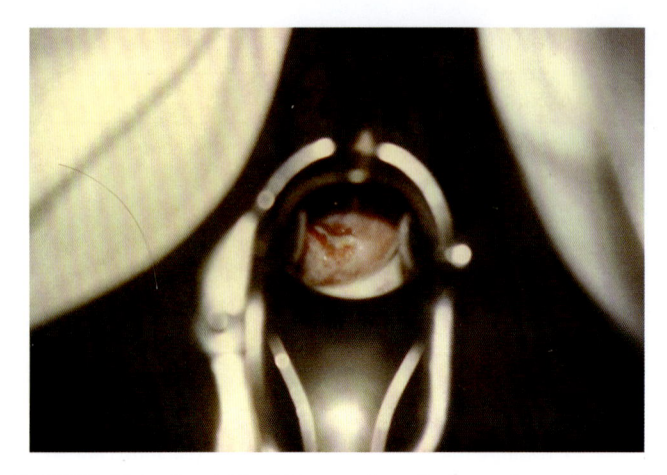

FIGURE 29.1. Cervicitis. Mucopurulent discharge from the cervix and eversion or ectropion of the cervix resulting in intermittent cervical bleeding are suggestive of cervicitis, which may be caused by chlamydia or gonorrheal infection. (*Source:* Centers for Disease Control and Prevention.)

Treatment

Chlamydia is usually treated with azithromycin or doxycycline. Alternative antibiotic therapies include erythromycin base, erythromycin ethylsuccinate, ofloxacin, and levofloxacin. Clinicians should inform patients that gastrointestinal side effects with erythromycin may be significant. Those patients with persistent symptoms, who are suspected to be nonadherent to a treatment plan, or who may have become reinfected should have a **test of cure** performed (repeated testing) 3 to 4 weeks after initial treatment is completed.

Because of the risk of reinfection, any woman with chlamydial infection should be retested 3 months after treatment or when she presents for her medical visit in the 12-month period following initial treatment. Patients undergoing treatment for chlamydia should be instructed to abstain from sexual intercourse until treatment is completed and all sexual partners are treated.

Neisseria gonorrhoeae (Gonorrhea)

Infections with *N. gonorrhoeae*, a Gram-negative intracellular diplococcus, are the second most common STI in the United States. In 2015, it was estimated that there were over 800,000 cases in the United States, and 395,216 of those were reported. The emergence of **antimicrobial-resistant strains**, an increased frequency of asymptomatic infections, and changing patterns of sexual behavior have all contributed to an overall rise in its incidence. In 2014–2015, the rate of gonorrhea increased in all regions of the United States, with a larger increase among men than women.

The highest rates of infection are seen in adolescents and young adults. *N. gonorrhoeae* infection can lead to PID with resultant risks of infertility caused by adhesion formation, tubal damage, and hydrosalpinx formation. Studies also suggest that infection with *N. gonorrhoeae* may facilitate transmission of HIV. Infections with *N. gonorrhoeae* are easily acquired by women and can involve the genital tract, rectum, and pharynx. Sexually active women 24 years and younger should be screened for gonorrhea annually, as should sexually active women age 25 years and older if they are at increased risk. Additional risk factors include inconsistent condom use among persons who are not in mutually monogamous relationships, previous or coexisting STIs, and exchanging sex for money or drugs. Gonorrhea is considered a reportable disease in all states, and sexual partners of infected individuals must be tested and treated.

Diagnosis

Signs and symptoms appear within 3 to 5 days of infection, but asymptomatic infections are common in both men and women. In men, infection is characterized by **urethritis**, a mucopurulent or purulent discharge from the urethra. In women, signs and symptoms are often mild enough to be overlooked and can include purulent discharge from the urethra, Skene duct, cervix, vagina, or anus.

Anal intercourse is not always a prerequisite to anal infection. A greenish or yellow discharge from the cervix indicative of cervicitis should alert the physician to the possibility of either *N. gonorrhoeae* or *C. trachomatis* infection. Infection of the Bartholin glands can lead to secondary infections, abscesses, or cyst formation. When the gland becomes swollen and painful, incision and drainage are appropriate, placement of a Word catheter should be considered.

The laboratory diagnosis of *N. gonorrhoeae* infection in women is made by testing endocervical, vaginal, or urine specimens. Specimens can be tested by culture, nucleic hybridization, or NAAT. Culture is the most widely used testing modality for specimens obtained from the pharynx or rectum, insofar as there are no nonculture tests that are FDA-cleared for the testing of these specimens. Male urethral specimens may be tested by Gram stain in symptomatic men but are not recommended as definitive testing for women or asymptomatic men. All patients who are tested for gonorrhea should also be tested for other STIs, including chlamydia, HIV, and syphilis.

Treatment

Aggressive therapy for patients with either suspected or confirmed *N. gonorrhoeae* should be undertaken to prevent the serious sequelae of untreated disease. Because of the emergence of quinolone-resistant strains of *N. gonorrhoeae*, these antimicrobials are no longer used for the treatment of these infections. The recommended treatment regimen is intramuscular (IM) ceftriaxone plus an oral dose of azithromycin administered together on the same day. If ceftriaxone is not available, the second-line treatment regimen is an oral dose of cefixime plus an oral dose of azithromycin. If the patient has a severe penicillin allergy, the following regimens are recommended: gemifloxacin, single oral dose plus azithromycin, single oral dose; or gentamicin, single IM dose plus azithromycin, single oral dose. Due to the high likelihood of concurrent chlamydial infection, patients should be treated for chlamydia as well, if chlamydial infection is not ruled out by NAAT.

Pelvic Inflammatory Disease

PID involves infection of the upper genital tract (endometrium, fallopian tubes, ovaries, and pelvic peritoneum) as a result of direct spread of pathogenic organisms along mucosal surfaces after initial infection of the cervix. The predominant organisms responsible for PID are *C. trachomatis* and *N. gonorrhoeae.*

Other organisms that have been isolated from the fallopian tubes of patients with PID include *Mycoplasma, Streptococcus, Staphylococcus, Haemophilus, Escherichia coli, Bacteroides, Peptostreptococcus, Clostridium,* and *Actinomyces.* Timing of cervical infection in relation to the menstrual cycle is important; the endocervical mucus resists upward spread, especially during the progesterone-dominant part of the cycle. Oral contraceptives mimic this effect, which explains, in part, their action in limiting PID.

The presence of motile sperm or strings from an intrauterine contraceptive device (IUD) can facilitate penetration of organisms through this protective barrier. The very small increased risk of PID with an IUD exists primarily in the first 3 weeks after IUD insertion and the risk drops to the baseline population risk for the following years after insertion. Tubal ligation usually provides a barrier to spread, although, in some cases, small microchannels facilitate continued spread. The relative mobility of the fallopian tube probably contributes to the rapid and widespread extension of infection.

Risk Factors

The greatest risk factor for PID is prior PID. Other risk factors include adolescence, having multiple sexual partners, not using condoms, and infection with any of the causative organisms. Between 10% and 40% of women with untreated chlamydial or gonorrheal infections of the cervix will develop acute PID.

Early diagnosis and treatment of PID help to prevent infertility and ectopic pregnancy. Infertility, which is due to scarring of damaged fallopian tubes and intraperitoneal adhesions, occurs in approximately 15% of patients after a single episode of salpingitis, increasing to 75% after three or more episodes. The risk of ectopic pregnancy is increased 7 to 10 times in women with a history of salpingitis.

Diagnosis

Symptoms of PID may be as nonspecific as vaginal discharge or abnormal vaginal bleeding. Patients suspected of having PID should be differentiated from those with ectopic pregnancy, septic incomplete abortions, acute appendicitis, diverticular disease, and adnexal torsion. More pronounced signs include muscular guarding, cervical motion tenderness, or rebound tenderness. A purulent cervical discharge is often seen, and the adnexa are usually moderately to exquisitely tender with a mass or fullness potentially palpable. Fever or chills may also be present, and the white blood cell count is usually elevated (Box 29.2). Peritoneal involvement can include **perihepatitis (Fitz-Hugh-Curtis syndrome)**, which is a result of infection ascending via the right paracolic gutter leading to localized fibrosis and scarring of the anterior surface of the liver and adjacent peritoneum.

BOX 29.2 Clinical Criteria for Diagnosis of Acute Salpingitis

Presence of one or more of the following:
1. Cervical motion tenderness
2. Uterine tenderness
3. Adnexal tenderness

plus

One or more of the following:
1. Temperature >101°F (>38.3°C)
2. Cervical or vaginal mucopurulent discharge
3. Abundant white blood cells on microscopy of vaginal fluid
4. Elevated erythrocyte sedimentation rate
5. Elevated C-reactive protein
6. Laboratory documentation of cervical infection with *Neisseria gonorrhoeae* or *Chlamydia trachomatis*

Centers for Disease Control and Prevention. Sexually Transmitted Diseases Treatment Guidelines 2015. https://www.cdc.gov/STI/tg2015/default.htm Accessed February 2017.

It is probably caused by chlamydial infection more often than by gonorrheal infection, with which it was originally described (Fig. 29.2). In severe cases or in patients with one or more prior episodes of PID, **tubo-ovarian abscesses (TOAs)** may form. Patients with TOA are acutely ill, often presenting with high fever, tachycardia, severe pelvic and abdominal pain, and nausea and vomiting.

Because PID may not be associated with specific signs and symptoms, empiric treatment for PID is recommended for sexually active young women who appear to have no other cause of illness and who are found to have uterine tenderness, adnexal tenderness, or cervical motion tenderness on pelvic examination. Women who are diagnosed with PID should also undergo testing for chlamydial, HIV, and gonorrheal infection.

Treatment

The 2015 CDC recommendation for uncomplicated gonorrhea includes combination therapy with ceftriaxone 250 mg IM and azithromycin 1 g orally as a single dose. Single-dose injectable cephalosporin regimens (other than ceftriaxone 250 mg IM) that are safe and generally effective against uncomplicated urogenital and anorectal gonococcal infections include ceftizoxime (500 mg IM), cefoxitin (2 g IM with probenecid 1 g orally), and cefotaxime (500 mg IM). However, many patients require hospitalization for adequate care. The decision for hospitalization may be based on specific criteria (Box 29.3). The focus of inpatient management is high-dose intravenous (IV) antibiotic therapy with an antimicrobial spectrum that covers aerobic and anaerobic organisms. In the case of a TOA that does not respond to antibiotics, surgical drainage or even hysterectomy, depending on the reproductive status and desires of the patient, may be warranted. Interventional radiology provides

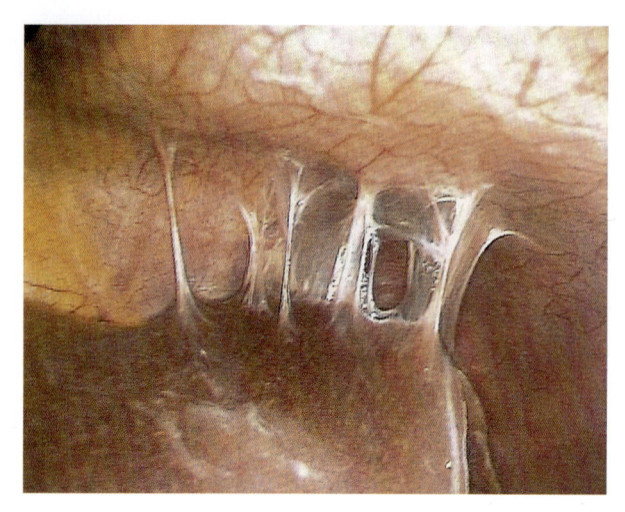

FIGURE 29.2. Perihepatitis (Fitz-Hugh–Curtis syndrome). Adhesions between the liver and diaphragm are evidence of perihepatitis caused by chlamydial infection. (From Overton C, Davis C, McMillan L, Shaw RW. *An Atlas of Endometriosis.* 3rd ed. London: Informa UK; 2007:9.4.)

> **BOX 29.3 Suggested Criteria for Hospitalization for Pelvic Inflammatory Disease**
>
> - Surgical emergencies (e.g., appendicitis) cannot be excluded.
> - The patient is pregnant.
> - The patient has not responded clinically to oral antimicrobial therapy.
> - The patient is unable to follow or tolerate an outpatient oral regimen.
> - The patient has a severe illness, nausea and vomiting, or high fever.
> - The patient has a TOA.
>
> Centers for Disease Control and Prevention. Sexually Transmitted Diseases Treatment Guidelines 2015. https://www.cdc.gov/STI/tg2015/default.htm Accessed February 2017.

a potential alternative technique of abscess drainage. Rupture of a TOA with septic shock is a life-threatening complication, with mortality approaching 10%. These patients must be treated surgically.

Genital Herpes

Genital herpes is caused by infection with herpes simplex virus (HSV), a DNA virus. This highly contagious condition affects more than 50 million persons in the United States. There are two types of HSV:

- HSV-1 is associated with cold sore lesions of the mouth but is increasingly the cause of genital lesions, particularly among adolescent and young women.
- HSV-2 is still the most common cause of genital infections, although an increasing proportion of new genital herpes infections among women may be due to HSV-1. Women infected with HSV-1 remain at risk for acquiring HSV-2 infection. If left untreated, lesions spontaneously heal in 2 to 3 weeks.

Screening recommendation: Type-specific HSV serologic testing should be considered for women presenting for an STI evaluation (especially for women with multiple sex partners).

Diagnosis

Up to 75% of primary infections (occurring in patients with no evidence of HSV-1 or HSV-2 antibodies) go unrecognized by either the patient or provider. First-episode infections are typically the most severe, with recurrent episodes being milder. Symptoms of an initial infection often include a flu-like syndrome and frequent neurologic involvement, occurring 2 to 3 days following infection.

Painful vesicles appear on the vulva, vagina, cervix, perineum, and perianal skin, often extending onto the buttocks, 3 to 7 days after exposure. These vesicles lyse and progress to shallow, painful ulcers with a red border. The lesions of herpes simplex infections are distinguishable from the ulcers found in chancroid, syphilis, or granuloma inguinale by their appearance and extreme tenderness.

They typically resolve in approximately 1 week (Fig. 29.3). Dysuria caused by vulvar lesions or urethral and bladder involvement may lead to urinary retention. Patients with primary lesions may require hospitalization for pain control or management of urinary complications. Aseptic meningitis with fever, headache, and meningismus occurs in some patients 5 to 7 days after the appearance of the genital lesions.

After primary infection, the HSV migrates via nerve fibers to remain dormant in the dorsal root ganglia. Recurrences are triggered by unknown stimuli, resulting in the virus traveling down the nerve fiber to the affected area. Recurrent lesions are usually less painful than those of a primary infection and persist for 2 to 5 days. Recurrent lesions may occur in women who already have antibodies to the same serotype. They can be unilateral rather than bilateral and present as fissures or vulvar irritation, as opposed to being vesicular in appearance. Infections with HSV-1 are less likely to cause recurrences than HSV-2, a characteristic that may be a consideration when suppressive therapy is being contemplated.

Most HSV-1 and HSV-2 infections in women are asymptomatic. The classic presentation of a painful cluster of vesicles and ulcers occurs in only a small proportion of women. When symptomatic, most patients have atypical presentations such as abrasions, fissures, and itching without obvious lesions. Viral shedding can occur for up to 3 weeks after lesions appear. Definitive diagnosis must be confirmed with reliable laboratory testing.

Tests

The laboratory tests used most often are viral culture and polymerase chain reaction (PCR). Culture is highly specific;

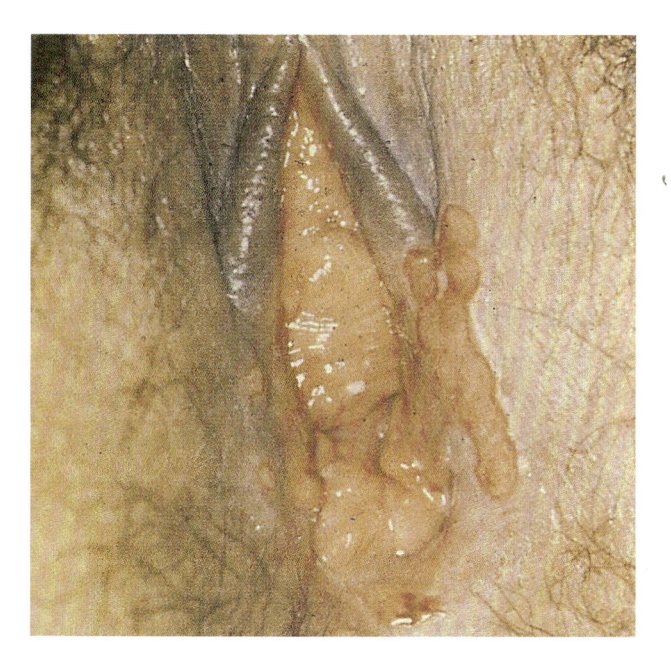

FIGURE 29.3. Genital herpes. The linear appearance of these painful herpetic erosions on the labia is a result of coalescence of several closely grouped vesicles. (*Source:* Centers for Disease Control and Prevention.)

however, it is not very sensitive, with a false-negative rate of 25% with primary infection and as high as 50% in a recurrent infection. PCR testing, though expensive, has a higher sensitivity and is increasingly used in many settings as the definitive test for HSV infection. In addition to these viral detection methods, the detection of type-specific antibodies to HSV-1 and HSV-2 in the blood also can help to establish the diagnosis. These tests may yield false-negative results when administered in the early stages of infection, as the median time from infection to seroconversion is 22 days. Approximately 20% of patients may remain seronegative after 3 months, particularly if they have received antiviral therapy. Type-specific testing may be useful in the following scenarios: (1) recurrent genital or atypical symptoms with negative HSV cultures, (2) clinical diagnosis of genital herpes in the absence of laboratory diagnosis, and (3) a partner with genital herpes.

Treatment
Antiviral drugs are the mainstay of treatment. Oral medication can reduce the duration of viral shedding and shorten the initial symptomatic disease course, but it does not affect the long-term course of the disease.

There is nothing available that eradicates the latent virus from the dorsal root ganglion or affects the risk, frequency, or severity of recurrences after the drug is discontinued. Treatments for first-episode genital herpes include **acyclovir**, **famciclovir**, and **valacyclovir**. Treatment is usually prescribed for 7 to 10 days but can be given longer if new lesions persist. These therapies do not decrease the likelihood of recurrence. Lesions should be kept clean and dry, and analgesics (e.g., acetaminophen or ibuprofen) should be provided as needed. Warm water baths can provide symptomatic relief during the first few days. Topical lidocaine may also prove beneficial but can result in local allergic reactions. Severe episodes may require hospitalization for parenteral analgesia and IV antiviral therapy. Such therapy is generally recommended for immunosuppressed or otherwise compromised patients.

Recurrences may also be treated with oral antiviral therapy. **Episodic therapy** decreases the duration of the episode (lesion, pain, and viral shedding) and is most effective when the patient initiates the therapy at prodrome, or at the beginning of the episode. Treatment regimens for recurrences are usually of a shorter duration than those administered for first episodes (i.e., 3–5 days). Episodic therapy is recommended for patients with infrequent symptomatic recurrences. Patients with frequent occurrences may be offered daily **suppressive therapy**, which prevents 80% of recurrences and results in a 48% reduction in viral transmission between sexual partners.

It should also be recommended for women with HSV-2 whose sexual partners do not have HSV or who have HSV-1 infection. Such discordant couples should also be advised that consistent use of condoms decreases but does not eliminate the risk of transmission. Patient request for suppressive therapy for herpes is also a consideration for outbreak prevention.

Pregnant women with a history of genital herpes should be carefully screened throughout the prenatal course for evidence of outbreaks, though routine antepartum genital HSV cultures in asymptomatic patients with recurrent disease are not recommended. Pregnant women with recurrences should be offered suppression therapy beginning at 36 weeks gestation. All women should be asked early in pregnancy about symptoms of genital herpes, including prodromal symptoms. Women with a history of herpes should be examined for external herpetic lesions when they present for evaluation in labor and delivery. Cesarean delivery to prevent neonatal transmission is indicated for women with active lesions or a typical herpetic prodrome (e.g., burning or vulvar pain) at the time of delivery.

Human Papillomavirus

HPV occurs in up to 80% of sexually active women by the age of 50 years. Transmission occurs through contact with infected genital skin, mucous membranes, or body fluids from a partner with either overt or subclinical HPV infections. HPV is species specific and only infects humans. Most infections are transient, but the proportion of women whose infections resolve decreases with age. HPV infections are typically asymptomatic and are identified only when DNA hybridization testing is done on Pap smears. Unlike other STIs, sequelae of HPV infection may take years to develop. More than 100 HPV subtypes have been identified, with at least 40 identified in genital infections. HPV viral types are routinely classified into low-risk and high-risk categories.

"Low-risk" subtypes, such as 6 and 11, are associated with genital condyloma. Subtypes such as 16, 18, 31, 33, 45, 52, and 58 are called "high risk" because of their association with cervical dysplasia and cervical cancer. Of the high-risk subtypes, HPV 16 and 18 together account for approximately two-thirds of cervical cancer cases, whereas low-risk HPV subtypes rarely lead to cancer.

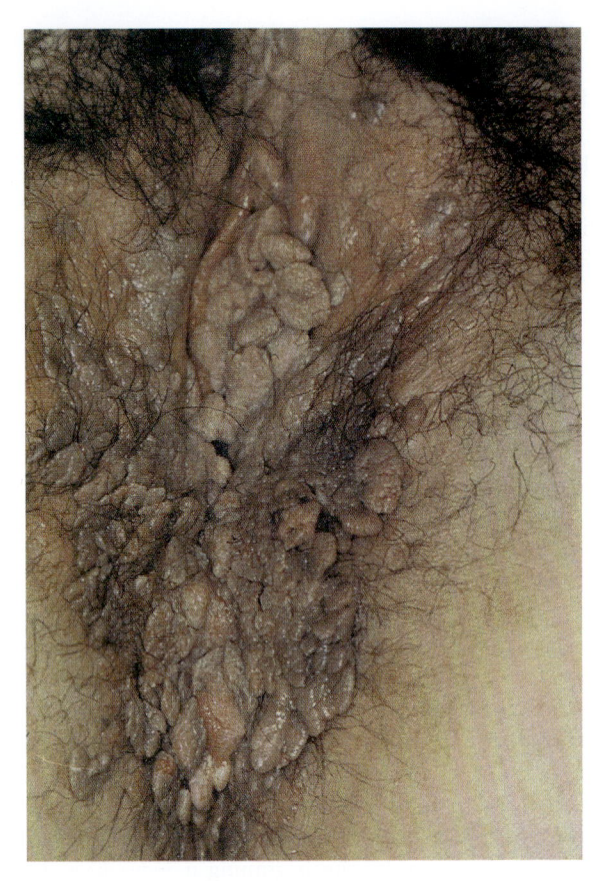

FIGURE 29.4. Condyloma acuminata. (From Wilkinson EJ, Stone IK. *Atlas of Vulvar Disease.* Baltimore, MD: Williams & Wilkins; 2003:9.3.)

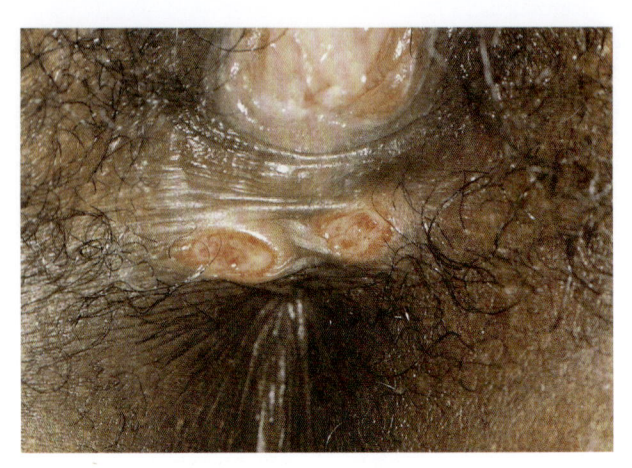

FIGURE 29.5. Syphilis chancres. Note the punched-out appearance and rolled edges. (From Wilkinson EJ, Stone IK. *Atlas of Vulvar Disease.* Baltimore, MD: Williams & Wilkins; 2003:8.46.)

Condyloma Acuminata

Condyloma acuminata (genital or venereal warts) are soft, fleshy growths caused by HPV infection that may arise from the vulva, vagina, cervix, urethral meatus, perineum, and anus (Fig. 29.4). They may occasionally also be found on the tongue or oral cavity. These distinctive lesions may be single or multiple and generally cause few symptoms. They are often accompanied by other STIs. Because HPV is spread by direct skin-to-skin contact, symmetrical lesions across the midline are common.

Diagnosis

The diagnosis of condyloma acuminata is based on physical examination, but it may be confirmed through biopsy of the warts. Thorough inspection of the external genitalia and anogenital region should be performed during the routine gynecologic examination, especially in patients with known cervical or vaginal lesions. Because the condyloma lata of syphilis may be confused with genital warts, the clinician must be able to distinguish the two types of lesions in patients at high risk for both infections (see Fig. 29.5).

Treatment

Management options include chemical treatments, cautery, and immunologic treatments. Patient-applied products include podofilox, imiquimod, and sinecatechins; these treatments should not be used during pregnancy. Treatments that are administered by a health care provider include application of trichloroacetic acid, application of podophyllin resin in tincture of benzoin, cryosurgery, surgical excision, laser surgery, or intralesional interferon injections. Lesions exceeding 2 cm respond best to cryotherapy, cautery, or laser treatment.

Lesions are more resistant to therapy in patients who are pregnant, have diabetes, smoke, or are immunosuppressed. In patients with extensive vaginal or vulvar lesions, cesarean delivery is sometimes recommended to avoid vaginal lacerations and/or problems with suturing tissues with extensive warts. There is a slight risk of transmission to the infant, which can cause subsequent development of laryngeal papillomata. Studies do not conclusively confirm a benefit to cesarean delivery in decreasing transmission to the infant.

Cervical Dysplasia

The relationship between infection with high-risk subtypes of HPV and cervical dysplasia and cancer is now well established. The diagnosis and management of these conditions is covered in Chapter 47.

A quadrivalent **HPV vaccine (Gardasil)** protects against HPV genotypes 6, 11, 16, and 18 (the strains of HPV that cause 90% of genital warts and 70% of cervical cancers). A newer 9-valent HPV vaccine was licensed by the U.S. FDA in 2014, and includes HPV genotypes 6, 11, 16, 18, 31, 33, 45, 52, and 58. This new vaccine provides additional prevention of cervical and vulvar neoplasia.

The American College of Obstetricians and Gynecologists (College) currently recommends routine HPV vaccination for females and males aged 9 to 26 years.

The vaccine is a protective tool and is not a substitute for cancer screening; women should be advised to follow current cervical cytologic screening guidelines regardless of their vaccination status.

Syphilis

In the United States, the incidence of syphilis declined 89.7% in the 1990s and reached its lowest rate in 2000. Beginning in 2001, the rate of syphilis began to increase, especially among men who have sex with men. Rates in women also increased, although not as steeply. In addition, after a 14-year decline, the rate of congenital syphilis in the United States increased to 12.4 per 100,000 live births in 2015. In 2004, the incidence of primary and secondary syphilis among women was 0.8 cases per 100,000 population. This rose to 1.4 in 2015. One reason suggested for the rise in syphilis rates overall is the increasing use of nonpenicillin antibiotics to treat penicillin-resistant gonorrhea; in the past, penicillin treatment of gonorrhea provided treatment for coexisting syphilis. Another reason may be disparities in access to care among some populations.

Treponema pallidum, the causative organism of syphilis, is one of a small group of spirochetes that are virulent in humans. Because this motile anaerobic spirochete can rapidly invade intact moist mucosa, the most common sites of entry for women are the vulva, vagina, and cervix. Transplacental spread may occur at any time during pregnancy and can result in congenital syphilis (see Chapter 24).

Stages

Syphilis can be a long-term disease with several stages.

Primary Stage

Primary syphilis, the first stage of the disease, is characterized by the appearance of a chancre at the site of entry approximately 10 to 60 days after infection with T. pallidum. The chancre has a firm, punched-out appearance and has rolled edges (Fig. 29.5). Because it is small and painless, the chancre may be missed during routine physical examination. Adenopathy or other mild systemic symptoms may also be present. The chancre heals spontaneously within 3 to 6 weeks. Serologic testing results at this stage of syphilis are generally negative.

Secondary Stage

Between 4 and 8 weeks after the primary chancre appears, manifestations of **secondary syphilis** develop. These include skin rash that often appears as rough, red, or brown lesions on the palms of the hands and soles of the feet. Other symptoms include lymphadenopathy, fever, headache, weight loss, fatigue, muscle aches, and patchy hair loss. Highly infective secondary eruptions, called *mucocutaneous mucous patches*, occur in 30% of patients during this stage. In moist areas of the body, flat-topped papules may coalesce, forming condyloma lata (Fig. 29.6). These may be distinguished from venereal warts by their broad base and flatter appearance. In untreated individuals, this stage resolves spontaneously in 2 to 6 weeks, and the disease enters the **latent stage**.

Latent Stage

During the early latent stage (1 year after secondary syphilis), the patient has no signs or symptoms of the disease, although serologic tests are positive. Relapse of symptoms is possible. Late latent syphilis (>1 year after secondary syphilis) is less contagious than early latent cases.

Tertiary Stage

One-third of untreated cases can progress to the **tertiary stage** of the disease in which transmission of the infection is highly

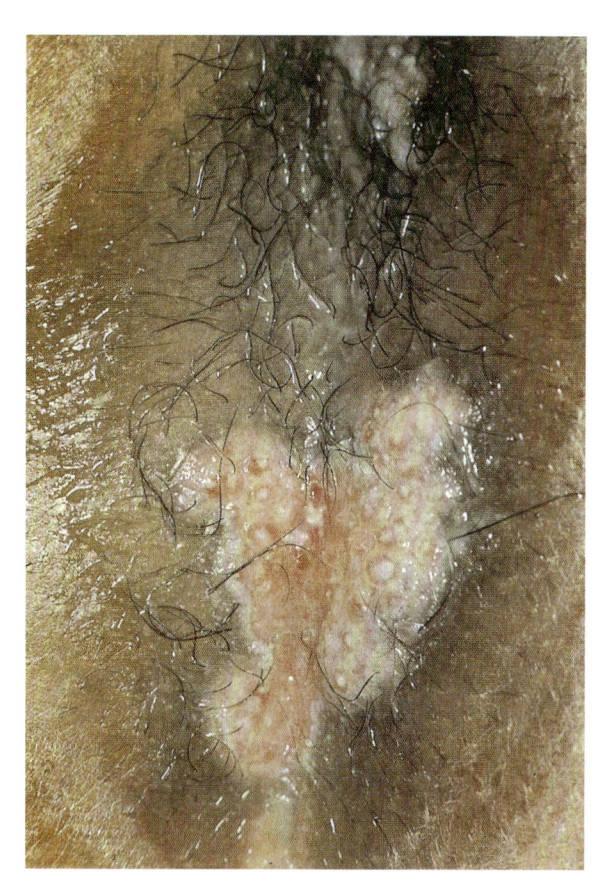

FIGURE 29.6. Condyloma lata in a patient with syphilis. (From Wilkinson EJ, Stone IK. *Atlas of Vulvar Disease*. Baltimore, MD: Williams & Wilkins; 2003:8.47.)

unlikely; however, severe damage to the central nervous and cardiovascular systems develops, along with ophthalmic and auditory abnormalities. Destructive, necrotic, granulomatous lesions, called **gummas**, may develop 1 to 10 years after infection.

Diagnosis

Syphilis is diagnosed by identifying motile spirochetes on dark-field microscopic examination and direct fluorescent antibody tests of material from primary or secondary lesions or lymph node aspirates. Presumptive diagnosis is possible with nontreponemal tests (the Venereal Disease Research Laboratory [VDRL] and rapid plasma reagin [RPR]) and treponemal tests (e.g., fluorescent treponemal antibody absorption and *T. pallidum* particle agglutination [Box 29.4]). The use of only one serologic test is insufficient; false-positive nontreponemal test results are sometimes associated with medical conditions unrelated to syphilis. A woman with a positive treponemal test will usually have this positive result for life, irrespective of treatment or activity of the disease. When neurosyphilis is suspected, a lumbar puncture, with a VDRL performed on the spinal fluid, is required.

Treatment

Syphilis is treated with benzathine penicillin G. The patient should be monitored using quantitative VDRL titers and

> **BOX 29.4 Types of Serologic Tests for Syphilis**
>
> **Nontreponemal**
> - VDRL
> - RPR card test
>
> **Treponemal**
> - Fluorescent treponemal antibody absorption
> - *Treponema pallidum* particle agglutination
> - Microhemagglutination assay for antibodies to *Treponema pallidum*

examinations at 3, 6, and 12 months. The patient should abstain from sexual intercourse until lesions are completely healed.

Human Immunodeficiency Virus and Acquired Immune Deficiency Syndrome

Acquired immune deficiency syndrome (AIDS) is the advanced manifestation of infection by HIV, an RNA retrovirus. The virus targets "helper" T cells (those with the CD4 marker) and monocytes. Depletion of these CD4 cells is an important manifestation of HIV infection.

Two types of HIV have been identified. HIV-1 is the most common type in the United States, whereas HIV-2 is more common in West African countries. The progression of HIV-1 infection varies from individual to individual. In addition to depletion in the number of CD4 cells, HIV-1 may weaken the immune function of these cells. Both lead to immune system compromise that leaves the body vulnerable to serious, often life-threatening infections from other bacteria, viruses, and parasites.

The American College of Obstetricians and Gynecologists recommends that females aged 13 to 64 years be tested for HIV at least once in their lifetime and annually thereafter based on factors related to risk.

Etiology

It is estimated that 1.2 million individuals in the United States are living with HIV or AIDS. AIDS is now the top cause of death in reproductive-age women worldwide. The rate of HIV and AIDS diagnosis decreased for female adults and adolescents in the United States from 2010 to 2015, from a rate of 5.4 to 3.2 per 100,000 adult females in 2015. Even with this decline, AIDS as a cause of death is still disproportionately higher among African-American and Hispanic reproductive-age women.

The three primary methods of contracting the virus are (1) intimate sexual contact, (2) use of contaminated needles or blood products, and (3) perinatal transmission from mother to child. HIV transmission in pregnancy has been greatly reduced as a result of routine screening in the first trimester as well as aggressive therapy at the time of delivery.

Viral loads are obtained at the time of labor, and guide the mode of delivery offered to reduce the risk of transmission.

Diagnosis and Management

The screening test is an enzyme-linked immunosorbent assay, and tests for antibodies against HIV 1/2, and HIV P24 antigen. Although rare, false-positive tests are possible and are more common in multiparous women and women taking oral contraceptives. Confirmation is achieved with an HIV 1/2 antibody differentiation assay.

Management of HIV focuses on prevention and chemotherapy. Prevention emphasizes the use of latex condoms and safe sex practices. Per current CDC guidelines, drug therapy for HIV infection generally includes two nucleoside reverse transcriptase inhibitors along with a third drug from one of these drug classes: integrase strand transfer inhibitor, non-nucleoside reverse transcriptase inhibitors, a protease inhibitor plus a pharmacokinetic booster.

In nonpregnant women, therapy is recommended for all symptomatic patients. Initiation of therapy for the asymptomatic patient with HIV is controversial. Factors involved in the decision making include the viral load and the CD4 cell count. Results are monitored with plasma HIV RNA levels. Instead of monotherapy, combination therapies of at least three agents have been recommended. In nonpregnant women, selection of medications should take into account any possibility of a planned or unplanned pregnancy.

Other Sexually Transmitted Diseases

C. trachomatis serotypes L1, L2, and L3 cause **lymphogranuloma venereum (LGV)**, a disease that has increased in prevalence in the Netherlands and other European countries. When transmitted via vaginal intercourse, LGV presents with inguinal or femoral lymphadenopathy in women. When transmitted anally, symptoms of anal bleeding, purulent anal discharge, constipation, and anal spasms may occur. A self-limiting genital or rectal vesicle or papule sometimes forms at the site of entry of the bacterium. LGV is a systemic infection that, if untreated, can cause secondary infection of rectal or anal lesions, which may lead to abscesses or fistulas.

Donovanosis, previously called **granuloma inguinale**, is caused by sexual transmission of the Gram-negative bacterium *Klebsiella granulomatis*. Although fewer than 100 new cases are reported each year in the United States, it is endemic in Papua New Guinea, central Australia, India, the Caribbean, and western Africa. The ulcerative lesions are vascular and bleed easily on contact. The disease is diagnosed clinically and can be confirmed by special stains of specimens taken from the lesions or from biopsy.

Chancroid, another STI characterized by genital ulcers, usually occurs in discrete outbreaks. Ten percent of individuals diagnosed with chancroid are also infected with HSV or *T. pallidum*. It is also a cofactor for HIV transmission. The causative bacterium, *Haemophilus ducreyi*, is difficult to culture. PCR is often used to confirm the diagnosis, which is made by clinical criteria and ruling out syphilis and HSV through testing of the ulcer secretions. Although rare in the United States, it is endemic in many developing countries. As a result, high-risk patients with painful ulcers should have this diagnosis considered.

Molluscum contagiosum is caused by the DNA poxvirus molluscum contagiosum virus. It is a highly contagious viral skin infection that can be transmitted through sexual contact. It is characterized by small, painless pearly papules that appear on the genital region, inner thighs, and buttocks. The papules usually resolve spontaneously within 6 months to 1 year. Cryotherapy or topical preparations, such as podophyllotoxin cream or iodine and salicylic acid, are used to treat the disease and prevent transmission.

Parasitic infections include **pediculosis pubis (pubic lice)** and **scabies**. Pubic lice are usually transmitted by sexual contact; some cases in which the lice have been transmitted through contact with infested clothing or bedding have been reported. The etiologic agent is the crab louse, *Phthirus pubis*. Scabies, caused by skin infestation of the human itch mite, can be transmitted via these same routes. The predominant symptom of both conditions is itching of the pubic area. Pubic lice or nits can sometimes be detected on pubic hair. Itching due to scabies infection may be delayed several weeks as the individual becomes sensitized to the antigens released by the parasites; however, itching may occur within 24 hours following reinfection. Pubic lice and scabies are treated with topical medications. The insecticide permethrin is first-line therapy for both pubic lice and scabies. Lindane is approved by the FDA but is not recommended as a first-line treatment due to its potential neurotoxicity.

CLINICAL FOLLOW-UP

The patient needs testing for the presence of an STI because of both her symptoms and her boyfriend's documented infection. She agrees to testing for not just chlamydia, but also gonorrhea, syphilis, HIV, and trichomoniasis. Testing for both herpes and hepatitis is also offered, but the patient declines these tests. Her test results are all negative except for chlamydia. She is treated with doxycycline, and her symptoms resolve. She is instructed to use condoms to prevent STIs. She is retested in 3 months, and her culture is negative. She remains asymptomatic.

thePoint® Visit http://thePoint.lww.com/activate for an interactive USMLE-style question bank and more!

CHAPTER 30

Pelvic Support Defects, Urinary Incontinence, and Urinary Tract Infection

This chapter deals primarily with APGO Educational Topic Areas:

TOPIC 36 SEXUALLY TRANSMITTED INFECTIONS AND URINARY TRACT INFECTIONS

TOPIC 37 PELVIC ORGAN PROLAPSE AND URINARY INCONTINENCE

Students should be able to distinguish normal and abnormal pelvic anatomy and support structures. They should understand the different types of urinary incontinence and prolapse and outline a basic approach to their initial evaluation and management. They should describe both medical and surgical options for treatment. Additionally, students should be able to outline evaluation and management of urinary tract infections (UTIs).

CLINICAL CASE

A 64-year-old multiparous woman presents with urinary incontinence. She describes passing small amounts of urine when she coughs or lifts heavy objects. This started several months ago and has resulted in her having to wear a pad to avoid wetting her clothes. Her older sister said that she should have surgery to "pin up her bladder." Physical examination is normal. During the office visit, there is no evidence of urine loss when she is asked to cough with her bladder full.

● INTRODUCTION

Pelvic support defects are conditions that reflect a loss of connective tissue support of the reproductive tract organs. They include loss of support of the uterus, paravaginal tissue, bladder wall, and urethra and urethrovesical angle as well as the distal rectum. **Pelvic organ prolapse** is a disorder in which organs have lost their support and descend through the urogenital hiatus. In order to identify patients who would benefit from treatment, the physician should be familiar with the types of pelvic support defects, the symptoms related to each, and the therapeutic options available.

● PELVIC SUPPORT DEFECTS

Pelvic support defects are more common among women of advancing age, because tissues become less resilient, and accumulated stresses have an additive effect. Possible risk factors include genetic predisposition, parity (particularly vaginal birth), menopause, advancing age, prior pelvic surgery, connective tissue disorders, and factors associated with elevated intra-abdominal pressure (e.g., obesity and chronic constipation with excessive straining). Loss of pelvic support can have both medical and social implications that necessitate evaluation and intervention. Signs include cervical hypertrophy, excoriation, ulceration, and bleeding. Life-threatening symptoms, such as ureteral obstruction, systemic infection, incarceration, and evisceration, are uncommon. Most women with a pelvic support defect on physical examination are asymptomatic; physical findings do not correlate with specific pelvic symptoms.

Causes

The pelvic organs are supported by a complex interaction of muscles (levator muscles), fasciae (urogenital diaphragm and endopelvic fascia), and ligaments (uterosacral and cardinal ligaments). Each of these structures can lose its ability to provide support through birth trauma, chronic elevations of intra-abdominal pressure (e.g., in obesity, chronic cough, and repetitive heavy lifting), intrinsic weaknesses, or atrophic changes caused by aging or estrogen loss. Historically, pelvic support disorders were believed to result solely from attenuation or stretching of pelvic connective tissue. More recent findings demonstrate that breaks or tears of site-specific connective tissue result in identifiable anatomic defects in pelvic support.

Types

Loss of adequate support for the pelvic organs may be manifest by descent or prolapse of the uterus, urethra (urethral detachment, or **urethrocele**), bladder (**cystocele**), or rectum (**rectocele**). A true hernia at the top of the vagina allowing the small bowel to herniate through (**enterocele**) can also occur. These anatomic defects are illustrated in Figure 30.1.

A useful concept that can help in understanding these disorders is to visualize the anterior vaginal wall as a hammock. With good support, the hammock is pulled tight, allowing the bladder to rest on the hammock. When support is lost, the hammock sinks, as if someone were now sitting in the hammock. The bladder now forces the anterior vaginal wall down and out, creating an anterior wall defect, or cystocele. A similar force

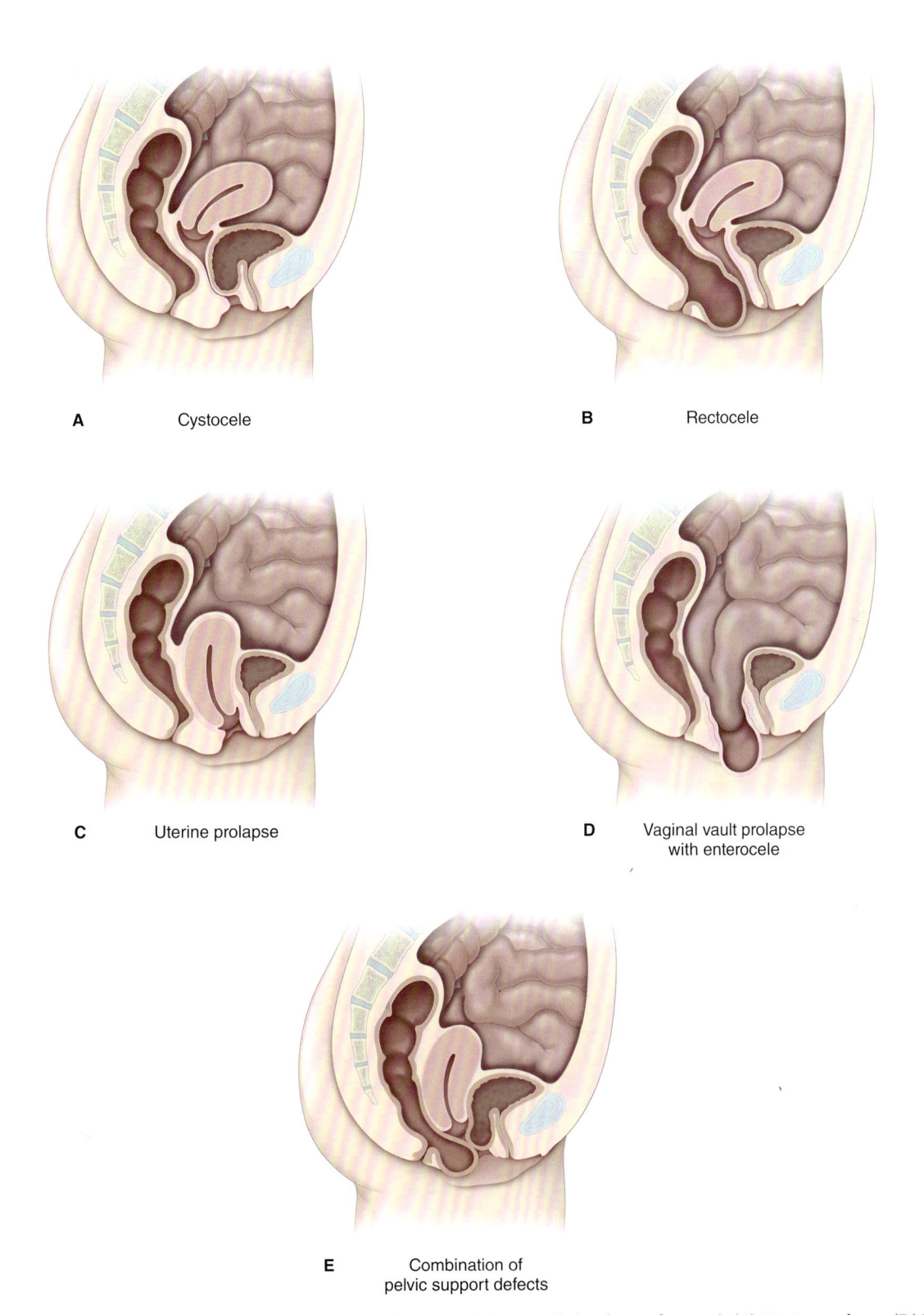

FIGURE 30.1. Pelvic support defects. (A) Cystocele (prolapse of bladder). (B) Rectocele (prolapse of rectum). (C) Uterine prolapse. (D) Uterine prolapse with enterocele (herniation of small bowel). (E) Combination of defects. (Used with permission from the American College of Obstetricians and Gynecologists. *Urogynecology: An Illustrated Guide for Women*. Washington, DC: ACOG; 2004.)

occurs in creating a rectocele, a posterior wall defect. The posterior vaginal wall loses the lateral support, and, thus, the pressure from the rectum forces the posterior vaginal wall in an upward direction. Loss of support for the uterus can lead to varying degrees of uterine prolapse. When the cervix descends beyond the vulva, it is termed **procidentia**. Loss of tissue support can also result in prolapse of the vaginal vault in patients who have had a hysterectomy. Although loss of support may affect any of the pelvic organs individually, multiple organ involvement is most common.

Evaluation

Patients with pelvic relaxation may have symptoms that include urinary or fecal loss or retention; vaginal pressure or heaviness; abdominal, low back, vaginal, or perineal pain or discomfort; a mass sensation; difficulty walking, lifting, or sitting; difficulty with sexual relations; and anxiety or fear related to the condition.

A comprehensive physical examination includes the evaluation of specific anatomic sites with measurements that define the severity of prolapse. Landmarks evaluated include the urethra, vagina (including the anterior and posterior vaginal walls, paravaginal wall, and vaginal apex), perineum, and anal sphincter.

Pelvic Organ Prolapse Quantification

The POP-Q (Pelvic Organ Prolapse Quantification) examination is a classification of pelvic support that measures six specific points in the vagina relative to the hymen. The findings are used to define a stage of prolapse (Fig. 30.2):

- Stage 0: No prolapse. The cervix (or vaginal cuff, if the patient has had a hysterectomy) is at least as high as the vaginal length.
- Stage I: The leading part of the prolapse is >1 cm above the hymen.
- Stage II: The leading edge is ≤1 cm above or below the hymen.
- Stage III: The leading edge is >1 cm beyond the hymen, but less than or equal to the total vaginal length.
- Stage IV: Complete eversion.

Urinary Incontinence

A common complaint of patients with a cystocele or urethrocele is urinary incontinence.

When the bladder loses its support, the mobility of the urethra increases as it pulls away from its attachment to the pubic symphysis. This is exacerbated when intra-abdominal pressure increases repetitively (e.g., when the patient performs the Valsalva maneuver, coughs, sneezes, or lifts heavy objects). Incontinence does not occur in all patients, and the degree of incontinence is often not commensurate with the degree of pelvic relaxation.

The presence of urethral hypermobility is sometimes assessed by the Q-tip test. With the patient in the lithotomy position, a cotton-tipped swab lubricated with lidocaine jelly is placed into the bladder and pulled back until resistance is met. Then the patient is asked to bear down. If there is urethral hypermobility, the end of the swab rotates upward, suggesting that the urethral–vesicular junction (UVJ) is being deflected downward by the intra-abdominal pressure. If the angle of the Q-tip rotation is greater than 30°, it is considered a positive test. The Q-tip test does not predict incontinence, but provides more detail to the physical examination, and is the only validated method for measurement of the anterior, posterior, and apical pelvic compartments. It may also be used to predict the success of treatment options that work by stabilizing the urethra. Although widely used, it has limited value in predicting the presence of genuine stress incontinence and/or success of incontinence surgery. More reliable and clinically useful information is available with sophisticated urodynamic testing.

Of note, some patients with stage III or IV prolapse do not present with incontinence, because they have a kink (i.e., functional obstruction) in the outflow tract that can simulate continence. On occasion, such patients may develop hydronephrosis or hydroureter due to this obstruction. A renal ultrasound is helpful to evaluate this scenario.

History

Most pelvic relaxation disorders are the result of structural failure of the tissues involved, but other contributing factors should be considered in the complete care of the patient. Questions that should be asked include the following:

- Has there been a change in intra-abdominal pressure? If yes, what is the cause?
- Does the patient have a chronic cough or constipation that has precipitated her symptoms?
- Is a neurologic process (such as diabetic neuropathy) complicating the patient's presenting complaint?

These issues as well as others should be considered prior to the selection of a diagnostic or therapeutic plan.

Differential Diagnosis

The presumptive diagnosis of a pelvic support defect is based on the evaluation of the structural integrity of pelvic support by physical examination. Other considerations include UTI, which may cause urgency, and urethral diverticulum or Skene gland abscesses, both of which can mimic a cystourethrocele and, in the case of diverticula, may be a cause of incontinence. These conditions can be identified by the patient's symptoms, careful "milking" of the urethra, or cystoscopy. It is occasionally difficult to differentiate between a high rectocele and an enterocele. This distinction may be facilitated through rectal examination or the identification of the small bowel in the hernia sac. It is common for the diagnosis of an enterocele to not be confirmed until surgical repair is being performed.

Treatment

Women with prolapse who are asymptomatic or mildly symptomatic can be observed at regular intervals, unless new, bothersome symptoms develop. The option of nonsurgical management should be discussed with all women with prolapse.

Nonsurgical alternatives include pessaries, pelvic floor exercises, and symptom-directed management. A variety of surgical procedures can also be considered.

Pessaries

Pessaries are removable devices made of rubber, plastic, or silicone. They can be utilized as first-line therapy for most cases of prolapse regardless of prolapse stage or site of predominant prolapse. Pessary devices are available in various shapes and sizes

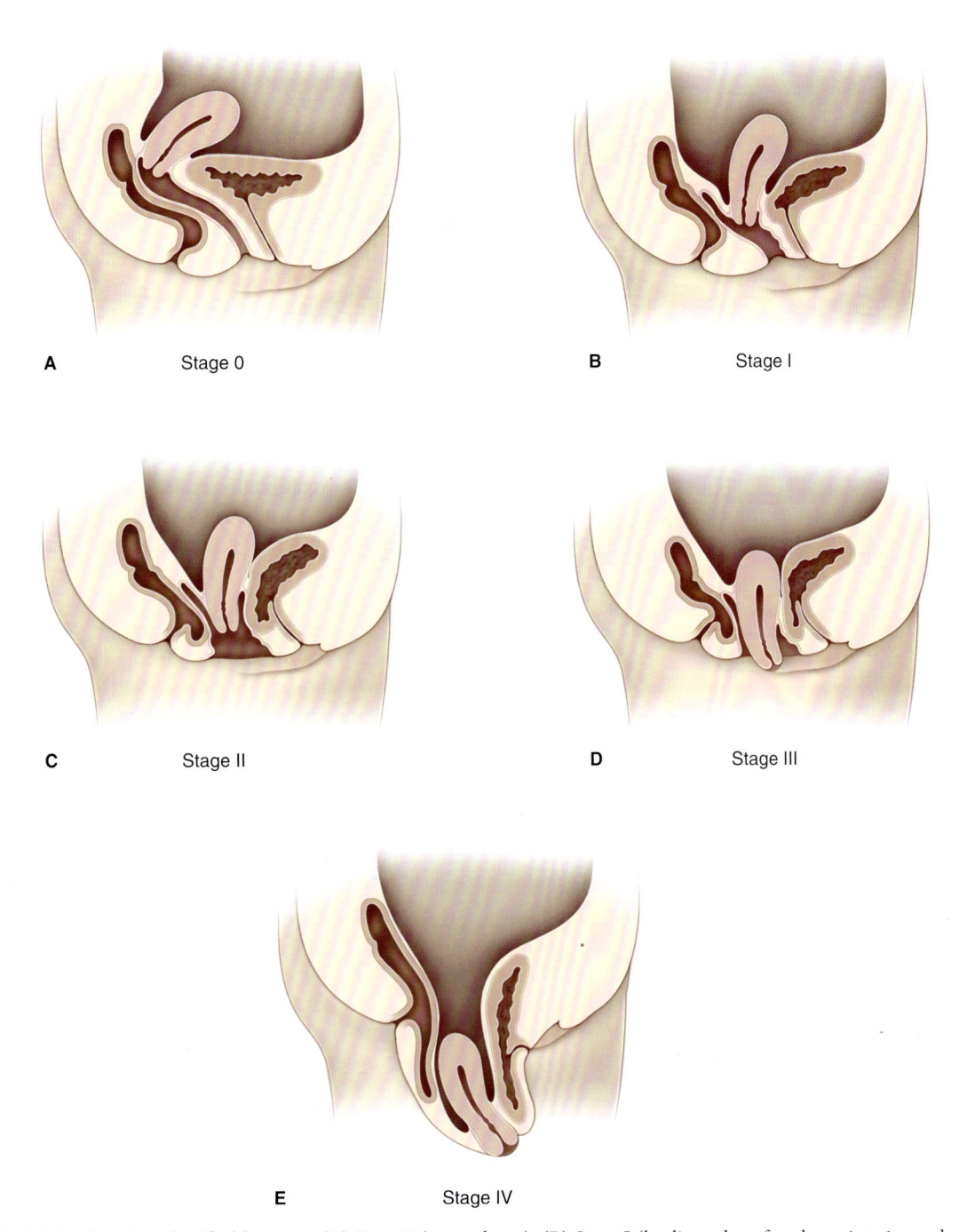

FIGURE 30.2. Pelvic relaxation classified by stage. (A) Stage 0 (no prolapse). (B) Stage I (leading edge of prolapse is > 1 cm above the hymen). (C) Stage II (leading edge of prolapse is ≤1 cm below the hymen). (D) Stage III (leading edge of prolapse is >1 cm beyond hymen, but less than or equal to the total vaginal length). (E) Stage IV (complete eversion).

as shown in Figure 30.3 and can be categorized as supportive (e.g., ring, Smith, Hodge, or Gehrung) or space-occupying (e.g., donut, Gellhorn, or cube).

Surgery

Surgical treatments for prolapse when the uterus is present include hysterectomy and uterine suspension. If the uterus has been removed, procedures include sacral colpopexy (attachment of the vaginal cuff to the sacral promontory) and fixation of the cuff to the uterosacral or sacrospinous ligament. **Colpocleisis** (complete obliteration of the vaginal lumen) can be offered to women who are at high risk for complications with reconstructive procedures and who do not desire vaginal intercourse.

Many women with advanced prolapse, particularly prolapse involving the anterior vagina, will not have symptoms of urinary incontinence. Approximately 40% of women without

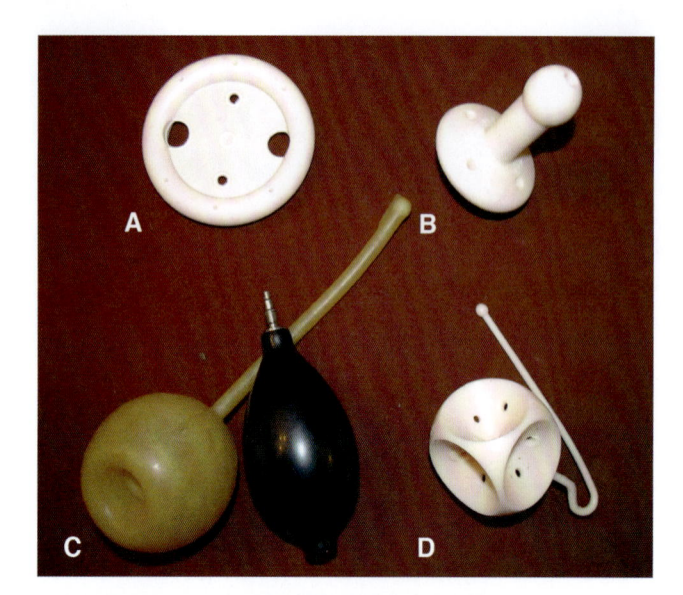

FIGURE 30.3. Examples of commonly used pessaries. (A) Ring pessary (for mild prolapse with mild cystocele). (B) Gellhorn pessary (for third-degree prolapse/procidentia). (C) Inflatoball (for mild cystocele/rectocele associated with procidentia/prolapse). (D) Cube pessary (for stress urinary incontinence, uterine prolapse, cystocele, and rectocele).

stress urinary incontinence develop symptoms of stress incontinence after surgical correction of pelvic organ prolapse. The potential risks and benefits of performing a prophylactic anti-incontinence procedure at the time of prolapse repair should be discussed with each surgical candidate.

URINARY INCONTINENCE

The prevalence of urinary incontinence appears to increase gradually during young adult life, has a broad peak around middle age, and then steadily increases in older adults. Urinary incontinence has been shown to affect women's social, clinical, and psychological well-being. It is estimated that less than one-half of all incontinent women seek medical care, even though the condition can often be treated.

Types

Several types of urinary incontinence have been identified, and a patient may have more than one type (Table 30.1).

Urge Incontinence (Detrusor Overactivity)

The normal voiding "reflex" is initiated when stretch receptors within the **detrusor muscle**, the layer of muscle that lines the interior bladder wall, send a signal to the brain. The brain then decides if it is socially acceptable to void. The detrusor muscle contracts, elevating the bladder pressure to exceed the urethral pressure. The external urethral sphincter, under voluntary control, relaxes, and voiding is completed.

Normally, the detrusor muscle allows the bladder to fill in a low-resistance setting. The volume increases within the bladder, but the pressure within the bladder remains low. Patients with an overactive detrusor muscle have uninhibited detrusor contractions. These contractions cause a rise in the bladder pressure that overrides the urethral pressure, and the patient will leak urine without evidence of increased intra-abdominal pressure. Idiopathic detrusor overactivity has no organic cause, but has a neurogenic component.

A patient with detrusor overactivity presents with the feeling that she must run to the bathroom frequently and urgently. This may or may not be associated with **nocturia**. These symptoms may occur spontaneously, after bladder surgery to correct stress incontinence, or after extensive bladder dissection during pelvic surgery. Urge incontinence is more common in older women and those with comorbidities such as bladder abnormalities, an altered bladder microbiome, and neurologic disorders.

Stress Urinary Incontinence

Normal physiology and anatomy allow for increased abdominal pressure to be transmitted along the entire urethra. In addition, the endopelvic fascia that extends beneath the urethra allows for the urethra to be compressed against the endopelvic fascia, thus maintaining a closed system and maintaining the bladder neck in a stable position.

TABLE 30.1 CHARACTERISTICS OF URINARY INCONTINENCE

Characteristic	Stress Incontinence	Urge Incontinence	Overflow Incontinence
Associated symptoms	None (occasional pelvic pressure)	Urgency, nocturia	Fullness, pressure, frequency
Amount of loss	Small, spurt	Large, complete emptying	Small, dribbling
Duration of loss	Brief, corresponds to stress	Moderate, several seconds	Often continuous
Associated event	Cough, laugh, sneeze, physical activity	None, change in position, running water	None
Position	Upright, sitting; rare when supine or asleep	Any	Any
Cause	Structural (cystocele, urethrocele)	Loss of bladder inhibition	Obstruction, loss of neurologic control

In patients with stress incontinence, increased intra-abdominal pressure is transmitted to the bladder, but not to the urethra (specifically, UVJ), due to loss of integrity of the endopelvic fascia. The bladder neck descends, the bladder pressure is elevated above the intraurethral pressure, and urine is lost. Patients with stress incontinence present with loss of urine during activities that cause increased intra-abdominal pressure, such as coughing, laughing, or sneezing. Stress incontinence is the most common form in young women.

Mixed Incontinence

Some patients may have symptoms of both urge incontinence and stress incontinence. These patients present a significant diagnostic challenge and benefit from the use of appropriate evaluation. This clinical scenario may be treated as stress or as detrusor instability, although it is not clear which approach offers a better outcome.

Overflow Incontinence

In this form of incontinence, the bladder does not empty completely during voiding due to an inability of the detrusor muscle to contract. This may occur because of an obstruction of the urethra or a neurologic deficit that causes the patient to lose the ability to perceive the need to void. Urine leaks out of the bladder when the bladder pressure exceeds the urethral pressure. Overflow incontinence may also occur with bladder outlet obstruction. These patients experience continuous leakage of small amounts of urine.

Other Incontinence

In patients who have had a recent delivery, pelvic surgery, or radiation, involuntary leakage of fluid should suggest the possibility of **fistulae** between the vagina and the bladder (**vesicovaginal**), urethra (**urethrovaginal**), or ureter (**ureterovaginal**). A communication between the bladder and the uterus (**vesicouterine**) may also be found on rare occasions. A fistula may also occur between the rectum and vagina (**rectovaginal fistula**), resulting in the passage of flatus or feces from the vagina (Fig. 30.4).

Evaluation

The basic evaluation for urinary incontinence includes a history, physical examination, direct observation of urine loss, measurement of **postvoid residual** (**PVR**) **volume** urine culture, and urinalysis. The goal of initial testing is to rule out UTI, neuromuscular disorders, and pelvic support defects, all of which are associated with urinary incontinence. The patient should be asked about her fluid intake, the relationship between her symptoms and fluid intake and activity, and medications. A voiding diary may be helpful in this evaluation process.

Urodynamic Testing

Urodynamic testing may also be useful. These tests measure the pressure and volume of the bladder as it fills and the flow rate as it empties. In **single-channel urodynamic testing**, the patient voids and the volume is recorded. A urinary catheter is then placed, and the PVR urine is recorded. The bladder is filled in a retrograde fashion. The patient is asked to note the first sensation that her bladder is being filled. She then is asked to note when she has a desire to void and when she can no longer hold her urine. Normal values are 100 to 150 cc for first sensation, 250 cc for first desire to void, and 500 to 600 cc for maximum capacity. In **multichannel urodynamic testing**, a transducer is placed in the vagina or rectum to measure intra-abdominal pressure. A transducer is placed in the bladder, and electromyogram pads are placed along the perineum. This form of testing provides an assessment of the entire pelvic floor, and an uninhibited bladder contraction can be clearly documented.

Cystourethroscopy

Cystourethroscopy, in which a slender, lighted scope is introduced into the bladder, is used to identify bladder lesions and foreign bodies, as well as urethral diverticula, fistulas, urethral strictures, and intrinsic sphincter deficiency. It is not routinely indicated as part of the surgical procedure for incontinence.

Treatment

Often, treatments are more effective when used in combination.

Nonsurgical Treatment Options

Lifestyle interventions that may help modify incontinence include weight loss, caffeine reduction, fluid management, reduction of physical exertion (e.g., work and exercise), cessation of smoking, and relief of constipation.

Pelvic muscle training (Kegel exercises) can be extremely effective in treating some forms of incontinence, especially stress incontinence. These exercises strengthen the pelvic floor and, thus, decrease the degree of urethral hypermobility. The patient is instructed to repeatedly tighten her pelvic floor muscles as though she were voluntarily stopping a urine stream. Biofeedback techniques and weighted vaginal cones are available

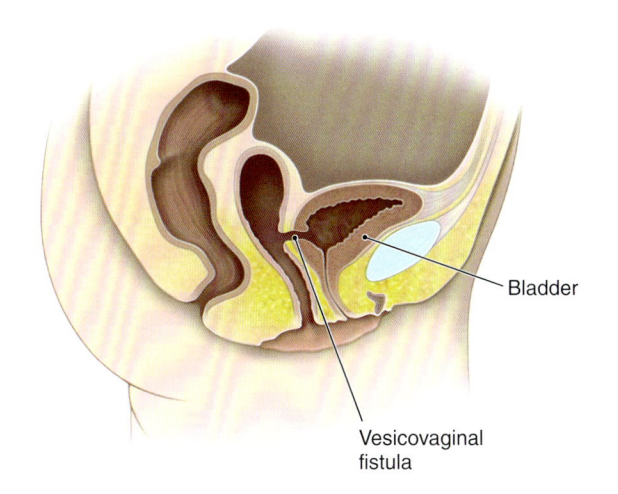

FIGURE 30.4. Vesicovaginal fistula. (Used with permission from the American College of Obstetricians and Gynecologists. *Urogynecology: An Illustrated Guide for Women.* Washington, DC: ACOG; 2004.)

to assist patients in learning the proper technique. When performed correctly, these exercises have success rates of about 85%. Success is defined as a decreased number of episodes of incontinence; however, once the patient stops the exercise regimen, incontinence typically recurs. Other treatments for stress incontinence include various pessaries and continence tampons that can be placed vaginally to aid in urethral compression.

Behavioral training is aimed at increasing the patient's bladder control and capacity by gradually increasing the amount of time between voids. This type of training is most often used to treat urge incontinence but may also be successful in treating stress incontinence and mixed incontinence. It may be augmented by biofeedback.

A number of pharmacologic agents appear to be effective for treating frequency, urgency, and urge incontinence. The response to treatment is variable and unpredictable, with side effects occurring commonly. Generally, drugs improve symptoms of detrusor overactivity by inhibiting the contractile activity of the bladder. These agents can be broadly classified into anticholinergic agents, tricyclic antidepressants, musculotropic drugs, and a variety of other less commonly used drugs.

Surgical Treatment Options

Many surgical treatments have been developed for stress urinary incontinence, but only a few—**retropubic colposuspension** and **sling procedures**—continue to be recommended based on sound evidence (Fig. 30.5A, B). The aim of retropubic colposuspension is to suspend and stabilize the anterior vaginal wall and, thus, the bladder neck and proximal urethra in a retropubic position. This prevents their descent and allows for urethral compression against a stable suburethral layer. In the **Burch procedure**, which can be performed abdominally or laparoscopically, two or three nonabsorbable sutures are placed on each side of the midurethra and bladder neck. Another procedure, performed transvaginally, uses tension-free tape placed at the midurethra to elevate the urethra back into place. The success of tension-free vaginal tape has led to the introduction of other products with modified techniques of applying a midurethral sling (i.e., retropubic "top-down") and transobturator approaches. These procedures, when performed along with surgery for pelvic organ prolapse, decrease the risk of postsurgery stress urinary incontinence.

In addition to retropubic colposuspensions and sling procedures, **bulking agents**, such as collagen, carbon-coated beads, and fat, can be used for the treatment of stress incontinence with intrinsic sphincter deficiency (see Fig. 30.5C). These materials are injected transurethrally or periurethrally around the bladder neck and proximal urethra, thereby providing a "washer" effect. These agents are usually used as second-line therapy in particular circumstances (e.g., after surgery has failed; when stress incontinence persists with a nonmobile bladder neck; or among older, debilitated women for whom any form of operative treatment may be hazardous).

Midurethral slings for stress urinary incontinence afford shorter operative and recovery times with comparable efficacy, and are therefore more cost-effective.

Success rates vary depending on the skill of the surgeon and the technique used. Tension-free vaginal tape and the Burch

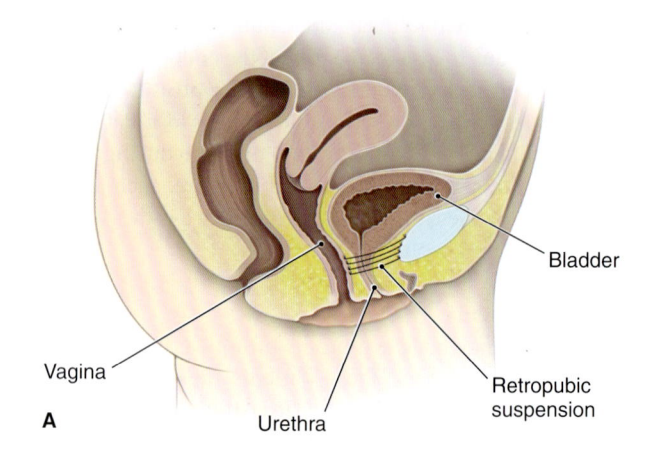

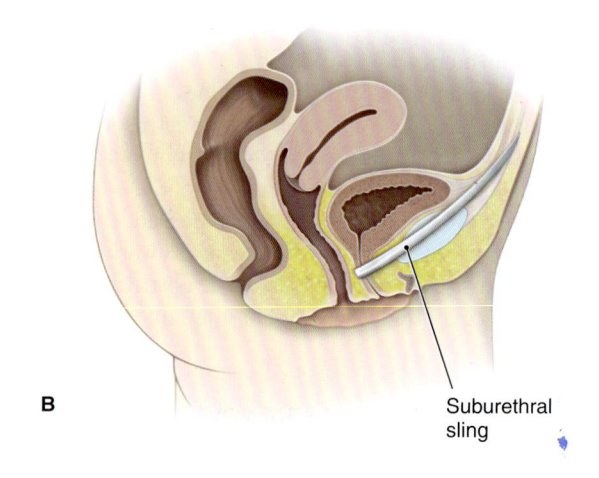

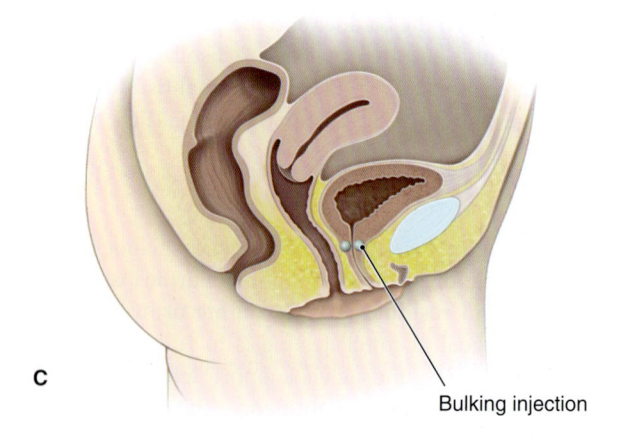

FIGURE 30.5. Surgical procedures for the treatment of incontinence. (A) Retropubic colposuspension. (B) Sling procedure. (C) Bulking agents. (Used with permission from the American College of Obstetricians and Gynecologists. Surgery for stress urinary incontinence. *Patient Education Pamphlet AP166*. Washington, DC: American College of Obstetricians and Gynecologists; 2017.)

retropubic colposuspension have success rates of 85% at 5 years. Because data beyond 5 years are limited, patients should be made aware that surgery is not necessarily a permanent solution. Evidence suggests that the cure rate of stress incontinence with Burch colposuspension may decrease over 10 to 12 years, reaching a plateau at 69%.

Other suboptimal outcomes include partial continence only as well as urinary retention caused by overcorrection (making the sling too tight). Up to 10% of patients require at least one additional surgery to cure their stress incontinence.

URINARY TRACT INFECTIONS

An estimated 11% of the U.S. women report at least one physician-diagnosed UTI per year, and the lifetime probability that a woman will have a UTI is 60%. Most UTIs in women ascend from bacterial contamination of the urethra. Except in immunosuppressed patients and those with tuberculosis, infections are rarely acquired by hematogenous or lymphatic spread. The relatively short female urethra, exposure of the meatus to vestibular and rectal pathogens, and sexual activity that may induce trauma or introduce other organisms all increase the potential for infection (Box 30.1). Estrogen deficiency contributes to ascending contamination by causing a decrease in urethral resistance to infection. This increased susceptibility may explain the 20% prevalence of asymptomatic bacteriuria in women over age 65 years.

Of first infections, 90% are caused by *Escherichia coli*. The remaining 10% to 20% of UTIs are caused by other microorganisms, occasionally colonizing the vagina and periurethral area. *Staphylococcus saprophyticus* frequently causes lower UTIs. *Proteus*, *Pseudomonas*, *Klebsiella*, and *Enterobacter* species all have been isolated in women with cystitis or pyelonephritis. These bacteria are frequently associated with structural abnormalities of the urinary tract, indwelling catheters, and renal calculi. *Enterococcus* species have also been isolated in women with structural abnormalities. Gram-positive isolates, including group B streptococci, are increasingly isolated along with fungal infections in women with indwelling catheters.

Clinical History

Patients with **lower UTIs** typically present with symptoms of frequency, urgency, nocturia, and/or dysuria. The symptoms found vary somewhat with the site of the infection (i.e., symptoms of bladder or trigone irritation include urgency, frequency, and nocturia, whereas urethral irritation tends to lead to frequency and dysuria). Some patients may report suprapubic pain or discomfort of the urethra and bladder base. Fever is uncommon in women with uncomplicated lower UTI.

Upper UTI, or *acute pyelonephritis*, frequently occurs with a combination of fever and chills, flank pain, and varying degrees of dysuria, urgency, and frequency (Box 30.2).

Laboratory Evaluation

Evaluation of the patient suspected of having a UTI should start with urinalysis. A standard urinalysis will detect pyuria,

---

BOX 30.1 Risk Factors for Urinary Tract Infection

Premenopausal Women
- History of UTI
- Frequent or recent sexual activity
- Diaphragm contraception use
- Use of spermicidal agents
- Increasing parity
- Diabetes mellitus
- Obesity
- Sickle cell trait
- Anatomic congenital abnormalities
- Urinary tract calculi
- Neurologic disorders or medical conditions requiring indwelling or repetitive bladder catheterization

Postmenopausal Women
- Vaginal atrophy
- Incomplete bladder emptying
- Poor perineal hygiene
- Rectocele, cystocele, urethrocele, or uterovaginal prolapse
- Lifetime history of UTI
- Type 1 diabetes mellitus

From the American College of Obstetricians and Gynecologists. Treatment of urinary tract infections in nonpregnant women. ACOG Practice Bulletin No. 91. Washington, DC: American College of Obstetricians and Gynecologists; 2008; 111(3):785–794 (Reaffirmed 2016). Used with permission.

BOX 30.2 Urinary Tract Infections: Key Definitions

- *Asymptomatic bacteriuria*: Considerable bacteriuria in a woman with no symptoms
- *Cystitis*: Infection that is limited to the lower urinary tract and occurs with symptoms of dysuria and frequent and urgent urination and, occasionally, suprapubic tenderness
- *Acute pyelonephritis*: Infection of the renal parenchyma and pelvicalyceal system accompanied by significant bacteriuria, usually occurring with fever and flank pain
- *Relapse*: Recurrent UTI with the same organism after adequate therapy
- *Reinfection*: Recurrent UTI caused by bacteria previously isolated after treatment and a negative intervening urine culture result, or a recurrent UTI caused by a second isolate.

From the American College of Obstetricians and Gynecologists. Treatment of urinary tract infections in nonpregnant women. ACOG Practice Bulletin No. 91. Washington, DC: American College of Obstetricians and Gynecologists; 2008; 111(3):785–794 (Reaffirmed 2016). Used with permission.

defined as 10 leukocytes per milliliter, but pyuria alone is not a reliable predictor of infection; however, pyuria and bacteriuria together on microscopic examination markedly increase the probability of UTI. Treatment of a symptomatic lower UTI with pyuria or bacteriuria does not require a urine culture. However, if clinical improvement does not occur within 48 hours, or in the case of recurrence, a urine culture is useful to help tailor treatment.

A urine culture should be performed in all cases of upper UTIs, with the urine obtained as a "clean-catch midstream" sample. This involves cleansing the vulva and catching a portion of urine passed during the middle of uninterrupted voiding. Urine obtained from catheters or suprapubic aspiration may also be used.

"Dipstick" tests for infection based on the detection of leukocyte esterase are useful as screening tests; however, women with symptoms but negative test results should have a urine culture or urinalysis or both performed because false-negative results are common.

Cultures of urine samples that show colony counts of more than 100,000 for a single organism generally indicate infection. Colony counts as low as 10,000 for *E. coli* are associated with infection when symptoms are present. If a culture report indicates multiple organisms, contamination of the specimen should be suspected.

Treatment

Once infection is confirmed by urinalysis or culture, antibiotic therapy should be instituted. *Three days of therapy is comparable to longer durations of therapy, with eradication rates exceeding 90%.* Recommended agents for 3-day therapy include trimethoprim–sulfamethoxazole, trimethoprim, ciprofloxacin, levofloxacin, and gatifloxacin. Alternative agents include nitrofurantoin, fluoroquinolones, and ciprofloxacin.

In cases of acute pyelonephritis, treatment should be initiated immediately. The choice of drug should be based on the knowledge of resistance in the community. Once the urine and susceptibility culture results are available, therapy is altered as needed. Most women can be treated on an outpatient basis initially or given intravenous fluids and one parenteral dose of an antibiotic before being discharged and given a regimen of oral therapy.

Patients who are severely ill, have complications, are unable to tolerate oral medications or fluids, and are pregnant, or who the clinician suspects will be noncompliant with outpatient therapy should be hospitalized and should receive empiric broad-spectrum parenteral antibiotics.

Recurrence

Women with frequent recurrences of previously documented UTIs may be empirically treated without recurrent testing for pyuria. *Management of recurrent UTIs should start with a search for known risk factors associated with recurrence.* These include biologic or genetic factors, frequent intercourse, long-term spermicide use, diaphragm use, a new sexual partner, young age at first UTI, and a maternal history of UTI. Behavioral changes, such as using a different form of contraception instead of spermicide, should be advised.

The first-line intervention for the prevention of the recurrence of cystitis is prophylactic or intermittent antimicrobial therapy.

For women with frequent recurrences, continuous prophylaxis with once-daily treatment with nitrofurantoin, norfloxacin, ciprofloxacin, trimethoprim, trimethoprim–sulfamethoxazole, or another agent has been shown to decrease the risk of recurrence by 95%. Drinking cranberry juice has been shown to decrease symptomatic UTIs, but the length of therapy and the concentration required to prevent recurrence long term are not known. Recurrence is common in postmenopausal women; the hypoestrogenic state with associated genitourinary atrophy likely contributes to the increased prevalence.

Screening for and treatment of asymptomatic bacteriuria is not recommended in nonpregnant, premenopausal women. Specific groups for whom treatment of asymptomatic bacteriuria is recommended include all pregnant women, women undergoing a urologic procedure in which mucosal bleeding is anticipated, and women in whom catheter-acquired bacteriuria persists 48 hours after catheter removal. Treatment of asymptomatic bacteriuria in women with diabetes mellitus, older institutionalized patients, older patients living in a community setting, patients with spinal cord injuries, and patients with indwelling catheters is not recommended.

CLINICAL FOLLOW-UP

This patient's history is strongly suggestive of genuine stress incontinence, despite her not losing urine when coughing on the examination table. She is scheduled to undergo urodynamic testing, which can provide more sensitive evaluation of voiding function. The patient is shown to have a normal voiding pattern, but there is also evidence of genuine stress incontinence with no evidence of urge incontinence. She is instructed in performing Kegel exercises every day for 6 weeks. Upon return, her incontinence is significantly improved, and she no longer needs to wear a pad.

CHAPTER 31
Endometriosis

This chapter deals primarily with APGO Educational Topic Area:

TOPIC 38 ENDOMETRIOSIS

Students should be able to discuss pathogenesis and common sites affected by endometriosis. They should outline a basic approach to the diagnosis of endometriosis, using common symptoms and physical examination findings, and to the management of endometriosis.

CLINICAL CASE

A 32-year-old gravida 0 woman presents with symptoms of cyclic lower abdominal pain, dysmenorrhea, and inability to conceive after trying unprotected intercourse for the past year. Her partner had a semen analysis performed, and it is reported to be normal. The patient's abdominal pain generally starts 1 to 2 days before her menses and lasts for the first day or so of menstrual flow. This pain has gradually worsened since the past 2 years and is no longer well-controlled with nonsteroidal anti-inflammatory medications. The patient has recently begun experiencing deep-thrust dyspareunia. The patient's periods have been regular with occasional episodes of midcycle spotting.

INTRODUCTION

Endometriosis is the presence of endometrial glands and stroma in any extrauterine site and may be suspected based on history, symptoms, and physical examination as well as laboratory and imaging information. Like the endometrial tissue from which it is derived, endometrial implants and cysts respond to the hormonal fluctuations of the menstrual cycle. Laparotomy or laparoscopy may reveal lesions consistent with endometriosis, but because lesions may be small, atypical, or caused by pathology other than endometriosis, only proven tissue biopsy is diagnostic.

It is estimated that 7% to 10% of women in the general population have endometriosis. Pelvic endometriosis is present in 6% to 43% of women undergoing sterilization, 12% to 32% of women undergoing laparoscopy for pelvic pain, and 21% to 48% of women undergoing laparoscopy for infertility. Endometriosis usually occurs in women of reproductive age and is less frequently found in postmenopausal women. Endometriosis occurs more often in women who have never had children. Many women with endometriosis are asymptomatic, and diagnosis is discovered only when surgery is performed for other indications.

Some evidence suggests that endometriosis may have a genetic component. Women with first-degree relatives with endometriosis have a 7- to 10-fold increased risk of developing endometriosis. The proposed mechanism of inheritance is polygenic and multifactorial.

PATHOGENESIS

The exact mechanisms by which endometriosis develops are not clearly understood. Three major theories are commonly cited:

1. Direct implantation of endometrial cells, typically by means of **retrograde menstruation** (Sampson theory): This mechanism is consistent with the occurrence of pelvic endometriosis and its predilection for the ovaries and pelvic peritoneum, as well as for sites such as an abdominal incision or episiotomy scar. (Many women experience some degree of retrograde menstruation without developing endometriosis.)
2. **Vascular and lymphatic dissemination** of endometrial cells (Halban theory): Distant sites of endometriosis can be explained by this process (i.e., endometriosis in locations such as lymph nodes, the pleural cavity, and kidney).
3. **Coelomic metaplasia** of multipotential cells in the peritoneal cavity (Meyer theory): Under certain conditions, these cells can develop into functional endometrial tissue. This could even occur in response to the irritation caused by retrograde menstruation. The early development of endometriosis in some adolescents before the onset of menstruation lends credence to this theory.

It is probable that more than one theory is necessary to explain the diverse nature and locations of endometriosis. Underlying all these possibilities is a yet undiscovered immunologic factor that would explain why some women develop endometriosis, whereas others with similar characteristics do not.

PATHOLOGY

Endometriosis is most commonly found on the ovaries and is typically bilateral. Other common pelvic structures involved include the pouch of Douglas or posterior cul-de-sac (particularly the uterosacral ligaments and rectovaginal septum), the round ligament, the fallopian tubes, and the sigmoid colon (Fig. 31.1 and Table 31.1). On rare occasions, distant endometriosis is found in abdominal surgical scars, the umbilicus, and various organs outside the pelvic cavity, including the lungs, brain, and upper ureters.

The gross appearance of endometriosis varies considerably and includes the following forms:

- Small (1 mm), clear, or white lesions
- Small, dark red ("mulberry"), or brown ("powder burn") lesions
- Cysts filled with dark red or brown hemosiderin-laden fluid ("chocolate" cysts)
- Dark red or blue "domes" that may reach 15 to 20 cm in size

Reactive fibrosis frequently surrounds these lesions, which gives a puckered appearance. More advanced disseminated disease causes further fibrosis and may result in dense adhesions.

SIGNS AND SYMPTOMS

Women with endometriosis demonstrate a wide variety of symptoms. The nature and severity of symptoms may not match either the location or extent of the disease. Women with grossly extensive endometriosis may have few symptoms, whereas those with minimal gross endometriosis may have severe pain. Endometriosis may also be asymptomatic. The pain associated with endometriosis is thought to depend more on the depth of invasion of the implants rather than on the number or extent of the superficial implants.

The classic symptoms of endometriosis include progressive dysmenorrhea and deep dyspareunia. Some patients experience chronic, unremitting pelvic discomfort along with dysmenorrhea and dyspareunia. Chronic pelvic pain may be related to the adhesions and pelvic scarring found in association with endometriosis.

Dysmenorrhea and Dyspareunia

Dysmenorrhea caused by endometriosis is not directly related to the amount of visible disease. In many women with endometriosis, the dysmenorrhea worsens over time. Endometriosis should be considered a possible etiology in patients who present with

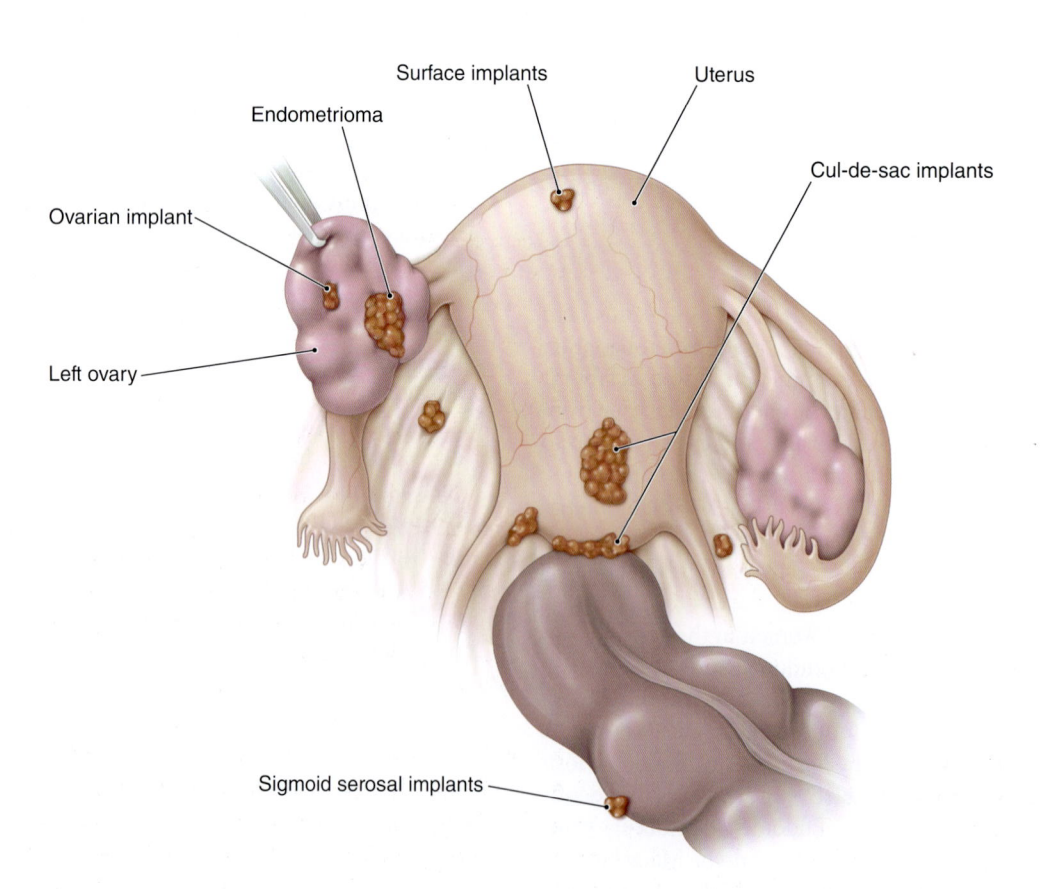

FIGURE 31.1. Locations of endometrial implants.

TABLE 31.1	SITES OF ENDOMETRIOSIS
Site	Frequency (Percentage of Patients)
Most common	60
• Ovary (often bilateral)	
• Pelvic peritoneum over the uterus	
• Anterior and posterior cul-de-sacs	
• Uterosacral ligaments	
• Fallopian tubes	
• Pelvic lymph nodes	
Infrequent	10–15
• Rectosigmoid	
• Other gastrointestinal tract sites	
• Vagina	
Rare	5
• Umbilicus	
• Episiotomy or surgical scars	
• Kidney	
• Lungs	
• Arms	
• Legs	
• Nasal mucosa	

dysmenorrhea that does not respond to oral contraceptives or nonsteroidal anti-inflammatory drugs (NSAIDs). Dyspareunia is often associated with uterosacral or deep posterior cul-de-sac involvement with endometriosis. The dyspareunia is typically reported on deep penetration, although there is no correlation between dyspareunia and the extent of endometriosis.

Infertility

Infertility is more frequent in women with endometriosis, although a cause-and-effect relationship has not been established. With extensive disease, pelvic scarring and adhesions that distort pelvic anatomy may cause infertility secondary to tubal distortion, but the cause of infertility in women with minimal endometriosis is unclear. Prostaglandins and autoantibodies have been implicated, but these relationships remain unproven. In some cases, infertility may be the only complaint, and endometriosis is discovered at the time of laparoscopic evaluation as part of the infertility workup. The presence of endometriosis in asymptomatic infertility patients varies between 30% and 50%.

Other Symptoms

Other, less common symptoms of endometriosis include gastrointestinal (GI) symptoms, such as rectal bleeding and **dyschezia** (painful bowel movements), in patients with endometrial implants on the bowel and urinary symptoms such as hematuria in patients with endometrial implants on the bladder or ureters. Occasionally, patients may present with an acute abdominal emergency, which may be associated with the rupture or torsion of an endometrioma.

Other Signs

Pelvic examination may reveal the "classic" sign of uterosacral nodularity associated with endometriosis, but it is often absent even when substantial gross endometriosis is discovered at surgery. The uterus may be relatively fixed and retroflexed in the pelvis because of extensive adhesions. Ovarian endometriomas may be tender, palpable, and freely mobile in the pelvis, or adhered to the posterior leaf of the broad ligament, the lateral pelvic wall, or the posterior cul-de-sac (see Fig. 31.2).

DIFFERENTIAL DIAGNOSIS

Depending on the symptoms, the differential diagnosis will change. In patients with chronic abdominal pain, diagnoses such as chronic pelvic inflammatory disease, pelvic adhesions, GI dysfunction, and other etiologies of chronic pelvic pain should be considered. In patients with dysmenorrhea, both primary dysmenorrhea and secondary dysmenorrhea should be considered. In patients with dyspareunia, differential diagnoses include chronic pelvic inflammatory disease, ovarian cysts, and symptomatic uterine retroversion. Sudden abdominal pain may be caused by a ruptured endometrioma as well as by ectopic pregnancy, acute pelvic inflammatory disease, adnexal torsion, and rupture of a corpus luteum cyst or ovarian neoplasm.

DIAGNOSIS

Endometriosis should be suspected in patients with the previously described symptoms. Many symptomatic women have normal findings on pelvic examination. The diagnosis of endometriosis can be suspected by direct visualization during laparoscopy or laparotomy and confirmed by tissue biopsy. Because endometriosis has various gross appearances, tissue biopsy and confirmation of endometrial glands and stroma are required for diagnosis. The presence of two or more of the following histologic features is used as the threshold criteria for the diagnosis by a pathologist:

- Endometrial epithelium
- Endometrial glands
- Endometrial stroma
- Hemosiderin-laden macrophages

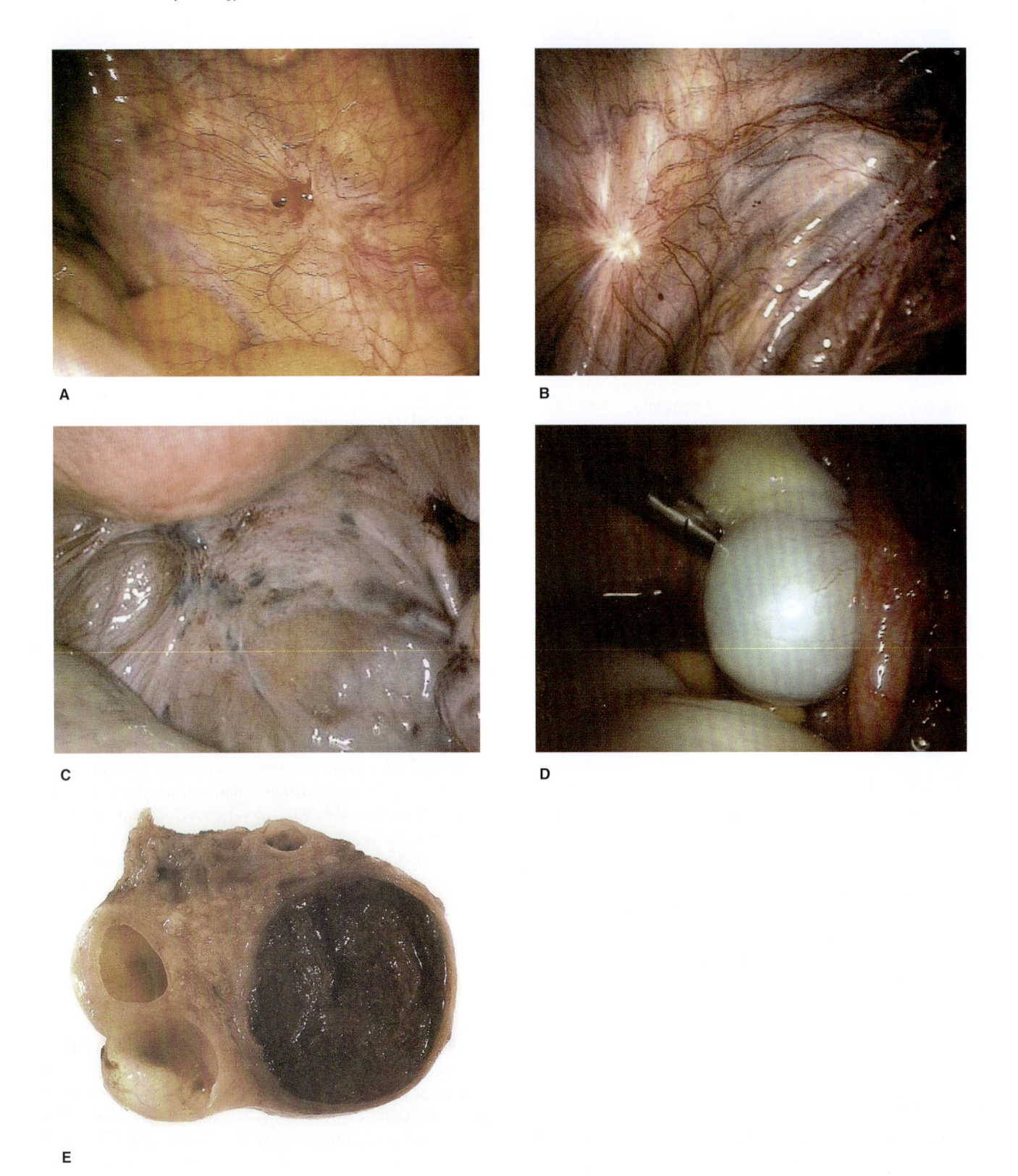

FIGURE 31.2. Endometrial implants. (A) clear lesion on the ovarian fossa; (B) white endometriotic deposit on the left uterosacral ligament; (C) "powder burn" lesion on the uterosacral ligaments; (D) right ovarian endometrioma; (E) chocolate cyst in an ovary containing other smaller fibrous-filled cavities. (From Overton C, Davis C, McMillan L, Shaw RW. *An Atlas of Endometriosis.* 3rd ed. London, U.K.: Informa UK; 2007:3.2, 4.2, 5.3, 5.4, 9.55.)

Because tissue confirmation of the diagnosis of endometriosis requires a surgical procedure, investigators have searched for a noninvasive alternative. Increased serum CA-125 levels have been correlated with moderate to severe endometriosis. However, because CA-125 levels may be elevated in many conditions (e.g., uterine fibroids, ovarian epithelial cancer, and pelvic inflammation) and nongynecologic sources (including cirrhosis and pancreatic and lung cancers) as well as in smokers, the clinical utility of using it as a diagnostic marker is limited.

Imaging

Imaging studies, such as ultrasonography, magnetic resonance imaging (MRI), and computed tomography, appear to be useful only in the presence of a pelvic or adnexal mass. Ultrasonography may be used to visualize ovarian endometriomas, which typically appear as cysts containing low-level, homogeneous internal echoes consistent with old blood. MRI may detect deeply infiltrating endometriosis that involves the uterosacral ligaments and the cul-de-sac but lacks sensitivity in detecting rectal involvement.

Classification

Once endometriosis is diagnosed, its extent and severity should be documented. The most widely accepted classification system has been established by the American Society for Reproductive Medicine (Fig. 31.3). Although this classification scheme has limitations, it provides a uniform system for recording findings and comparing the results of various therapies.

● TREATMENT

Available therapies include expectant, hormonal, surgical, and combination medical-and-surgical treatment. The choice of treatment depends on the patient's individual circumstances, which include (1) the presenting symptoms and their severity, (2) the location and severity of endometriosis, and (3) the desire for future childbearing. No treatment provides a permanent cure. Total abdominal hysterectomy with bilateral salpingo-oophorectomy is associated with a 10% risk of recurrent symptoms and a 4% risk of additional endometriosis. Reasonable goals for management of endometriosis include reduction in pelvic pain, minimizing surgical intervention, and preserving fertility.

Expectant Management

Patients can be treated expectantly (i.e., without either medical or surgical therapy) in some selected cases, including in those with limited disease whose symptoms are minimal or nonexistent and those who are attempting to become pregnant. Because endometriosis responds to estrogen and progesterone, older patients with mild symptoms may opt to wait until the natural decrease in levels of these hormones that occurs with menopause.

Medical Therapy

Because the glands and stroma of endometriosis respond to both exogenous and endogenous hormones, suppression of endometriosis is based on a medication's potential ability to induce atrophy of the endometrial tissue. This treatment approach is optimal for patients who are currently symptomatic, have documented endometriosis beyond minimal disease, and desire pregnancy in the future. The patient should be aware that recurrence after the completion of medical therapy is common and that medical therapy does not affect adhesions and fibrosis caused by the endometriosis. Medical therapy may often be instituted empirically without a definitive surgical diagnosis of endometriosis, if the patient's symptoms are consistent with the disease and appropriate, thorough physical examination and workup have been performed to rule out other causes of pain, including gynecologic, GI, and urologic causes.

Oral Contraceptives

Because of their ease of administration and relatively low level of side effects, combined oral contraceptives used in conjunction with NSAIDs are often the first line of treatment for pain associated with endometriosis. Oral contraceptive therapy induces a decidual reaction in the functioning endometriotic tissue. Continuous therapy, in which the oral contraceptive regimen is taken continuously without the 7 days of inactive pills that induce withdrawal bleeding, can also be prescribed to prevent secondary dysmenorrhea.

Progesterone therapy, in the form of subcutaneous depot medroxyprogesterone acetate (DMPA) or implants, suppresses gonadotropin release and, in turn, ovarian steroidogenesis; it also directly affects the uterine endometrium and endometrial implants. DMPA has been associated with an increased risk of bone mineral loss, although bone mineral density returned to pretreatment levels 12 months after treatment (see Chapter 26). Daily oral medroxyprogesterone is an option for women who are trying to become pregnant insofar as it does not offer a reliable contraceptive effect.

Other Pharmacologic Agents

Danazol is a medication that suppresses both luteinizing hormone (LH) and follicle-stimulating hormone (FSH) midcycle surges. In the absence of LH and FSH stimulation, the ovary no longer produces estrogen, which induces amenorrhea and endometrial atrophy. Side effects of danazol, which occur in a minority of patients, are related to its hypoestrogenic and androgenic properties and include acne, spotting and bleeding, hot flushes, oily skin, growth of facial hair, decreased libido, atrophic vaginitis, and deepening of the voice. Some of these side effects do not resolve with the discontinuation of therapy. Lipoprotein metabolism is also altered; serum high-density lipoprotein levels increase significantly, whereas low-density lipoprotein levels decrease.

Comparable symptom relief can be achieved with fewer effects using gonadotropin-releasing hormone (GnRH)

American Society for Reproductive Medicine
Revised Classification of Endometriosis

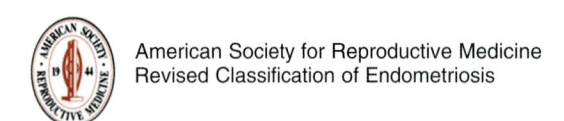

Patient's name _____ Date _____

Stage I (minimal) — 1–5
Stage II (mild) — 6–15
Stage III (moderate) — 16–40
Stage IV (severe) — >40

Laparoscopy _____ Laparotomy _____ Photography _____
Recommended treatment _____

Total _____ Prognosis _____

Peritoneum	Endometriosis	<1 cm	1–3 cm	>3 cm
	Superficial	1	2	4
	Deep	2	4	6
Ovary	R Superficial	1	2	4
	Deep	4	16	20
	L Superficial	1	2	4
	Deep	4	16	20
	Posterior cul-de-sac obliteration	Partial		Complete
		4		40
	Adhesions	<1/3 Enclosure	1/3–2/3 Enclosure	>2/3 Enclosure
Ovary	R Filmy	1	2	4
	Dense	4	8	16
	L Filmy	1	2	4
	Dense	4	8	16
Tube	R Filmy	1	2	4
	Dense	4*	8*	16
	L Filmy	1	2	4
	Dense	4*	8*	16

*If the fimbriated end of the fallopian tube is completely enclosed, change the point assignment to 16. Denote appearance of superficial implant types as red [(R), red, red-pink, flamelike, vesicular blobs, clear vesicles], white [(W), opacifications, peritoneal defects, yellow-brown], or black [(B), black, hemosiderin deposits, blue]. Denote percent of total described as R__%, W__%, and B__%. Total should equal 100%.

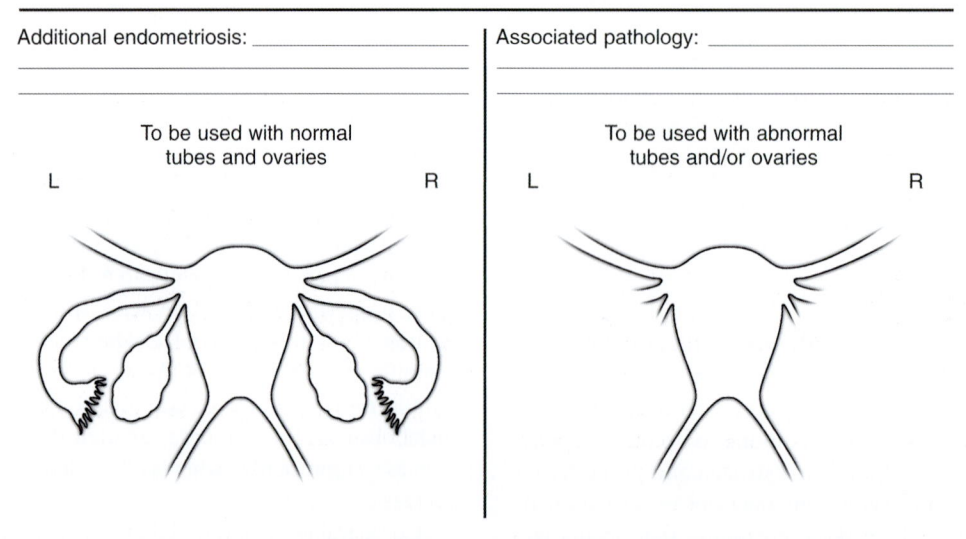

Additional endometriosis: _____   Associated pathology: _____

To be used with normal tubes and ovaries

To be used with abnormal tubes and/or ovaries

FIGURE 31.3. Revised American Society for Reproductive Medicine classification of endometriosis. (Reprinted from American Society for Reproductive Medicine. Revised American Society for Reproductive Medicine classification of endometriosis: 1996. *Fertil Steril.*; 1997;67(5):817–821, with permission from the American Society for Reproductive Medicine.)

Examples & Guidelines

Stage I (minimal)

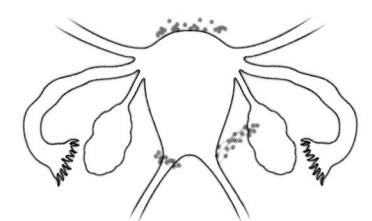

Peritoneum
  Superficial endo — 1–3 cm   −2
R. ovary
  Superficial endo — <1 cm   −1
  Filmy adhesions — <1/3   −1
Total points   4

Stage II (mild)

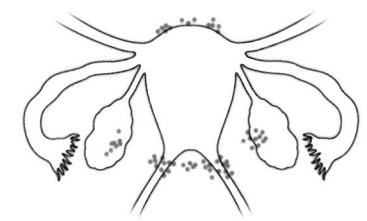

Peritoneum
  Deep endo — >3 cm   −6
R. ovary
  Superficial endo — <1 cm   −1
  Filmy adhesions — <1/3   −1
L. ovary
  Superficial endo — <1 cm   −1
Total points   9

Stage III (moderate)

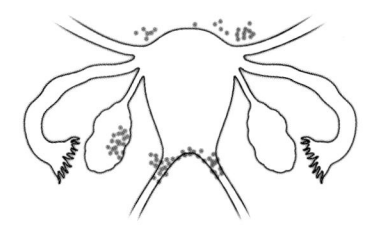

Peritoneum
  Deep endo — >3 cm   −6
Cul-de-sac
  Partial obliteration   −4
L. ovary
  Deep endo — 1–3 cm   −16
Total points   26

Stage III (moderate)

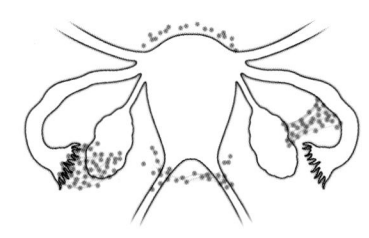

Peritoneum
  Superficial endo — >3 cm   −4
R. tube
  Filmy adhesions — <1/3   −1
R. ovary
  Filmy adhesions — <1/3   −1
L. tube
  Dense adhesions — <1/3   −16*
L. ovary
  Deep endo — <1 cm   −4
  Dense adhesions — <1/3   −4
Total points   30

Stage IV (severe)

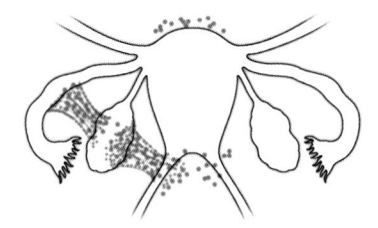

Peritoneum
  Superficial endo — >3 cm   −4
L. ovary
  Deep endo — 1–3 cm   −32†
  Dense adhesions — <1/3   −8†
L. tube
  Dense adhesions — <1/3   −8†
Total points   52

*Point assignment changed to 16.
†Point assignment doubled.

Stage IV (severe)

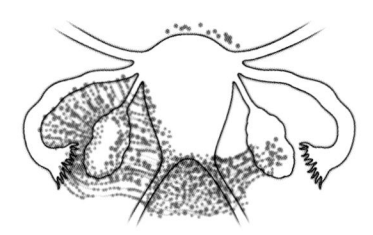

Peritoneum
  Deep endo — >3 cm   −6
Cul-de-sac
  Complete obliteration   −40
R. ovary
  Deep endo — 1–3 cm   −16
  Dense adhesions — <1/3   −4
L. tube
  Dense adhesions — >2/3   −16
L. ovary
  Deep endo — 1–3 cm   −16
  Dense adhesions — >2/3   −16
Total points   114

---

*Determination of the stage or degree of endometrial involvement is based on a weighted point system. Distribution of points has been arbitrarily determined and may require further revision or refinement as knowledge of the disease increases.

To ensure complete evaluation, inspection of the pelvis in a clockwise or counterclockwise fashion is encouraged. Number, size, and location of endometrial implants, plaques, endometriomas, and/or adhesions are noted. For example, five separate 0.5-cm superficial implants on the peritoneum (2.5 cm total) would be assigned 2 points. (The surface of the uterus should be considered peritoneum.) The severity of the endometriosis or adhesions should be assigned the highest score only for peritoneum, ovary, tube, or cul-de-sac. For example, a 4-cm superficial and a 2-cm deep implant of the peritoneum should be given a score of 6 (not 8). A 4-cm deep endometrioma of the ovary associated with more than 3 cm of superficial disease should be scored 20 (not 24).

In those patients with only one adnexa, points applied to disease of the remaining tube and ovary should be multiplied by two.

†Points assigned may be circled and totaled. Aggregation of points indicates stage of disease (minimal, mild, moderate, or severe).

The presence of endometriosis of the bowel, urinary tract, fallopian tube, vagina, cervix, skin, etc., should be documented under "additional endometriosis." Other pathology such as tubal occlusion, leiomyomata, uterine anomaly, etc, should be documented under "associated pathology." All pathology should be depicted as specifically as possible on the sketch of pelvic organs, and means of observation (laparoscopy or laparotomy) should be noted.

FIGURE 31.3. (*cont.*)

agonists. GnRH agonists downregulate the pituitary gland and cause marked suppression of LH and FSH. However, the side effects are less severe than those of danazol, because androgenic side effects are eliminated. However, the hypoestrogenic effect produced by GnRH agonists may cause hot flushes and night sweats and a slight increase in the risk of bone density loss. If a patient develops side effects while taking a GnRH agonist, if the therapy is required for longer than 6 months, or if repeated treatments are required, **add-back therapy** consisting of low-dose combination oral contraceptives, low-dose hormone therapy, or medroxyprogesterone should be considered. Norethindrone acetate 5 mg has been extensively studied and is also approved for this use by the Food and Drug Administration. Add-back therapy is often started with GnRH agonist therapy because it does not affect the drug's control of pelvic pain and mitigate the vasomotor and bone density side effects. Aromatase inhibitor therapy is also emerging as an alternative for the pain associated with endometriosis and may be considered for some patients.

Surgical Therapy

The surgical management of endometriosis can be classified as either conservative or extirpative.

Conservative Surgery

Conservative surgery includes excision, cauterization, or ablation (by laser or electrocoagulation) of visible endometriotic lesions; normalization of anatomy; and preservation of the uterus and other reproductive organs to allow for a possible future pregnancy. Conservative surgery is often undertaken at the time of the initial laparoscopy performed for pain or infertility. If extensive disease is found, conservative surgery involves lysis of adhesions; removal of active endometriotic lesions; and, possibly, reconstruction of reproductive organs. Success rates of conservative surgery appear to correlate with the severity of the disease at the time of surgery as well as with the skill of the surgeon. Medical therapy can be instituted before surgery to reduce the amount of endometriosis and after surgery to facilitate healing and prevent recurrence. Pregnancy rates following electrical energy or argon laser range from 34% to 75%. Pregnancy rates after carbon dioxide laser vaporization range from 25% to 100% for stage 2 disease, from 19% to 66% for stage 3 disease, and from 25% to 50% for stage 4 disease.

Extirpative Surgery

Extirpative surgery for endometriosis is reserved only for cases in which the disease is so extensive that conservative medical or surgical therapy is not feasible, or when the patient has completed her family and wishes definitive therapy. Definitive surgery includes total abdominal hysterectomy, bilateral salpingo-oophorectomy, lysis of adhesions, and removal of endometriotic implants. One or both ovaries may be spared if they are uninvolved, and the endometriosis can be resected completely. Approximately one-third of women treated conservatively will have recurrent endometriosis and require additional surgery within 5 years. Ovarian conservation at the time of hysterectomy carries an increased risk of recurrent endometriosis requiring additional surgery. After bilateral oophorectomy, estrogen therapy may be initiated immediately, with little risk of reactivating residual disease.

CLINICAL FOLLOW-UP

This patient's history is typical for endometriosis, and the patient was offered empiric treatment with an oral contraceptive, a gonadotropin-releasing hormone agonist, or diagnostic laparoscopy. Because of the patient's desire to achieve pregnancy in the shortest amount of time, she elected to undergo laparoscopic evaluation, which documented mild to moderate pelvic endometriosis with tubal scarring.

CHAPTER 32

Dysmenorrhea and Chronic Pelvic Pain

This chapter deals primarily with APGO Educational Topic Areas:

TOPIC 39   CHRONIC PELVIC PAIN

TOPIC 46   DYSMENORRHEA

Students should be able to define chronic pelvic pain as well as primary and secondary dysmenorrhea and list common etiologies. They should be able to outline a basic approach to initial evaluation and management of these disorders. They should also appreciate the associated psychological and social issues.

CLINICAL CASE

A 17-year-old virginal woman complains of cyclic, sharp, crampy, lower abdominal pain that begins on the first day of her menstrual flow and lasts 2 to 3 days. Her periods are regular and heavy with clots. Pelvic examination is normal.

INTRODUCTION

Dysmenorrhea is defined as painful menstruation. This is often sufficiently severe that it prevents a woman from performing normal activities. It may also be accompanied by other symptoms, including diarrhea, nausea, vomiting, headache, and dizziness. Dysmenorrhea may be because of a clinically identifiable cause (**secondary dysmenorrhea**) or by an excess of prostaglandins, leading to painful uterine muscle activity (**primary dysmenorrhea**). The term **chronic pelvic pain** refers to noncyclic pelvic pain (not solely associated with menstruation) that lasts for 6 months or more. For most patients, diagnosis of dysmenorrhea or chronic pelvic pain is made by careful evaluation through history and physical examination. In some instances, evaluation using other modalities, including laparoscopy, may be needed. Once the diagnosis is established, therapies may be instituted.

DYSMENORRHEA

Primary and secondary dysmenorrhea are a source of recurrent disability for a significant number of women in their early reproductive years. It is uncommon for primary dysmenorrhea to occur during the first three to six menstrual cycles, when regular ovulation is not yet well established. The incidence of primary dysmenorrhea is greatest in women in their late teens to early twenties and declines with age. Secondary dysmenorrhea becomes more common as a woman ages, because it accompanies the rising prevalence of causal factors. Childbearing does not affect the occurrence of either primary or secondary dysmenorrhea.

Etiology

Primary Dysmenorrhea

Primary dysmenorrhea is caused by excess **prostaglandin F$_{2\alpha}$** (**PGF$_{2\alpha}$**) produced in the endometrium. Prostaglandin production in the endometrium normally increases under the influence of progesterone, reaching a peak at, or soon after, the start of menstruation. With the onset of menstruation, formed prostaglandins are released from the shedding endometrium. In addition to the increase in prostaglandins from endometrial shedding, necrosis of endometrial cells provides increased substrate arachidonic acid from cell walls for prostaglandin synthesis. Prostaglandins are potent smooth muscle stimulants that cause intense uterine contractions, resulting in intrauterine pressures that can exceed 400 mm Hg and baseline intrauterine pressures in excess of 80 mm Hg (normal baseline is about 20 mm Hg). PGF$_{2\alpha}$ also causes contractions in smooth muscle elsewhere in the body, resulting in nausea, vomiting, and diarrhea (Table 32.1). Besides PGF$_{2\alpha}$, prostaglandin E$_2$ (PGE$_2$) is also produced in the uterus. PGE$_2$, a potent vasodilator and inhibitor of platelet aggregation, has been implicated as a cause of primary menorrhagia.

Secondary Dysmenorrhea

Secondary dysmenorrhea is caused by structural abnormalities or disease processes that occur outside the uterus, within the uterine wall, or within the uterine cavity (Box 32.1). Common causes of secondary dysmenorrhea include **endometriosis** (the presence of endometrial glands and stroma outside of the uterus), **adenomyosis** (the presence of ectopic endometrial tissue within the myometrium), adhesions, **pelvic inflammatory disease** (**PID**), and **leiomyomata** (uterine fibroids).

Diagnosis

Patients with primary dysmenorrhea present with recurrent, month-after-month, spasmodic lower abdominal pain that

TABLE 32.1 PAIN AND ASSOCIATED SYSTEMIC SYMPTOMS IN PRIMARY DYSMENORRHEA

Symptom	Estimated Incidence (%)
Pain: spasmodic, colicky, labor like; sometimes described as an aching or heaviness in lower middle abdomen; may radiate to the back and down the thighs; starts at the onset of menstruation; lasts hours to days	100
Associated symptoms	
Nausea and emesis	90
Tiredness	85
Nervousness	70
Dizziness	60
Diarrhea	60
Headache	50

BOX 32.1 Causes of Secondary Dysmenorrhea

Extrauterine Causes
- Endometriosis
- Tumors (benign and malignant)
- Inflammation
- Adhesions
- Psychogenic (rare)
- Nongynecologic

Intramural Causes
- Adenomyosis
- Leiomyomata

Intrauterine Causes
- Leiomyomata
- Polyps
- Intrauterine contraceptive devices
- Infection
- Cervical stenosis and cervical lesions

occurs on the first 1 to 3 days of menstruation. **Dyspareunia** is generally not found in patients with primary dysmenorrhea and, if present, should suggest a secondary cause.

Symptoms

In patients with primary dysmenorrhea, the pain is often diffusely located in the lower abdomen and suprapubic area, with radiation around or through to the back. The pain is described as "coming and going," or similar to labor. This pain is frequently accompanied by moderate-to-severe nausea, vomiting, and diarrhea. Fatigue, low backache, and headache are also common. Patients often assume a fetal position in an effort to gain relief, and many report having used a heating pad or hot water bottle in an effort to decrease their discomfort (a therapy that is enjoying resurgence in use).

In patients with secondary dysmenorrhea, the pain often lasts longer than the menstrual period. It may start before menstrual bleeding begins, become worse during menstruation, then persist after menstruation ends. Secondary dysmenorrhea often starts later in life than primary dysmenorrhea.

History

The specific complaints that an individual patient reports are determined by the underlying abnormality. Therefore, a careful medical history often suggests the underlying problem and helps direct further evaluations. Complaints of heavy menstrual flow combined with pain suggest uterine changes such as adenomyosis, leiomyomata, or polyps. Pelvic heaviness or a change in abdominal contour should raise the possibility of large leiomyomata or intra-abdominal neoplasia. Fever, chills, and malaise suggest infection. A coexisting complaint of infertility may suggest endometriosis or chronic PID or its sequelae.

Assessment

For patients with dysmenorrhea, the physical examination is directed toward uncovering possible causes of secondary dysmenorrhea. A pelvic examination may reveal asymmetry or irregular enlargement of the uterus, suggesting leiomyomata. Uterine leiomyomata are easily recognizable on bimanual examination by the irregular contour of the uterus and rubbery solid consistency of the fibroids. Adenomyosis may cause a tender, symmetrically enlarged, "boggy" uterus. Adenomyosis is supported by the exclusion of other causes of secondary dysmenorrhea, but definitive diagnosis can be made only by histologic examination of a hysterectomy specimen. Painful nodules in the posterior cul-de-sac and restricted motion of the uterus should suggest endometriosis (see Chapter 31). Restricted motion of the uterus is also found in cases of pelvic scarring from adhesions or inflammation. Thickening and tenderness of the adnexal structures caused by inflammation may suggest this diagnosis as the cause of secondary dysmenorrhea. Cultures or other tests of the cervix for *Neisseria gonorrhoeae* and *Chlamydia trachomatis* should be obtained if infection is suspected. In some patients, a final diagnosis may not be established without invasive procedures, such as laparoscopy.

In evaluating the patient thought to have primary dysmenorrhea, the most important differential diagnosis is that of secondary dysmenorrhea. Although the patient's history is often characteristic, primary dysmenorrhea should not be diagnosed without a thorough evaluation to eliminate other possible causes. Physical finding of patients with primary dysmenorrhea should be normal. There should be no palpable abnormalities of the uterus or adnexa, and no abnormalities should be found on speculum or abdominal examinations. Patients examined while experiencing symptoms often appear pale and diaphoretic, but the abdomen is soft and nontender, and the uterus is normal.

Therapy

Primary dysmenorrhea is an appropriate diagnosis for patients with dysmenorrhea in whom no other clinically identifiable cause is apparent. Patients with primary dysmenorrhea generally experience exceptional pain relief through the use of **nonsteroidal anti-inflammatory drugs** (**NSAIDs**), which are prostaglandin synthetase inhibitors. Other useful components of therapy for primary dysmenorrhea include the application of heat; exercise; psychotherapy and reassurance; and, on occasion, endocrine therapy (i.e., oral contraceptives to induce anovulation and pain relief [see Chapter 26]).

Nonsteroidal Anti-inflammatory Drugs

Ibuprofen, naproxen, and mefenamic acid are commonly prescribed NSAIDs for primary dysmenorrhea. For a time, selective cyclooxygenase inhibitors were becoming the NSAID of choice because of their targeted action. However, these drugs are now rarely used because of their potential association with life-threatening cardiovascular and gastrointestinal (GI) effects. Studies suggest that continuous low-level topical heat therapy can provide pain relief comparable to that offered by NSAID therapy without the systemic side effects that may occur with these drugs. Therapy with NSAIDs is generally so successful that, if some response is not evident, the diagnosis of primary dysmenorrhea should be reevaluated.

Combined Oral Contraceptives

Combined oral contraceptives can be useful in patients who do not desire childbearing and who do not have contraindications to their use. They work by suppressing ovulation and stabilizing estrogen and progesterone levels, with a resultant decrease in endometrial prostaglandins and spontaneous uterine activity. Oral contraceptives may be taken in the traditional 28-day cycle, or in an extended fashion that increases the interval between menses. The continuous use of oral contraceptives to eliminate menses can often eliminate dysmenorrhea altogether. Depot medroxyprogesterone acetate (Depo Provera), long-acting implantable progesterone contraceptives (Nexplanon), and progesterone intrauterine delivery systems (Mirena), although not designed for treatment of dysmenorrhea, have all been shown to decrease it.

Presacral Neurectomy

In the rare patient who does not respond to medical and other therapies and whose pain is so severe as to be incapacitating, **presacral neurectomy** may be a consideration. The procedure involves surgical disruption of the "presacral nerves," the superior hypogastric plexus, which is found in the retroperitoneal tissue from the fourth lumbar vertebra to the hollow over the sacrum. The risk of intraoperative complications, including injury to adjacent vascular structures and long-term sequelae such as chronic constipation, limits the use of this surgical procedure.

Therapy for Secondary Dysmenorrhea

For secondary dysmenorrhea, when a specific diagnosis is possible, therapy directed at the underlying condition is most likely to succeed. Specific treatments for many of these diagnoses are discussed in their respective chapters. When definitive therapy cannot be used—for example, in the case of a patient with adenomyosis who wishes to preserve fertility—symptomatic therapy in the form of analgesics or modification of the menstrual cycle may be effective.

CHRONIC PELVIC PAIN

Chronic pelvic pain is a common disorder that represents significant disability and utilization of resources. Estimates suggest that 15% to 20% of women aged 18 to 50 years have some level of chronic pelvic pain that lasts longer than 1 year. Although there is no generally accepted definition of chronic pelvic pain, one proposed definition is noncyclic pain lasting for more than 6 months that localizes to the anatomic pelvis, anterior abdominal wall at or below the umbilicus, the lumbosacral back, or the buttocks and is of sufficient severity to cause functional disability or lead to medical care.

Chronic pelvic pain may be caused by diseases of the reproductive, genitourinary, and GI tracts (Box 32.2 and Table 32.2). Other potential somatic sources of pain include the pelvic bones, ligaments, muscles, and fascia. Sometimes there is no clear etiology for the pain.

Assessment

The successful evaluation and treatment of chronic pelvic pain require time and a patient, caring physician. Effective management of this disease is dependent on a good physician–patient relationship, and the therapeutic effects of the relationship itself should not be overlooked. Taking the history and physical examination offer a time in which the physician may both gather information and establish a trusting rapport. The evaluation should begin with the presumption that there is an organic cause for the pain. Even in patients with obvious psychosocial stress, organic pathology can and does occur. Only when other reasonable causes have been ruled out should psychiatric diagnoses such as somatization, depression, or sleep and personality disorders be entertained.

History

As with the evaluation of any pain, attention must be paid to the description and timing of the symptoms involved. The history should include a thorough medical, surgical, menstrual, and sexual history. Specific questions regarding associated symptoms, provocative and palliative factors, and timing may help delineate the organ system from which the pain originates. Inquiries should be made into the patient's home and work status, social history, and family history (past and present). The

BOX 32.2 Gynecologic Conditions That May Cause or Exacerbate Chronic Pelvic Pain, by Level of Evidence

Level A[1]
- Endometriosis[2]
- Gynecologic malignancies (especially late stage)
- Ovarian retention syndrome (residual ovary syndrome)
- Ovarian remnant syndrome
- Pelvic congestion syndrome
- PID[2]
- Tuberculous salpingitis

Level B[3]
- Adhesions[2]
- Benign cystic mesothelioma
- Leiomyomata[2]
- Postoperative peritoneal cysts

Level C[4]
- Adenomyosis
- Atypical dysmenorrhea or ovulatory pain
- Adnexal cysts (nonendometriotic)
- Cervical stenosis
- Chronic ectopic pregnancy
- Chronic endometritis
- Endometrial or cervical polyps
- Endosalpingiosis
- Intrauterine contraceptive device
- Ovarian ovulatory pain
- Residual accessory ovary
- Symptomatic pelvic relaxation (genital prolapse)

[1] Level A: good and consistent scientific evidence of causal relationship to chronic pelvic pain.
[2] Diagnosis frequently reported in published series of women with chronic pelvic pain.
[3] Level B: limited or inconsistent scientific evidence of causal relationship to chronic pelvic pain.
[4] Level C: Based more on tradition and expert opinion than upon empiric evidence.

---

patient should be questioned about sleep disturbances and other signs of depression as well as a past history of physical and sexual abuse. Studies have found a significant correlation between a history of abuse and chronic pain. If a history of abuse is obtained, the patient should also be screened for any current physical or sexual abuse.

Physical Examination

Physical examination of patients with chronic pain is directed toward uncovering possible causative pathologies. The patient should be asked to indicate the location of the pain as a guide to further evaluation and to provide some indication of the character of the pain. If the pain is localized, the patient will point to a specific location with a single finger; if the pain is diffuse, the patient will use a sweeping motion of the whole hand. Maneuvers that duplicate the patient's complaint should be noted, but undue discomfort should be avoided to minimize guarding, which would limit a thorough examination. **Carnett sign** or tensing of the abdominal wall while raising the legs or chin in the supine position can help identify myofascial pain, which should increase with these maneuvers involving the rectus muscles. Visceral pain will decrease or remain unchanged with these maneuvers. In addition, care should be taken to examine for muscle spasm pain induced by the obturator internus muscle (abduct and internally rotate leg against pressure) and the levator ani muscles (tighten pelvic floor as if to stop urine or Kegel exercise).

Differential Diagnosis

Many of the same conditions that cause secondary dysmenorrhea may cause chronic pain states. As in the evaluation of patients with dysmenorrhea, cervical cultures should be obtained if infection is suspected. For most patients, a reasonably accurate differential diagnosis can be established through the history and physical examination. The wide range of differential diagnoses possible in chronic pelvic pain lends itself to a multidisciplinary approach, which might include psychiatric evaluation or testing. Consultation with social workers, physical therapists, gastroenterologists, anesthesiologists, orthopedists, and others should be considered. The use of imaging technologies or laparoscopy may also be required to determine a diagnosis. However, in approximately one-third of patients with chronic pelvic pain who undergo laparoscopic evaluation, no identifiable cause is found. Nevertheless, two-thirds of these patients have potential causes identified where none was apparent before laparoscopy.

Conditions That Increase the Risk of Chronic Pelvic Pain

Common disorders in women with chronic pelvic pain are PID, irritable bowel syndrome (IBS), interstitial cystitis, endometriosis, and adhesions. However, it is sometimes difficult to pinpoint a specific cause of chronic pelvic pain. Many women with chronic pelvic pain have more than one disease that might lead to pain.

Pelvic Inflammatory Disease

Approximately 18% to 35% of women who have had PID will develop chronic pelvic pain. The exact mechanism is unknown, but may involve chronic inflammation, adhesive disease, and the coexistence of psychosocial factors. PID is discussed in more detail in Chapter 29.

Irritable Bowel Syndrome

IBS occurs in 50% to 80% of women with chronic pelvic pain. The diagnosis of IBS is defined by the **Rome III criteria**: symptoms of recurrent abdominal pain or discomfort and a marked change in bowel habit for at least 6 months, with symptoms experienced on at least 3 days of at least 3 months. Two or more of the following must apply: (1) pain is relieved by a bowel

TABLE 32.2 NONGYNECOLOGIC CONDITIONS THAT MAY CAUSE OR EXACERBATE CHRONIC PELVIC PAIN, BY LEVEL OF EVIDENCE

Level of Evidence	Urologic	Gastrointestinal	Musculoskeletal	Other
Level A[a]	Bladder malignancy Interstitial cystitis[b] Radiation cystitis Urethral syndrome	Carcinoma of the colon Constipation Inflammatory bowel disease Irritable bowel syndrome[b]	Abdominal wall myofascial pain (trigger points) Chronic coccygeal or back pain[b] Faulty or poor posture Fibromyalgia Neuralgia of iliohypogastric, ilioinguinal, and/or genitofemoral nerves Pelvic floor myalgia (levator ani or piriformis syndrome) Peripartum pelvic pain syndrome	Abdominal cutaneous nerve entrapment in surgical scar Depression[b] Somatization disorder
Level B[c]	Uninhibited bladder contractions (detrusor dyssynergia) Urethral diverticulum	—	Herniated nucleus pulposus Low back pain[b] Neoplasia of spinal cord or sacral nerve	Celiac disease Neurologic dysfunction Porphyria Shingles Sleep disturbances
Level C[d]	Chronic urinary tract infection Recurrent, acute cystitis Recurrent, acute urethritis Stone/urolithiasis Urethral caruncle	Colitis Chronic intermittent bowel obstruction Diverticular disease	Compression of lumbar vertebrae Degenerative joint disease Hernias: ventral, inguinal, femoral, Spigelian Muscular strains and sprains Rectus tendon strain Spondylosis	Abdominal epilepsy Abdominal migraine Bipolar personality disorders Familial Mediterranean fever

[a] Level A: good and consistent scientific evidence of causal relationship to chronic pelvic pain.
[b] Diagnosis frequently reported in published series of women with chronic pelvic pain.
[c] Level B: limited or inconsistent scientific evidence of causal relationship to chronic pelvic pain.
[d] Level C: causal relationship to chronic pelvic pain based on expert opinions.

movement, (2) onset of pain is related to a change in frequency of stool, or (3) onset of pain is related to a change in the appearance of stool. IBS is often usefully subcategorized for purposes of treatment depending on the predominant complaint: pain, diarrhea, constipation, or alternating constipation and diarrhea. The pathophysiology of the syndrome is not clearly identified, but factors proposed to be involved include altered bowel motility, visceral hypersensitivity, psychosocial factors (especially stress), an imbalance of neurotransmitters (especially serotonin), and infection (often indolent or subclinical). A history of childhood sexual or physical abuse is highly correlated with the severity of symptoms experienced by those with IBS.

Interstitial Cystitis

Interstitial cystitis is a chronic inflammatory condition of the bladder that is often characterized by pelvic pain, urinary urgency and frequency, and dyspareunia. The proposed etiology is a disruption of the **glycosaminoglycan** layer that normally coats the mucosa of the bladder. The interstitial cystitis symptom index predicts the diagnosis of interstitial cystitis and may be used to help determine whether cystoscopy is indicated. Further evaluation can be done with bladder distention with water or intravesical potassium sensitivity testing.

THERAPY

Patients with chronic pelvic pain offer a therapeutic challenge. If possible, care should be directed at a specific cause. The use of analgesics should be on a fixed time schedule that is independent of symptoms.

Medical Therapy

Suppression of ovulation may be useful as either a therapeutic modality or a diagnostic tool to assist in ruling out ovarian or menstrual processes. **Gonadotropin-releasing hormone agonists** cause a central downregulation of the ovarian hormones and have been used in the treatment of endometriosis. These agents may also help relieve some of the symptoms of IBS, interstitial cystitis, and pelvic congestion syndrome (in which engorged pelvic blood vessels are purported to cause pelvic aching and pain), all of which are hormonally mediated to some extent.

Patients with symptoms characteristic of IBS should be referred to a gastroenterologist for further evaluation. The use of a food diary to identify and eliminate foods that are associated with symptoms, combined with the nurturing physician–patient relationship to avoid "doctor shopping" and episodic care, is the mainstay of treatment. Limiting caffeine, alcohol, fatty foods, and gas-producing vegetables is often helpful. Lactose or wheat gluten intolerance may be identified by the diary. If constipation is a major symptom, the consumption of 20 to 30 g of fiber or the use of osmotic laxatives such as lactulose is often useful. When diarrhea is a major symptom, antidiarrheals can be useful. Gas pain and cramping may be treated with antispasmodics such as dicyclomine and hyoscyamine.

Treatments for interstitial cystitis include dietary modification, intravesical agents, and oral agents aimed at decreasing inflammation and pain signals. As with IBS, caffeine, alcohol, artificial sweeteners, and acidic foods should be eliminated. **Dimethyl sulfoxide** is the only drug approved for direct bladder instillation to treat interstitial cystitis, although many physicians treat with a combination of anti-inflammatory and analgesic medications. Oral agents include antihistamines, tricyclic antidepressants, and **pentosan polysulfate sodium**, a glycosaminoglycan analog that may help reestablish the disrupted mucosa of the bladder.

Surgical Therapies

Surgical therapies, such as **hysterectomy**, should be performed only after nongynecologic causes have been ruled out. Hysterectomy is very effective in relieving pain arising from the uterus and may also improve symptoms in women without identifiable uterine pathology.

Other Therapies

Alternate treatment modalities such as transcutaneous electrical nerve stimulation, biofeedback, nerve blocks, laser ablation of the uterosacral ligaments, and presacral neurectomy may be used, as appropriate. Adding psychotherapy to medical treatment of chronic pelvic pain appears to improve response over that of medical treatment alone and should be considered. In some cases, the goal of treatment may not be a cure, that is, elimination of the chronic pain but, rather, successful management of the symptoms to allow maximal function and quality of life.

FOLLOW-UP

Patients being treated for pelvic pain (dysmenorrhea or chronic pain states) should be carefully monitored for success and the possibility of complications from the therapy. Patients on oral contraceptives for the first time should be asked to return for follow-up after 2 months and again after 6 months. Once successful therapy is established, routine periodic health maintenance visits should continue. Patients with chronic pelvic pain should be encouraged to return for follow-up on a periodic basis, rather than only when pain is present, thus avoiding reinforcing pain behavior as a means to an end.

CLINICAL FOLLOW-UP

This patient's history is typical of primary dysmenorrhea. Based on this determination, the patient was started on nonsteroidal anti-inflammatory therapy. The patient experienced immediate improvement in her cramps and coincidentally noted a slight reduction in her menstrual flow.

---

thePoint®   Visit http://thePoint.lww.com/activate for an interactive USMLE-style question bank and more!

CHAPTER 33

Disorders of the Breast

This chapter deals primarily with APGO Educational Topic Area:

TOPIC 40 DISORDERS OF THE BREAST

Students should be able to describe normal versus abnormal findings. They should outline a basic approach to patients with common breast complaints and breast cancer including evaluation and initial management.

CLINICAL CASE

A 26-year-old patient presents with a 2- to 3- cm smooth, painless, freely movable mass in her left breast. She reports that the mass becomes somewhat tender but does not change during her menstrual cycle and has grown slowly over the past year. The patient initially found the mass during breast self-examination.

INTRODUCTION

Diseases of the breast encompass a diverse spectrum of pathology, from benign breast disease to breast cancer. It is imperative that women's health care providers understand the evaluation, treatment, and surveillance of breast-related complaints. Providers must ensure appropriate breast cancer screening for all patients, whether at high or low risk. In order to properly evaluate, treat, and follow breast-related complaints, a multidisciplinary approach is often necessary. Although referral to a specialist is sometimes necessary, the obstetrician–gynecologist is often the first person a woman consults for breast-related signs and symptoms.

ANATOMY

The adult female breast is actually a modified sebaceous gland, located within the superficial fascia of the chest wall (Fig. 33.1). Histologically, the breast is composed primarily of lobules or glands, milk ducts, connective tissue, and fat. The relative amounts of these tissue types vary considerably with age. In younger women, the breast consists predominantly of glandular tissue. With age, the glands involute and are replaced by fat, a process accelerated by menopause. Differences in palpable consistency and in radiographic density between the glands and fat are key modifiers of breast cancer detection programs.

Architecturally, the breast is organized into 12 to 20 lobes, with a disproportionate amount of the glandular or lobular tissue in the upper outer quadrants of each breast. This disproportionate distribution of glandular tissue accounts for why breast cancer most commonly arises in the upper outer quadrant. The lobules consist of clusters of secretory cells arranged in an alveolar pattern and surrounded by myoepithelial cells. These glands drain into a series of collecting milk ducts that course through the breast, ultimately coalescing into approximately 5 to 10 collecting ducts that lead to and drain at the nipple. Typically, cancer begins at these terminal duct–lobular units of the breast and follows the path of those ducts.

Congenital anomalies of the breast can include absence of the breast as well as accessory breast tissue located anywhere along the "milk lines," which extend from the axilla to the groin. Extra nipples (**polythelia**) are more common than true accessory breasts (**polymastia**).

The breast has a rich blood supply and lymphatic system, which support milk production and overall breast health. The blood supply comes from perforating branches of the internal mammary artery, the lateral thoracic artery, the thoracodorsal artery, the thoracoacromial artery, and various intercostal perforating arteries. The lymphatic vessels lead to several superficial and deep nodal chains throughout the trunk and neck, including those located in the axilla, deep to the pectoralis muscles, and caudal to the diaphragm (Fig. 33.2). The ipsilateral lymph node and, occasionally, the internal mammary nodes are the most common route of metastasis.

Breast tissue is very sensitive to hormonal changes, especially the glandular cells. The transition from the immature, pediatric breast to the mature, adult breast is orchestrated by the changes in circulating levels of estrogen and progesterone that accompany puberty. **Estrogen** is primarily responsible for the growth of adipose tissue and lactiferous ducts. Conversely, **progesterone** stimulation leads to lobular growth and alveolar budding.

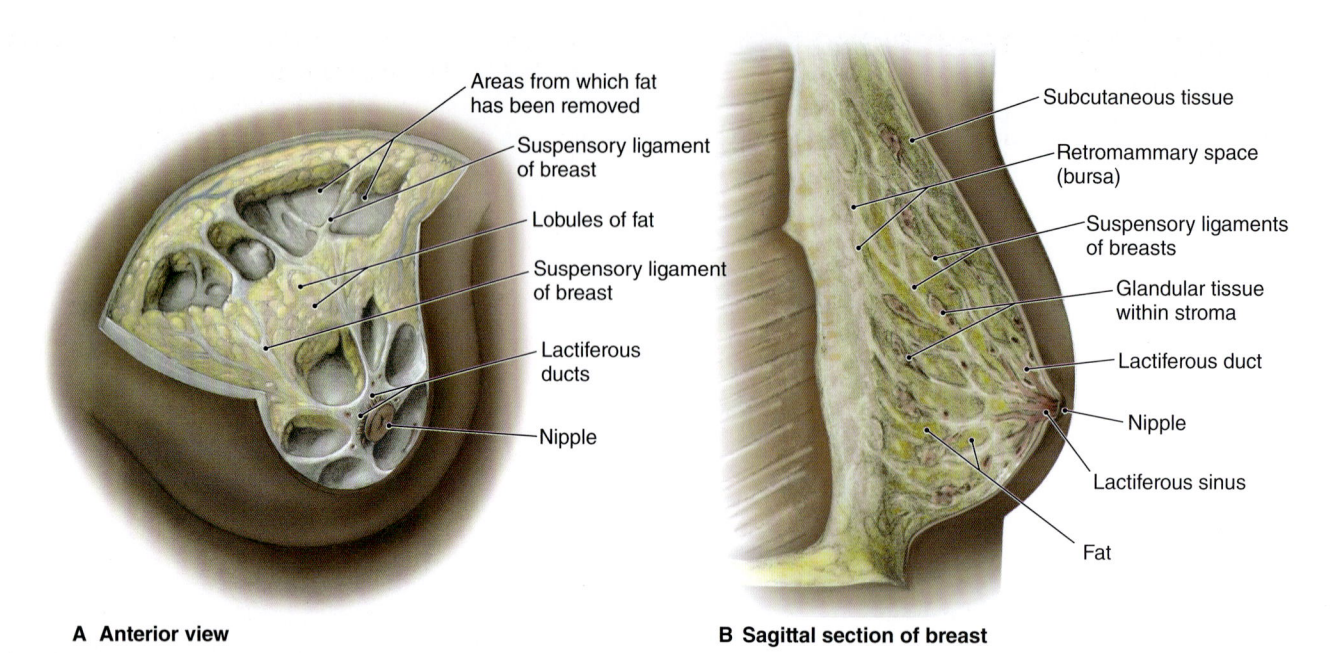

FIGURE 33.1. Anatomy of the breast. (From Agur A, Dalley AF. *Grant's Atlas of Anatomy.* 12th ed. Baltimore, MD: Lippincott Williams & Wilkins; 2008:5.)

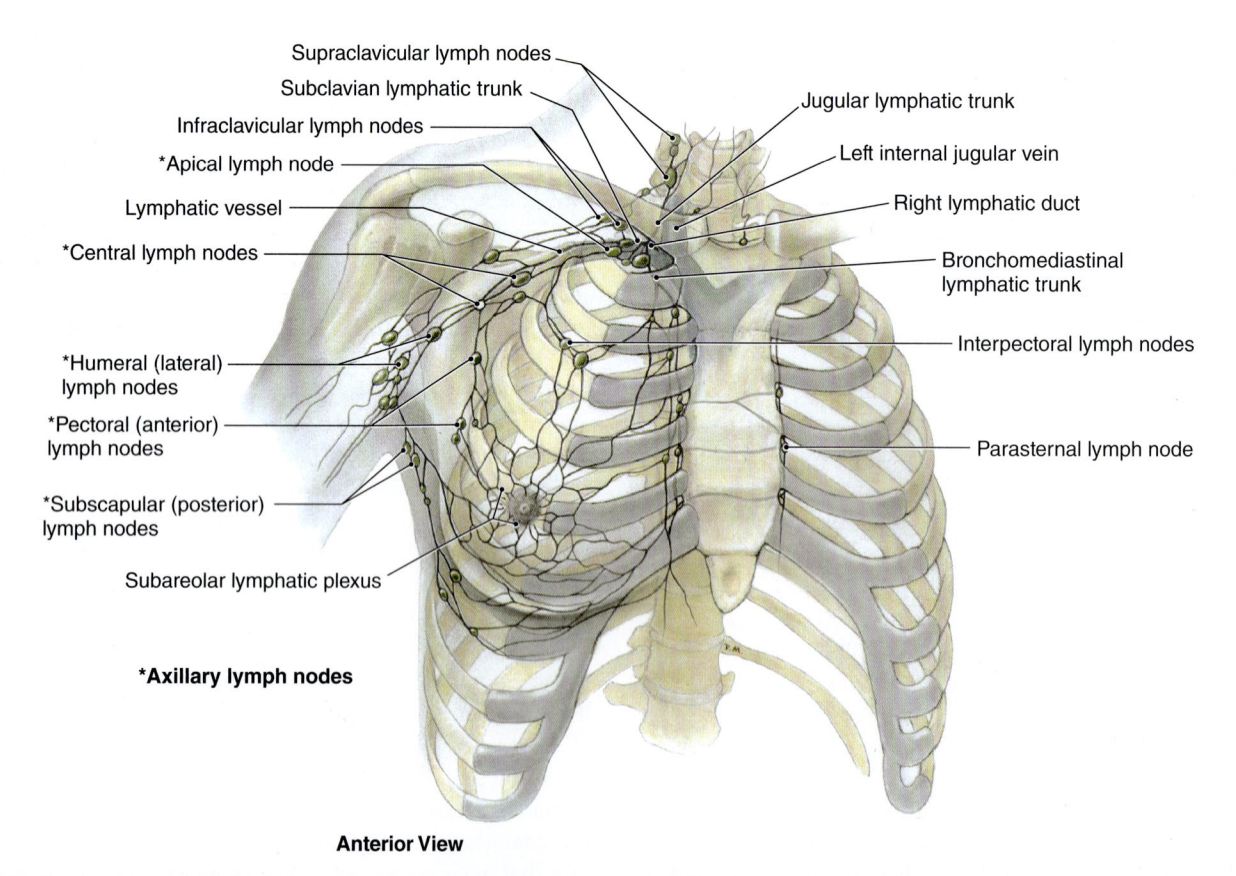

FIGURE 33.2. Lymphatic drainage of the breast. (From Agur A, Dalley AF. *Grant's Atlas of Anatomy.* 12th ed. Baltimore, MD: Lippincott Williams & Wilkins; 2008:5.)

EVALUATION OF BREAST SIGNS AND SYMPTOMS

A timely evaluation of the patient who presents with a breast complaint is important if for no other reason than to relieve patient anxiety. A systematic approach to evaluating a breast-related complaint will efficiently yield the proper diagnosis. The two most common presenting complaints related to the breast are pain and concern about a mass.

Physicians should be aware of the different etiologies of breast pain and be able to offer reassurance, follow-up, and potential treatment. One study has found that breast cancer was diagnosed in 6% of patients with breast complaints (most commonly a mass). Therefore, it is important that breast signs and symptoms be properly evaluated.

Patient History

The patient interview is considered the single most important step in the initial evaluation of any disease process. In the case of complaints related to the breast, questions that will aid in deciding the next step include the location of complaints, duration of symptoms, how a mass was first discovered, presence or absence of nipple discharge, any changes in size, and association with menstrual cycle. In addition, the clinician should ask about the presence of risk factors that would increase the likelihood of malignancy (Box 33.1).

Physical Examination

A complete breast examination should evaluate both breasts in a systematic fashion, both axillae and the entire chest wall. The best time to perform a breast examination is in the follicular phase of the menstrual cycle. If the initial examination fails to yield a dominant mass, the options (based on the patient's risk factors) include either performing a repeat examination in 3 months or referral to a specialized breast care clinic.

Diagnostic Testing

After performing a complete history and physical examination, a number of modalities can be used to help locate and characterize a breast mass.

Mammography
Mammography is an x-ray technique used to study the breast. Mammography is able to detect lesions approximately 2 years before they become palpable (Fig. 33.3).

Mammography can be done either as a screening or as a diagnostic test. During a screening mammogram, the patient stands or sits in front of the x-ray machine. Two smooth plastic plates are placed around the breast and subsequently compressed to allow for complete visualization of the tissue. A standard four-image screening mammogram involves two craniocaudal and two mediolateral images. Images are formed either on standard radiographic film or by digital means (digital radiography). Digital radiographic techniques offer more possibilities of "postprocessing" of the image to enhance detection but are more expensive. Digital mammography has become more widely available though no direct superiority has been proven for either technique. Digital mammogram may be preferred for women with more dense breast tissue. In each method, the images are evaluated for defects suspicious of cancer, microcalcifications, distortion of the normal architecture, and any discrete nonpalpable lesion. Lobular carcinoma is more difficult to detect with routine screening mammography.

In collaboration with the National Cancer Institute (NCI) and the Food and Drug Administration (FDA), the American

BOX 33.1 Risk Factors for Breast Cancer

- Age
- Personal history of breast cancer
- History of atypical hyperplasia (ductal or lobular) on past biopsies
- Inherited genetic mutations (*BRCA1* and *BRCA2*)
- High breast tissue density
- First-degree relatives with breast or ovarian cancer diagnosed at an early age
- Early menarche (age <12 years) or late cessation of menses (age >55 years)
- No term pregnancies
- Late age at first live birth (>30 years)
- Never breastfed
- Radiation exposure (chest)
- Recent and long-term oral contraceptive use
- Postmenopausal obesity
- Personal history of endometrial or ovarian cancer
- Ashkenazi Jewish heritage

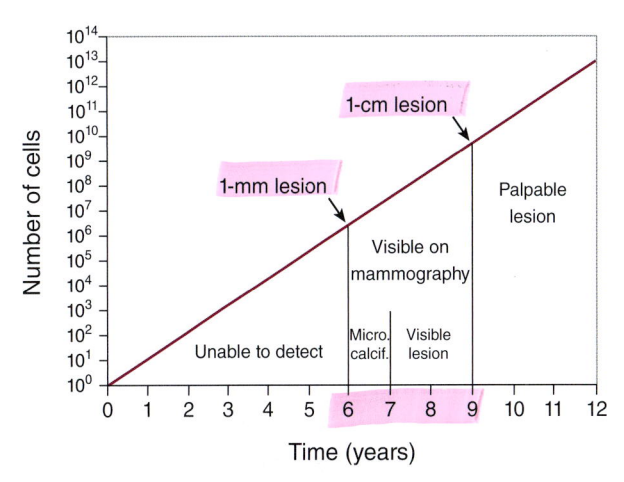

FIGURE 33.3. Mammographic and clinical detection of a breast mass. With a presumed doubling time of 100 days, breast cancer may be detected by mammography significantly earlier than it can be identified clinically. Micro calcif., microcalcification.

College of Radiology has standardized the reporting of mammographic results through a system known as the Breast Imaging Reporting and Data System (BI-RADS). This system helps clearly communicate the final assessment and recommendations to referring physicians (Table 33.1).

A diagnostic mammogram is done to supplement an abnormal screening mammogram or if a woman has a breast complaint and/or palpable mass. In women older than 40 years, mammography is often used as the first-line study in evaluating a patient presenting with a breast mass, even if not palpable on clinical breast examination (CBE). Spot compressions and magnified views are used to further localize any lesions, along with providing dimensions of the surrounding tissue (Fig. 33.4). The contralateral breast should also be imaged in cases of a clinically apparent mass. If possible, the lymph nodes are also imaged to search for unrecognized abnormalities.

Ultrasonography

Ultrasonography has come to play an important role in the evaluation of breast lesions. It is useful in evaluating inconclusive mammographic findings, in evaluating the breasts of young women and others with dense tissue, allowing better differentiation between a solid and cystic mass, and in guiding tissue core-needle biopsies. An anechoic defect found on ultrasound is consistent with a simple cyst and can be drained for symptomatic relief. In women younger than 30 years (especially adolescents), ultrasonography is the most common initial modality to evaluate a breast mass because the breast is mainly composed of glandular tissue.

Magnetic Resonance Imaging

Magnetic resonance imaging (MRI) can be a useful adjunct to diagnostic mammography.

The use of MRI for screening the general population is limited by the cost of the examination, lack of standard examination technique, and inability to detect microcalcifications. However, MRI is being used as an adjunct for early detection of breast cancer in women at very high risk, and it may also be used as part of postcancer breast diagnosis for further evaluation of breast involvement.

Fine-Needle Aspiration Biopsy

Fine-needle aspiration is useful in determining if a palpable lump is a simple cyst. The procedure is performed in the office with or without the aid of local anesthesia. The suspected mass is stabilized between two fingers of one hand and aspirated using a 22- to 24-gauge needle. Clear aspirated fluid does not need to undergo pathologic evaluation, and the patient may return for a CBE within 4 to 6 months if the mass disappears. If it reappears, the patient is managed with diagnostic mammography and ultrasonography. Bloody aspirated fluid should be evaluated cytologically, and the patient should undergo diagnostic mammography and ultrasonography.

Core-Needle Biopsy

In a **core-needle biopsy**, a large needle (14–16 gauge) is used to obtain samples from larger, solid breast masses. Three to six samples of tissue approximately 2 cm long are obtained and are evaluated for abnormal cells in relation to the surrounding breast tissue taken in the sample.

TABLE 33.1 AMERICAN COLLEGE OF RADIOLOGY BREAST IMAGING REPORTING AND DATA SYSTEM

BI-RADS Classification	Summary Recommendations	Explanation
0	Need additional imaging evaluation	A mammogram with a lesion that needs additional imaging, such as spot compression films, magnifications, and additional views
1	Negative	Breast appears normal
2	Benign findings	Negative mammogram but interpreter wishes to describe a finding
3	Probably benign finding	A mammogram with a lesion highly likely to be benign; follow-up is suggested to establish mammographic stability
4A	Low suspicion of malignancy	A lesion needing intervention
4B	Intermediate suspicion	Malignancy possible
4C	Moderate concern	No classic signs but malignancy expected
5	Highly suggestive of malignancy	A lesion with a high probability of being cancer—appropriate referral to a breast surgeon is needed
6	Known biopsy-proven malignancy	Appropriate action should be taken

BI-RADS, Breast Imaging Reporting and Data System.
Modified from Sickles EA, D'Orsi CJ, Bassett LW. ACR BI-RADS® mammography. In: *ACR BI-RADS® Atlas, Breast Imaging Reporting and Data System*. Reston, VA: American College of Radiology; 2013.

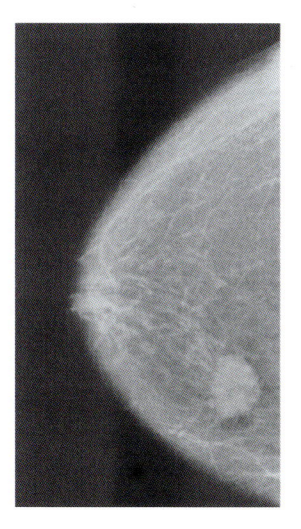

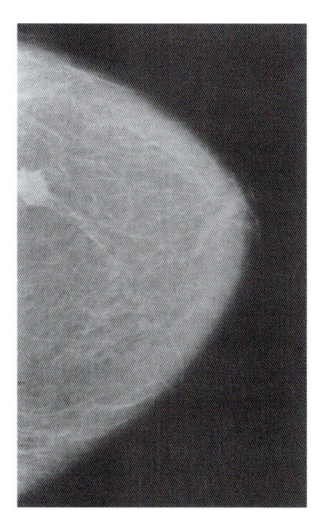

FIGURE 33.4. Bilateral film screen mammograms showing typical carcinoma in each breast, illustrating the importance of bilateral mammography in the workup of a clinically apparent mass. (Berek JS, Hacker NF. *Berek & Hacker's Practical Gynecologic Oncology*. 4th ed. Philadelphia, PA: Lippincott Williams & Wilkins; 2009.)

Diagnosis Algorithm

If a breast mass is found through a CBE, breast self-examination (BSE), or by a partner, the clinician must clearly document the finding and assign appropriate follow-up care. Figure 33.5 presents a practical algorithm for the evaluation and follow-up of a patient with a breast mass.

BENIGN BREAST DISEASE

Benign breast disease includes a large number of conditions that can significantly affect a woman's quality of life. With accurate diagnosis, many benign breast conditions can be effectively treated with medications or other measures. Women presenting with a breast mass should also be evaluated for their risk of breast cancer.

Mastalgia

Mastalgia, or breast pain, can be divided into three categories: cyclic, noncyclic, and extramammary (nonbreast) pain. **Cyclic mastalgia** begins with the luteal phase of the menstrual cycle and resolves after the onset of menses. The pain is generally bilateral and often involves the upper outer quadrants of the breast. **Noncyclic mastalgia** is not associated with the menstrual cycle and includes such etiologies as tumors, mastitis, cysts, and a history of trauma or breast surgery. In some women, noncyclic mastalgia is idiopathic, and no cause is found. Noncyclic pain has also been associated with some medications, including hormonal medications; antidepressants, such as sertraline and amitriptyline; and antihypertensive drugs, in addition to others. If the onset of mastalgia is associated with the start of hormonal therapy, stopping or reducing the hormones may be beneficial. **Extramammary pain** can be caused by a number of conditions, such as chest wall trauma, rib fractures, shingles, and fibromyalgia. Treatment for musculoskeletal disorders includes anti-inflammatory drugs, but more serious causes of chest pain, such as angina, need to be ruled out.

Medical Therapy

The only medication approved by the FDA for treating mastalgia is danazol, but it has significant side effects. Other hormonal therapies that may decrease pain include bromocriptine and gonadotropin-releasing hormone agonists, but these drugs also have side effects that limit their widespread use. Lisuride maleate is a dopamine agonist that has shown pain-reducing effects, and it has fewer side effects than bromocriptine. Selective estrogen receptor modulators (SERMs), such as tamoxifen, also have a role in treating severe mastalgia, though this is an off-label use of the medications. These medications act as estrogen antagonists in the breast. Side effects of tamoxifen include an increased risk of endometrial hyperplasia and deep venous thrombosis as well as hot flushes and vaginal bleeding. One study concluded that side effects are reduced when the medication is given in smaller doses. Tamoxifen should be used only for cases of severe mastalgia that does not respond to other therapies. Raloxifen, also an SERM, has been shown to decrease the incidences of breast cancer in high-risk women. Unlike tamoxifen, it does not stimulate the endometrium. Hot flashes and increased risk of venous thrombosis are similar to tamoxifen.

Some women with cyclic mastalgia have reported a decrease in pain with oral contraceptives or the injectable contraceptive medroxyprogesterone acetate.

Other Therapies

Nonpharmacologic measures to help relieve breast pain include a properly fitting brassiere or a sports bra worn throughout the day or during exercise, weight reduction, and regular exercise. Although no studies have demonstrated the efficacy of these measures, they are worth recommending to patients and may help relieve pain. Some patients report decreased mastalgia with decreased caffeine and vitamin E supplements but definitive studies have mixed results on effectiveness.

Nipple Discharge

Nipple discharge is usually benign but may be an early sign of endocrine dysfunction or cancer. The color, consistency, and whether the discharge is bilateral or unilateral can yield important clues about its cause. A nonspontaneous, nonbloody, bilateral nipple discharge is usually attributed to fibrocystic changes of the breast or **ductal ectasia,** a condition characterized by dilation of the mammary ducts, periductal fibrosis, and inflammation. Ductal ectasia is seen in adolescent women as well as in perimenopausal women. Green, yellow, or brown sticky discharge can be due to ductal ectasia or fibrocystic changes of the breast. Milky discharge is common during childbearing, but it can also be associated with other endocrinologic abnormalities (hyperprolactinemia or hypothyroidism) and medications (oral contraceptives and tricyclic antidepressants). Purulent

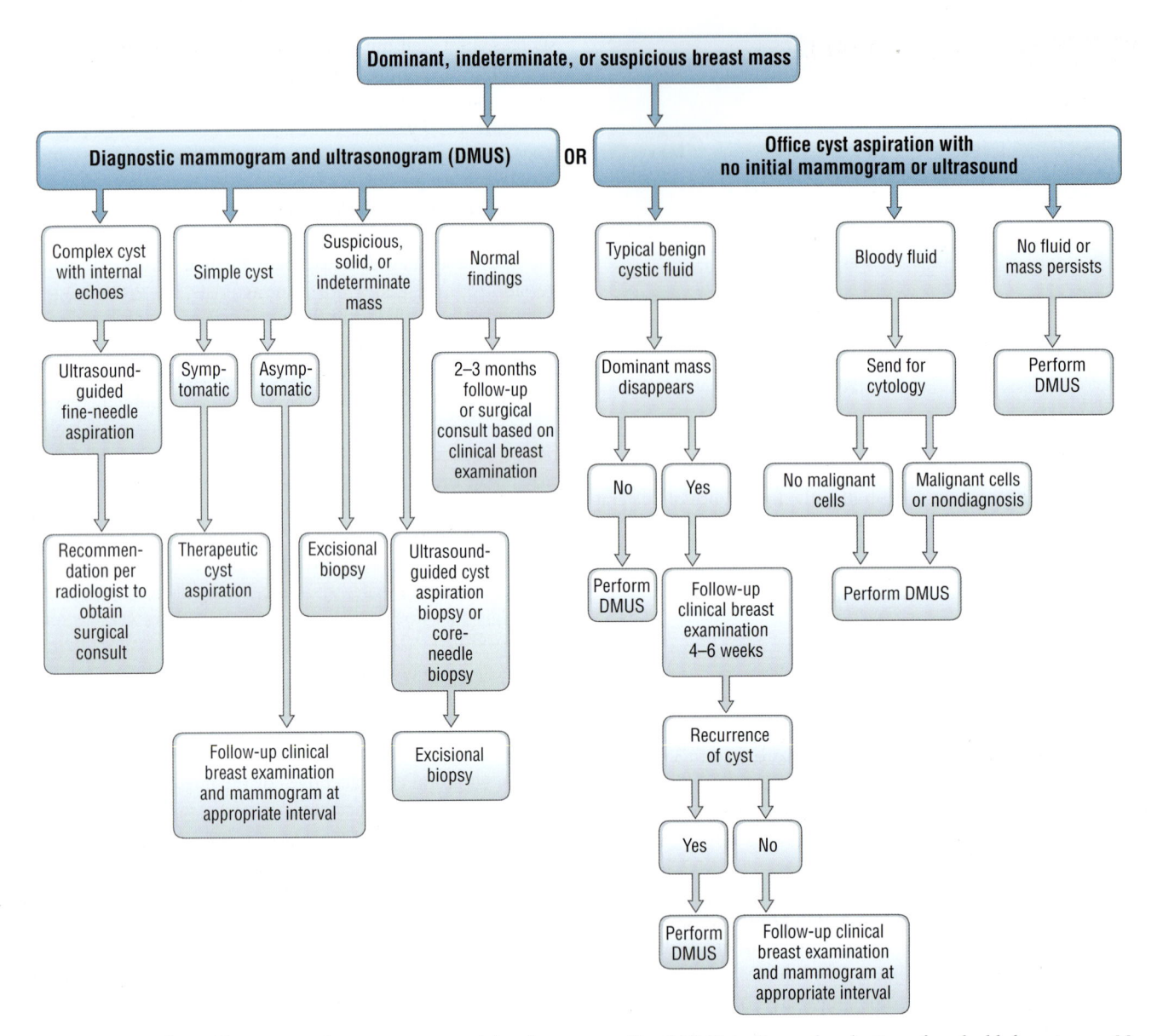

FIGURE 33.5. Workup of dominant, indeterminate, or suspicious breast mass. (Pruthi S. Detection and evaluation of a palpable breast mass. *Mayo Clin Proc.* 2001;76(6):641–647.)

discharge may indicate an infectious etiology and may be due to mastitis or a breast abscess.

Bloody, unilateral nipple discharge may be caused by an invasive ductal carcinoma, intraductal papilloma, or intraductal carcinoma. Patients with nipple discharge of this type usually require ductography and ductal excision. Breast ductography is an imaging technique that can reveal the location of an intraductal lesion. A new technique that employs fiberoptic technology, fiberoptic ductoscopy, allows the direct visualization of the breast ducts as well as sampling of ductal cells. However, this modality is not widely available.

Breast Masses

The most worrisome finding for patients and clinicians is an unexplained breast mass. Some characteristics of breast masses that suggest malignancy include size greater than 2 cm, immobility, poorly defined margins, firmness, skin dimpling or color changes, retraction or change in the nipple (e.g., scaling), bloody nipple discharge, and ipsilateral lymphadenopathy. The growth rate of a tumor in the breast is thought to be constant from the time of its origin. It is estimated that it takes an average of 5 years for a tumor to reach palpable size.

Benign Breast Masses

A variety of benign breast masses are found on clinical or self-breast examinations, screening mammograms, or incidentally. Table 33.2 summarizes the three morphologic categories and their associated risk of developing invasive breast cancer.

TABLE 33.2 BENIGN BREAST LESIONS

Morphlogic Category (with Relative Risk of Developing Invasive Breast Cancer)	Examples of Pathologic Lesions
Nonproliferative (1.0)	Fibrocystic changes Cysts Fibrosis Adenosis Lactational adenomas Fibroadenomas
Proliferative without atypia (1.5–2.0)	Epithelial hyperplasia Sclerosing adenosis Complex sclerosing lesions (radial scar) Papillomas
Proliferative with atypia (8.0–10.0)	Lobular carcinoma in situ Ductal carcinoma in situ

Modified from Kumar V, Abbas AK, Nelson F, eds. *Robbins and Cotran Pathologic Basis of Disease*. 7th ed. Philadelphia, PA: Elsevier Saunders; 2005.

Nonproliferative Lesions

Fibrocystic changes of the breast are a spectrum of features that can be observed in the normal breast. Lobules of the breast may dilate and form cysts of varying sizes. The cyst walls are lined by flattened atrophic epithelium or may be modified through apocrine metaplasia. If these cysts rupture, the resulting scarring and inflammation may lead to fibrotic changes, which make the breast feel firm. An increase in the number of glands with associated lobular growth is known as **adenosis**. In this case, the architecture of the lobule remains unchanged. In some lactating women, a palpable lactation adenoma may arise secondary to an exaggerated hormonal response.

Simple fibroadenomas are common tumors found in women in their late teens and early twenties. These masses are solid, round, rubbery, and mobile on examination. The tumors do have structural and glandular components in the mass. Although they do not have malignant potential, they can enlarge in pregnancy and cause discomfort.

Proliferative Lesions without Atypia

These lesions are commonly found on mammography and do not usually cause a palpable mass. Histologically, they represent proliferation of cells of the ductal or lobular epithelium. The cells themselves are normal, that is, nonmalignant.

In a normal breast, only myoepithelial cells and a single layer of luminal cells rest on the basement membrane. If there are more than two cell layers, the abnormality is known as **epithelial hyperplasia**. If there is increased fibrosis within the expanded lobule with distortion and compression of the epithelium, the lesion is termed **sclerosing adenosis**. A **radial scar** (or complex sclerosing lesion) is a nidus of tubules entrapped in a densely hyalinized stroma surrounded by radiating arms of epithelium. The lesion mimics an invasive carcinoma. Finally, **papillomas** are intraductal growths composed of abundant stroma and lined by both luminal and myoepithelial cells. Solitary intraductal papillomas are found in the major lactiferous ducts of women, typically between the ages of 30 and 50 years, and cause a serous or serosanguinous drainage.

Proliferative Lesions with Atypia

When malignant cells replace the normal epithelium lining the ducts or lobules, the lesion is known as a carcinoma in situ. The basement membrane remains intact, and, therefore, the cells cannot metastasize.

There are two major types of carcinoma in situ: **lobular carcinoma in situ** (**LCIS**) and **ductal carcinoma in situ** (**DCIS**). LCIS is characterized by obliteration of the lumina of the glandular acini by a uniform population of small, atypical cells. In DCIS, the ducts are filled with atypical epithelial cells. Women with DCIS are at increased risk for developing invasive cancer or a recurrence of the DCIS lesion. For these reasons, DCIS should be evaluated with core-needle biopsy followed by surgical biopsy or excision. Management of LCIS and its related condition, atypical lobular hyperplasia, consists of excisional biopsy. Following treatment of both LCIS and DCIS, preventive therapy with SERMs such as tamoxifen has been shown to reduce the risk of invasive breast cancer in these patients.

BREAST CANCER

Breast cancer is the second most common malignancy in women, ranking only behind skin cancer. In addition, it is the second leading cause of cancer-related death in women. According to the American Cancer Society, an estimated 266,120 women would be diagnosed with and 40,920 women would die of breast cancer in 2018. The steady increase in the incidence of breast cancer can be attributed to the increased use of mammography screening, which has enabled the detection of smaller invasive lesions and the earlier diagnosis of in situ lesions. Advances in treatment have also helped maintain the downward trend in overall breast cancer mortality.

Nevertheless, breast cancer is a serious health concern in the United States. It is estimated that the United States spends approximately $8.1 billion annually on treating breast cancer. The lifetime risk of developing breast cancer in the United States is approximately 12.1% (1 in 8), while the lifetime risk of dying from breast cancer is 2.7% (1 in 37). The age-adjusted death rate was 21.3 per 100,000 women per year in 2012.

Risk Factors

Numerous studies have documented factors that increase the relative risk of breast cancer (see Box 33.1).

Age and Race

Age is the single largest risk factor for developing breast cancer. The majority of breast cancer cases occur in women over the age of 50 years. Stratified studies relate risk with age (by decades) and show that the risk of developing breast cancer increases as a woman gets older. For example, a woman has a 1.4% chance of being diagnosed with breast cancer between the ages of 40 and 49 years, compared with 3.7% between the ages of 60 and 69 years. When stratified by race, white women are more likely to be diagnosed with breast cancer compared with age-matched women of African-American descent, Latin, and Asians.

Family History and Genetics

Women who have first-degree relatives (parent, sibling, and offspring) with breast cancer have a higher risk than the general population. If a woman younger than 40 years is diagnosed with breast cancer, evaluating for genetic mutations that predispose individuals to cancer is reasonable. The two most commonly discussed genetic mutations linked to breast cancer are the *BRCA1* and *BRCA2* gene mutations.

BRCA1 is a gene located on the 17q21 chromosome. This mutation is associated with nearly half of the early-onset breast cancers and approximately 90% of hereditary ovarian cancers. *BRCA2* is a gene located on the 13q12-13 chromosome. This mutation has a lower incidence of early-onset breast cancers (35%) and much lower risk of ovarian cancer, compared with *BRCA1*.

Reproductive and Menstrual History

In general, women who have an early age of menstrual onset (before the age of 12 years) and transition through menopause after the age of 55 years are at increased risk for breast cancer. Delayed childbearing and nulliparity also increase the chance of breast cancer.

Radiation Exposure

Breast tissue of young women (along with the bone marrow and infant thyroid) is highly susceptible to the cancer-causing effects of ionizing radiation. Women who have received a sufficiently large dose of radiation (radiation therapy to treat Hodgkin disease or an enlarged thymus gland) are at risk for **radiation-induced breast cancer**. The relationship between dose of radiation and risk of cancer is directly linear, although the threshold is unclear. Thus far, epidemiologic studies have not detected a significant increase in cancer risk below a cumulative dose of about 20 cGy. To put this dose into perspective, a typical mammogram results in a breast tissue dose of about 0.3 cGy. The time needed for a radiation-induced lesion to develop is about 5 to 10 years from exposure.

Breast Changes

It is believed that women with dense breast tissue are at increased risk for breast cancer. In addition, histologic biopsies finding atypical hyperplasia or LCIS greatly increase the risk of breast cancer.

Other Factors

Being overweight after menopause has been linked to an increased risk of breast cancer. A possible mechanism in this relationship is that the increased peripheral conversion of androstenedione to estrone stimulates breast cancer development. Lack of exercise throughout life is linked to the increased risk of breast cancer through the associated risk of obesity.

Women who consume 2 to 4 alcoholic drinks per week have a 30% greater risk of dying from breast cancer than women who never drink. The exact mechanism of action is unclear, but researchers speculate that alcohol consumption stimulates the growth and progression of breast cancer by inducing angiogenesis and increasing the expression of vascular endothelial growth factor.

Breast Cancer Risk Assessment Tool: The Gail Model

The NCI has developed a computer-based tool to allow clinicians to estimate a woman's risk of developing invasive breast cancer over the next 5 years and in their lifetime (up to age 90 years). The tool is based on a mathematical model of breast cancer risk calculation called the Gail model. Seven risk factors are used in the calculations: a history of LCIS or DCIS, age, age at onset of menstruation, age at the time of the first live birth, number of first-degree relatives with breast cancer, history of breast biopsy, and race/ethnicity. The usefulness of the Gail model is limited in patients with second-degree relatives with breast cancer (e.g., paternal transmission) and is falsely increased in patients with multiple breast biopsies. A family history of breast cancer is the strongest predictor of risk among the factors used in the model.

Women at high risk, defined as a 5-year risk of 1.7% or more, can be referred for possible prophylactic therapy. Current prophylactic options include chemoprevention with the SERMs tamoxifen and raloxifene and prophylactic mastectomy. Because all of the options are associated with significant side effects, individualized risk assessment should be performed to determine whether a patient is a candidate for breast cancer risk reduction and, if so, which option is best.

Histologic Types of Breast Cancer

Malignant tumors of the breast may arise from any of the major components of the breast. The American Joint Committee on Cancer (AJCC) classifies most breast malignancies into one of three histologic categories according to their corresponding cells of origin: ductal, lobular, and nipple.

About 70% to 80% of breast cancers are invasive ductal carcinomas. These are most common among women in their fifties and have a tendency to spread to regional lymph nodes. Invasive lobular carcinomas comprise 5% to 15% of breast cancers. This type is often multifocal and bilateral. Table 33.3 summarizes the differences between the two processes. Paget disease of the nipple presents as a superficial skin lesion similar to eczema.

Breast Cancer Staging

The AJCC stages breast malignancies according to the TNM system that describes characteristics of the primary tumor, involvement of regional lymph nodes, and distant metastasis. **T** = primary **T**umor; **N** = regional lymph **N**odes; **M** = distant

TABLE 33.3 MAJOR DIFFERENCES BETWEEN DCIS AND LCIS

	DCIS	LCIS
Structure involved	Ducts	Lobules
Type of subsequent cancer	Ductal	Ductal or lobular
Breast at risk for invasive cancer	Ipsilateral breast	Either breast
Laterality	Unilateral	Often bilateral
Number of sites of origin	Unicentric	Multicentric

DCIS, ductal carcinoma in situ; LCIS, lobular carcinoma in situ.

TABLE 33.4 TREATMENT OF BREAST CANCER BY STAGE

Stage	Surgery	Adjuvant Treatment
0	Total mastectomy or breast conservation therapy (includes lumpectomy and breast irradiation)	
I	Total mastectomy or breast conservation therapy (includes lumpectomy and breast irradiation) ± sentinel node biopsy/axillary lymph node dissection	Chemotherapy >1 cm ± tamoxifen
II	Modified radical mastectomy or breast conservation therapy (includes lumpectomy and breast irradiation)/axillary lymph node dissection	Chemotherapy >1 cm ±Tamoxifen Radiation therapy of the supraclavicular nodes ± chest wall, mastectomy performed if ≥4 positive nodes
III	Modified radical mastectomy or breast conservation therapy (includes lumpectomy and breast irradiation)/axillary lymph node dissection	Chemotherapy ± neoadjuvant chemotherapy ±Tamoxifen Radiation therapy of the supraclavicular nodes ± chest wall, if mastectomy performed Radiation therapy of the breast (inflammatory breast cancer)
IV	Surgery for local control	±Chemotherapy ±Hormonal agents

Modified from Gemigani ML. Breast cancer. In: Barakat RR, Bevers MW, Gershenson DM, Hoskins WJ, eds. *The Memorial Sloan-Kettering & MD Anderson Cancer Center Handbook of Gynecologic Oncology.* 2nd ed. London: Martin Dunitz Publishers; 2002:297–319.

Metastasis. Surgical stage helps determine the appropriate types of therapy (Table 33.4).

In addition to stage, receptor status is another important indicator of breast cancer prognosis. Expression of estrogen or progesterone receptors positively affects prognosis. The **Her2/neu** (or **c-erb-B2**) is an oncogene encoding a membrane-bound growth factor receptor. Overexpression confers a poor prognosis and is noted in 20% to 30% of invasive ductal cancers.

Breast Cancer Treatment

Breast cancer poses both a local regional risk (i.e., to the breast and regional lymph nodes) and a systemic risk.

Surgical Therapy

The surgical treatment is **lumpectomy (breast conservation therapy)** or **mastectomy**. Both procedures are aimed at achieving local control. Mastectomy is removal of all breast tissue and the nipple areolar complex with preservation of the pectoralis muscles. A modified radical mastectomy also includes removal of the axillary lymph nodes. Radiation therapy is used in conjunction with mastectomy for later stages of breast cancer and to accompany lumpectomy and partial mastectomy for early stages of breast cancer. Radiation is an essential component of lumpectomy. The combination of lumpectomy and radiation yields outcomes that are equal to those of radical mastectomy.

Breast reconstruction should be an option for all women who desire it. Reconstruction can be achieved by several methods, including the insertion of a saline implant under the pectoral muscle or by using a rectus muscle to replace the lost tissue. To prepare for a saline implant, a tissue expander is placed beneath the muscle. Saline is injected into the expander over a period of weeks to months until the space is large enough to accommodate the implant. Breast reconstruction can take place immediately after surgery or it can be delayed for several months. Radiation therapy can be given if breast reconstruction has taken place.

Medical Therapy

Adjuvant (systemic) therapy is used in the treatment of all stages of breast cancer, regardless of lymph node status. Adjuvant therapy includes chemotherapeutic drugs that kill cancer cells and hormonal therapies such as tamoxifen that act as estrogen antagonists. Tamoxifen and raloxifen are used to treat women with estrogen receptor–positive breast cancer. It can be used in conjunction with chemotherapy. It is also given as a 5-year course of preventive treatment following surgery. **Aromatase inhibitors (AIs)** prevent the production of estrogen in postmenopausal women. AIs are used to extend survival in women with metastatic cancer, as primary adjuvant therapy, and in conjunction with tamoxifen to prevent cancer recurrence.

Another drug used to treat breast cancer is trastuzumab. It acts on membrane-bound protein produced by Her2/neu. If a patient's cancer is found to overexpress the Her2/neu protein, trastuzumab can be given as adjuvant therapy. Trastuzumab is associated with significant side effects, including heart failure, respiratory problems, and life-threatening allergic reactions.

Follow-Up

Obstetrician–gynecologists are in the unique position of providing care for women who have been treated for breast cancer. For some women, the continuation of care spans many years. Once the initial treatment has been completed, the obstetrician–gynecologist often takes on the role of screening and surveillance. For the first 2 years, follow-up appointments occur every 3 to 6 months and then annually after that. Annual mammography and physical examinations should continue indefinitely. Most breast cancer recurrences will occur within 5 years of primary therapy.

SCREENING GUIDELINES

For the general population, breast cancer surveillance involves a combination of CBEs and radiographic imaging. In 2009, the U.S. Preventative Service Task Force (USPSTF) found insufficient evidence for teaching BSEs. The American College of Obstetricians and Gynecologists (College) supports the practice of BSE only in high-risk patients and for breast self-awareness in low-risk patients.

The value of CBE in detecting breast cancer has also been studied. Pooled data from multiple studies support the use and effectiveness of CBE. Multiple reviews have supported the combination of CBE and mammography for breast cancer screening for women ages 50 to 69 years. In 2009, the USPSTF concluded that the current evidence is insufficient to assess the additional benefits and harms of CBE beyond screening mammography in women 40 years or older.

The value of mammography increases with age. The USPSTF found sufficient evidence to demonstrate that mammogram screening every 1 to 3 years significantly reduced mortality from breast cancer. Controversy exists over screening intervals in younger women, in whom the incidence of breast cancer remains low. The College currently recommends that mammography not be performed annually after the age of 40 years, whereas the USPSTF recommends that the decision to start regular, biennial screening mammography before age 50 years should be an individual one and take patient context into account, including the patient's values regarding specific benefits and harms. The USPSTF concluded that the current evidence is insufficient to assess the additional benefits and harms of screening mammography in women 75 years or older, though many patients and practitioners continue to recommend the practice.

These screening standards do not apply to women with inherited genetic mutations placing them at increased risk for developing breast cancer. In this population, breast cancer occurs at a younger age and is missed by screening mammography nearly 50% of the time. Current recommendations for *BRCA* carriers include monthly BSEs beginning at the age of 18 to 20 years, annual CBEs, and screening mammograms beginning after age 25 years (or 5–10 years before the age of diagnosis in the affected relative). MRI is recommended as a supplement to mammography, not a replacement.

CLINICAL FOLLOW-UP

This patient's history and findings are consistent with fibrocystic change. Physical examination suggested a cystic mass, and aspiration with a small-gauge needle yields a quantity of straw-colored fluid and resolution of the mass. Follow-up 1 month later fails to find any recurrence.

CHAPTER 34

Gynecologic Procedures

This chapter deals primarily with APGO Educational Topic Area:

TOPIC 41 GYNECOLOGIC PROCEDURES

Students should be able to describe preoperative, perioperative, and postoperative care to optimize outcomes for gynecologic surgical patients. They should be able to outline indications, the consent process, and complications of standard inpatient and outpatient gynecologic procedures and imaging.

CLINICAL CASE

A 34-year-old woman is referred for the evaluation of an abnormal Pap smear, which was reported as "ASCUS (atypical squamous cells of undetermined significance) with positive high-risk human papillomavirus present." A colposcopy is performed, which was satisfactory and showed no lesions. Endocervical curettage was performed and was reported as showing a high-grade lesion.

● IMAGING STUDIES

Gynecologic imaging plays an important role in the diagnostic evaluation of women for a variety of reproductive health conditions. Although the ability to image various parts and organs of the body has dramatically enhanced clinicians' diagnostic capabilities, these methods do not replace a careful and thoughtful history and physical evaluation. However, they can add more detail, which assists in both medical and surgical management. The effective use of these modalities requires that the physician be familiar with the benefits and limitations of each method.

Ultrasonography

Ultrasonography remains the most common modality for evaluation of the female pelvis. It uses high-frequency sound reflections to identify different body tissues and structures. Short bursts of low-energy sound waves are sent into the body. When these waves encounter the interface between two tissues that transmit sound differently, some of the sound energy is reflected back toward the sound source. The returning sound waves are detected, and the distance from the sensor is deduced using the elapsed time from transmission to reception. An image is then created and displayed on a monitor. Ultrasonography is safe for pregnant and nonpregnant patients.

Most ultrasonography produces two-dimensional images. Three-dimensional studies can be used for volume calculation and to provide detail about the surfaces of particular structures. In gynecology, three-dimensional ultrasonography is especially useful in the evaluation of müllerian abnormalities (see Chapter 4). Four-dimensional ultrasonography, which shows movement, is also available and has proven helpful in evaluating such things as fetal cardiac abnormalities.

Two kinds of probes are used in gynecologic ultrasonography: transabdominal and transvaginal (Fig. 34.1). Owing to a lower frequency used, a transabdominal probe has an increased depth of penetration, which allows for the assessment of large uterine or adnexal masses. However, in obese patients, it may not allow proper imaging of pelvic structures. A transvaginal probe can be placed internally; thus, it often gives improved views of the cervix, uterus, ovaries, and tubes. Also, it has a higher frequency and shorter depth of penetration, which result in enhanced resolution.

Uses of Ultrasonography

One of the most valuable uses of ultrasonography in gynecology is for evaluating masses. The imaging technique helps distinguish between cystic and solid adnexal masses. Although magnetic resonance imaging (MRI) and computed tomography (CT) can also be used for evaluation of ovarian cysts, ultrasonography is far less costly; for this purpose, experts consider it superior to either MRI or CT. It is also possible to delineate leiomyoma (fibroid) size and number using ultrasonography.

Use of the endometrial stripe thickness for evaluation of postmenopausal bleeding has been studied extensively. Following menopause, the endometrium becomes atrophic, and its thickness decreases, remaining relatively constant without hormonal stimulation. Ultrasonographic evaluation of the endometrial stripe involves measuring the thickest portion of the endometrial echo in the sagittal plane. The significance of an endometrial thickness of greater than 4 mm in an asymptomatic, postmenopausal patient has not been established, and this finding need not routinely trigger evaluation.

FIGURE 34.1. Transabdominal (A) and transvaginal (B) ultrasonography.

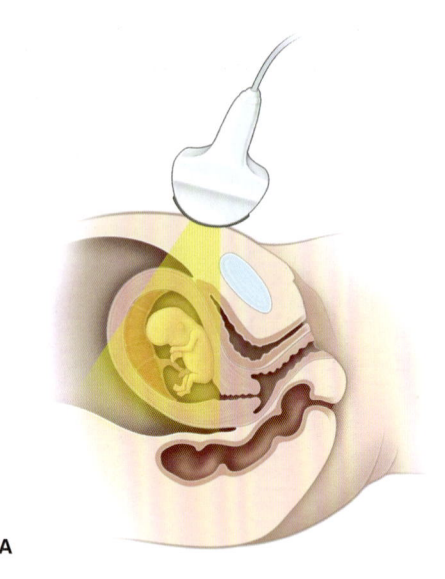

The primary imaging test of the uterus for the evaluation of abnormal uterine bleeding (AUB) is transvaginal ultrasonography. If transvaginal ultrasonographic images are not adequate or further evaluation of the cavity is necessary, then sonohysterography (SHG) or hysteroscopy (preferably in the office setting) is recommended. Saline infusion during ultrasonography (**SHG**) can aid in the visualization of the endometrial cavity and can often identify intrauterine polyps or submucosal leiomyomas (Fig. 34.2). In this technique, saline is infused via a transcervically inserted catheter. The saline acts as a contrast agent to delineate the endometrium and intracavity masses. The primary role of SHG is in the diagnosis of the cause of AUB.

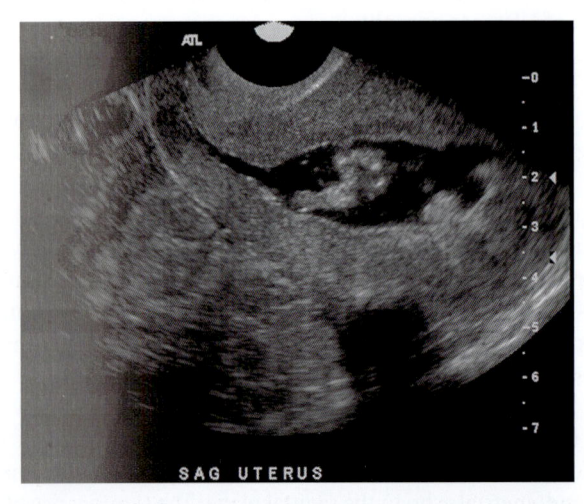

FIGURE 34.2. Sonohysterogram showing several polyps. (Used with permission from American College of Obstetricians and Gynecologists. *Precis: Gynecology.* 4th ed. Washington, DC: ACOG; 2011.)

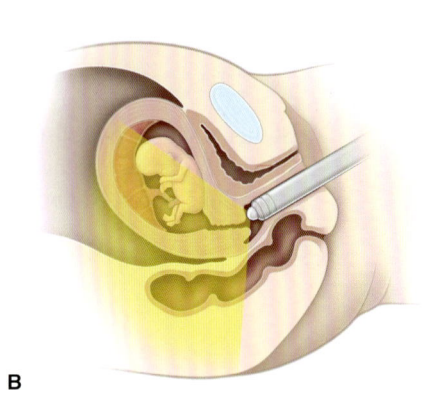

Computed Axial Tomography

Computed axial tomography (**CAT**, or **CT**) scanning uses computer algorithms to construct cross-sectional images based on x-ray information. With the use of oral or intravenous (IV) contrast agents, CT scanning can help evaluate pelvic masses, identify lymphadenopathy, and plan radiation therapy.

CT involves slightly greater radiation exposure than a conventional single-exposure radiograph but provides significantly more information. The radiation dose of an abdominal CT is still below that thought to cause fetal harm. Nevertheless, because of CT's increased risk of fetal effects, MRI (see below) or ultrasonography should be used for imaging instead of CT whenever possible during pregnancy.

Magnetic Resonance Imaging

MRI is based on the magnetic characteristics of various atoms and molecules in the body. Because of the variations in chemical composition of body tissues (especially the content of hydrogen, sodium, fluoride, and phosphorus), MRI can distinguish between types of tissues, such as blood and fat. This distinction is useful in visualizing lymph nodes, which are usually surrounded by fat; in characterizing adnexal masses; and in locating hemorrhage within organs. MRI is also useful for visualizing the endometrium, myometrium, and cystic structures in the ovaries. Emerging areas of clinical applicability include assessment of lesions in the breast and staging of cervical cancer. In pregnant patients requiring imaging beyond ultrasound, an MRI is preferred over a CT.

Breast Imaging

Mammography is an x-ray procedure used to evaluate breast concerns and screen for breast cancer. It is performed by passing

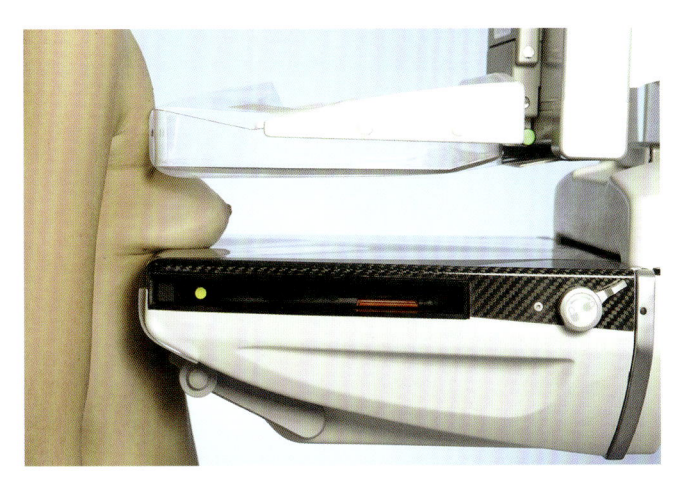

FIGURE 34.3. Mammogram.

a small amount of radiation through compressed breast tissue (Fig. 34.3). Because mammography has a high false-positive rate (10% per screening in postmenopausal women and as high as 20% per screening in obese or premenopausal women), additional testing may be required. Digital mammography allows better visualization of heterogeneously dense or extremely dense breast tissue than conventional mammography.

Ultrasonography is also used to evaluate cystic or solid breast masses and guide aspiration of cysts. MRI may also be used as an imaging technique for breast tissue and has been recommended as an adjunct in selected high-risk women. Ultrasonography may be an option for additional screening in women at high risk who are candidates for MRI screening but cannot receive MRI because of gadolinium contrast allergy, claustrophobia, or other barriers.

Hysterosalpingography

Hysterosalpingography (**HSG**) is most often used to evaluate the patency of the fallopian tubes in women who may be infertile. This procedure is done in a radiologic suite. After a radiopaque contrast material is injected transcervically, fluoroscopy (live x-ray) is used to determine whether contrast material spills into the peritoneal cavity (Fig. 34.4). HSG can also be used to define the size and shape of the uterine cavity and to detect developmental abnormalities, such as a unicornuate, septate, and didelphic uterus (see Chapter 4). It also can demonstrate most endometrial polyps, submucous myomata, and intrauterine adhesions that are significant enough to have important reproductive consequences. It is also carried out to confirm the efficacy of transcervically placed sterilization devices (e.g., Essure).

● PROCEDURES

Gynecologic procedures include diagnostic procedures, such as biopsy and colposcopy, as well as procedures used as treatment modalities. Some procedures, such as laparoscopy and hysteroscopy, can be performed for both diagnosis and treatment and are

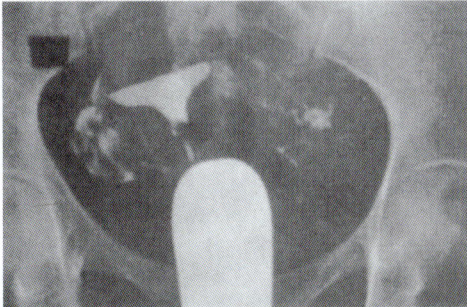

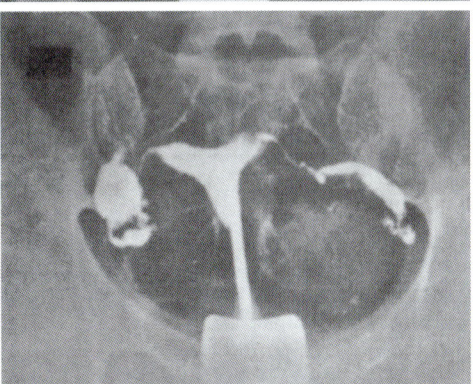

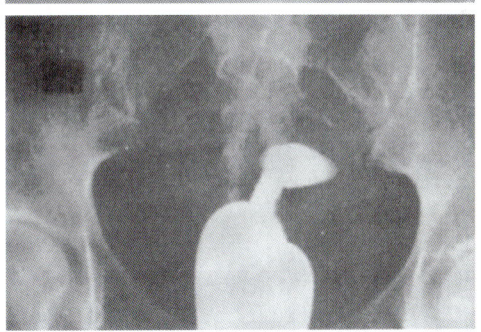

FIGURE 34.4. Hysterosalpingography.

chosen specifically for this reason. For all invasive procedures (and some imaging studies), the informed consent process is a necessity and must precede the start of the procedure. Some form of "time out," which includes positive identification of the patient and planned procedure, should be performed with all participating parties in the room prior to commencing the procedure.

Genital Tract Biopsy

Biopsies of the vulva, vagina, cervix, and endometrium are frequently necessary in gynecology. These procedures are usually comfortably performed in the office; they require either no anesthesia or local anesthesia.

Vulvar Biopsy

Vulvar biopsies are performed to evaluate visible lesions, persistent pruritus, burning, or pain. A circular, hollow metal instrument 3 to 5 mm in diameter, called a **punch**, is used to remove a small disk of tissue for evaluation (Fig. 34.5). For hemostasis,

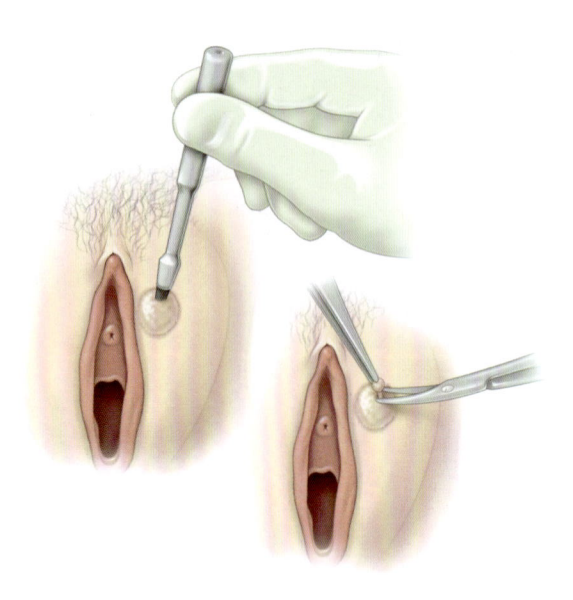

FIGURE 34.5. Biopsy of vulvar lesion. The punch is rotated in place to incise tissue.

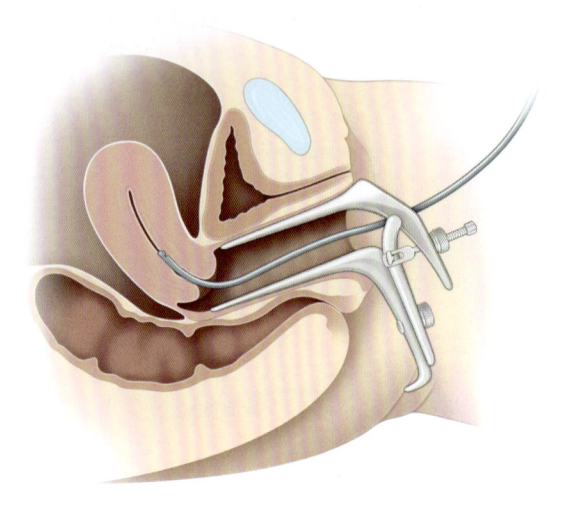

FIGURE 34.6. Endometrial biopsy. (Figure adapted from the American College of Obstetricians and Gynecologists, © 2008.)

local pressure or coagulants (styptics) such as Monsel solution (ferric subsulfate) are often used. Sutures are rarely necessary. Local anesthesia is required for this type of biopsy.

Vaginal Biopsy

Vaginal biopsy is performed to assess suspicious masses and to evaluate the vagina in the presence of cervical abnormalities. Women who have had a prior hysterectomy for cervical cancer should continue to have Pap tests every 3 years for 20 years performed on the vaginal cuff; if a result is abnormal, a vaginal biopsy may be required. Vaginal biopsy is performed with pinch biopsy forceps. Local anesthesia is rarely required.

Cervical Biopsy

Cervical biopsy is performed with biopsy forceps and, perhaps, a colposcope for visualization. No anesthesia is necessary. Indications for cervical biopsy include chronic cervicitis, suspected neoplasm, and ulcer. It may also be performed as an adjunct to colposcopy during the evaluation of selected cytologic abnormalities.

Endometrial Biopsy

Endometrial biopsy (EMB) is generally used to evaluate AUB, such as menorrhagia, metrorrhagia, and menometrorrhagia. EMB is accomplished with a small diameter catheter with a mild suction mechanism (Fig. 34.6). Various types are available. Anesthesia is not necessary, but many patients are more tolerant of EMB when given ibuprofen (400–800 mg) 1 hour prior to the procedure.

Colposcopy

Colposcopy is performed to evaluate abnormal cytology (Pap) results. It facilitates detailed evaluation of the surface of the cervix, vagina, and vulva when premalignancy or malignancy is suspected based on history, physical examination, or cytology. Cervical biopsy of suspicious lesions is frequently performed during colposcopy. Chapter 47 provides more detail about colposcopy.

Cryotherapy

Cryotherapy is a technique that destroys tissue by freezing. A hollow metal probe (cryoprobe) is placed on the tissue to be treated. The probe is then filled with a refrigerant gas (nitrous oxide or carbon dioxide) that causes it to cool to an extremely low temperature (between −65°C and −85°C), freezing the tissue that is in contact with the probe. Cryotherapy is most often used to treat cervical intraepithelial neoplasia (CIN) and other benign lesions such as condyloma. The formation of ice crystals within the cells of the treated tissue leads to tissue destruction and subsequent sloughing. Patients who have had cryotherapy of the cervix can expect to have a watery discharge for several weeks as the tissues slough and healing occurs. Although cryotherapy is inexpensive, well tolerated, and generally effective, it is less precise than other methods of tissue destruction, such as laser ablation and electrosurgery. Cryotherapy and laser vaporization should be used only after rigorously excluding invasive cancer. Destructive therapies do not yield histologic specimens and are not used when this is a consideration.

Laser Vaporization

Highly energetic coherent light beams (produced by light amplification by stimulated emission of radiation [LASER]) may be directed onto tissues, facilitating tissue destruction or incision, depending on the specific wavelength of light used and the power density of the beam. Infrared wavelength (from a CO_2 laser) is the most common type of laser used in gynecologic procedures. Yttrium-aluminum-garnet, argon, or potassium-titanyl-phosphate lasers, all of which have different effects on tissues, are also used. Some can be used in the presence of saline or water. The type of laser is selected according to the indication or desired effect of the surgery. Although expensive, the great precision that laser offers makes it a useful tool in specific clinical settings.

Laser therapy is used to treat vaginal and vulvar lesions, such as condyloma, vaginal intraepithelial neoplasia, and vulvar intraepithelial neoplasia. Laser is also used to treat other dermatologic vulvar disorders, including molluscum contagiosum and lichen sclerosis atrophy. Prior to the development of the loop electrosurgical excision procedure (LEEP, see below), laser ablation and conization were common treatment modalities for CIN ablation and cervical conization.

Dilation and Curettage

Dilation and curettage (D&C) is a procedure in which the cervix is dilated using a series of graduated dilators, followed by curettage (scraping) of the endometrium, for both diagnostic (histologic) and therapeutic reasons. D&C is usually performed under anesthesia in the operating room. Some common indications for D&C include AUB, incomplete or missed abortion, inability to perform EMB in the office, postmenopausal bleeding, and suspected endometrial polyp(s). With the availability of newer imaging procedures, D&C is now less commonly performed. In some settings, smaller cannulae with self-contained suction devices are used in the office setting for diagnostic (EMB) or therapeutic (incomplete abortions or "menstrual extractions") indications—similar to D&C.

Hysteroscopy

Hysteroscopy is the visualization of the endometrial cavity using a narrow telescope-like device (Fig. 34.7) attached to a light source, camera, and distension medium (often normal saline). It is used to view lesions such as polyps, intrauterine adhesions (synechiae), septa, and submucous myomas. Special instruments allow directed resection of such abnormalities. Hysteroscopy may be performed in the inpatient setting under general anesthesia; however, it can also be performed in the office as a diagnostic procedure or in conjunction with either endometrial ablation or SHG.

Procedures for nonreversible sterilization have been designed to be used in conjunction with the hysteroscope. In these procedures, metal coils (Essure) are inserted into the ostium of each fallopian tube under direct visualization. Scarring of the tubal ostia then occurs. To confirm that the tubes are occluded, an HSG must be performed 3 months later.

Endometrial Ablation

Endometrial ablation is used to destroy the uterine lining. The procedure is used to treat AUB in premenopausal women with normal endometrial cavities who do not wish to become pregnant. It is not a method of sterilization; therefore, women who undergo ablation must use some other form of birth control. Various ablation devices are available; they may use heat, cold, or electrosurgical energy. Some, but not all, of the available techniques involve direct visualization of the endometrium with a hysteroscope. Many women opt for endometrial ablation because it is a minor procedure, thus avoiding major surgery in the form of a hysterectomy. The procedure can be performed in either the surgical suite or the office. In the office, a combination of nonsteroidal anti-inflammatory drugs, a local anesthetic, and an anxiolytic is used to provide pain relief. To date, ideal regimens for using local anesthetic agents have not been determined. Success is not assured—hysterectomy rates associated with endometrial ablation are at least 24% within 4 years following the procedure.

Pregnancy Termination

Pregnancy termination refers to the planned interruption of pregnancy before viability and is often referred to as **induced abortion**. It is generally accomplished surgically through dilation of the cervix and evacuation of the uterine contents, performed under local anesthesia. In the first and early second trimester, removal of the products of conception uses either a suction or a sharp curette. Suction curettes are often preferred because they are less likely to cause uterine damage, such as endometrial scarring or perforation. In the second trimester, destructive grasping forceps may be used to remove the pregnancy through a dilated cervix (called **dilation and evacuation**).

Alternatively, in the first trimester (within 9 weeks of the first day of the last menstrual period), pregnancy can be terminated using medication rather than surgical techniques. Medication abortion may be carried out using one of the following methods:

- Mifepristone and misoprostol pills
- Mifepristone pills and vaginal misoprostol
- Methotrexate and vaginal misoprostol
- Vaginal misoprostol alone

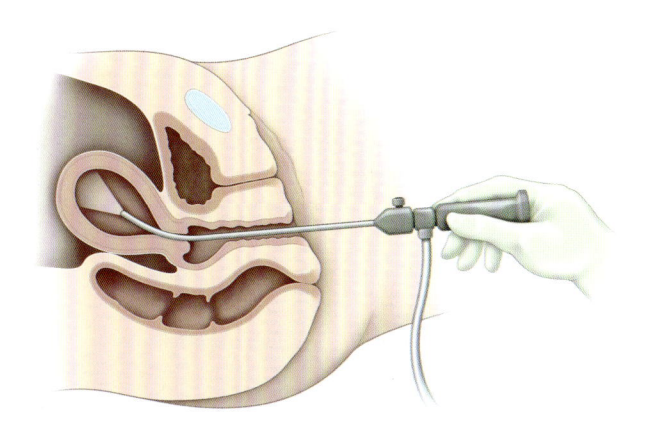

FIGURE 34.7. Hysteroscopy. (Figure adapted from the American College of Obstetricians and Gynecologists, © 2006.)

A woman who is still pregnant after an attempted medical abortion needs to have a surgical abortion.

Cervical Conization

Conization is a surgical procedure in which a cone-shaped sample of tissue, encompassing the entire cervical transformation zone and extending up the endocervical canal, is removed from the cervix (Fig. 34.8). It may be required as the definitive diagnostic procedure in the evaluation of an abnormal Pap test when the colposcopic examination is inadequate or when colposcopic biopsy findings are inconsistent with Pap test results. Colposcopy-guided conization may also be used therapeutically in cases of CIN. Various techniques for conization are available, including cold knife (scalpel), laser excision, and electrosurgery (LEEP, also called *large loop excision of the transformation zone*). Laser excision and LEEP are often performed in the office. Long-term complications may include cervical insufficiency and stenosis.

Minimally Invasive and Robotic Surgery

Laparoscopy (also known as **minimally invasive surgery**) is the visualization of the pelvis and abdominal cavity using an endoscopic telescope, which is most often placed via an incision in the periumbilical region (Fig. 34.9). The procedure may be diagnostic or therapeutic. Laparoscopic evaluation and treatment may be performed for conditions such as chronic pelvic pain, endometriosis, infertility, pelvic masses, ectopic pregnancies, and congenital abnormalities. Sterilization (bilateral tubal ligation) using techniques such as bipolar cautery, clips, or bands can be accomplished easily via laparoscopy (see Chapter 27). During the procedure, carbon dioxide is used to distend the peritoneal cavity to provide visualization. Additional instruments with diameters of 5 to 15 mm may be inserted via other laparoscopic incisions. The number, length, and location of incisions depend on the instruments needed and the size of any tissue specimens that are to be removed. Transvaginal insertion of a uterine manipulator facilitates these maneuvers.

Robotic devices may be used to position and manipulate the viewing and operating devices. This technology allows for three-dimensional images and finer dexterity but at a trade-off for increased setup time and equipment costs. Clear superiority for robotic techniques has only been proven for a limited number of indications. Four randomized controlled trials compared robot-assisted surgery for benign gynecologic disease with laparoscopy, and none showed any benefit from using the robotic approach. Overall, the current literature shows conflicting evidence and is of poor quality. Based on the four trials and two large cohort studies, robot-assisted hysterectomy appears to have similar morbidity profiles to laparoscopic procedures but results in significantly higher costs.

After laparoscopy, the most common complaints include incisional pain and shoulder pain due to referred pain of diaphragmatic irritation from the gas used to provide visualization. Rare but serious complications include damage to major blood vessels, the bowel, and other intra-abdominal or retroperitoneal structures. However, when compared with laparotomy,

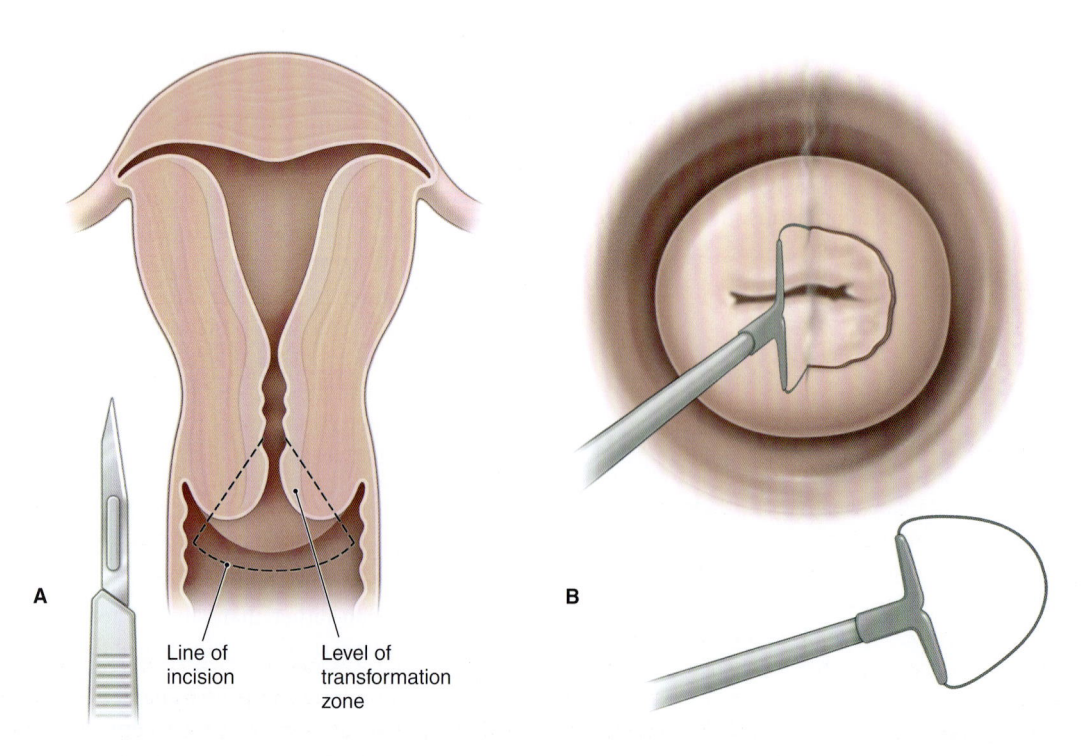

FIGURE 34.8. Conization of the cervix. **(A)** Cold-knife technique. **(B)** LLETZ/LEEP (large loop excision of the transformation zone/loop electrosurgical excision procedure) technique.

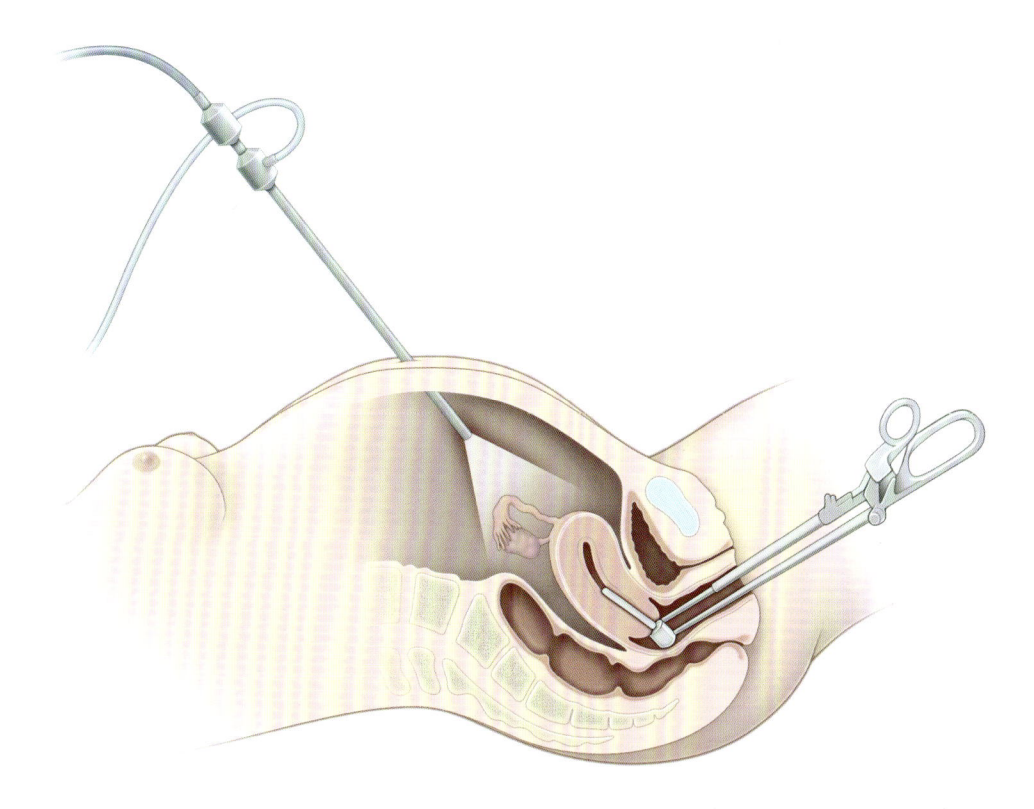

FIGURE 34.9. Laparoscopy. (Figure adapted from the American College of Obstetricians and Gynecologists, © 2008.)

laparoscopy has several advantages, including avoidance of long hospital stays, smaller incisions, quicker recovery, and decreased pain.

Hysterectomy

Hysterectomy, removal of the uterus, is still one of the most commonly performed surgical procedures. In the United States, more than 500,000 hysterectomies are completed annually. The indications for hysterectomy are numerous; they include AUB that has not responded to conservative management, pelvic pain, postpartum hemorrhage, symptomatic leiomyomas, symptomatic uterine prolapse, cervical or uterine cancer, and severe anemia from uterine hemorrhage.

Patients are often confused by inaccurate terms used to describe types of hysterectomy. To many patients, a "complete" hysterectomy means removal of the uterus, fallopian tubes, and ovaries, and a "partial" hysterectomy means removal of the uterus but not the tubes and ovaries. However, the correct term for the removal of both tubes and both ovaries is a **bilateral salpingo-oophorectomy**, and this procedure is not automatically part of a hysterectomy. Thus, it is important to determine exactly what procedure a patient may have had. Equally important is what a patient is expecting when a surgical procedure is planned. A **total hysterectomy** is the removal of the entire uterus, whereas a **supracervical** (or **subtotal**) **hysterectomy** removes the uterine corpus while leaving the cervix. The uterus may be removed by several different routes.

Abdominal Hysterectomy
Abdominal hysterectomy is performed via a laparotomy incision. The laparotomy incision can be either transverse, usually **Pfannenstiel**, or vertical. The decision to perform a laparotomy involves many factors—the skill of the surgeon, the size of the uterus, concern for extensive pathology (e.g., endometriosis or cancer), the need to perform adjunct surgery during the surgery (e.g., lymph node dissection, appendectomy, and omentectomy), and previous intra-abdominal scarring or surgeries.

Vaginal Hysterectomy
Vaginal hysterectomy is preferred if there is adequate uterine mobility (descent of the cervix and uterus toward the introitus), the bony pelvis is of an appropriate configuration, the uterus is not too large, and there is no suspected adnexal pathology. In general, vaginal hysterectomy is performed for benign disease. The advantage of vaginal surgery is less pain than with abdominal surgery, quicker return of normal bowel function, fewer febrile episodes or unspecified infections, and a shorter hospital stay. If indicated, a unilateral or bilateral salpingo-oophorectomy can be performed in conjunction with a vaginal hysterectomy.

Laparoscopic-Assisted Vaginal Hysterectomy
Laparoscopic-assisted vaginal hysterectomy (**LAVH**), with or without a bilateral salpingo-oophorectomy, is often performed for patients who desire minimally invasive surgery and may not have adequate descent of their uterus to undergo a vaginal

hysterectomy. LAVH can be accomplished by performing most or all of the procedures laparoscopically; then the uterus is removed through the vagina. The vaginal cuff can then be sutured transvaginally or laparoscopically.

Total Laparoscopic Hysterectomy

It is possible to perform a hysterectomy totally via the laparoscopic approach. This is usually accomplished with the assistance of a morcellator, which divides the uterus into multiple smaller specimens that can be removed through the ports. Recent concerns regarding morcellation and the spread of undiagnosed malignancy has greatly decreased and, in some institutions, prohibited its use. Even large uteri can be safely removed through small incisions. This approach is reserved for benign indications only because a histological evaluation is not practical after morcellation.

UROGYNECOLOGY PROCEDURES

Many gynecologists perform urogynecology procedures in the office and operating room. These procedures include the Q-tip test, urodynamic tests, cystoscopy, transvaginal tape (sling), and the Burch procedure. A description of these procedures can be found in Chapter 30.

PREOPERATIVE, INTRAOPERATIVE, AND POSTOPERATIVE CONSIDERATIONS

Preoperative Considerations

Any surgical procedure carries risks. Naturally, more invasive procedures carry higher risks. Before patients sign preoperative surgical consent forms, they should be counseled on the risks of infection, hemorrhage, and damage to surrounding structures (bowel, bladder, blood vessels, and other anatomic structures). Many hospitals require that patients also sign a consent form for a blood transfusion in case of an emergency. Some patients refuse to sign such consents for blood transfusion for personal or religious reasons, and this should be clearly documented in the chart. A discussion with the patient regarding the safety of the blood used for transfusion should address the risk of acquiring human immunodeficiency virus, hepatitis B and C viruses, and other blood-borne pathogens.

Preoperative testing, which could include blood work, urinalysis, other laboratory tests (e.g., glucose, creatinine, hemoglobin, and coagulation parameters), pregnancy testing, electrocardiogram, and imaging studies (e.g., CT and MRI), should be individualized based on the patient's age (especially in pediatric patients), concurrent medical problems, route of anesthesia, and surgical procedure planned.

Minor procedures are now more commonly performed in the office setting for patient convenience, avoidance of general anesthesia, and improved reimbursement. In addition, not all patients are surgical candidates, and nonsurgical therapeutic options should always be considered. Patients may have such significant medical problems (e.g., poorly controlled diabetes, heart disease, and pulmonary disease) that they might not safely tolerate anesthesia or surgery.

Intraoperative Considerations

Several intraoperative and perioperative issues should be considered. Prophylactic antibiotics are indicated for many gynecologic surgeries and should be administered within 1 hour of skin incision. Often, a Foley catheter is inserted prior to surgery to prevent the bladder from becoming distended during the procedure. A preoperative pelvic examination of the anesthetized patient can prove useful.

Postoperative Considerations

Postoperatively, a nurse and a member of the anesthesia team assess the patient in the postanesthesia care unit. The patient is either discharged home or admitted to the hospital, depending on the type of procedure performed and the condition of the patient. An operative note must be documented in the chart immediately postoperatively, outlining the preoperative diagnosis, postoperative diagnosis, procedure, surgeon(s), type of anesthesia, amount and type of IV fluid administered, any other fluids given (transfusions or other products), urine output (if indicated), findings, pathology specimens sent, complications, and a statement of patient's condition upon completion of the procedure. This note should generally document steps made to ensure patient safety such as a preoperative "time out"; deep vein thrombosis (DVT) prophylaxis, as indicated; and sponge and instrument counts at the end of the case. Postoperative orders for inpatient stays should include a notation of the procedure performed, the name of the attending physician and service, frequency of vital signs, parameters for calling the physician, diet, activity, IV fluids, pain medications, resumption of any home medications (e.g., antihypertensives, diabetic drugs, and antidepressants), antiemetic medications, DVT prophylaxis, Foley catheter, incentive spirometer, and any necessary laboratory studies.

During a postoperative hospitalization, the patient should be seen at least daily. Careful assessment and monitoring of pain, bladder and bowel function, nausea and vomiting, and vital signs are routine. Early ambulation can reduce the risk of thromboembolism. The most common surgical complications are fever, urinary tract infection (UTI), surgical site drainage and bleeding, minor separation of skin incisions, hemorrhage, pneumonia, ileus, and minor surgical site infection(s). Less common postoperative complications include skin and subcutaneous wound separation, fascial dehiscence or evisceration, bowel perforation, urinary tract injury, severe hemorrhage requiring reoperation, DVT, pulmonary embolism (PE), abscess, sepsis, fistulas, and anesthetic reactions.

Postoperative Complications

Fever is defined as two oral temperatures of ≥38°C at 4-hour intervals. Primary sources of fever include the respiratory and urinary tracts, the incision(s), thrombophlebitis, and any medications or transfusions. **Atelectasis** occurs when patients do not take large inspiratory breaths due to abdominal discomfort. Use of an incentive spirometer can minimize the risk of atelectasis and pneumonia. Use of an indwelling urinary catheter should be minimized, because placement for more than 24 hours increases the risk of UTI (cystitis or pyelonephritis). Ambulatory status affects breathing (hypoventilation when supine) and possible thrombosis (DVT or PE). The wound should be assessed for any signs of infection. If there are no easily visible incisions as with vaginal surgery, a pelvic examination and/or imaging of the pelvis may be needed in selected situations, but is not routinely performed. If the fever resolves after withdrawal of a medication, then a presumptive diagnosis of drug reaction can be made. If the patient has received blood products, the possibility of a reaction to antigens in the transfusion should be investigated as a cause of the fever. Antibiotics should be ordered only when infection is suspected; antipyretics are preferred when only fever is present.

CLINICAL FOLLOW-UP

Based on this patient's discrepancy between the relatively benign Pap findings and those of the endocervical curettage, further evaluation is required. Because the main area of concern is the endocervical canal, the patient is scheduled for a deep, narrow cold-knife conization.

thePoint® Visit http://thePoint.lww.com/activate for an interactive USMLE-style question bank and more!

CHAPTER 35
Human Sexuality

This chapter deals primarily with APGO Educational Topic Area:

TOPIC 56 SEXUALITY AND MODES OF SEXUAL EXPRESSION

Students should be able to describe normal female sexual physiology. They should identify the influence of physical, medical, psychological, and societal factors on the female sexual response. They should be able to outline an initial approach to evaluation of different forms of female sexual dysfunction.

CLINICAL CASE

A 23-year-old G5P5 woman presents because she has lost interest in intercourse with her husband. A review of her past history finds that she was married at an early age, conceiving her first child soon after. She had "difficult pregnancies" with her last two pregnancies, and was unable to get a planned tubal ligation after her last pregnancy. Her last pregnancy ended roughly 6 months ago. She reports trouble losing her pregnancy-related weight gain despite reporting little appetite.

INTRODUCTION

An estimated 35% to 45% of women perceive they have some type of sexual problem—most commonly low sexual desire. Illness, medical and surgical treatment; lack of knowledge to manage this life experience; and emotional and physical stresses contribute to the frequency and severity of sexual problems. Physicians should be able to identify sexual disorders and know whether to offer treatment or refer such patients to a specialist.

Determinants of healthy sexuality are complex and multifactorial. Intrapersonal factors include the sense of one's self as a sexual being, one's overall health status, a general perception of well-being, and the quality of an individual's previous sexual experiences. For partnered individuals, this same list applies to the partner. Interpersonal aspects include the duration and overall quality of the relationship, communication styles, and the number and type of ongoing life events and stressors. Examples of generally "positive" life events, which nevertheless can contribute to sexual dysfunction, include the birth of a child and retirement.

Sexuality involves a broad range of expressions of intimacy and is fundamental to self-identification, with strong cultural, biologic, and psychological components. The obstetrician–gynecologist has an important role in assessing sexual function, because many women view their sexuality as an important quality-of-life issue. Moreover, gynecologic disease processes and therapeutic interventions have the potential to affect sexual response. The clinician should not make assumptions or judgments about the woman's behavior and, when counseling patients, should keep in mind the possibility of cultural and personal variation in sexual practices.

SEXUAL IDENTITY

At the most basic level, the experience of sexuality begins with an individual's genotype and phenotype. From this basic biologic underpinning, children develop a gender identity during early childhood. Eventually, each individual develops a sense of self as a sexual being and a sexual orientation. Each of these latter components is fluid and can vary over time and with particular circumstances. For example, some individuals who consider themselves heterosexual periodically engage in sexual encounters with same-sex partners.

HUMAN SEXUAL RESPONSE

In evaluating sexual problems, it is useful to consider the mechanisms of sexual response in women. Sexual function and dysfunction are perhaps the supreme examples of a necessary blending of mind and body. This interaction is crucial to the understanding of the assessment and management of sexual problems. The dualistic approach common to more traditional models of sexual response limits the understanding of female sexuality insofar as it suggests that dysfunction is psychological and/or biologic. Newer approaches are more holistic in their representations of female sexual response.

Traditional Model

Intimacy-based sexual response models that take other factors into consideration are replacing the traditional Masters and Johnson and Kaplan models of the human sexual response cycle.

The traditional cycle depicts a linear sequence of events: desire, arousal, plateau of constant high arousal, peak intensity arousal and release (orgasm), possible repeated orgasms, and then resolution (Fig. 35.1). However, the sexual response cycle in women is complex, and events do not always occur in a predictable sequence, as they usually do in men.

Neither the stimuli to which the response occurs nor the nature of the "cyclicity" is evident in the traditional model. The usefulness of this model for depicting women's sexuality is limited by the following considerations:

- Women are sexual for many reasons—sexual desire, as in sexual thinking and fantasizing, may be absent initially.
- Sexual stimuli are integral to women's sexual responses.
- The phases of women's desire and arousal overlap.
- Nongenital sensations and a number of emotions frequently overshadow genital sensations in terms of importance.
- Arousal and orgasm are not separate phenomena.
- The intensity of arousal (even if orgasm occurs) is highly variable from one occasion to another.
- Orgasm may not be necessary for satisfaction.
- The outcome of the experience strongly influences the motivation to repeat it.
- Dysfunctions may overlap (e.g., desire and arousal disorders, and orgasm and arousal disorders).

Intimacy-Based Model

An alternative sexual response model depicts an intimacy-based motivation, integral sexual stimuli, and the psychological and biologic factors that govern the processing of those stimuli (i.e., determining the woman's arousability) (Fig. 35.2).

A woman's primary motivation for sexual response often is to be closer to her partner. If sexual arousal is experienced, the stimuli continue, the woman remains focused, and the sexual arousal is enjoyed, she may then sense sexual desire to continue the experience for the sake of the sexual sensations. A psychological and physically positive outcome heightens emotional intimacy with her partner, thereby strengthening the motivation. Any spontaneous desire (i.e., sexual thinking, conscious sexual wanting, and fantasizing) may augment the intimacy-based cycle. Spontaneous desire is particularly common early in relationships or when partners have been apart, is sometimes related to the menstrual cycle, and is extremely variable among women.

Physiology of Female Sexual Response

Systemically, the physiologic components of the female sexual response (Box 35.1) are mediated by increased activity of the autonomic nervous system and include tachycardia, skin flushing, and vaginal lubrication. Several neurotransmitters have been linked to the sexual response cycle. Norepinephrine,

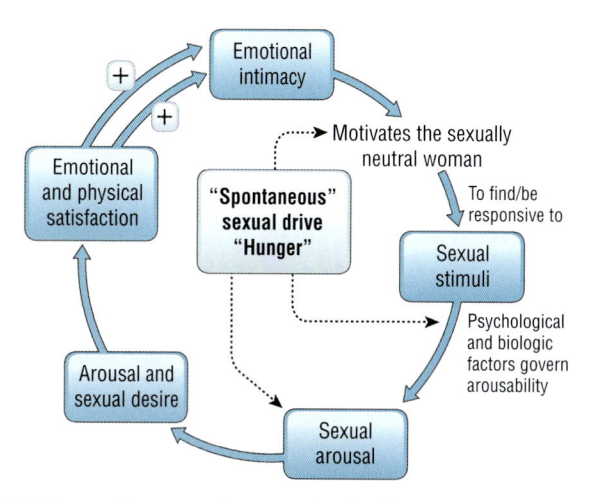

FIGURE 35.2. Negative and positive feedback loops of sexual function. (From Basson R. Female sexual response: the role of drugs in the management of sexual dysfunction. *Obstet Gynecol.* 2001;98(2):350–353.)

BOX 35.1 Components of Subjective Sexual Arousal in Women

- Mental sexual excitement—proportional to how exciting the woman finds the sexual stimulus and context
- Vulvar congestion—direct awareness (tingling and throbbing) is highly variable
- Pleasure from stimulating the engorging vulva
- Vaginal congestion—the woman's direct awareness is highly variable
- Pleasure from stimulating congested anterior vaginal walls and Halban fascia
- Increased and modified lubrication—wetness is usually not directly arousing to the woman
- Vaginal nonvascular smooth muscle relaxation—the woman is usually not aware of this
- Pleasure from stimulating nongenital areas of the body
- Other somatic changes—blood pressure level, heart rate, muscle tone, respiratory rate, and temperature

---

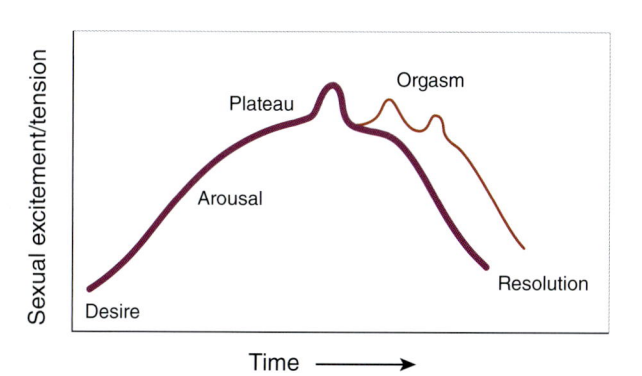

FIGURE 35.1. Traditional sexual response cycle of Masters and Johnson and Kaplan. (From Basson R. Female sexual response: the role of drugs in the management of sexual dysfunction. *Obstet Gynecol.* 2001;98(2):350–353.)

dopamine, oxytocin, and serotonin via 5-hydroxytryptamine (5-HT) 1A and 2C are thought to have positive sexual effects, and serotonin via most other receptors, prolactin, and γ-aminobutyric acid (GABA) are thought to affect the cycle negatively.

Throbbing and tingling and feelings of urgency for more genital contact and vaginal entry are far less consistent for sexually healthy women than are the equivalent sensations in men. Sexually healthy women typically experience these confirmatory sexual stimuli indirectly by the enjoyment of manual or oral stimulation or genital stimulation with a vibrator, which are enhanced when there is vulvar engorgement.

The measurement most commonly used for vaginal congestion is the vaginal pulse amplitude. The upper portion of the vagina dilates via a mechanism that is poorly understood. Figure 35.3 demonstrates some of the physiologic changes seen in sexual response phases. The duration of each phase varies with each individual and for a given individual at different times in her life, and phases can also overlap. Moreover, the state of subjective arousal is itself cognitively appraised. Women consider the appropriateness of being sexual in a particular situation and evaluate their safety. This moment-to-moment emotional and cognitive feedback modulates the experience of arousal. The value of the phases depicted, then, lies in their use in identifying the physiologic events that occur during intimate encounters leading to climax. Clinically, the provider can inquire, during the initial interview and in the course of ongoing therapy, about whether these responses exist.

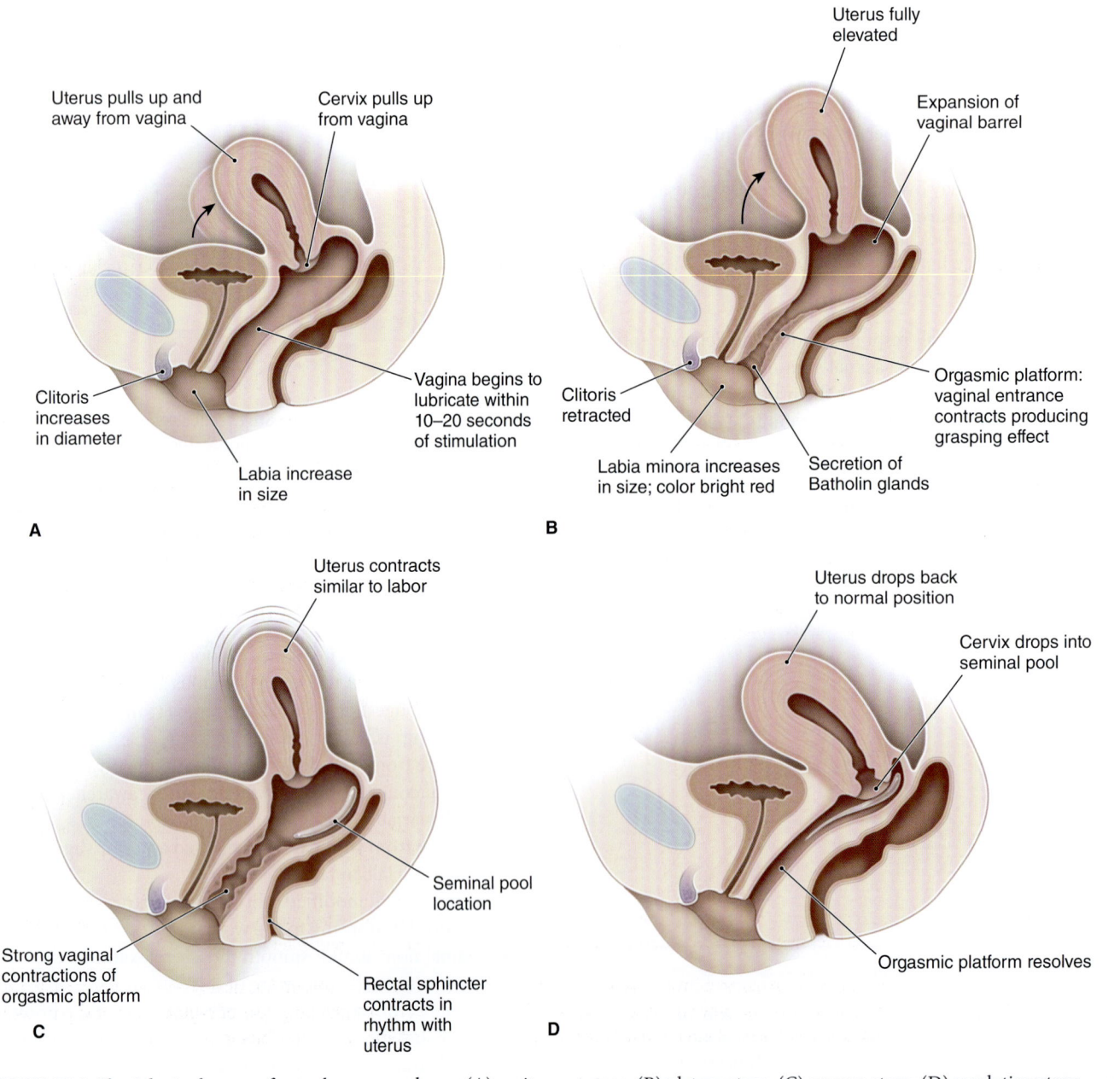

FIGURE 35.3. Physiologic changes of sexual response phases: (A) excitement stage; (B) plateau stage; (C) orgasm stage; (D) resolution stage.

SEXUAL DYSFUNCTION

There is uncertainty as to what exactly constitutes a sexual disorder. The definition of "sexual disorder" is made more complex because what is considered "disordered" varies with time and culture. The World Health Organization's International Statistical Classification of Diseases and Related Problems (ICD-10) suggests that sexual dysfunctions are "the various ways in which an individual is unable to participate in a sexual relationship the way he or she would wish." Table 35.1 lists the categories of sexual dysfunction as recognized by the *Diagnostic and Statistical Manual of Mental Disorders: DSM-5*, which limits its definitions to mental disorders. These definitions continue to be revised and updated to address contextual and other factors.

FACTORS AFFECTING SEXUALITY

The relationship between an overall sense of personal well-being and sexual function is complex.

Depression

Approximately one-third of the women presenting with sexual dysfunction are clinically depressed. Among individuals in whom depression has already been diagnosed, the type and progress of ongoing therapy and prescribed medication should be noted.

Medications

The commonly prescribed selective serotonin reuptake inhibitors, such as fluoxetine, paroxetine, sertraline, and escitalopram, can be associated with decreased sexual desire. The clinical observation that is helpful when evaluating the contribution of medications to female sexual dysfunction is that antidepressants that activate dopaminergic, (central) noradrenergic, and 5-HT1A and 5-HT2C receptors may augment sexual response, whereas those that activate other 5-HT receptors, prolactin, and GABA reduce sexual response. The medications least likely to interfere with sexual response are nefazodone, mirtazapine, bupropion, venlafaxine, and buspirone.

Further complicating this picture is that depression itself causes a decrease in sexual desire. Other medications that can be associated with female sexual dysfunction are included in Box 35.2.

Medical Conditions

Medical conditions that affect energy and well-being may indirectly affect sexual desire and response, particularly those that

TABLE 35.1 CATEGORIES OF SEXUAL DYSFUNCTION

Disorder	Diagnostic and Statistical Manual of Mental Disorders (DSM-5)	Commentary
Female sexual interest/arousal disorder	Reduced or absent interest in sexual activity including lack of erotic thoughts and cues. No interest in initiating sexual activity or responding to same from partner. Absent or reduced sensations (genital and nongenital) during sexual activity. The disturbance causes marked distress or interpersonal difficulty	It is necessary to take into account the interpersonal context. There may be a "desire discrepancy" where a woman has a lower desire for sex than does her partner. If patient identifies as "asexual," the diagnosis of female sexual interest/arousal disorder is not made
Female orgasmic disorder	Marked delay in, infrequency of, or absence of orgasm following a normal excitement phase; or marked reduced intensity of orgasm. The disturbance causes distress or interpersonal difficulty	The clinical usefulness of these definitions is limited for the following reasons: • Women with female orgasmic disorder often have female sexual interest/arousal disorder • It is often the intensity of orgasm that has markedly diminished and is causing distress—especially with women who have neurologic disorders or sudden premature loss of androgen production
Genitopelvic pain/penetration disorder	Recurrent or persistent genital pain associated with sexual intercourse (dyspareunia). The disturbance causes marked distress or interpersonal difficulty	Penile–vaginal movement of intercourse may be impossible because of the pain caused by partial or complete penile entry
	Recurrent or persistent involuntary spasm of the musculature of the outer third of the vagina that interferes with sexual intercourse (vaginismus)	Muscular "spasm" has never been documented. Reflexive muscle tightening, fear of vaginal entry, and pain with its attempt are characteristic

Data from the American Psychiatric Association. *Diagnostic and Statistical Manual of Mental Disorders: DSM-5.* Washington, DC: APA; 2013.

are associated with the loss of estrogen and/or androgen production (Box 35.3). Estrogen is thought to have both a direct effect (by supporting vulvar and vaginal congestion) and an indirect effect (by influencing mood) on female sexual response. There is likewise a strong consensus that androgens are needed for sexual response in women, although the limitations of widely available laboratory assays have made it difficult to establish a direct correlation between specific androgen levels and women's sexual desire.

Psychological Factors

Psychological factors commonly affect sexual response in women as well (Box 35.4). Psychological factors continuously modulate any arousal experienced from sexual stimuli and influence the woman's motivation to seek or respond to those sexual stimuli—compounding any negative effects from biologic factors.

MANAGEMENT

A woman's sexuality is influenced by her health and emotional well-being; likewise, healthy sexual functioning promotes physical and emotional well-being. However, studies suggest that fewer than one half of patients' sexual concerns are recognized by their physicians. The obstetrician–gynecologist has a paramount role in assessing sexual function and managing sexual dysfunction to ensure the well-being of his or her patients. Beginning with screening a patient for sexual dysfunction, taking her history, and assessing sexual dysfunction risk factors, the physician establishes a diagnosis if dysfunction is present and treats the patient or refers her for treatment, as appropriate.

Screening for Sexual Dysfunction

Discussions of sexuality are accomplished best in a confidential and supportive setting. Mutual trust and respect in the patient–clinician relationship will allow appropriate discussion of questions and concerns about sexuality. A nonjudgmental and respectful approach by the clinician, as well as awareness by the clinician of his or her own biases, is essential for effective care.

BOX 35.2 Medications Commonly Affecting Sexual Response

- Selective estrogen receptor modulators (such as raloxifene, tamoxifen, and phytoestrogens)
- Codeine-containing analgesics
- Alcohol (chronic abuse)
- Cyproterone acetate
- Medroxyprogesterone (high doses)
- Some β-blockers used for hypertension or migraine prevention
- Anticonvulsants taken for epilepsy (but not necessarily for other conditions)
- Oral contraceptives

BOX 35.3 Conditions Commonly Affecting Sexual Response

Conditions associated with loss of adrenal androgen production and/or loss of estrogen production
- Bilateral salpingo-oophorectomy
- Chemotherapy-induced menopause
- Gonadotropin-releasing hormone–induced menopausal symptoms
- Premature ovarian failure
- Oral estrogen therapy (may cause androgen insufficiency)
- Oral contraceptives (may cause androgen insufficiency)
- Addison disease
- Hypopituitary states
- Hypothalamic amenorrhea
- Chronic renal failure
- Chronic cardiac failure
- Chronic neurologic conditions
- Chronic renal disease
- Arthritis
- Hyperprolactinemia
- Hypothyroid and hyperthyroid states
- Conditions interfering with autonomic function and/or somatic genital nerve function
- Diabetes mellitus
- Multiple sclerosis
- Spinal cord injury
- Radical pelvic surgery
- Past Guillain-Barré syndrome

BOX 35.4 Psychological Factors Commonly Affecting Sexual Response

- Past negative sexual experiences, including abuse
- Knowledge of a likely unsatisfactory or painful outcome (e.g., dyspareunia)
- Decreasing self-image (e.g., from chronic infertility)
- Potent nonsexual distractions
- Lack of physical privacy
- Feelings of shame, naiveté, or embarrassment
- Partner sexual dysfunction
- Lack of safety from pregnancy and sexually transmitted diseases
- Orientation concerns
- Fear of physical safety

Patients are more likely to develop trusting relationships with their health care practitioners when the issue of confidentiality has been addressed directly. A confidential relationship, in turn, can facilitate the open disclosure of health histories and behaviors. The use of broad, open-ended questions in a routine history gathering can help disclose problems that require further exploration. Inquiry about the partner's sexual function and level of satisfaction may elicit more specific information and give an indication of the couple's level of communication.

Studies have suggested that directed screening for dysfunction can be as simple as three questions in the review of systems: "Are you sexually active (expressive, involved)?" "Do you have any sexual concerns (problems, troubles)?" and "Do you have any pain associated with sex?" If any of the responses suggest that a dysfunction may be present, further, more open-ended questions are in order. Questioning patients about their sexual desire, especially about responsive desire and the components of arousal, can point to management options about which patients and their partners can be counseled. Simply providing information, confirming that many women have the same concerns, and explaining how one aspect of dysfunction leads to another can be therapeutic.

The clinician should not make assumptions about the woman's choice of partner. Although most women report that their sexual partners are men, some women only have sex with other women, and others may have partners of both sexes. The use of terms such as "partner" instead of "husband" and "sexual activity" instead of "intercourse" and an understanding of nonheterosexual sexuality—including that of lesbians, bisexual women, and transgendered individuals—will assist in open communication and assessment of the patient's problem.

Additional History

The patient's history is the crucial part of an assessment for sexual dysfunction. The duration of the dysfunction and whether it has evolved over months or years should be clarified. Long-term problems are particularly difficult to evaluate and manage, and a concomitant in-depth psychological assessment may be needed. The context of the patient's life when the dysfunction began is needed, addressing psychological, biologic, and relationship factors. Her medical history and past sexual experiences are recorded, including medications and any substance abuse. The woman's developmental history also may be needed, particularly if her dysfunction is lifelong.

Deliberate inquiries should be made to assess the quality of the interpersonal relationship between the patient and her partner, including mutual satisfaction with their sexual relationship. The perceived importance of physical intimacy for a given couple depends largely on whether they are satisfied with that aspect of their relationship. Among couples who are not experiencing sexual dysfunctions, each partner will estimate that the sexual component of their relationship accounts for approximately 10% of their overall happiness. In couples experiencing sexual difficulties, however, the sexual aspects are estimated as accounting for approximately 60% of the overall relationship quality. This dramatic shift in perception underscores the importance that physical intimacy holds within the context of the overall relationship.

Risk Factors

Women often disclose sexual disorders during visits for routine gynecologic care, whereas some patients present with a complaint involving a sexual issue or of a specific sexual dysfunction. Other patients neither express a sexually related complaint nor have a medical problem with a commonly associated sexual issue. Still other patients have a medical problem or have had a medical or surgical therapy that is known to be associated with sexual issues or problems (Box 35.5).

In addition, sexual function may be affected by biologic and psychological aspects of reproduction and the life cycle (Box 35.6). The mechanisms governing the interplay between psychological responses to reproductive events and the biologic changes themselves are not well understood. However,

---

BOX 35.5 Medical Risk Factors for Sexual Disorders

- Depression, with or without antidepressants
- Breast cancer that required chemotherapy
- Radical hysterectomy for cancer of the cervix
- Multiple sclerosis
- Hypertension
- Diabetes
- Sexual abuse

BOX 35.6 Biologic and Psychological Risk Factors for Sexual Disorders

- Healthy pregnancy
- Complicated pregnancy where intercourse and orgasm are precluded
- Postpartum considerations
- Recurrent miscarriage
- Therapeutic abortion
- Infertility
- Perimenopause
- Natural menopause
- Premature menopause (idiopathic and iatrogenic)
- Use of oral contraceptives

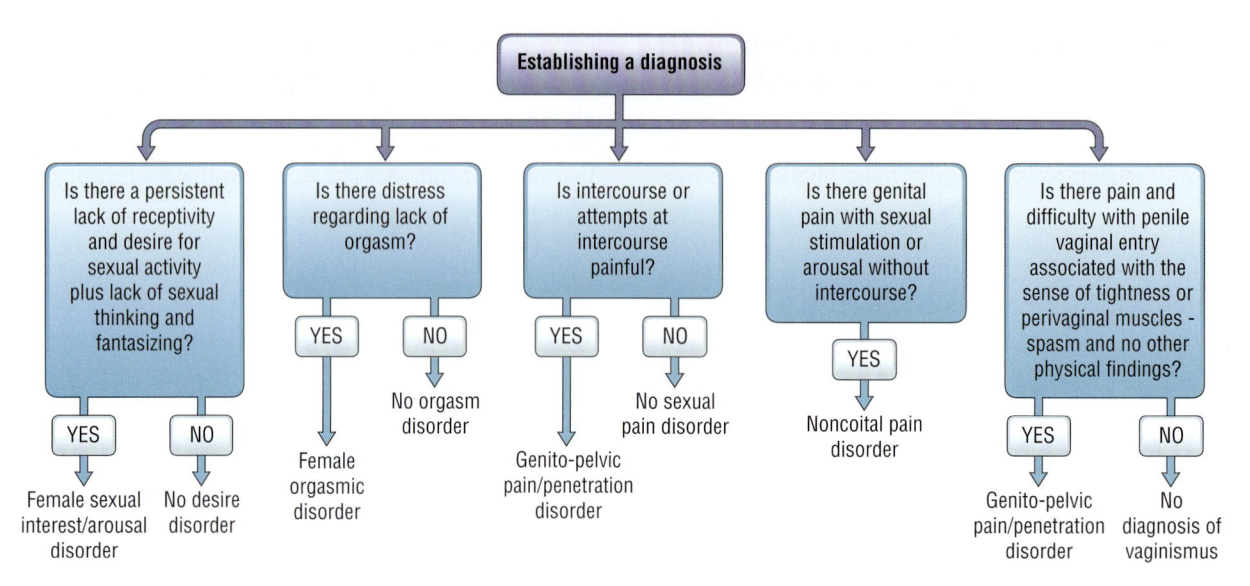

FIGURE 35.4. Algorithm for establishing a diagnosis of female sexual dysfunction.

women's past sexual experiences, self-image, support from and attraction to their sexual partners, sufficiency of their knowledge of sexuality, and sense of control are all typically important factors.

Establishing a Diagnosis

For each of the various dysfunctions, it is important to establish whether it is lifelong or acquired and to distinguish between dysfunctions that are situational and those that are global or generalized (Fig. 35.4). If the woman's sexual response is healthy in some circumstances, physical organic factors are not involved in a dysfunction. It is, therefore, important to ask patients about their sexual response with masturbation, with viewing or reading erotica, and with being with individuals other than their regular partners—even if this activity does not involve physical sexual interaction.

● TREATMENT

Some sexual problems can be managed by the primary physician, whereas others are best referred to a sex therapist. A detailed, sensitive, and respectful assessment will help establish a dialogue with the patient. It is difficult to distinguish between assessment and treatment, because the physician often provides information during the assessment that is therapeutic. Management may be within the scope of the obstetrician–gynecologic practice, or a referral may be appropriate, depending on the nature and the extent of the problem, and the physician's comfort with addressing the issues. Box 35.7 shows interventions that commonly occur in gynecologic offices. Largely, the decision should be based on whether or not the physician has adequate resources

---

BOX 35.7 Primary Care Treatments for Sexual Dysfunction

- Giving nonjudgmental and respectful information (e.g., of women's sexual response cycles)
- Normalizing nonpenetrative sex to both partners
- Screening for depression and sexual side effects of antidepressants
- Screening for medication-associated female sexual dysfunction and advising alternative medications
- Replacing estrogen locally or systemically
- Replacing testosterone (formulations for women are currently being developed)
- Prescribing flibanserin, a multifunctional serotonin agonist-antagonist approved by the Food and Drug Administration in 2015 for the treatment of hypoactive sexual desire disorder in premenstrual women
- Treating hyperprolactinemia, hypothyroidism, or hyperthyroidism
- Possibly using vasoactive drugs for genital arousal disorder in the future
- Applying the model of women's responsive desire to the individual patient experiencing low desire, empowering her and her partner to make the necessary changes

---

to approach sexual dysfunction from an integrated perspective, rather than merely a biologic one. Psychology, pharmacology, partner intimacy, and alternative therapies are some of the other factors that must be addressed in treating sexual dysfunction. Referrals to mental health practitioners, marriage or relationship counselors, or sex therapists may be appropriate. Box 35.8 shows when and why to refer patients.

BOX 35.8 When to Refer Patients with Sexual Dysfunction

The decision to refer a patient depends on a number of factors, including:
- Expertise of the obstetrician–gynecologist
- Complexity of the sexual dysfunction
- Presence or absence of partner sexual dysfunction
- Availability of a psychologist, psychiatrist, or sex therapist
- Motivation of the patient (and partner) to undergo more detailed assessment before therapeutic interventions

More detailed assessments and management may be available from:
- Physicians with extra training and expertise in sexuality—psychiatrists, family practitioners, gynecologists, and urologists
- Psychologists
- Sex therapists and abuse counselors
- Physiotherapists (regarding hypertonic pelvic muscle–associated dyspareunia)
- Relationship counselors
- Support groups (e.g., for women with past histories of breast cancer, women with vulvar vestibulitis syndrome–associated chronic dyspareunia, and women with interstitial cystitis–associated dyspareunia)

CLINICAL FOLLOW-UP

The most common cause of reduced libido is depression. Social stresses, the demands of a household with multiple small children, and the possibility of fears about future pregnancy all suggest depression in this patient. A screening questionnaire confirms the suspicion, and with medication, social support, and counseling, her libido would be expected to resolve shortly. However, as mentioned previously, antidepressants may also decrease libido as a side effect. Ongoing follow-up between patient and provider is important.

---

thePoint® Visit http://thePoint.lww.com/activate for an interactive USMLE-style question bank and more!

CHAPTER 36
Sexual Assault and Domestic Violence

This chapter deals primarily with APGO Educational Topic Areas:

TOPIC 57 SEXUAL ASSAULT
TOPIC 58 DOMESTIC VIOLENCE

Students should be able to identify the risk factors for sexual assault and appropriately screen for domestic violence. They should appreciate the prevalence of violence against women and children. They should be able to outline the initial management of a victim of sexual assault, addressing both medical and psychosocial issues.

CLINICAL CASE

A 20-year-old G1P1 college student presents for evaluation after being forced to have unprotected sexual intercourse by her date. Her last menstrual period was about 3 weeks ago; she has no medical problems and is taking no medication. She appears anxious and "nervous" and has trouble collecting her thoughts. Her urine pregnancy test is negative.

INTRODUCTION

Sexual assault and domestic violence pose obvious immediate and often enduring long-term health and emotional risks. The compassionate and thoughtful care of victims and their families is an important goal of everyone involved in health care.

SEXUAL ASSAULT

Sexual assault is defined legally as involving any genital, oral, or anal penetration by a part of the accused's body or by an object, using force or without consent.

Criminal sexual assault, or rape, is often further characterized to include acquaintance rape, date rape, statutory rape, child sexual abuse, unwanted kissing, touching, fondling, and incest. These terms generally relate to the age of the victim and her relationship to the abuser. Local law defines the details of each of these characterizations.

Each year, some 365,000 women in the United States experience sexual assault, rape, or attempted rape. An estimated one in five women have experienced sexual assault in their lifetimes and one in seventy-one men will be raped. However, most do not file a complaint or report, and, therefore, its true prevalence is unknown. Rape is the most underreported crime. According to the National Sexual Violence Resource, 63% of adult sexual assaults are not reported and only 12% of child sexual abuse is reported. The 2009 U.S. National Crime Victimization Survey estimates that only 55% of rapes and sexual assaults were reported. When a male is raped, less than 10% are thought to be reported, and female–male and female–female rape are not included in this survey. Inconsistent definitions of rape, overreporting, underreporting, and false reporting create controversial statistical disparities and the concern that many rape statistics are unreliable or misleading. Because of the complex problems caused by sexual assault, treatment is best managed by a multidisciplinary team that fulfills the following roles:

- **Care for the victim's emotional needs**, acute and (if possible within the constraints of the health care system) long term
- **Evaluation and treatment of medical needs**, acute and follow-up
- **Collection of forensic specimens** and preparation of a record acceptable for health care and in the legal process

Definitions and Types of Sexual Assault

Sexual assault occurs in all age, racial, and socioeconomic groups; the very young, handicapped, and the very old are particularly vulnerable. Although the act may be committed by a stranger, in many cases it is committed by an acquaintance.

Some situations have been defined as variants of sexual assault. **Marital rape** is defined as forced coitus or related sexual acts within a marital relationship without the consent of a partner; it often occurs in conjunction with and as part of physical abuse in cases of domestic or intimate partner violence.

Date rape or **acquaintance rape** is another manifestation of intimate partner violence. In this situation, a woman may voluntarily participate in sexual play, but coitus occurs, often forcibly, without her consent. Date rape often goes unreported, because the woman may think that she contributed to the act by participating up to a point or that she will not be believed. Lack of consent may also occur in situations in which cognitive function is impaired by flunitrazepam, alcohol, or other drugs; sleep; injury with unconsciousness; or developmental delay.

All states have statutory rape statutes criminalizing sexual intercourse with a girl younger than a specific age, because she is defined, by statute, as being incapable of consenting. Many states also have laws addressing **aggravated criminal sexual assault**, which has the following attributes: weapons are used, lives are endangered, or physical violence is inflicted; the act is committed in relationship to another felony; or the woman is older than 60 years, physically handicapped, or mentally retarded.

Management

The medical and health consequences of sexual assault are both short and long term. All patients should be screened for a history of sexual assault. Most women with a history of sexual assault will not have reported it to a nonpsychiatric physician. Yet, women with a history of assault are more likely to present with chronic pelvic pain, dysmenorrhea, vaginismus, nonspecific vaginitis, menstrual cycle disturbances, and sexual dysfunction than are women without such a history. Adults abused as children are four to five times more likely to have abused alcohol and illicit drugs. They are also twice as likely to smoke, be physically inactive, and be severely obese. Survivors are more likely to have had 50 or more intercourse partners.

Clinicians evaluating women in the acute phase of a sexual assault have a number of responsibilities, both medical and legal (Box 36.1). Specific responsibilities are determined by the patient's needs and state law. Clinicians should be familiar with state rape and assault laws and comply with any legal requirements regarding reporting and the collection of evidence. They must also be aware that every state and the District of Columbia require physicians to report child abuse, including sexual assault. Additionally, physicians should be aware of local protocols regarding the use of specially trained sexual assault forensic examiners or sexual assault nurse examiners.

The clinician should provide medical and counseling services as well as inform the patient of both her medical and legal rights. Many jurisdictions and several clinics have developed a sexual assault assessment kit, which lists the steps necessary and the items to be obtained so that as much information as possible can be prepared for forensic purposes. Many health care facilities have nurses who are trained to collect needed samples and information. If these individuals are available, it is appropriate to request their assistance. Rape crisis counselors and centers can also provide valuable support. In addition, the clinician must assess and treat all injuries, perform STD screening, and provide prophylaxis against infectious diseases and unintended pregnancy.

Initial Care

When a woman who has experienced sexual assault communicates with the physician's office, emergency department, or clinic before presenting for evaluation, she should be encouraged to come immediately to a medical facility and

---

BOX 36.1 Physician's Role in Evaluation of Sexual Assault Patients

Medical Issues
- Ensure that informed consent is obtained from patient
- Assess and treat physical injuries or triage and refer
- Obtain pertinent past gynecologic history
- Perform physical examination, including pelvic examination (with appropriate chaperone or support person present)
- Obtain appropriate specimens for sexually transmitted disease (STD) testing
- Obtain baseline serologic tests for hepatitis B virus, human immunodeficiency virus (HIV), and syphilis
- Provide appropriate infectious disease prophylaxis as indicated
- Provide or arrange for provision of emergency contraception as indicated
- Provide counseling regarding findings, recommendations, and prognosis
- Arrange follow-up medical care and referrals for psychosocial needs

Legal Issues[a]
- Provide accurate recording of events
- Document injuries
- Collect samples (pubic hair, fingernail scrapings, vaginal secretion and discharge samples, saliva, blood-stained clothing, or other personal articles) as indicated by local protocol or regulation
- Identify the presence or absence of sperm in the vaginal fluids and make appropriate slides
- Report to authorities as required
- Ensure security of chain of evidence

[a] Many jurisdictions have prepackaged "rape kits" for the initial forensic examination that provide specific containers and instructions for the collection of physical evidence and for written and pictorial documentation of the victim's subjective and objective findings. Hospital emergency rooms or the police themselves may supply the kits when called to respond or when bringing a patient to the hospital. Most often the emergency physician or specially trained nurse response team will perform the examination, but all physicians should be familiar with the forensic examination procedure. If called to perform this examination and the physician has no or limited experience, it may be judicious to call for assistance because any break in the technique in collecting evidence, or break in the chain of custody of evidence, including improper handling of samples or mislabeling, will virtually eliminate any effort to prosecute in the future.

American College of Obstetricians and Gynecologists. Sexual Assault, Committee Opinion #499. Washington, DC: American College of Obstetricians and Gynecologists; August 2011.

---

be advised not to change her clothes, bathe, douche, urinate, defecate, wash out her mouth, clean her fingernails, smoke, eat, or drink.

In recent years, there has been a trend toward the implementation of hospital-based programs to provide acute medical and evidentiary examinations by sexual assault nurse examiners or sexual assault forensic examiners. Physicians play a role in the policy and procedure development and implementation of these programs and serve as sources for referral, consultation, and follow-up. In some parts of the country, however, obstetrician–gynecologists will still be the first point of contact for evaluation and care following a sexual assault.

Emergency Evaluation

In an optimal situation, the woman is able to seek care in a facility where there is a trained multidisciplinary team. A team member should remain with the patient to help provide a sense of safety and security and, thereby, begin the therapeutic process, including, specifically, assurance of the patient's lack of guilt. The patient should be encouraged, in a supportive, nonjudgmental manner, to talk about the assault and her feelings. Treatment for life-threatening trauma needs to begin immediately. Such trauma is uncommon, although minor trauma is seen in one-fourth of the victims. Even in life-threatening situations, any sense of control that can be given the patient is helpful. Obtaining consent for treatment is not only a legal requirement but also an important aspect of the emotional care of the patient, by helping her regain control of her body and her circumstances.

Although patients are commonly reluctant, they should be encouraged to work with the police, because such cooperation is associated with improved emotional outcomes for victims. History taking about a sexual assault is necessary to gain medical and forensic information and is, as well, an important therapeutic activity. Recalling the details of the assault in the supportive environment of the health care setting allows the victim to begin to gain an understanding of what has happened and to start emotional healing (Box 36.2).

BOX 36.2 Documenting Patient History after Assault

Gynecologic History
- Menstrual history
- Method of contraception
- Date of last consensual sexual experience
- Obstetric history
- Gynecologic history, including infections
- Activities (e.g., bathing, douching, eating, and drinking since the assault) that could affect forensic evidence gathered

Details of Sexual Assault
- Location, timing, and nature of the sexual assault
- Use of force, weapons, or any substances that would impair the mental status of the victim
- Loss of consciousness
- Information about the assailant, including ejaculation and use of a condom, contraceptive, or lubricant

Physical Examination

Victims of sexual assault should be given a complete general physical examination, including a pelvic examination. Forensic specimens should be collected, and cultures or other tests for STDs should be obtained. When collecting forensic specimens, it is critical that the clinician follow the directions on the forensic specimen kit. If called on to perform a sexual assault examination, the physician who has no experience or limited experience should consider requesting assistance to ensure appropriate evidence collection. These specimens are kept in a health professional's possession or control until turned over to an appropriate legal representative. This ensures that the correct specimen reaches the forensic laboratory and is called the **chain of evidence**.

Initial laboratory tests should include cultures or other tests from the vagina, anus, and pharynx for STDs. Collection of serum for rapid plasma reagin (RPR) for syphilis, hepatitis antigens, and HIV is needed. Urinalysis, culture, and sensitivity, as well as a pregnancy test for menstrual age women (regardless of contraceptive status) are collected. **Antibiotic prophylaxis** should be offered when indicated (Table 36.1). **Emergency contraception** should be offered and is described in Chapter 26.

Note that rape and sexual assault are legal terms that should not be used in medical records. Rather, the health care provider should only report the findings and not state a conclusion.

Posttreatment Evaluation

Within 24 to 48 hours of disclosure and initial treatment, victims should be contacted by phone or seen for a **posttreatment evaluation**. At this time, emotional or physical problems are managed and follow-up appointments arranged. Potentially serious problems, such as suicidal ideation, rectal bleeding, and evidence of pelvic infection, may go unrecognized by the victim during this time because of fear or continued cognitive dysfunction. Specific questions must be asked to ensure that such problems have not arisen.

Subsequent Care

The patient's HIV status should be tested within 72 hours of the initial assault and then repeated at 6 weeks, 3 months, and 6 months. Regardless of whether nonoccupational postexposure prophylaxis is initiated, the physician should provide HIV risk reduction and primary prevention counseling.

At a 1-week follow-up visit, a general review of the patient's progress is made and any specific new problems addressed. The next routine visit is at 6 weeks, when a complete evaluation, including physical examination, repeat tests for STDs, and a repeat RPR is performed. Another visit at 12 to 18 weeks may be indicated for repeat HIV titers, although the current understanding of HIV infection does not allow an estimate of the risk of exposure for sexual assault victims. Each victim should receive as much counseling and support as is necessary, with referral to a long-term counseling program if needed.

If the physician is not directly involved in the acute care of the victim, it is helpful for him or her to obtain records of the patient's emergency evaluation. These enable the physician to be certain that all appropriate testing was performed and to

TABLE 36.1 TESTING AND MEDICAL PROPHYLAXIS FOR SEXUAL ASSAULT PATIENTS

Sexually Transmitted Disease Infections	Prophylaxis
Gonococcal infection	For patients with uncomplicated genital, rectal, and pharyngeal gonorrhea, dual therapy for gonococcal infections is recommended by the CDC with combination therapy with: • Ceftriaxone 250 mg as a single intramuscular dose PLUS Azithromycin 1 g orally in a single oral dose OR, if ceftriaxone is not available: • Cefixime, 400 mg, single oral dose PLUS Azithromycin, 1 g, single oral dose* If the patient has a severe penicillin allergy: • Gemifloxacin, 320 mg, single oral dose PLUS Azithromycin, 2 g, single oral dose OR • Gentamicin, 240 mg, single intramuscular dose PLUS Azithromycin, 2 g, single oral dose* *If azithromycin is not available or if the patient is allergic to azithromycin, doxycycline (100 mg orally twice a day for 7 days) may be substituted as the second antimicrobial. Note: • Dose of azithromycin is increased to 2 g when used with the alternative antibiotics, gemifloxacin or gentamicin. • Dual therapy with gentamicin and azithromycin or azithromycin alone should be used during pregnancy testing should be done at initial examination; if vaginal discharge, malodor, and itching are present, examination for bacterial vaginosis and candidiasis should be conducted
Chlamydia trachomatis infection Trichomoniasis Bacterial vaginosis	• Ceftriaxone, 125 mg intramuscularly in a single dose PLUS Metronidazole, 2 g orally in a single dose PLUS Azithromycin, 1 g orally single dose OR • Doxycycline, 100 mg twice daily orally for 7 days Note: Testing for chlamydia and *Trichomonas vaginalis* should be done at initial examination; if vaginal discharge, malodor, and itching are present, examination for bacterial vaginosis and candidiasis should be conducted.
Syphilis	• Routine prophylaxis is not currently recommended • Serologic tests should be conducted at initial evaluation and repeated 6, 12, and 24 weeks after the assault
Hepatitis B	• Postexposure hepatitis B vaccination (without hepatitis B immune globulin) administered at the time of initial examination if not previously vaccinated • Follow-up doses should be administered at 1–2 and 4–6 months after first dose • Serologic tests should be conducted at initial evaluation
HIV infection	<72 hours postexposure with an individual known to have HIV: • 28-day course of highly active retroviral therapy; consultation with an HIV specialist is recommended (serologic tests should be conducted at initial evaluation and repeated 6, 12, and 24 weeks after the assault) 72 hours postexposure to an individual of unknown HIV status or >72 hours postexposure: • Individualized assessment
Herpes simplex virus infection	• Routine prophylaxis is not currently recommended but should be individualized if there is a report of a genital lesion on assailant • A 7- to 10-day course of acyclovir, famciclovir, or valacyclovir may be offered; however, there are no data on the efficacy of this treatment
Human papillomavirus infection	• There is no preventive, postexposure treatment recommended at this time (see Chapter 47 for routine prevention guidelines)
Pregnancy	• Emergency contraception; first dose should be given within 72 hours of the assault (see Chapter 26)
Injuries	If more than 10 years since last immunization: • Tetanus toxoid booster, 0.5 mL intramuscularly

Adapted from Workowski KA, Levine WC; Centers for Disease Control and Prevention. Sexually Transmitted Diseases Treatment Guidelines 2010. *MMWR Recomm Rep.* 2012;61(31);590–594; del Rio C, Hall G, Holmes K, et al. Oral Cephalosporins No Longer a Recommended Treatment for Gonococcal Infections recommendations from the U.S. Department of Health and Human Services.

provide the patient with full results. Patients may be disturbed to learn that the results of their forensic evaluation are usually not provided to their physician. In this situation, it is helpful to refer the patient to local legal or police authorities, who can also be helpful in answering patients' questions.

Emotional Issues

A woman who is sexually assaulted loses control over her life during the period of the assault. Her integrity and sometimes her life are threatened. She may experience intense anxiety, anger, or fear.

Rape Trauma Syndrome

After the assault, a **rape trauma syndrome** commonly occurs, comprising an acute phase and a delayed phase. This rape trauma syndrome is similar to a grief reaction in many respects. As such, it can only be resolved when the victim has emotionally worked through the trauma and personal loss related to the event and replaced it with other life experiences. An inability to think clearly or remember things such as her past medical history, termed **cognitive dysfunction**, is a particularly distressing aspect of the syndrome. The involuntary loss of cognition may raise fears of "being crazy" or of being perceived as "crazy" by others. It is also frustrating for the health care team, unless it is recognized that this is an involuntary, temporary, and understandable reaction to the sexual assault and not a willful action.

Acute Phase (Immediate Response)
The acute phase of rape trauma syndrome may last for hours or days and is characterized by distortion or paralysis of the individual's coping mechanisms. Outward responses vary from complete loss of emotional control to an apparently well-controlled behavior pattern. Signs may include generalized pain throughout the body; headache; eating and sleep disturbances; and emotional symptoms, such as depression, anxiety, and mood swings.

Delayed (or Organization) Phase
The delayed phase of rape trauma syndrome is characterized by flashbacks, nightmares, and phobias as well as somatic and gynecologic symptoms. Often occurring months or years after the event, it may involve major life adjustments.

Posttraumatic Stress Disorder

Those who have experienced physical and sexual assault are also at great risk for developing posttraumatic stress disorder. Clusters of symptoms may not appear for months or even years after a traumatic experience. These symptoms include the following:

- Reliving the event
- Experiencing flashbacks, recurring nightmares, and, more specifically, intrusive images that appear at any time
- Extreme emotional or physical reactions, including shaking, chills, palpitations, or panic reactions accompanying vivid recollections of the attack

Avoiding reminders of the event constitutes another symptom in posttraumatic stress disorder. These women become emotionally numb, withdrawing from friends and family and losing interest in everyday activities. There may be an even deeper reaction of denial of awareness that the event actually happened.

Symptoms such as easy startling, being hypervigilant, irritability, sleep disturbances, and lack of concentration are part of a third symptom cluster known as **hyperarousal**. These women often will have a number of co-occurring conditions, such as depression, dissociative disorders (losing conscious awareness of the present, or "zoning out"), addictive disorders, and many physical symptoms.

● CHILD SEXUAL ASSAULT

Ninety percent (90%) of child victimization is by parents, family members, or family friends; "stranger rape" is relatively uncommon in children. It is extremely important to know who the perpetrator is and how the child sustained the injury so that the child can be removed from an unsafe environment. Box 36.3 shows behavioral and physical signs and symptoms commonly associated with child sexual abuse.

Assessment/Examination

Because the assessment of a child for sexual abuse involves specific skills and has the potential for legal challenge, the individual who undertakes this evaluation should have significant experience in this area. This assessment is usually done by pediatricians and is beyond the skills of most general gynecologists. Awareness of and sensitivity to the issues, special needs, and circumstances of the child are important for obstetrician–gynecologists who are consulted to treat an injury to the pelvic floor. In many cities, a child abuse team consisting of trained experts including physicians, social workers, and counselors is available to perform the assessment.

BOX 36.3 Signs of Child Sexual Assault

- Night terrors
- Changes in sleeping habits
- Clinging
- Sexual acting out
- Aggression
- Regression
- Eating disturbances
- Recurrent somatic complaints of abdominal pain
- Headaches
- Vaginal pain
- Dysuria
- Encopresis
- Enuresis
- Hematochezia
- Vaginal erythema
- Vaginal discharge or bleeding

The sexual abuse evaluation begins with an interview of the caretaker and the child. Unless the child refuses to leave the caretaker, the child should be interviewed privately to obtain specific details of the abuse. Questioning should be nondirective to elicit spontaneous responses such as time and location of the abuse, description of the scene, name and description of the perpetrator, and type of sexual acts. The child's statements should be recorded verbatim; electronic interviews are helpful so that the child does not have to describe the abuse repeatedly. Good documentation of the interview is critical in the prosecution of sexual abuse cases because, in many instances, the patient's statement is the only evidence that the abuse occurred. Documentation of the specific names the child uses for her genitalia is recommended to help others understand the context of her statements.

The urgency of an evaluation of sexual abuse depends on how soon after the event the child is brought in for care. If the child presents within 72 hours of the last episode of abuse, the physician should immediately arrange for evaluation of the child and focus on collection of forensic evidence. However, fewer than 10% of child sexual abuse cases are reported within 72 hours. In cases that are reported after 72 hours, the patient should be referred to the nearest sexual abuse center, where more resources are available to conduct the evaluation.

Management

In the treatment of a child who is the victim of sexual abuse, management should focus (as applicable) on treatment of injuries, treatment of STDs, prevention of pregnancy, protection against further abuse, and psychological support for the patient and her family. Approximately 5% of abused children will acquire a sexually transmitted infection (STI); the clinician must decide if culturing for STIs is appropriate by evaluating the individual situation and taking into account community standards. Superficial injuries (e.g., bruises, edema, and local irritation) resolve within a few days and require only meticulous perineal hygiene. In some patients with extensive skin abrasions, broad-spectrum antibiotics may be given as prophylaxis. Small vulvar hematomas can usually be controlled by pressure or an ice pack, and even massive swelling of the vulva usually subsides promptly when cold packs and external pressure are applied. More extensive penetrative vaginal and anal injuries require thorough radiographic and anesthetic examination to rule out intra-abdominal penetration.

DOMESTIC VIOLENCE

Domestic violence is reported by over 25% of women at some time during their lives and is a significant source of illness and injury to women.

Definition

Domestic violence refers to the violence perpetrated within the context of family or intimate relationships. Family members include parents, siblings, and other blood relatives as well as legal relatives such as step-parents, in-laws, and guardians. Violence that occurs between current or former partners is referred to as **intimate partner violence** and includes male abuse by female partners and violence between partners in lesbian, gay, bisexual, and transgendered relationships.

Domestic violence may involve one or more of these presentations:

- **Physical abuse**, such as hitting, slapping, kicking, and choking, is the most obvious form of physical abuse. It should be suspected when there is evidence of trauma, especially to the head and neck or trunk associated with a history of violence, or when an explanation of the trauma does not seem appropriate (Table 36.2). Unfortunately, pregnancy appears to be a period of greater risk of inflicted trauma.
- **Sexual abuse** is another presentation of domestic violence.
- **Emotional**, **financial**, or **psychological abuse**, **neglect**, or **threat** and is often traumatic and/or long-standing. Examples include undermining of self-worth, deprivation of sleep or emotional support, repetitive unpredictability of response to life situations, threats, destruction of personal property or the killing of pets, lies, manipulation of friends, and interference in the workplace. Domestic violence is usually cyclic and repetitive, with periods of calm alternating with periods of rapidly increasing tensions or violence, the latter often increasing in severity with each iteration of the cycle.
- **Reproductive and sexual coercion** are forms of abuse as well. This behavior includes explicit attempts to impregnate a partner against her will, control outcomes of a pregnancy, coerce a partner to have unprotected sex, and interfere with contraceptive methods.

TABLE 36.2 INDICATORS OF PHYSICAL ABUSE IN DOMESTIC VIOLENCE

Area of Injury	Descriptions
Head and neck	Bruises, abrasions, strangle marks, black eye, broken nose, orbital ridge, or jaw, pulled hair, permanent hearing loss, facial lacerations
Trunk	Evidence of blunt trauma, including bruises (especially breasts and abdomen), fractured collarbones, and ribs
Skin	Multiple lesions in various stages of healing, "rug rash" abrasions, burns (cigarette, lighter, liquid splash), bites
Extremities	Evidence of restraint, including muscle strains, spiral fractures, rope or restraint burns, "crescent moon"–shaped fingernail marks or bruises in the shape of a hand or blunt instrument

Screening: Risk Factors

Recognition is the first, most important, and most often a missed issue. When domestic violence is suspected, compassionate and thoughtful discussion with the possible victim, as well as attention to any physical injury, is requisite. All patients should be asked about past or present violence in their lives as part of the routine health history. Although all women are at risk for abuse, certain life experiences and circumstances may place some women at greater risk (Box 36.4).

The clinician's role is (1) to know the signs and symptoms of intimate partner violence, (2) to ask all patients about the past or present exposure to violence, (3) to intervene and refer as appropriate, and (4) to assess the patient's risk of danger (Box 36.5).

BOX 36.4 Identifying the Abused Woman

No true stereotype exists, but certain risk factors are found among victims:
- Younger women, especially those in long, difficult relationships
- History of violence or dysfunctional family of origin
- Dysfunctional past relationships
- Pregnancy, especially if unintended
- Relationships in transitions (i.e., separation and divorce)
- Any situation where the partner is overly attentive, especially if he repeatedly answers for her
- STDs
- Substance abuse

Clinical clues that the patient is or has been abused:
- Unexplained, multiple, and recurring injuries
- Elusive pain and other somatic complaints
- Specific problems in pregnancy
- Poor compliance, hostility, passivity, minimal response
- Psychological changes, especially depression, anxiety, panic attacks, sleep and eating disorders
- Compulsive sexual behaviors, seductive behavior with examiners (not sexual, but to gain attention)
- Self-destructive, high-risk behaviors (poor self-care, substance abuse, self-neglect and self-injury, and suicidal ideation)
- Increased use of prescription narcotics and tranquilizers
- Frequent visits and increased use of the health care system
- Extensive medical records documenting unresolved problems
- Unusual disclosure style (too detailed, not credible, cannot explain injuries in a satisfactory way, and cannot explain why instructions have not been followed)
- Difficulty in tolerating examination

Difficulty in tolerating other medical situations that recreate traumatic experiences (isolation, injection of medications, restraints and immobilization, and surgery)

Counseling

If the patient will be returning to an unsafe home, safety planning should be conducted, and referrals to service agencies in the community should be provided. Women can be encouraged to call a woman's shelter for more help with a safety plan and be assured that such calls would be anonymous. Box 36.6 details suggested steps for patients when they are ready to leave an abusive situation.

BOX 36.5 The RADAR Model of the Physician's Approach to Domestic Violence

R: Remember to ask routinely about partner violence (past and present) in your own practice

A: Ask directly about violence with such questions as, "At any time, has a partner hit, kicked, or otherwise hurt or frightened you?" Interview your patient in private at all times.

D: Document information about "suspected domestic violence" or "intimate partner violence" in the patient's chart, and file reports when required by law

A: Assess your patient's safety. Is it safe to return home? Find out if any weapons are kept in the house, if the children are in danger, and if the violence is escalating

R: Review options with your patients. Know about the types of referral options (e.g., shelters, support groups, and legal advocates)

Massachusetts Medical Society. *Partner Violence: How to Recognize and Treat Victims of Abuse.* 4th ed. Waltham, MA: Massachusetts Medical Society; 2004.

BOX 36.6 Making an Exit Plan to Leave an Abusive Relationship

- Pack a bag in advance and leave it at a neighbor's or friend's house. Include cash or credit cards and extra clothes for yourself and your children. Take each child's favorite toy or plaything.
- Hide an extra set of car and house keys outside of the house in case you have to leave quickly.
- Take important papers, such as the following:
  - Birth certificate (including children's)
  - Health insurance cards and medicine
  - Deed or lease to the house or apartment
  - Checkbook and extra checks
  - Social security number or green card/work permit
  - Court papers or orders
  - Driver's license or photo identification
  - Pay stubs

Used with permission from American College of Obstetricians and Gynecologists. *Guidelines for Women's Health Care.* 4th ed. Washington, DC: American College of Obstetricians and Gynecologists; 2014. P.542

CLINICAL FOLLOW-UP

A sense of emotional dysfunction is common in the immediate period following a sexual assault. The possibility that both the confusion and the sexual assault could be connected with a substance or substances ingested with or without the patient's knowledge could be involved and should be explored when the prospect is seriously considered. A complete history and physical examination is needed, along with STD testing, evidence collection, antibiotic prophylaxis, and emotional support.

---

thePoint®   Visit **http://thePoint.lww.com/activate** for an interactive USMLE-style question bank and more!

V Reproductive Endocrinology and Infertility

CHAPTER 37
Reproductive Cycles

This chapter deals primarily with APGO Educational Topic Area:

TOPIC 45 NORMAL AND ABNORMAL UTERINE BLEEDING

Students should be able to describe endocrinologic and physiologic characteristics of a normal menstrual cycle.

CLINICAL CASE

A 42-year-old woman presents with concerns that there may be something wrong with her "hormones" and she fears that she may be going through menopause. Her menstrual periods began at the age of 13 years and were moderately regular except when interrupted for her two pregnancies. Periods lately have been roughly 32 days apart, are preceded by breast tenderness and bloating, and generally have 3–4 days of flow. She underwent a tubal ligation following the birth of her last child. The patient's concern centers on a lack of energy, loss of libido, and moderate weight gain. She reports that this is how all the other women in her family "went through the change."

INTRODUCTION

In the female reproductive cycle, ovulation is followed by menstrual bleeding in a cyclic, predictable sequence, if pregnancy does not occur. This recurring process is established during puberty (average age of menarche is 12 years) and continues until the years prior to menopause (average age is 51 years). Regular ovulatory cycles are usually established by the third year after menarche, and continue until the perimenopause. Therefore, between ages 15 and 45 years, a woman has approximately 30 years of ovulatory reproductive cycles. The reproductive cycles may be interrupted by conditions, including pregnancy, lactation, illness, gynecologic disorders, and endocrine disorders, and exogenous factors, such as hormone-based contraceptives and various other medications.

The duration of an adult reproductive cycle, from the beginning of one menses (Day 1) to the beginning of the next menses (Day 1), averages approximately 28 days (±7 days) and comprises three distinct phases. The **follicular phase** begins with the onset of menses (the first day of the menstrual cycle) and ends on the day of the **luteinizing hormone (LH) surge**. **Ovulation** occurs within 30 to 36 hours of the LH surge. The **luteal phase** begins on the day of the LH surge and ends with the onset of menses. The follicular and luteal phases each last approximately 14 days in regularly menstruating reproductive age women; however, variability in cycle length is more frequent at the extremes of reproductive ages. The duration of the luteal phase remains relatively constant, whereas the duration of the follicular phase can vary.

HYPOTHALAMIC–PITUITARY–GONADAL AXIS

Hypothalamic–pituitary–gonadal axis refers to the complex interactions between the hypothalamus, pituitary, and ovaries that regulate the reproductive cycle. These interactions are based on the interplay of the hormones released by these structures: gonadotropin-releasing hormone (GnRH); the gonadotropins **follicle-stimulating hormone (FSH)** and LH; and the ovarian sex steroid hormones, estrogen and progesterone. Through stimulatory and inhibitory actions, these hormones directly and indirectly stimulate oocyte development and ovulation, endometrial development to facilitate embryo implantation, and menstruation. Feedback loops between the hypothalamus, pituitary, and ovaries are presented in Figure 37.1. Disruption of any of these communication and feedback loops results in alterations of hormone levels, which can lead to disorders of the reproductive cycle; ultimately, ovulation, reproduction, and menstruation can be affected.

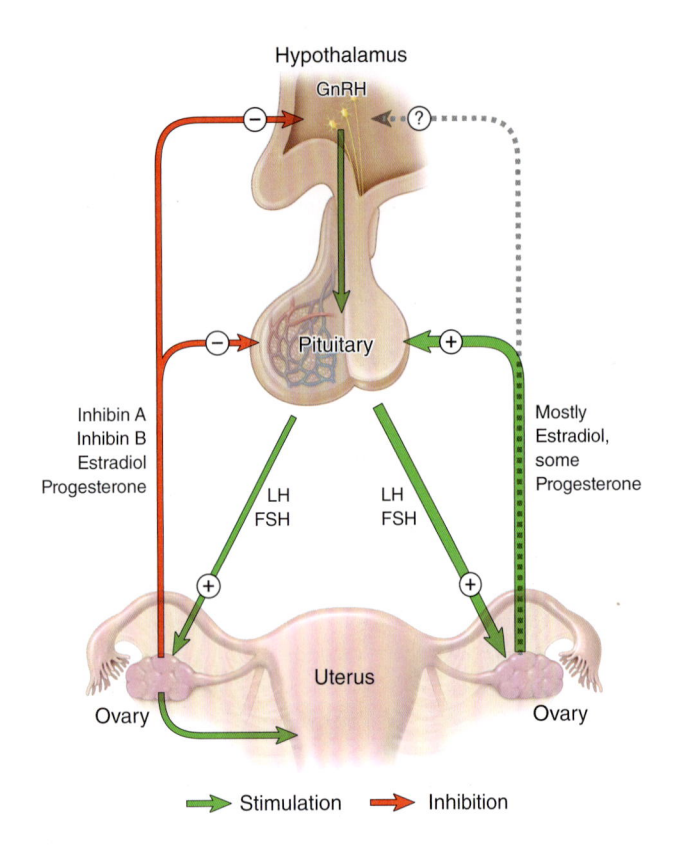

FIGURE 37.1. The reproductive cycle requires complex interactions and feedback between the hypothalamus, pituitary, and ovaries, which are simplified in this diagram. GnRH, gonadotropin-releasing hormone; FSH, follicle-stimulating hormone; LH, luteinizing hormone.

Hypothalamic Gonadotropin-Releasing Hormone Secretion

The **GnRH** is secreted in a pulsatile fashion from the arcuate nucleus of the hypothalamus. GnRH reaches the anterior pituitary through the hypothalamic–pituitary portal vascular system. The pulsatile secretion of GnRH stimulates and modulates pituitary gonadotropin secretion. Due to its remote location and a half-life of 2 to 4 minutes, GnRH cannot be directly measured; therefore, measurements of LH pulses are used to indicate GnRH pulsatile secretion. Ovarian function requires the pulsatile secretion of GnRH in a specific pattern that ranges from 60-minute to 4-hour intervals. Therefore, the hypothalamus serves as the pulse generator of the reproductive cycle. Coordinated GnRH release is stimulated by various neurotransmitters and catecholamines as well as by the inherent pulsatility of the GnRH neurons.

Pituitary Gonadotropin Secretion

The pituitary gonadotropins FSH and LH are glycoprotein hormones secreted by the anterior pituitary gland. FSH and LH are also secreted in pulsatile fashion in response to the pulsatile release of GnRH; the magnitude of secretion and the rates of secretion of FSH and/or LH are determined largely by the levels of ovarian steroid hormones, **estrogen** and **progesterone**, and other ovarian factors (such as inhibin, activin, and follistatin).

When a woman is in a state of relative estrogen deficiency, as in the early follicular phase, the principal gonadotropin secreted is FSH. The ovary responds to FSH secretion with estradiol production, with subsequent negative feedback on the pituitary inhibiting FSH secretion and positive feedback facilitating LH secretion.

Ovarian Steroid Hormone Secretion

At birth, the human ovary contains approximately 1 to 2 million primordial follicles. Each follicle contains an oocyte that is arrested in prophase of the first meiotic division. A large number of these inactive primordial follicles undergo a degenerative process known as **atresia** during childhood; thus, at menarche, 300,000 to 500,000 oocytes remain.

The immature oocyte is encircled by a single layer of **granulosa cells**, followed by a thin basement membrane that separates the follicle from the surrounding ovarian stroma. Early follicular maturation occurs independently of gonadotropins, the granulosa cells proliferate into multiple layers, and the surrounding stromal cells differentiate into **theca cells**. Granulosa cells produce estrogens, including estrone and **estradiol**, the latter being the more potent of the two. Theca cells produce androgens, which serve as the precursors required for granulosa cell estrogen production. Androgens (androstenedione and testosterone) enter the granulosa cells by diffusion and are converted to estrogen. The two-cell theory of estrogen synthesis is diagrammed in Figure 37.2.

During follicular development, FSH binds to FSH receptors on the granulosa cells, causing cellular proliferation and increased binding of FSH, thereby increasing production of estradiol. Estradiol stimulates the proliferation of LH receptors on theca and granulosa cells, and LH stimulates the theca cells to produce androgens. Greater androgen production leads to increased estradiol production. Rising estrogen levels influence the pituitary gland through negative feedback and result in suppression of FSH and LH secretion. In the late follicular phase, peak estradiol concentrations from the dominant follicle have positive feedback on the pituitary, which stimulates the midcycle surge of LH secretion that is necessary for ovulation. With ovulation, the dominant ovarian follicle releases its oocyte and transitions to a progesterone-secreting ovarian cyst, the **corpus luteum**. The process of follicular maturation is presented in Figure 37.3.

● REPRODUCTIVE CYCLE

As discussed, the reproductive cycle is divided into three phases: Menstruation and the follicular phase, ovulation, and the luteal phase. These three phases refer to the status of the ovary during the reproductive cycle. In contrast, when referring to the endometrium, the phases of the menstrual cycle are termed the **proliferative and secretory phases.**

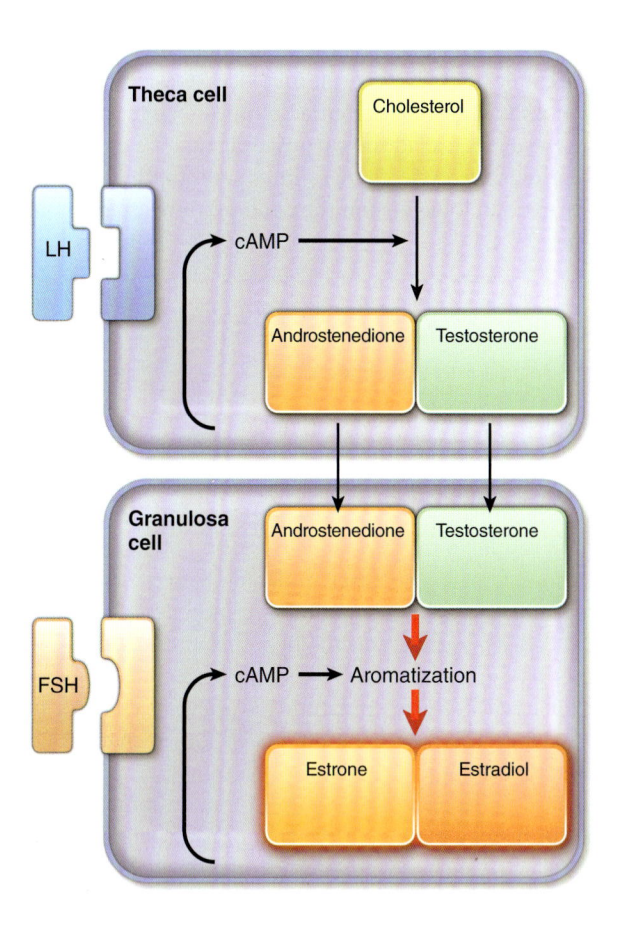

FIGURE 37.2. The two-cell theory of estrogen production. cAMP, cyclic adenosine monophosphate; LH, luteinizing hormone; FSH, follicle-stimulating hormone.

Phase I: Menstruation and the Follicular Phase

The first day of menstrual bleeding is considered day 1 of the menstrual cycle. When conception does not occur, the involution of the corpus luteum and, hence, the decline of progesterone and estrogen levels cause menstruation. Normal menstruation lasts 3 to 7 days, during which women lose 20 to 60 mL of dark, nonclotting (previously clotted) blood. Menstruation consists of blood and desquamated superficial endometrial tissues. Prostaglandins in the secretory endometrium and menstrual blood produce contractions of the uterine vasculature and musculature, which in turn cause endometrial ischemia and uterine cramping. These prostaglandin-associated uterine contractions also aid in expulsion of the menstrual blood and tissue. Rising estrogen levels in the early follicular phase induce endometrial healing, which leads to cessation of menstruation.

At the end of the luteal phase, serum concentrations of estradiol, progesterone, and LH reach their lowest levels. In response to low hormone levels, FSH begins to rise in the late luteal phase before the onset of menstruation to recruit the next cohort of follicles. Thus, during menstruation, follicular growth has already been initiated for the new reproductive cycle. Estradiol levels rise during the follicular phase, causing a decline in FSH. LH remains low in the early follicular phase, but increasing estrogen levels have positive feedback on LH release, and LH starts to rise by the midfollicular phase. Although several follicles begin the maturation process, only the follicle with the greatest number of granulosa cells and FSH receptors and the highest estradiol production becomes the dominant follicle; the nondominant follicles undergo atresia.

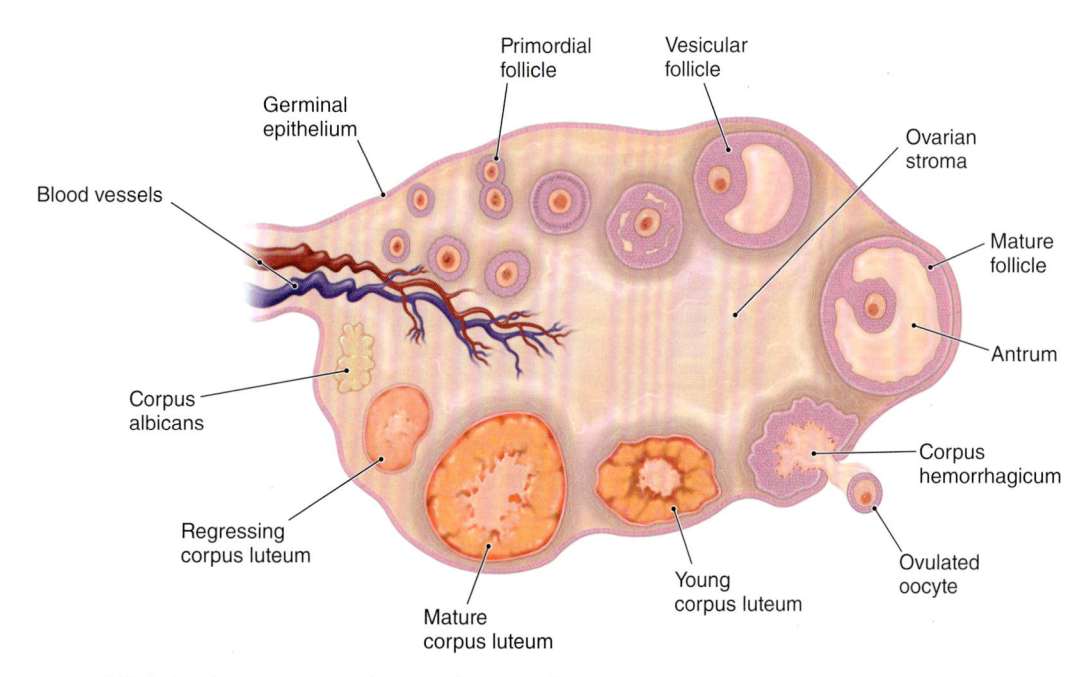

FIGURE 37.3. Ovarian follicle development during the reproductive cycle.

Phase II: Ovulation

As the dominant follicle secretes an increasing amount of estradiol, there is marked positive feedback to the pituitary gland to secrete LH. By days 11 to 13 of the cycle, the LH surge occurs, which triggers ovulation. The LH surge begins 34 to 36 hours prior to ovulation, and peak LH secretion occurs 10 to 12 hours prior to ovulation. With the LH surge, the granulosa and theca cells undergo distinct changes and begin production of progesterone. Meiosis of the primary follicle resumes after the LH surge and the first polar body is released; the oocyte then arrests in metaphase of the second meiotic division until fertilization occurs. During ovulation, the oocyte is expelled from the follicle, and the follicle is converted into the corpus luteum.

Some women experience a twinge of pain ("**mittelschmerz**") at the time of ovulation and can precisely identify the time of ovulation. Other women do not experience this brief discomfort but can recognize characteristic symptoms that occur due to progesterone production after ovulation.

Phase III: Luteal Phase

The luteal phase of the menstrual cycle is characterized by an alteration in the balance of sex steroid secretion from predominance of estrogen to predominance of progesterone. The process of follicular development has led to increased numbers of LH receptors on the granulosa and theca cells. The midcycle LH surge stimulates these LH receptors and converts the enzymatic machinery of these cells to produce and secrete progesterone; this process is called **luteinization**. Progesterone has negative feedback on pituitary secretion of FSH and LH; therefore, both hormones are suppressed during the luteal phase. The corpus luteum also produces estradiol in a pattern that parallels progesterone secretion.

The production of progesterone begins approximately 24 hours before ovulation and rises rapidly thereafter. Maximal progesterone production occurs 3 to 4 days after ovulation. The lifespan of the corpus luteum ends approximately 9 to 11 days after ovulation; if conception does not occur, the corpus luteum undergoes involution (a progressive decrease in size), and progesterone production sharply declines. This withdrawal of progesterone releases FSH from negative feedback; thus, FSH levels begin to rise prior to menstruation and the initiation of a new cycle.

The carefully orchestrated sequence of estrogen production and then progesterone production is essential for proper endometrial development to allow implantation of an embryo. If the oocyte becomes fertilized and implantation occurs, the resulting zygote begins secreting human chorionic gonadotropin, which sustains the corpus luteum for another 6 to 7 weeks. Adequate progesterone production by the corpus luteum is necessary to sustain early pregnancy. By 9 to 10 weeks of pregnancy, placental steroidogenesis is well established, and the placenta assumes progesterone production.

The corpus luteum measures approximately 2.5 cm in diameter, has a characteristic deep yellow color, and can be seen on gross inspection of the ovary if surgery is performed during the luteal phase of the cycle. As the function of the corpus luteum declines, it decreases in volume and loses its yellow color. After a few months, the corpus luteum becomes a white fibrous streak within the ovary, called the **corpus albicans**.

Reproductive cycle changes in gonadotropins, steroid hormones, ovarian follicles, and the endometrium are summarized in Figure 37.4.

CLINICAL MANIFESTATIONS OF HORMONAL CHANGES

Hormonal changes induced by the hypothalamic–pituitary–gonadal axis and the adrenal gland trigger puberty, and hormones continue to exert a cyclic influence until a woman reaches menopause. At that time, the lack of cyclic ovarian function results in the permanent cessation of menstruation.

Various female structures undergo changes in response to the reproductive cycle hormones: The endometrium and endocervix, breasts, vagina, and the hypothalamus. Changes in the endocervix and breasts can be directly observed. Daily assessment of basal body temperature can identify changes in the hypothalamic thermoregulation center. Other changes can be assessed by cytologic examination of a sample from the vaginal epithelium or histologic evaluation of an endometrial biopsy. A careful history may identify symptoms associated with hormone effects, such as abdominal bloating, fluid retention, mood and appetite changes, and uterine cramps at the onset of menstruation.

Endometrium

Within the uterus, the endometrium undergoes dramatic histologic changes during the reproductive cycle. During menstruation, the entire endometrium is expelled, and only the basal layer remains. During the follicular phase, the rise in estrogen levels stimulates endometrial cell growth: The endometrial stroma thickens and the endometrial glands become elongated to form the proliferative endometrium. In an ovulatory cycle, the endometrium reaches maximal thickness at the time of ovulation.

When ovulation occurs, the predominant hormone shifts from estrogen to progesterone, and distinct changes occur within the endometrium at almost daily intervals. Progesterone causes differentiation of the endometrial components and converts the proliferative endometrium into a secretory endometrium. The endometrial stroma becomes loose and edematous, while blood vessels entering the endometrium become thickened and twisted. The endometrial glands, which were straight and tubular during the proliferative phase, become tortuous and contain secretory material within the lumen. With the withdrawal of progesterone at the end of the luteal phase, the endometrium breaks down and is sloughed during menses.

If ovulation does not occur, and estrogen continues to be produced, the endometrial stroma continues to thicken, and the endometrial glands continue to elongate. Endometrial thickness can be measured by several diagnostic tools (e.g., transvaginal

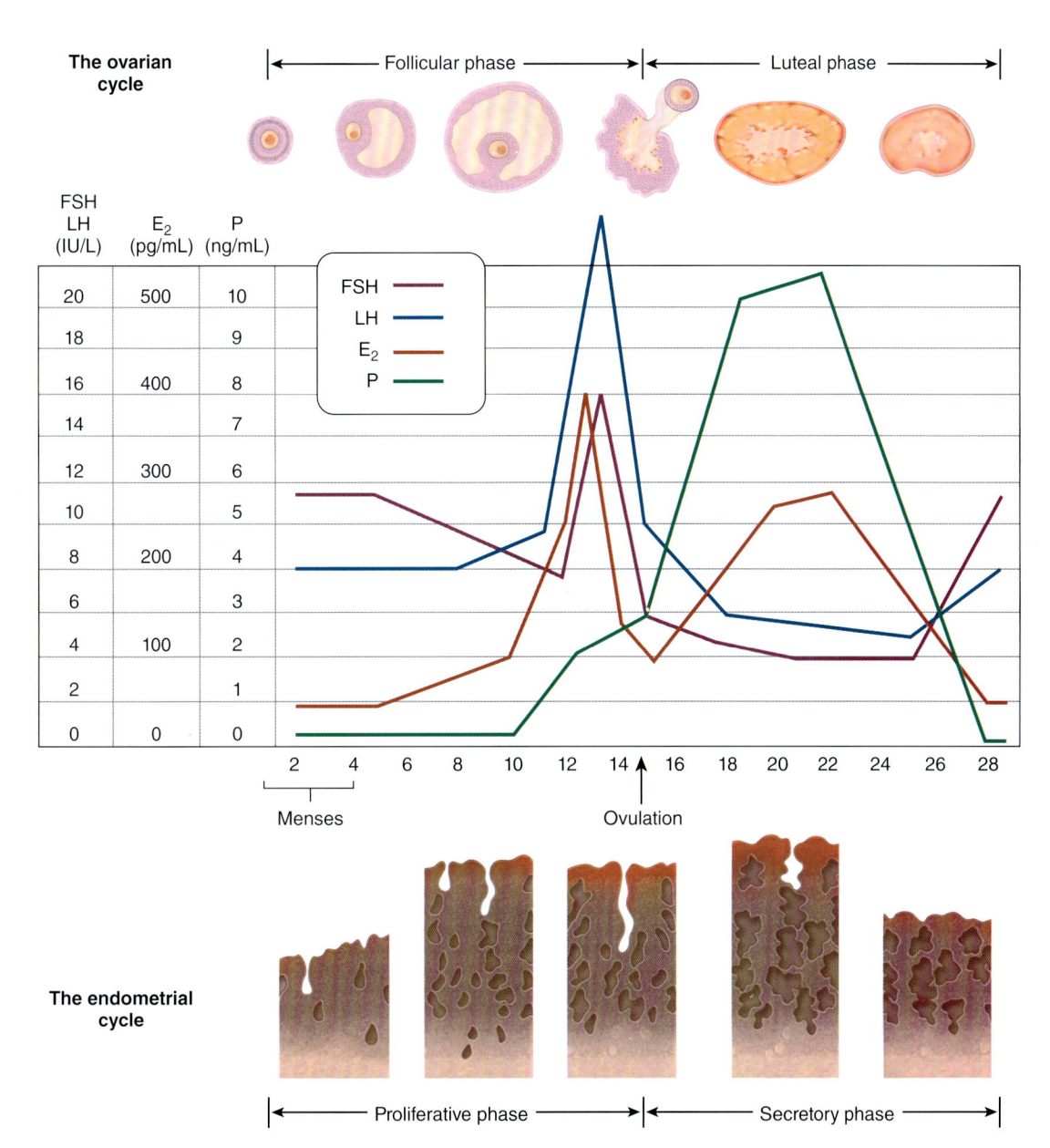

FIGURE 37.4. A summary of pituitary, ovarian, uterine, and vaginal changes during the reproductive cycle. FSH, follicle-stimulating hormone; LH, luteinizing hormone; E_2, estradiol; P, progesterone.

ultrasonography, sonohysterography), but only an endometrial biopsy will differentiate proliferative and secretory endometrium. The endometrium eventually outgrows its blood supply and sections of the endometrium slough intermittently. Without progesterone withdrawal to initiate desquamation of the entire endometrium, bleeding is acyclic and occurs outside of hormonal control irregularly and for prolonged periods of time. When women present with abnormal uterine bleeding, anovulatory bleeding is a common diagnosis (see Chapter 39).

Endocervix

The endocervix contains glands that secrete mucus in response to hormonal stimulation. Under the influence of estrogens, the endocervical glands secrete large quantities of thin, clear, watery mucus. Endocervical mucus production is maximal at the time of ovulation. This mucus facilitates sperm capture, storage, and transport and is rich in fructose. With ovulation, progesterone reverses the effect of estrogen on the endocervical mucus, and mucus production diminishes.

Some women monitor their cervical mucus to optimize the timing of intercourse when trying to conceive or in order to avoid conception. However, the timing of these changes is nonspecific and is one of the less effective methods of contraception recognized by the American College of Obstetricians and Gynecologists when compared with other methods, such as long-acting reversible contraceptives (intrauterine devices and implants).

Breasts

Estrogen exposure is necessary for pubertal breast development; however, reproductive cycle changes in the breast occur primarily due to progesterone effect. The ductal elements of the breast, nipple, and areola respond to progesterone secretion. Some women will notice more breast tenderness and fullness in the luteal phase due to progesterone-mediated changes.

Vagina

Estrogen promotes growth of the vaginal epithelium and maturation of the superficial epithelial cells of the mucosa. During sexual stimulation, the presence of estrogen aids vaginal transudation and lubrication, which facilitates intercourse. During the luteal phase of the reproductive cycle, the vaginal epithelium retains its thickness, but the secretions are markedly diminished.

Hypothalamic Thermoregulation Center

Progesterone is a hormone with thermogenic effects; under the influence of progesterone, the hypothalamus shifts the basal body temperature upward by 0.5°F to 1.0°F over the average preovulatory temperature. This shift occurs abruptly with the beginning of progesterone secretion and quickly returns to baseline with the decline in progesterone secretion. Therefore, these changes in basal body temperature reflect changes in plasma progesterone concentration.

Because the basal body temperature assumes basal conditions at rest, it should be performed immediately in the morning upon awakening, prior to any activity. Special thermometers with an expanded scale are available for this purpose. Identification of this characteristic biphasic curve provides retrospective, indirect evidence of ovulation; however, some ovulatory women do not demonstrate these changes.

CLINICAL FOLLOW-UP

Although there may be some familial element to when a woman undergoes menopause, this patient would seem to have a normal reproductive cycle with melasma that suggests that she continues to ovulate. She is reassured when told this information and that her prior tubal ligation would have no effect on the age of menopause. Further exploration of her history and symptoms suggested mild depression, which was further confirmed when a test of thyroid function returned normal values.

thePoint®   Visit http://thePoint.lww.com/activate for an interactive USMLE-style question bank and more!

CHAPTER 38
Puberty

This chapter deals primarily with APGO Educational Topic Area:

TOPIC 42   PUBERTY

Students should be able to describe the normal endocrinologic changes and normal sequence of events in puberty and identify any deviations. They should be able to outline a basic approach to evaluating the patient with precocious puberty and delayed puberty. They should discuss the complex psychological issues associated with puberty and abnormal puberty.

CLINICAL CASE

A 15-year-old girl is brought in by her mother because she has not yet started to menstruate. She is tall for her age but otherwise of normal body habitus. She had a growth spurt that began when she was about age 12 years and began breast development at age 13 years. Physical examination finds Tanner stage III breast development and stage III to IV pubic hair. She shaves her underarms.

INTRODUCTION

Puberty is an endocrine process that involves the physical, emotional, and sexual transition from childhood to adulthood. It occurs gradually in a series of well-defined events and milestones. When puberty is early or delayed, an understanding of the hormonal events of puberty and the sequence of physical changes is essential to diagnosis of a potential problem. Knowledge of the events of puberty is also key to understanding the process of reproduction.

NORMAL PUBERTAL DEVELOPMENT

A series of endocrine events initiate the onset of sexual maturation. The hypothalamic–pituitary–gonadal axis begins to function during fetal life and remains active during the first few weeks following birth, after which time the axis becomes quiescent secondary to enhanced negative feedback of estrogen. The hypothalamic–pituitary–gonadal axis again becomes active during puberty, triggering the production of gonadotropin-releasing hormone (GnRH). The gonadotropins control the production of sex steroids from the ovary, and higher levels cause the physical changes of puberty. At approximately age 10 to 11 years, **adrenarche**, the increase in production of androgens, occurs in the adrenal glands. Adrenarche involves the increased production of dehydroepiandrosterone, which can be converted to more potent androgens (testosterone and dihydrotestosterone).

The process of sexual maturation requires approximately 4 years. It takes place in an orderly, predictable sequence that includes growth acceleration, breast development (**thelarche**), pubic hair development (**pubarche**), maximum growth rate, **menarche**, and ovulation. The initial event is accelerated growth; however, this may be subtle, and breast budding is easier to detect as the first event. The sequence of breast development and pubic hair growth is quantified by the Tanner classification of sexual maturity (Fig. 38.1).

The ages at which some of these events occur are presented in Table 38.1. There is a strong relationship between body fat content and the onset of puberty. Mild (body mass index [BMI] 30–34.99) to moderate (BMI 35–39.99) obesity results in earlier puberty, whereas thinness results in later puberty. The onset of puberty is also marked by significant ethnic differences. Puberty usually begins earlier in African-American and Mexican American girls than in white girls, and much of this difference may result from differences in BMI (Table 38.1). In contrast, puberty tends to begin in Asian American girls later than in white girls. BMI may account for most of this difference, although as yet undefined genetic or environmental factors may be important. Also, socioeconomic conditions, nutrition, and access to preventive health care may influence the timing and progression of puberty.

ABNORMALITIES OF PUBERTAL DEVELOPMENT

The abnormalities of puberty include precocious puberty, primary amenorrhea, delayed sexual maturation, and incomplete sexual maturation.

The presence of any of these disorders requires investigation of both the hypothalamic–pituitary–gonadal axis and the

TABLE 38.1 ETHNICITY AND ONSET OF PUBERTY

Event	Mean Age (years)		
	Non-Hispanic Blacks	Mexican Americans	Non-Hispanic Whites
Thelarche	9.5	9.8	10.3
Pubarche	9.5	10.3	10.5
Menarche	12.2	12.5	12.5

Data from McDowell MA, Brody DJ, Hughes JP. Has age at menarche changed? Results from the National Health and Nutrition Examination Survey (NHANES) 1999–2004. *J Adoles Health*. 2007; 40(4): 227-231; Goldman MB, Troisi R, Rexrode KM. *Women and Health*, 2nd ed. Waltham, MA: Academic Press, 2013; Finer LB, Philbin JM. Trends in ages at key reproductive transitions in the United States, 1951–2010. *Women's Health Issues* 24(3): e271-e279.

reproductive outflow tract. The initial evaluation should begin with the measurement of pituitary gonadotropin (follicle-stimulating hormone [FSH] and luteinizing hormone [LH]) levels, which helps distinguish a hypothalamic–pituitary etiology from a gonadal etiology.

Precocious Puberty

Precocious puberty is the onset of secondary sexual characteristics prior to the age of 6 years in African-American girls and 7 years in white girls. Precocious puberty is caused by either GnRH-dependent or GnRH-independent sex hormone production (Box 38.1). GnRH-dependent or true (central) precocious puberty develops secondary to the early activation of the hypothalamic–pituitary–gonadal axis. The most common causes are idiopathic; other causes include infection, inflammation, and injury of the central nervous system. In idiopathic precocious puberty, the arcuate nucleus in the hypothalamus is prematurely activated. This causes early sexual maturation with early reproductive capability. The elevated estrogen levels produced affect the skeleton, resulting in short stature in adulthood secondary to premature closure of the epiphyseal plates. These individuals are at risk for early sexual activity and potential sexual abuse and may have psychosocial problems related to their early sexual development. Occasionally, GnRH-dependent precocious puberty results from neoplasms of the hypothalamic–pituitary stalk. In this situation, although sexual development begins early, the rate of sexual development is slower than usual. Transient inflammatory conditions of the hypothalamus may also result in GnRH-dependent precocious puberty; however, sexual development may begin and end abruptly. Laboratory studies show either an appropriate rise in gonadotropins or a steady gonadotropin level in the prepubertal range.

GnRH-independent sex hormone production, or precocious pseudopuberty (peripheral), results from sex hormone production (androgens or estrogens) independent of hypothalamic–pituitary stimulation. Ovarian cysts and tumors, McCune–Albright syndrome, adrenal tumors, and iatrogenic

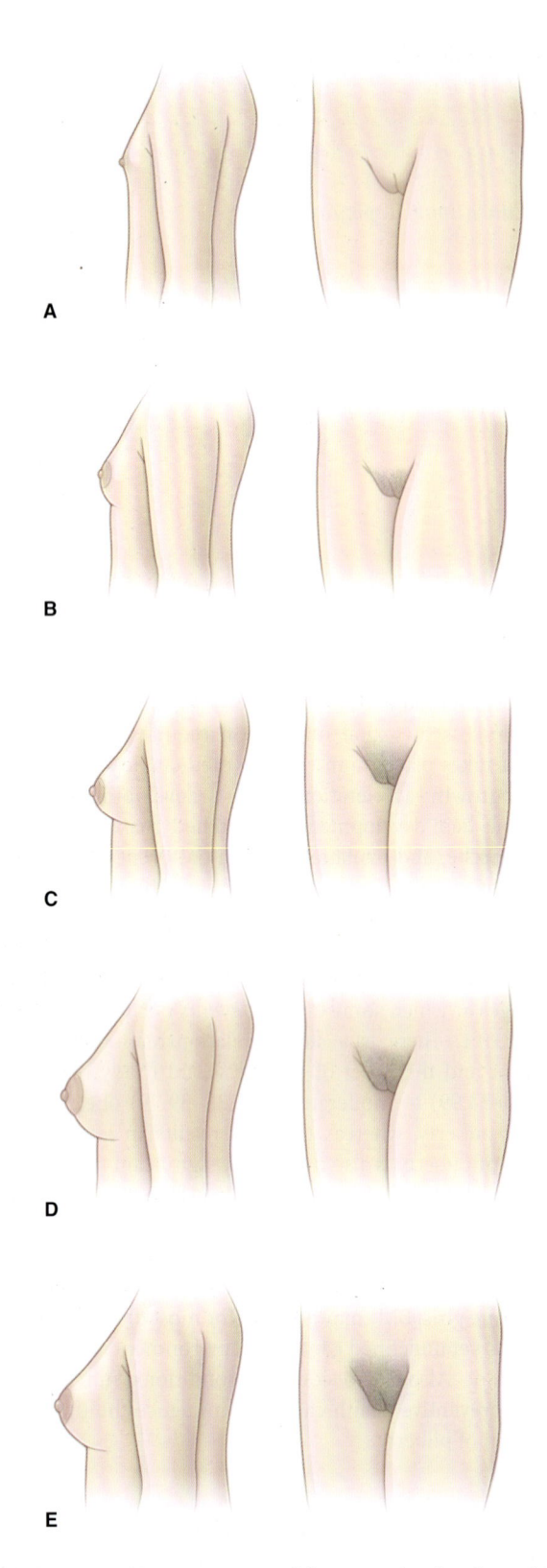

FIGURE 38.1. Tanner staging of breast and pubic hair development, which includes five stages. (Adapted from American College of Obstetricians and Gynecologists. *Precis: Reproductive Endocrinology.* 3rd ed. Washington, DC: ACOG; 2007.)

BOX 38.1 — Causes of Precocious Sexual Development

Gonadotropin-Releasing Hormone–Dependent (Central) Causes

Idiopathic origin
- Central nervous system tumors
- Hypothalamic hamartoma
- Craniopharyngiomata
- Gliomata
- Metastatic
- Arachnoid or suprasellar cysts

Central nervous system infection/inflammation
- Encephalitis
- Meningitis
- Granulomata

Central nervous system injury
- Irradiation
- Trauma
- Hydrocephalus

Gonadotropin-Releasing Hormone–Independent (Peripheral) Causes

Exogenous sex steroid administration
Primary hypothyroidism
Ovarian tumors
- Granulosa–theca cell
- Lipoid cell
- Gonadoblastoma
- Cystadenoma
- Germ cell

Simple ovarian cyst
McCune–Albright syndrome
Incomplete precocious sexual development
Premature thelarche
- Nonprogressive, idiopathic
- Progresses to precocious puberty

Premature adrenarche
- Idiopathic
- Congenital adrenal hyperplasia
- Precursor to polycystic ovary syndrome
- Adrenal or ovarian tumor (rare)

---

causes including hormone and alternative medicine ingestion can cause this condition. Some tumors, such as granulosa cell tumors, teratoma, and dysgerminomas, directly secrete sex hormones. Physical examination usually reveals a palpable pelvic mass and leads to further evaluation/imaging studies.

McCune–Albright syndrome (polyostotic fibrous dysplasia) is characterized by multiple bone fractures, café-au-lait spots, and precocious puberty. Premature menarche can be the first sign of the syndrome. The syndrome is thought to result from a defect in cellular regulation with a mutation in the α-subunit of the G protein that stimulates cyclic adenosine triphosphate formation, which causes affected tissues to function autonomously. This mutation causes the ovary to produce estrogen without the need for FSH stimulation, resulting in sexual precocity independent of the pituitary and hypothalamus.

Adrenal causes of precocious puberty include adrenal tumors and enzyme-secreting defects such as **congenital adrenal hyperplasia (CAH)**. Tumors are very rare and must secrete estrogen to cause early sexual maturation. The most common form of CAH, 21-hydroxylase deficiency, presents at birth with the finding of ambiguous genitalia. However, the nonclassical form, previously known as "late-onset CAH", tends to present at adolescence. In this disorder, the adrenal glands are unable to produce adequate amounts of cortisol as a result of a partial block in the conversion of 17-hydroxyprogesterone to deoxycortisol. Deficiency of the 21-hydroxylase enzyme leads to a shunting away from aldosterone and cortisol production in cholesterol biosynthesis toward the production of sex hormones, which results in precocious adrenarche. A pathognomonic finding for 21-hydroxylase deficiency is an elevated 17-hydroxyprogesterone level. Plasma renin is also measured to determine the amount of mineralocorticoid deficiency. Medical therapy is instituted as early as possible and is aimed at steroid/mineralocorticoid replacement, depending on the severity of the deficiency. In the nonclassical form of CAH, patients present with premature adrenarche, anovulation, and hyperandrogenism, appearing somewhat like patients with polycystic ovarian syndrome.

Iatrogenic causes, such as drug ingestion, must be considered in all children who present with precocious puberty. These children may exhibit increased pigmentation of the nipples and areola of the breast secondary to ingestion of oral contraceptives, anabolic steroids, and hair or facial creams. Many herbal or alternative medications carry unanticipated estrogenic effects.

Treatment

The main goals of treatment of precocious puberty are to arrest and diminish sexual maturation until a normal pubertal age as well as to maximize adult height. Therapy for GnRH-dependent precocious puberty involves administration of a GnRH agonist. Results occur rapidly and continue during the first year of treatment. Treatment for GnRH-independent precocious puberty attempts to suppress gonadal steroidogenesis.

Delayed Puberty

There is wide variation in normal pubertal development. An evaluation for primary amenorrhea should be considered for any adolescent who has not reached menarche by age 15 years or has not done so within 3 years of thelarche. Lack of breast development by age 13 years also should be evaluated. These findings should prompt the physician to initiate a workup to determine the cause of the delay. The most common causes of delayed puberty are shown in Box 38.2.

BOX 38.2 Causes of Delayed Puberty

Hypergonadotropic hypogonadism (FSH > 30 mIU/mL)
- Gonadal dysgenesis (Turner syndrome)

Hypogonadotropic hypogonadism (FSH + LH < 10 mIU/mL)
- Constitutional (physiologic) delay
- Kallmann syndrome
- Anorexia/extreme exercise
- Pituitary tumors/pituitary disorders
- Hyperprolactinemia
- Drug use

Anatomic causes
- Müllerian agenesis
- Imperforate hymen
- Transverse vaginal septum

FSH, follicle-stimulating hormone; LH, luteinizing hormone.

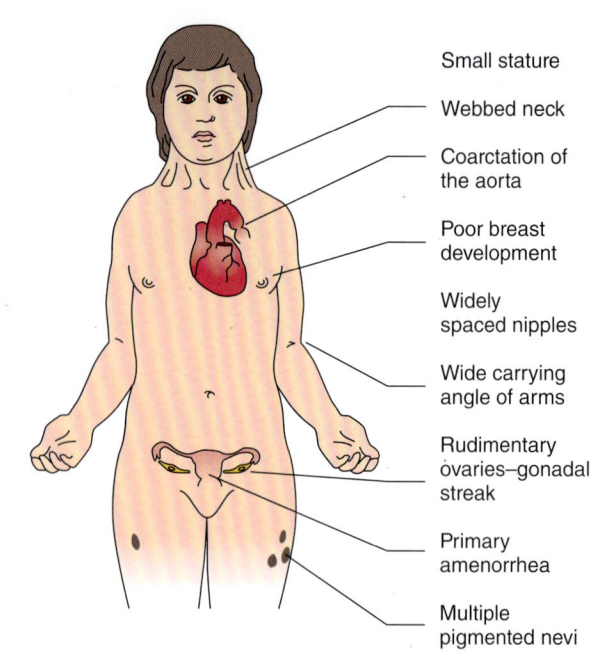

FIGURE 38.2. Clinical features of Turner syndrome. In Turner syndrome, there is an abnormality or absence of one of the X chromosomes in all cell lines. Patients have streak gonads with an absence of ovarian follicles. These patients typically present with primary amenorrhea, short stature, webbed neck (pterygium colli), shield chest with widely spaced nipples, high-arched palate, and an increased carrying angle of the elbow (cubitus valgus). (Modified from Rubin R, Strayer DS. *Rubin's Pathology*. 5th ed. Baltimore, MD: Lippincott Williams & Wilkins; 2008:195.)

Hypergonadotropic Hypogonadism

The most common cause of delayed puberty with an elevated FSH is gonadal dysgenesis, or Turner syndrome. In this condition, there is an abnormality in, or absence of, one of the X chromosomes in all cell lines (45X,O). Patients have streak gonads, with an absence of ovarian follicles; therefore, gonadal sex hormone production does not occur at puberty. These patients typically have primary amenorrhea, short stature, webbed neck (pterygium colli), shield chest with widely spaced nipples, high-arched palate, and an increased carrying angle of the elbow (cubitus valgus) as shown in Figure 38.2.

Estrogen administration should be initiated at the normal time of initiation of puberty, and growth hormone should be initiated very early (often prior to estrogen therapy) and aggressively to normalize adult height. Estrogen is necessary to stimulate breast development, genital tract maturation, and the beginning of menstruation. Low-dose estrogen is used to initiate secondary sexual maturation, and the dose is increased once breast budding and menarche occur. If an excessive amount of estrogen is administered initially, epiphyseal closure may begin, and long bone growth is truncated and adult height compromised. A delay in estrogen administration can lead to the development of osteoporosis in the teenage years. Progestins should not be given until the patient has reached Tanner stage IV, because premature progestin therapy may prevent the breast from developing completely, thus resulting in an abnormal contour (a more tubular breast).

Hypogonadotropic Hypogonadism

The arcuate nucleus of the hypothalamus secretes GnRH in cyclic bursts (or a pulsatile fashion), which stimulates the release of gonadotropins from the anterior pituitary gland. Dysfunction of the arcuate nucleus disrupts the short hormonal loop between the hypothalamus and pituitary. As a result, FSH and LH secretion does not occur. Consequently, the ovaries are not stimulated to secrete estradiol, and secondary sexual maturation is delayed.

The most common cause of this type of delayed puberty is constitutional (physiologic) delay. Other causes include Kallmann syndrome; anorexia, exercise, or stress; pituitary tumors/pituitary disorders; hyperprolactinemia; and drug use.

Constitutional delay of puberty represents approximately 20% of all cases of delayed puberty. It is thought to be a normal variant of the development process and trends can be seen within families. Children with constitutional delay usually have not only delay of secondary sexual maturation but also short stature with an appropriate delay of bone maturation.

Kallmann Syndrome

In **Kallmann syndrome**, the olfactory tracts are hypoplastic, and the arcuate nucleus does not secrete GnRH. Young women with Kallmann syndrome have little or no sense of smell and do not have breast development. This condition can be diagnosed on initial physical examination by challenging the olfactory function with known odors, such as coffee or rubbing alcohol. Once the condition is recognized and treated, the prognosis for successful secondary sexual maturation and reproduction is excellent. Secondary sexual maturation can be stimulated by the administration of exogenous hormones or by the administration of pulsatile GnRH. Patients typically can have normal reproductive function. Ovulation is induced by the administration of exogenous gonadotropin, and progesterone is given in the luteal phase to allow implantation of the embryo.

Other Causes

Other causes of hypothalamic amenorrhea include weight loss, strenuous exercise (such as vigorous dancing or long-distance running), anorexia nervosa, and bulimia. These conditions all result in suppressed gonadotropin levels with low estrogen levels. The correction of the underlying abnormality (such as weight gain in patients with weight loss) restores normal gonadotropin levels, stimulating ovarian steroidogenesis and the resumption of pubertal development.

Craniopharyngioma is the most common tumor associated with delayed puberty. This tumor develops in the pituitary stalk with suprasellar extension from nests of epithelium derived from Rathke pouch. Magnetic resonance imaging is the recommended modality to locate a (supra)sellar calcified cyst. Calcifications are present in approximately 70% of craniopharyngiomas.

Anatomic Causes

During fetal life, müllerian ducts develop and fuse in the female fetus to form the upper reproductive tract (i.e., the fallopian tubes, uterus, and upper vagina). The lower and midportion of the vagina develop from the canalization of the genital plate (see Chapter 4).

Müllerian Agenesis

Müllerian agenesis, or **Mayer–Rokitansky–Küster–Hauser syndrome**, is the most common cause of primary amenorrhea in women with normal breast development. In this syndrome, there is congenital absence of the vagina and, usually, an absence of the uterus and fallopian tubes. Ovarian function is normal, because the ovaries are not derived from müllerian structures; therefore, all the secondary sexual characteristics of puberty occur at the appropriate time. Physical examination leads to the diagnosis of müllerian agenesis. Renal anomalies (e.g., reduplication of the ureters, horseshoe kidney, and unilateral renal agenesis) occur in 40% to 50% of cases. Skeletal anomalies such as scoliosis occur in 10% to 15% of cases. Mayer–Rokitansky–Küster–Hauser syndrome is generally sporadic in expression, although occasional occurrences in families can be seen.

There are several therapeutic approaches to this condition. Nonsurgical approaches should be tried first, using dilators and pressure on the dimple between the urethra and the rectum twice a day. This tissue is quite pliable and, with increasing dilator size, a normal length vagina can be achieved. An artificial vagina may be created by repetitive pressure by vaginal dilators on the perineum or by surgical construction followed by a split thickness skin graft. After creation of a vagina, these women are able to have sexual intercourse. Sexually experienced patients may present with natural dilation of the vaginal dimple and occasionally require no additional dilation therapy. However, patients who successfully use dilation therapy may require continuation of dilation on an intermittent basis if they are not regularly engaging in vaginal intercourse. With the advances in assisted reproductive technologies, including in vitro fertilization and use of a surrogate mother (gestational carrier), it is possible for a woman with this condition to have a genetic child by using her oocytes.

Imperforate Hymen

The simplest genital tract anomaly is **imperforate hymen**. In this condition, the genital plate canalization is incomplete, and the hymen is, therefore, closed. Menarche occurs at the appropriate time, but, because there is obstruction to the passage of menstrual blood, it is not apparent. This condition presents with pain in the area of the uterus and a bulging, bluish-appearing vaginal introitus. Hymenotomy is the definitive therapy. This condition may be confused with a transverse vaginal septum. Transverse vaginal septa can occur along the vagina at any level and result in obstruction to outflow of menses. A vaginal septum can be resected and primarily repaired via a procedure called a "Z-vaginoplasty". Prolonged obstruction to menstruation can be associated with an increased incidence of endometriosis.

CLINICAL FOLLOW-UP

Although this girl is behind her peers in pubertal development, her sequence and stage seem appropriate, and menses should be anticipated at any time. Delays in onset of puberty may also be associated with low body weight, athletic training (female athlete triad), and eating disorders. A diagnosis of delayed puberty would not normally be assigned unless she fails to menstruate 5 years after the onset of thelarche.

---

thePoint® Visit **http://thePoint.lww.com/activate** for an interactive USMLE-style question bank and more!

CHAPTER 39
Amenorrhea and Abnormal Uterine Bleeding

This chapter deals primarily with APGO Educational Topic Areas:

TOPIC 43 AMENORRHEA

TOPIC 45 NORMAL AND ABNORMAL UTERINE BLEEDING

Students should be able to recognize abnormal patterns of bleeding, particularly amenorrhea and oligomenorrhea. They should be able to explain the pathophysiology and etiology of abnormal bleeding as well as outline a basic approach to evaluation and management of amenorrhea, oligomenorrhea, and other patterns of abnormal bleeding. They should be able to identify risk factors, common presenting signs and symptoms, physical examination findings, and consequences of lack of treatment.

CLINICAL CASE
A 19-year-old woman presents because her normally regular menstrual period is now 3 weeks overdue. She reports fatigue, bloating, and breast fullness similar to what she normally experiences prior to menses. She began menstruating at age 12 years and, after her first year, the periods have been regular every 28 to 32 days and are associated with mild menstrual pain.

● INTRODUCTION

Amenorrhea (absence of menstruation) and abnormal uterine bleeding (AUB) are the most common gynecologic disorders of reproductive-age women. Amenorrhea and AUB are discussed as separate topics in this chapter. However, the pathophysiology underlying amenorrhea and AUB is often the same.

AUB is a difference in frequency, duration, and amount of menstrual bleeding. A logical approach to terminology is to separate abnormal bleeding into two broad categories: Abnormal bleeding associated with ovulatory cycles, which usually have organic causes, and bleeding due to anovulatory causes, which is usually diagnosed through exclusion based on history.

● AMENORRHEA

Primary amenorrhea is defined as no menarche by 16 years of age. Although primary amenorrhea has been defined as no menarche by 16 years of age, many diagnosable and treatable disorders can and should be detected earlier. Thus, an evaluation for primary amenorrhea should be considered for any girl who has not reached menarche by 15 years of age or has not done so within 3 years of thelarche. Lack of breast development by 13 years of age also should be evaluated. If a menstruating woman has not menstruated for 3 to 6 months or for the duration of three typical menstrual cycles for the patient with oligomenorrhea, she is classified as having **secondary amenorrhea**.

The designation of primary or secondary amenorrhea has no bearing on the severity of the underlying disorder or on the prognosis for restoring cyclic ovulation. Terms often confused with these include **oligomenorrhea**, defined as bleeding that occurs less frequently than every 35 days, and **hypomenorrhea**, defined as a reduction in the number of days or the amount of menstrual flow. Amenorrhea not caused by pregnancy occurs in 5% or less of all women during their menstrual lives.

Causes of Amenorrhea

When endocrine function along the hypothalamic–pituitary–ovarian axis is disrupted or an abnormality develops in the genital outflow tract (obstruction of the uterus, cervix, or vagina or scarring of the endometrium), menstruation ceases. Causes of amenorrhea are divided into those arising from (1) pregnancy, (2) hypothalamic–pituitary dysfunction, (3) ovarian dysfunction, and (4) alteration of the genital outflow tract.

Pregnancy
Because pregnancy is the most common cause of amenorrhea, it is essential to exclude pregnancy in the evaluation of amenorrhea. A history of breast fullness, weight gain, and nausea suggests the diagnosis of pregnancy, which is confirmed by a positive β-human chorionic gonadotropin assay. It is important to rule out pregnancy to allay the patient's anxiety, avoid unnecessary testing, and avoid potential jeopardy to the pregnancy itself. Lastly, the diagnosis of ectopic pregnancy should be entertained in the presence of abnormal menses, abdominal symptoms, and a positive pregnancy test, insofar as this would necessitate medical or surgical intervention.

Hypothalamic–Pituitary Dysfunction
Release of hypothalamic gonadotropin-releasing hormone (GnRH) occurs in a pulsatile fashion, modulated by catecholamine secretion from the central nervous system and by

BOX 39.1	Causes of Hypothalamic–Pituitary Amenorrhea

Functional causes
- Weight loss
- Excessive exercise
- Obesity

Drug-Induced causes
- Marijuana
- Psychoactive drugs, including antidepressants

Neoplastic causes
- Prolactin-secreting pituitary adenomas
- Craniopharyngioma
- Hypothalamic hamartoma

Psychogenic causes
- Chronic anxiety
- Pseudocyesis
- Anorexia nervosa

Other causes
- Head injury
- Chronic medical illness

BOX 39.2	Causes of Ovarian Failure

Chromosomal causes (see Chapter 7)
- Turner syndrome (45,X gonadal dysgenesis)
- X chromosome long-arm deletion (46,XX q5)

Other causes
- Gonadotropin-resistant ovary syndrome (Savage syndrome)
- Premature natural menopause
- Autoimmune ovarian failure

feedback of sex steroids from the ovaries. When this pulsatile secretion of GnRH is disrupted or altered, the anterior pituitary gland is not stimulated to secrete follicle-stimulating hormone (FSH) and luteinizing hormone (LH). This results in an absence of folliculogenesis despite estrogen production, no ovulation, and a lack of corpus luteum with its usual production of estrogen and progesterone. Because of the lack of increased sex hormone production with minimal stimulation of the endometrium, there is no menstruation.

Alterations in catecholamine secretion and metabolism in sex steroid hormone feedback or an alteration of blood flow through the hypothalamic–pituitary portal plexus can disrupt the signaling process that leads to ovulation. This latter disruption can be caused by tumors or infiltrative processes that impinge on the pituitary stalk and alter blood flow.

The most common causes of hypothalamic–pituitary dysfunction are presented in Box 39.1. Most hypothalamic–pituitary amenorrhea is of functional origin and can be corrected by modifying causal behavior, by stimulating gonadotropin secretion, or by giving exogenous human menopausal gonadotropins.

The physician cannot differentiate hypothalamic–pituitary causes of amenorrhea from ovarian or genital outflow causes by medical history or even physical examination alone. However, there are some clues in the medical history and physical examination that would suggest a hypothalamic–pituitary etiology for amenorrhea. A history of any condition listed in Box 39.1 should cause the physician to consider hypothalamic–pituitary dysfunction. The definitive method to identify hypothalamic–pituitary dysfunction is to measure FSH, LH, and prolactin levels in the blood. In these conditions, FSH and LH levels are in the low range. The prolactin level is normal in most conditions but is elevated in prolactin-secreting pituitary adenomas.

Ovarian Dysfunction

In primary ovarian insufficiency, the ovarian follicles are either exhausted or are resistant to stimulation by pituitary FSH and LH. As the ovaries cease functioning, blood concentrations of FSH and LH increase. Women with primary ovarian insufficiency experience the symptoms and signs of estrogen deficiency. A summary of causes is presented in Box 39.2.

Alteration of the Genital Outflow Tract

Obstruction of the genital outflow tract prevents overt menstrual bleeding even if ovulation occurs. Most cases of outflow obstruction result from congenital abnormalities in the development and canalization of the müllerian ducts. Imperforate hymen and the absence of the uterus or vagina are the most common anomalies that result in primary amenorrhea. Surgical correction of an imperforate hymen allows for menstruation and fertility. Less commonly encountered anomalies, such as a transverse vaginal septum, are more difficult to correct, and, even with attempted surgical correction, menstruation and fertility are often not restored.

Asherman Syndrome

Scarring of the uterine cavity (**Asherman syndrome**) is the most frequent anatomic cause of secondary amenorrhea (Fig. 39.1). Women who undergo dilation and curettage (D&C) for retained products of pregnancy (especially when infection is present) are at risk for developing scarring of the endometrium. Cases of mild scarring can be corrected by surgical lysis of the adhesions performed by hysteroscopy and D&C. However, severe cases are often refractory to therapy. Estrogen therapy should be added to the surgical treatment postoperatively to stimulate endometrial regeneration of the denuded areas. In some cases, a balloon or intrauterine (contraceptive) device may be placed in the uterine cavity to help keep the uterine walls separated to prevent recurrence of adhesions.

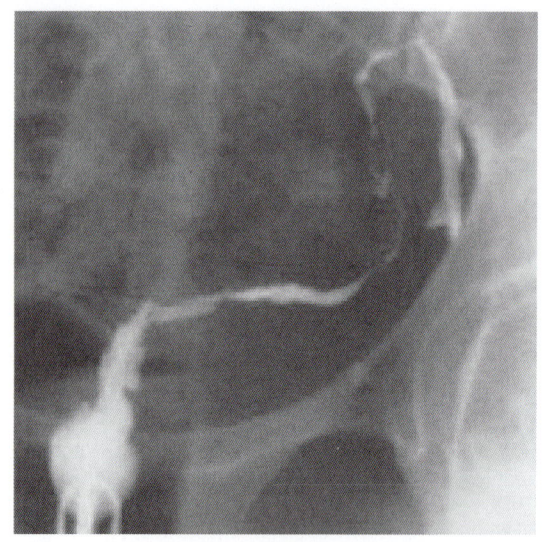

Laboratory studies used in the assessment of amenorrhea include pregnancy testing and measurement of levels of thyroid-stimulating hormone, prolactin, and FSH. Thyroid-stimulating hormone level is evaluated to rule out subclinical hypothyroidism. An elevated FSH level in women younger than 40 years may signify primary ovarian insufficiency. Once confirmed by repeat testing, elevated FSH levels should prompt evaluation of autoimmune antibodies. The American Society for Reproductive Medicine recommends completion of a chromosomal analysis, including premutation analysis for fragile X syndrome, in women in whom primary ovarian insufficiency is diagnosed.

The first step is to establish a cause for the amenorrhea. The **"progesterone challenge" test** is commonly used to determine whether or not the patient has adequate estrogen, a competent endometrium, and a patent outflow tract. A 10- to 14-day course of oral medroxyprogesterone acetate or micronized progesterone is expected to induce progesterone withdrawal bleeding within a week after completing the oral course. An injection of 100 mg of progesterone in oil can also be used. If bleeding does occur, estrogen effect on the endometrium is established, and the patient is presumed to be anovulatory or oligo-ovulatory. If withdrawal bleeding does not occur, the patient may be hypoestrogenic or have an anatomic condition such as Asherman syndrome or outflow tract obstruction.

Hyperprolactinemia associated with some pituitary adenomas (or other medical conditions) results in amenorrhea and **galactorrhea** (a milky discharge from the breasts). Approximately 80% of all pituitary tumors secrete prolactin, causing galactorrhea, and these patients are treated with either cabergoline (Dostinex) or the dopamine agonist bromocriptine (Parlodel). In approximately 5% of patients with hyperprolactinemia and galactorrhea, the underlying etiology is hypothyroidism. A low serum thyroxine level eliminates negative feedback signaling to the hypothalamic–pituitary axis. As a result, thyrotropin-releasing hormone (TRH) levels increase. Positive feedback signaling, which normally stimulates dopamine secretion, is also absent, causing a decrease in dopamine levels. Elevated TRH stimulates the release of prolactin from the pituitary gland. The reduced dopamine secretion results in elevated levels of thyroid-stimulating hormone and prolactin.

In patients who desire pregnancy, ovulation can be induced through the use of clomiphene citrate, human menopausal gonadotropins, pulsatile GnRH, or aromatase inhibitors. In patients who are oligo-ovulatory or anovulatory as commonly encountered with **polycystic ovary syndrome (PCOS)**, ovulation can usually be induced with clomiphene citrate. In patients with hypogonadotropic hypogonadism, ovulation can be induced with pulsatile GnRH or human menopausal gonadotropins. Women with genital tract obstruction require surgery to create a vagina or to restore genital tract integrity. Menstruation will never be established if the uterus is absent. Women with premature menopause may require exogenous estrogen therapy in order to treat or prevent the effects of the loss of endogenous estrogen production.

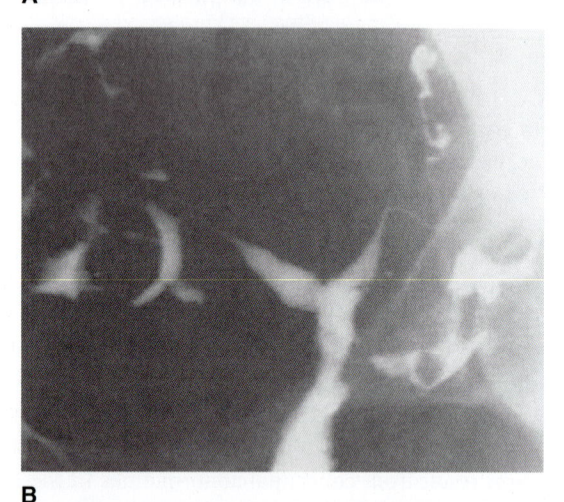

FIGURE 39.1. Asherman syndrome. (A) Hysterosalpingogram of a patient with Asherman syndrome. Note the thin sliver of endometrial cavity. (B) The same patient after hysteroscopic resection of intrauterine adhesions. Both fallopian tubes are now visualized. (Knockenhauer ES, Blackwell RE. Operative hysteroscopic procedures. In: Azziz R, Murphy AA, eds. *Practical Manual of Operative Laparoscopy and Hysteroscopy.* 2nd ed. New York: Springer-Verlag; 1997:290.)

Treatment of Amenorrhea

A thorough patient history should be taken including past medical illnesses; date of last menstrual period; history of amenorrhea; exercise (amount per day and per week); dietary history (restrictions, special diets); eating disorders; medications; illicit drug use; psychiatric history; and a history of conditions such as hirsutism, acne, and galactorrhea.

Physical examination should include Tanner staging; evaluation of genital tract anatomy; presence of hirsutism, acne, or both; and measurement of body mass index. The need for imaging studies, such as ultrasonography, MRI, and CT, will depend on the patient's medical history and whether the evaluation is for primary or secondary amenorrhea.

ABNORMAL UTERINE BLEEDING

Failure to ovulate results in either amenorrhea or irregular uterine bleeding. Irregular bleeding that is associated with anovulation and unrelated to anatomic lesions of the uterus is referred to as **anovulatory uterine bleeding**. It is most likely to occur in association with anovulation as found in PCOS, exogenous obesity, or adrenal hyperplasia.

Women with hypothalamic amenorrhea (hypothalamic–pituitary dysfunction) and no genital tract obstruction are in a state of relative estrogen deficiency. Estrogen is inadequate to stimulate growth and development of the endometrium. Therefore, there is inadequate endometrium for uterine bleeding to occur. In contrast, women with oligo-ovulation and anovulation with AUB have constant, noncyclic blood estrogen concentrations that slowly stimulate growth and development of the endometrium. Without the effect of ovulation, progesterone-induced changes do not occur. Initially, these patients have amenorrhea because of the chronic, constant estrogen levels, but, eventually, the endometrium outgrows its blood supply and sloughs from the uterus at irregular times and in unpredictable amounts.

When there is chronic stimulation of the endometrium from low plasma concentrations of estrogens, the episodes of uterine bleeding are infrequent and light. In contrast, with chronic stimulation of the endometrium from increased plasma concentrations of estrogens, the episodes of uterine bleeding can be frequent and heavy. Because amenorrhea and AUB both result from anovulation, it is not surprising that they can occur at different times in the same patient.

Luteal Phase Defect

Subtle alterations in the mechanisms of ovulation can produce abnormal cycles, even when ovulation occurs such as seen with the **luteal phase defect**. In cases of luteal phase defect, ovulation does occur; however, the corpus luteum of the ovary is not fully developed to secrete adequate quantities of progesterone to support the endometrium for the usual 13 to 14 days and is not adequate to support a pregnancy if conception does occur. The menstrual cycle is shortened, and menstruation occurs earlier than expected. Although this is not a classic anovulatory uterine bleeding, its clinical presentation of shortened cycles can present diagnostic and therapeutic challenges.

Midcycle Spotting

Another example of abnormal bleeding in patients who do ovulate is midcycle spotting, in which patients report bleeding at the time of ovulation. In the absence of demonstrable pathology, this self-limited bleeding can be attributed to the sudden drop in estrogen level that occurs at this time of the cycle, which destabilizes the endometrium.

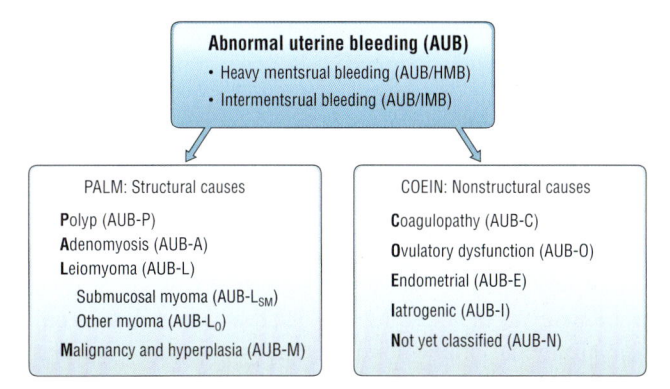

FIGURE 39.2. Basic PALM-COEIN (polyp; adenomyosis; leiomyoma; malignancy and hyperplasia; coagulopathy; ovulatory dysfunction; endometrial; iatrogenic; and not yet classified) classification system for the causes of abnormal uterine bleeding. This system, approved by the International Federation of Gynecology and Obstetrics, uses the term AUB paired with descriptive terms that describe associated bleeding patterns (heavy menstrual bleeding and irregular menstrual bleeding), or a qualifying letter (or letters), or both to indicate its etiology (or etiologies). (American College of Obstetricians and Gynecologists. *Diagnosis of Abnormal Uterine Bleeding in Reproductive-Aged Women. Practice Bulletin 128.* Washington, DC: American College of Obstetricians and Gynecologists; July 2012.)

Diagnosis of Abnormal Uterine Bleeding

"Diagnosis of AUB is given when vaginal bleeding is not regular, not predictable, and not associated with premenstrual signs and symptoms that usually accompany ovulatory cycles." These signs and symptoms include breast fullness, abdominal bloating, mood changes, edema, weight gain, and uterine cramps.

Before anovulatory uterine bleeding can be diagnosed, anatomic causes including neoplasia should be excluded. In a reproductive-aged woman, complications of pregnancy as a cause of irregular vaginal bleeding should be excluded. Other anatomic causes of irregular vaginal bleeding include uterine leiomyomata, inflammation or infection of the genital tract, hyperplasia or carcinoma of the cervix or endometrium, cervical and endometrial polyps, and lesions of the vagina (Fig. 39.2). Pelvic ultrasonography or sonohysterography may assist in diagnosing these lesions. Women with organic causes for bleeding may have regular ovulatory cycles with superimposed irregular bleeding.

Laboratory assessment for AUB should include a pregnancy test, complete blood count (CBC); measurement of TSH levels; and cervical cancer screening. Testing for *Chlamydia trachomatis* should be considered, especially in patients at high risk of infection.

If the diagnosis is uncertain based on history and physical examination alone, a woman may keep a basal body temperature chart for 6 to 8 weeks to look for the shift in the basal temperature that occurs with ovulation. An ovulation predictor kit may also be used. Luteal phase serum progesterone may also be measured. In cases of anovulation and abnormal bleeding, an endometrial biopsy may reveal endometrial hyperplasia. Because AUB results from chronic, unopposed estrogenic stimulation of the endometrium, the endometrium appears proliferative or, with prolonged estrogenic stimulation, hyperplastic. Without treatment, these women are at increased risk for endometrial cancer.

Treatment of Abnormal Uterine Bleeding

The risks to a woman with anovulatory uterine bleeding include anemia, incapacitating blood loss, endometrial hyperplasia, and carcinoma. Uterine bleeding can be severe enough to require hospitalization. Both hemorrhage and endometrial hyperplasia can be prevented by appropriate management.

The primary goal of treatment of anovulatory uterine bleeding is to ensure regular shedding of the endometrium and consequent regulation of uterine bleeding. If ovulation is achieved, conversion of the proliferative endometrium into secretory endometrium will result in predictable uterine withdrawal bleeding.

A progestational agent may be administered for a minimum of 10 days. The most commonly used agent is medroxyprogesterone acetate. When the progestational agent is discontinued, uterine withdrawal bleeding ensues within 7 to 10 days, thereby mimicking physiologic withdrawal of progesterone.

As an alternative, administration of oral contraceptives (OCs) suppresses the endometrium and establishes regular, predictable withdrawal cycles. No particular OC preparation is better than any of the others for this purpose. Women who take OCs as treatment for AUB often resume AUB after therapy is discontinued.

If a patient is being treated for a particularly heavy bleeding episode, once organic pathology has been ruled out, treatment should focus on two issues: (1) control of the acute episode and (2) prevention of future recurrences. Both high-dose estrogen and progestin therapy as well as combination treatment (OC pills, three pills per day for 1 week) and tranexamic acid have been advocated for management of heavy abnormal bleeding in the acute phase. Effective medical therapies include the levonorgestrel intrauterine system, OCs (monthly or extended cycles), progestin therapy (oral or intramuscular), tranexamic acid, and nonsteroidal anti-inflammatory drugs. If a patient is receiving IV conjugated equine estrogen, the health care provider should add progestin or transition to OCs. Unopposed estrogen should not be used as long-term treatment for chronic AUB. Uterine bleeding lasting an extended period of time that does not respond to medical therapy is often managed surgically with D&C, uterine artery embolization, endometrial ablation, or hysterectomy. Endometrial ablation should be considered only if other treatments have been ineffective or are contraindicated, and it should be performed only when a woman does not have plans for future childbearing and when the possibility of endometrial or uterine cancer has been reliably ruled out as the cause of the acute AUB.

CLINICAL FOLLOW-UP

A urine pregnancy test is positive and the patient reluctantly admits to unprotected intercourse.

CHAPTER 40
Hirsutism and Virilization

This chapter deals primarily with APGO Educational Topic Area:

TOPIC 44   HIRSUTISM AND VIRILIZATION

Students should be able to define hirsutism and virilization, distinguishing normal and abnormal variants of normal secondary sexual characteristics and describing the etiology and pathophysiology of both of these diagnoses. They should outline a basic approach to evaluation and management in these patients. They should identify associated diseases, common presenting signs and symptoms, and physical examination findings.

CLINICAL CASE

A 57-year-old woman presents with concerns about a growing problem of visible hair on her upper lip. She attained menopause at the age of 49 years and has not taken any hormonal therapy or herbal supplements. The hair has slowly appeared over the past year or so and gradually darkened. Upon questioning, she has noted some additional hair growth on her chin.

INTRODUCTION

Hirsutism is excess terminal hair in a male pattern of distribution. It is manifested initially by the appearance of midline terminal hair. Terminal hair is darker, coarser, and kinkier than vellus hair, which is soft, downy, and fine. Care must be taken to evaluate the possibility that excess terminal hair is familial, not pathological, in origin. A scale used for the evaluation of hirsutism is shown in Figure 40.1. When a woman is exposed to excess androgens, terminal hair first appears on the lower abdomen and around the nipples, next around the chin and upper lip, and finally between the breasts and on the lower back. Usually, a woman with hirsutism also has acne. For women in Western cultures, terminal hair on the abdomen, breasts, and face is considered unsightly and presents a cosmetic problem. As a result, at the first sign of hirsutism, women often consult their physician to seek a cause for the excess hair growth and seek treatment to eliminate it.

Virilization is defined as masculinization of a woman and is associated with a marked increase in circulating **testosterone**. As a woman becomes virilized, she first notices enlargement of the clitoris, followed by temporal balding, deepening of the voice, involution of the breasts, and a remodeling of the limb–shoulder girdle as well as hirsutism. Over time, she takes on a more masculine appearance. Hirsutism and virilization may be clinical clues to an underlying androgen excess disorder.

When evaluating and treating hirsutism and virilization, the sites of androgen production and the mechanisms of androgen action should be considered. Idiopathic (constitutional or familial) hirsutism, a diagnosis of exclusion, is the most common nonpathologic etiology, representing about one-half of all cases. The most common pathologic cause of hirsutism is polycystic ovarian syndrome (PCOS), followed by congenital adrenal hyperplasia (CAH). These conditions must be diagnosed by laboratory evaluations. Treatment of androgen excess should be directed at suppressing the source of androgen excess or blocking androgen action at the receptor site.

ANDROGEN PRODUCTION AND ANDROGEN ACTION

In women, **androgens** are produced in the adrenal glands, the ovaries, and adipose tissue, where there is extraglandular production of testosterone from androstenedione. The following three androgens may be measured when evaluating a woman with hirsutism and virilization:

1. **Dehydroepiandrosterone** (**DHEA**): a weak androgen secreted principally by the adrenal glands. This is generally measured as dehydroepiandrosterone sulfate (DHEA-S) because of its longer half-life, making it a more reliable measure.
2. **Androstenedione:** a weak androgen secreted in equal amounts by the adrenal glands and ovaries.
3. **Testosterone:** a potent androgen secreted by the adrenal glands and ovaries and produced in adipose tissue from the conversion of androstenedione.

The sites of androgen production and proportions produced are presented in Table 40.1. In addition, testosterone is also converted within hair follicles and within genital skin to **dihydrotestosterone** (**DHT**), which is an androgen even more potent than testosterone. This metabolic conversion is the result of the local action of 5α-reductase on testosterone at these sites. This is the basis for constitutional hirsutism, which is discussed later.

Adrenal androgen production is controlled by reciprocal feedback regulation through pituitary secretion of

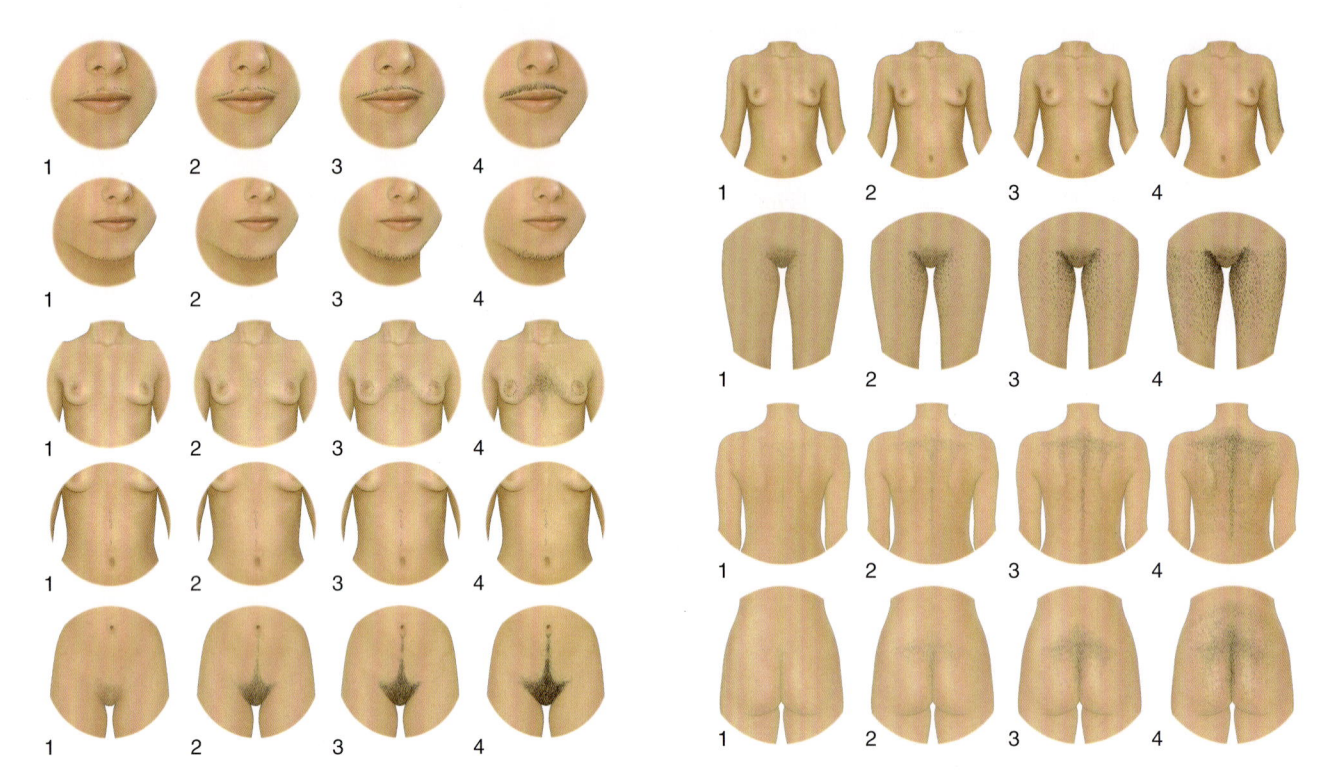

FIGURE 40.1. Modified Ferriman-Gallwey scale, a clinical tool for assessing the extent and distribution of hirsutism.

TABLE 40.1	SITES OF ANDROGEN PRODUCTION		
Site	DHEA-S (%)	Androstenedione (%)	Testosterone (%)
Adrenal glands	90	50	25
Ovaries	10	50	25
Extraglandular	0	0	50

DHEA-S, dehydroepiandrosterone sulfate.

adrenocorticotropic hormone (ACTH). ACTH stimulates the adrenal cortical production of cortisol. In the metabolic sequence of cortisol production, DHEA is one precursor hormone. In enzymatic deficiencies of adrenal steroidogenesis (21-hydroxylase deficiency and 11β-hydroxylase deficiency), DHEA accumulates and is further metabolized to androstenedione and testosterone. The flow of adrenal hormone production is shown in Figure 40.2.

Ovarian androgen production is regulated by luteinizing hormone (LH) secretion from the pituitary gland. LH stimulates theca lutein cells surrounding the ovarian follicles to secrete androstenedione and, to a lesser extent, testosterone. These androgens are precursors for estrogen production by granulosa cells of the ovarian follicles. In conditions of sustained or increased LH secretion, androstenedione and testosterone increase.

Extraglandular testosterone production occurs in adipocytes (fat cells) and depends on the magnitude of adrenal and ovarian androstenedione production. When androstenedione production increases, there is a dependent increase in extraglandular testosterone production. In obese women, the conversion of androstenedione to testosterone is increased. There is also an increase in estrone in obese women.

Testosterone is the primary androgen that causes increased hair growth, acne, and the physical changes associated with virilization. After testosterone is secreted, it is bound to a carrier protein—**sex hormone–binding globulin (SHBG)**—and primarily circulates in plasma as a bound steroid hormone. Bound testosterone is unable to attach to testosterone receptors and is, therefore, metabolically inactive. Only a small fraction (1%–3%) of testosterone is unbound (free). It is this small fraction of free hormone that results in testosterone's effects. The liver produces SHBG, and estrogens stimulate hepatic production of SHBG. As a result, greater estrogen production is associated with less free testosterone, whereas decreased estrogen production is associated with increased free testosterone. Therefore, measurement of total testosterone alone may not reflect the amount of biologically active testosterone.

Testosterone receptors are scattered throughout the body. For the purpose of this discussion, testosterone receptors are considered only in hair follicles, sebaceous glands, and genital skin. Free testosterone enters the cytosol of testosterone-dependent cells. There it is bound to a testosterone receptor and carried into the nucleus of the cell to initiate its metabolic action. When testosterone is excessive, increased hair growth, acne, and **rugation** (a fold, crease, or wrinkle) of the genital skin are seen. Some individuals have increased 5α-reductase within hair follicles, resulting in excessive local production of DHT.

Excess androgen production has several causes, including PCOS, testosterone-secreting tumors, adrenal disorders, and iatrogenic as well as idiopathic causes. Figure 40.3 presents a

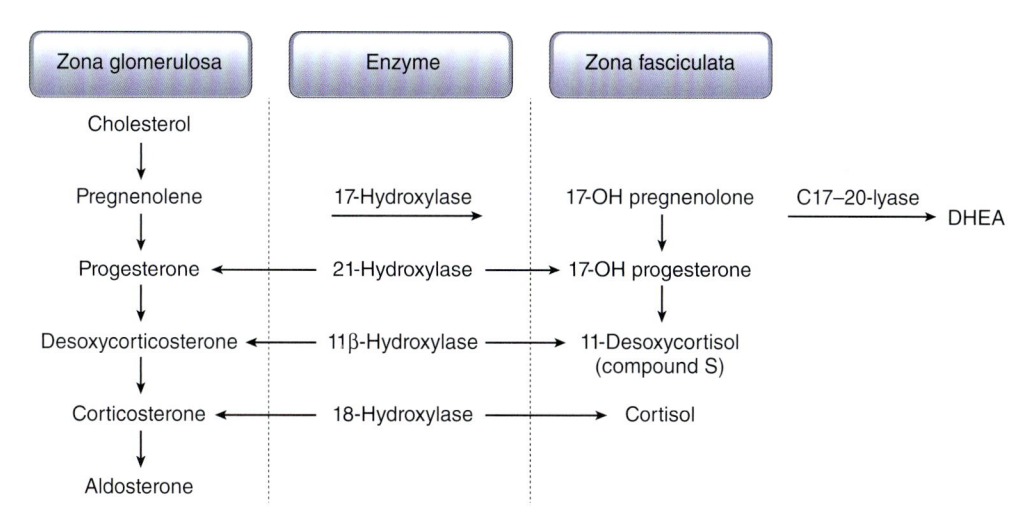

FIGURE 40.2. Flowchart of adrenal steroidogenesis. DHEA, dehydroepiandrosterone.

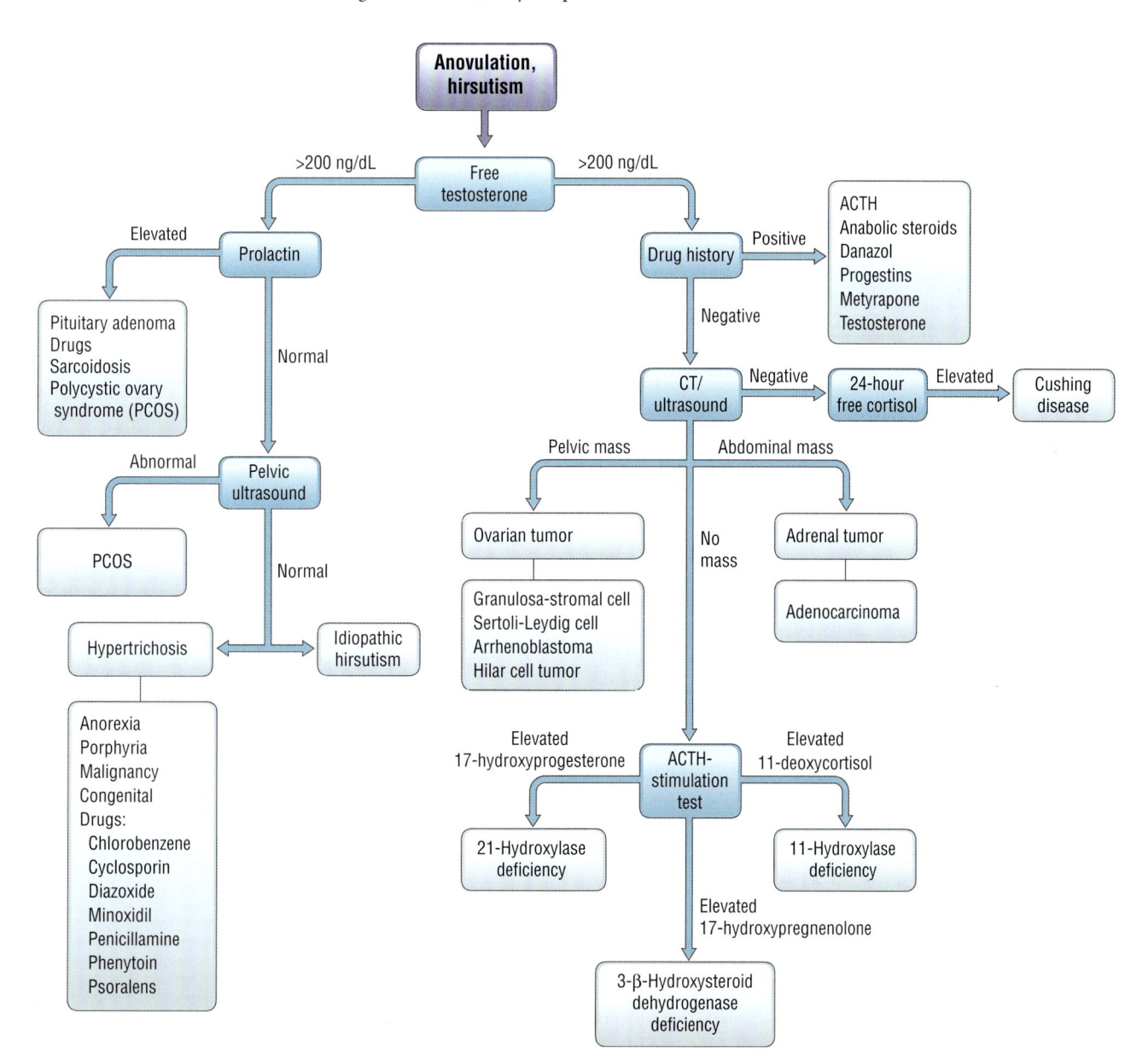

FIGURE 40.3. Scheme for the evaluation of hirsutism. ACTH, adrenocorticotropic hormone; CT, computed tomography.

scheme for the evaluation of hirsutism that encompasses the various etiologies that lead to this condition.

● POLYCYSTIC OVARY SYNDROME

PCOS is the most common cause of androgen excess and hirsutism in women. The etiology of this disorder is unknown. Some cases appear to result from a genetic predisposition, whereas others seem to result from obesity or other causes of LH excess.

Symptoms of PCOS include oligomenorrhea or amenorrhea, acne, hirsutism, and infertility. The disorder is characterized by chronic anovulation or extended periods of infrequent ovulation (**oligo-ovulation**). It is a syndrome primarily defined by excess androgen. The definition of PCOS has varied in the past.

The Rotterdam criteria, which supplanted the National Institutes of Health diagnostic criteria established in 1990 and 2000, incorporated the appearance of the ovary based on ultrasonography into the schema. Ultrasonography criteria for the diagnosis of polycystic ovaries were decided by expert consensus (Fig. 40.4). These criteria have been criticized for including more mild phenotypes, which increases the prevalence of PCOS and may complicate treatment decisions. The Androgen Excess Society criteria recognize **hyperandrogenism** as a necessary diagnostic factor, in combination with other symptoms of the syndrome.

Hyperandrogenism can generally be established on the basis of clinical findings (e.g., hirsutism, acne, or serum hormone measurement). To establish the diagnosis, the patient should have two of the following criteria:

- Oligo-ovulation or anovulation usually marked by irregular menstrual cycles
- Biochemical or clinical evidence of hyperandrogenism
- Polycystic-appearing ovaries on ultrasonography
- It is also important to rule out other endocrine disorders that can mimic PCOS, such as CAH, Cushing syndrome, and hyperprolactinemia.

Obesity

In many women with PCOS, obesity seems to be the common factor (seen in 50% of patients), and the acquisition of body fat coincides with the onset of PCOS. Stein and Leventhal first described PCOS patients as women with hirsutism, irregular cycles, and obesity. Originally called Stein–Leventhal syndrome, PCOS does not currently have obesity as one of its diagnostic criteria. In fact, approximately 20% of women with PCOS are not obese. PCOS is related to obesity by the following mechanism: LH stimulates the theca lutein cells to increase androstenedione production. Androstenedione undergoes aromatization to estrone within adipocytes. Although estrone is a weak estrogen, it has a positive-feedback action or stimulating effect on the pituitary secretion of LH. LH secretion is, therefore, stimulated by increased estrogen. With increasing obesity comes increased conversion of androstenedione to estrone. With the increased rise in androstenedione,

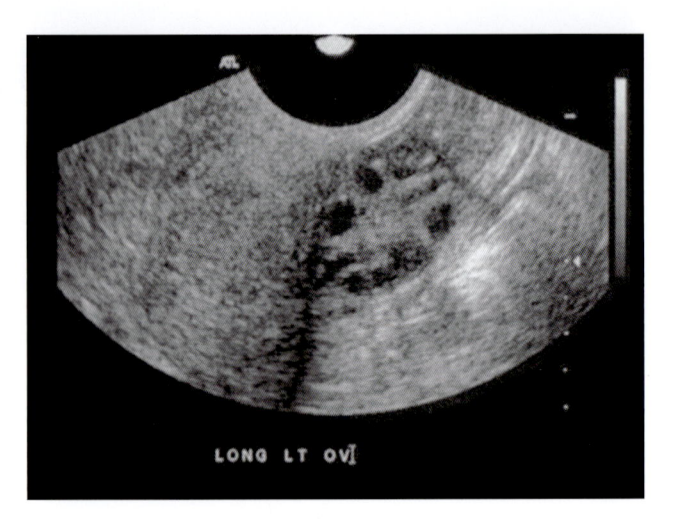

FIGURE 40.4. Ultrasound of polycystic ovary showing the characteristic "string-of-pearls" appearance of the cysts. (From Guzick DS. Polycystic ovary syndrome. *Obstet Gynecol.* 2004;103(1):187.)

there is coincident increased testosterone production, which causes acne and hirsutism (Fig. 40.5). In obesity, compensatory hyperinsulinemia may result in decreased levels of SHBG and, thus, more bioavailable circulating androgen serves as a trophic stimulus to androgen production in the adrenal gland and ovary. Insulin may also have direct hypothalamic effects, such as abnormal appetite stimulation and gonadotropin secretion. Hyperandrogenism, although central to the syndrome, may have multiple etiologies, some not related to insulin resistance.

Hormonal studies in women with PCOS show the following: (1) increased LH:FSH (follicle-stimulating hormone) ratio, (2) estrone in greater concentration than estradiol, (3) androstenedione at the upper limits of normal or increased, and (4) testosterone at the upper limits of normal or slightly increased.

Therefore, PCOS can be viewed as one of excess androgen and excess estrogen. The unopposed long-term elevated estrogen levels that characterize PCOS increase the risk of abnormal uterine bleeding, endometrial hyperplasia, and, in some cases, the development of endometrial carcinoma.

Metabolic Syndrome

The typical woman with PCOS has many of the signs of **metabolic syndrome** (syndrome X), which is defined by the presence of at least three of the following components:

- Waist circumference 35 inches or greater
- Triglyceride level 150 mg/dL or higher
- High-density lipoprotein cholesterol <50 mg/dL
- Blood pressure 130/85 mm Hg or higher
- Fasting glucose level 100 mg/dL or higher

Approximately 40% of patients with PCOS have impaired glucose tolerance, and 8% have overt type 2 diabetes mellitus. These patients should be screened for diabetes. Classic lipid abnormalities include elevated triglyceride levels, low high-density

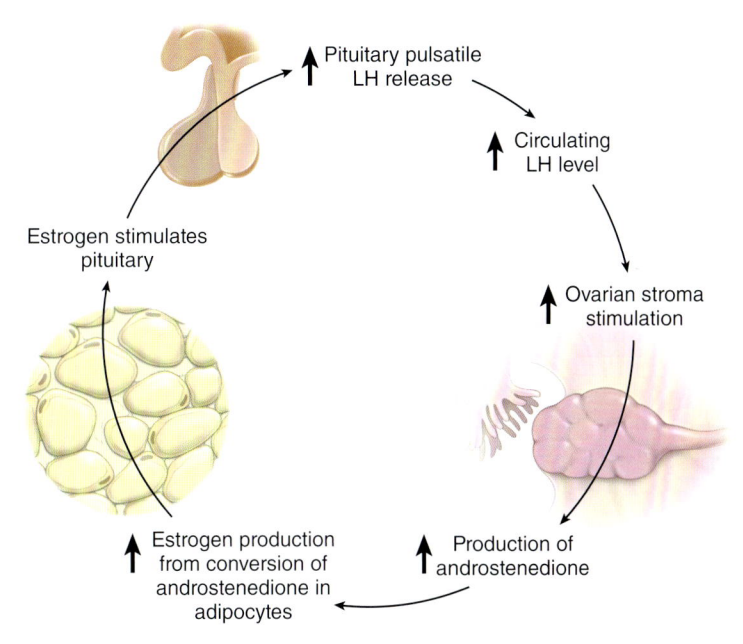

FIGURE 40.5. Proposed mechanism that demonstrates how obesity leads to polycystic ovary syndrome. LH, luteinizing hormone.

lipoprotein levels, and elevated low-density lipoprotein levels. Hypertension is also common in individuals with this condition. The combination of the preceding abnormalities potentially increases the risk of cardiovascular disease. The genetic contribution to PCOS remains uncertain, and there is currently no recommended genetic screening test.

HAIR-AN Syndrome

Acanthosis nigricans has also been found in a significant percentage of these patients. The HAIR-AN syndrome (*h*yper*a*ndrogenism, *i*nsulin *r*esistance, *a*canthosis *n*igricans) constitutes a defined subgroup of patients with PCOS. Administration of the insulin-sensitizing agent metformin in these patients also reduces androgen and insulin levels.

Treatment

PCOS is a functional disorder, the treatment of which should be targeted to interrupt the disorder's positive-feedback cycle. The most common therapy for PCOS is the administration of combination oral contraceptives, which suppresses pituitary LH production. Suppressing LH causes decreased production of androstenedione and testosterone. The ovarian contribution to the total androgen pool is thereby decreased. Acne clears, new hair growth is prevented, and there is decreased androgenic stimulation of existing hair follicles. By preventing unopposed estrogen exposure, oral contraceptives also prevent endometrial hyperplasia, and women have cyclic, predictable, withdrawal bleeding episodes.

If a woman with PCOS wishes to conceive, oral contraceptive therapy is not a suitable choice. If the patient is obese, a weight reduction diet designed to restore the patient to a normal weight should be encouraged. With body weight reduction alone, many women resume regular ovulatory cycles and conceive spontaneously. In some women, ovulation induction with clomiphene citrate is needed and is facilitated by weight reduction. If clomiphene citrate use fails to result in pregnancy, the recommended second-line intervention is either exogenous gonadotropins or laparoscopic ovarian surgery. Aromatase inhibitors, such as letrozole and anastrozole, have been proposed as both primary and secondary treatment for ovulation induction in these women, and results appear comparable to clomiphene from small trials. Insulin sensitizers (e.g., metformin alone or with clomiphene citrate) may be used to reduce insulin resistance, control weight, and facilitate ovulation. No antidiabetic agents are currently approved by the U.S. Food and Drug Administration for the treatment of PCOS-related menstrual dysfunction.

Hyperthecosis

Hyperthecosis is a more severe form of PCOS. In cases of hyperthecosis, androstenedione production may be so great that testosterone reaches concentrations that cause virilization. Women with this condition may exhibit temporal balding, clitoral enlargement, deepening of the voice, and remodeling at the limb–shoulder girdle. Hyperthecosis is often refractory to oral contraceptive suppression. It is also more difficult to successfully induce ovulation in women with this condition.

● OVARIAN NEOPLASMS

Several androgen-secreting ovarian tumors can cause hirsutism and virilization, including Sertoli–Leydig cell tumors and three rare neoplasms.

Sertoli–Leydig Cell Tumors

Sertoli–Leydig cell tumors (also called androblastoma and arrhenoblastoma) are ovarian neoplasms that secrete testosterone. These tumors constitute <0.4% of ovarian tumors and usually occur in women between the ages of 20 and 40 years. The tumor is most often unilateral (95% of cases) and may reach a size of 7 to 10 cm in diameter.

The history and physical examination give critical clues in diagnosing subjects who present with hirsutism and testosterone-secreting ovarian tumors. Testosterone-secreting tumors usually have a more rapid onset and more severe hirsutism with virilizing signs. Women with Sertoli–Leydig cell tumor have a rapid onset of acne, hirsutism (75% of patients), amenorrhea (30% of patients), and virilization. A characteristic clinical course of two overlapping stages comprises, first, the stage of defeminization, characterized by amenorrhea, breast atrophy, and loss of the subcutaneous fatty deposits responsible for the rounding of the feminine figure, and, second, the stage of masculinization, characterized by clitoral hypertrophy, hirsutism, and deepening of the voice. These changes may occur over 6 months or less.

Laboratory studies of this disorder show suppression of FSH and LH, low plasma androstenedione, and marked elevation of testosterone. An ovarian mass may be palpable on pelvic examination. Once the diagnosis is suspected, there should be no delay in surgical removal of the involved ovary. The contralateral ovary should be inspected, and if it is found to be enlarged, it should be bisected for gross inspection.

Following surgical removal of a Sertoli–Leydig cell tumor, ovulatory cycles return spontaneously, and further progression of hirsutism is arrested. If the clitoris has become enlarged, it does not revert to its pretreatment size. However, temporal hair is generally restored, and the body habitus becomes feminine once again. Terminal hair in a sexual distribution will not revert to vellus hair, but the growth and pigmentation will slow. Most patients will require mechanical removal of excess hair following removal of the ovarian tumor. The 10-year survival rates for this low-grade malignant ovarian tumor approximate 90% to 95%.

Uncommon Virilizing Ovarian Tumors

Gynandroblastoma is a rare ovarian tumor, having both granulosa cell and arrhenoblastoma components. The predominant clinical feature is masculinization, although estrogen production may simultaneously produce endometrial hyperplasia and irregular uterine bleeding. **Lipid (lipoid) cell tumors** are usually small ovarian tumors containing sheets of round, clear, pale staining cells with a differential histologic diagnosis of hilar cell tumors, stromal luteoma of pregnancy, and Sertoli–Leydig cell tumors. The clinical presentation is masculinization or defeminization associated with elevated 17-ketosteroids in many cases.

Hilar cell tumors arise from an overgrowth of mature hilar cells or from ovarian mesenchyme and are typically found in postmenopausal women. They are characterized clinically by masculinization, which supports the idea that hilar cells are the homologs of the interstitial or Leydig cells of the testis. Histologically, the tumors contain pathognomonic Reinke albuminoid crystals in most cases, and grossly, they are always small, unilateral, and benign. Treatment is surgical removal for these three rare tumors.

● ADRENAL ANDROGEN EXCESS DISORDERS

Adrenal disorders that cause an increase in androgen production can lead to hirsutism and virilization; the most common are CAH, Cushing syndrome, and adrenal neoplasms.

Congenital Adrenal Hyperplasia

CAH is caused by enzyme deficiencies that result in precursor (substrate) excess, thereby resulting in androgen excess. DHEA is a precursor for androstenedione and testosterone.

21-Hydroxylase Deficiency

The most common cause of increased adrenal androgen production is adrenal hyperplasia as a result of **21-hydroxylase deficiency**; 21-hydroxylase catalyzes the conversion of progesterone and 17α-hydroxyprogesterone (17-OH progesterone) to desoxycorticosterone and compound S. When 21-hydroxylase is deficient, there is an accumulation of progesterone and 17-OH progesterone, which are metabolized subsequently to DHEA. This disorder affects approximately 2% of the population and is caused by an alteration in the genes for 21-hydroxylase, which are carried on chromosome 6. The genetic defect is autosomal recessive and has variable penetrance.

In the most severe form of 21-hydroxylase deficiency, the newly born female infant is simply virilized (ambiguous genitalia) or is virilized and suffers from life-threatening salt wasting (Box 40.1). However, milder forms are more common and can appear at puberty or even later in adult life. A mild deficiency of 21-hydroxylase is frequently associated with terminal body hair, acne, subtle alterations in menstrual cycles, and infertility. These patients can also have sonographic evidence of polycystic-appearing ovaries.

When 21-hydroxylase deficiency manifests at puberty, adrenarche may precede thelarche. The history of pubic hair growth occurring before the onset of breast development may be a clinical clue to this disorder. The diagnosis of 21-hydroxylase deficiency is made by measuring increased 17-OH progesterone in plasma during the follicular phase (preferably measured while fasting). Patients with classic 21-hydroxylase deficiency will have significantly elevated plasma 17-OH progesterone levels, usually over 2,000 ng/dL. Those with less severe 21-hydroxylase deficiency may have mildly elevated basal levels, 200 ng/dL, and an increase to usually 1,000 ng/dL in response to ACTH stimulation. DHEA-S and androstenedione will also be elevated and contribute to the hirsutism and virilizing signs.

> **BOX 40.1** Manifestations of 21-Hydroxylase Deficiency
>
> **Severe**
> - Newborn female infant
> - Virilized (ambiguous genitalia), or virilized and has life-threatening salt wasting
>
> **Mild**
> - Frequently associated with terminal body hair, acne, subtle alterations in menstrual cycles, and infertility
> - Patients can also have sonographic evidence of polycystic-appearing ovaries
>
> **Manifested at puberty**
> - Adrenarche may precede thelarche
> - History of pubic hair growth occurring before the onset of breast development may be a clinical clue

11β-Hydroxylase Deficiency

A less common cause of adrenal hyperplasia is **11β-hydroxylase deficiency**. The enzyme 11β-hydroxylase catalyzes the conversion of desoxycorticosterone to cortisol. A deficiency in this enzyme also results in increased androgen production. The clinical features of 11β-hydroxylase deficiency are mild hypertension and mild hirsutism. The diagnosis of 11β-hydroxylase deficiency is made by demonstrating increased plasma desoxycorticosterone.

Treatment

Treatment of CAH is aimed at restoring normal cortisol levels. In CAH, cortisol production is reduced as a result of enzymatic block. This decreased cortisol production results in a compensatory increase in ACTH secretion, which is the body's attempt to stimulate cortisol production. This increased ACTH production results in the oversecretion of precursor molecules proximal to the enzymatic block, which results in overproduction of androgens. In patients with a high-grade enzymatic block, inadequate amounts of glucocorticoids and mineralocorticoids are made, resulting in salt loss, which can be life threatening. Nonclassic CAH can be managed easily by supplementing glucocorticoids. Usually, prednisone 2.5 mg daily (or its equivalent) suppresses adrenal androgen production to within the normal range. When this therapy is instituted, facial acne usually clears promptly, ovulation is restored, and there is no new terminal hair growth.

Medical therapy for adrenal and ovarian disorders cannot resolve hirsutism. It can only suppress new hair growth. Hair that is present must be controlled by shaving, bleaching, using depilatory agents, electrolysis, or laser hair ablation.

Cushing Syndrome

Cushing syndrome is an adrenal disease resulting in adrenal excess. As a result of an adrenal neoplasm or an ACTH-producing tumor, the patient demonstrates signs of corticosteroid excess that include truncal obesity, moonlike facies, glucose intolerance, skin thinning with striae, osteoporosis, proximal muscle weakness in addition to evidence of hyperandrogenism, and menstrual irregularities.

Adrenal Neoplasms

Androgen-secreting adrenal adenomas cause a rapid increase in hair growth associated with severe acne; amenorrhea; and, sometimes, virilization. In androgen-secreting adenomas, DHEA-S is usually elevated above 6 mg/mL. The diagnosis of this rare tumor is established by computed axial tomography or magnetic resonance imaging of the adrenal glands. Adrenal adenomas must be removed surgically.

CONSTITUTIONAL HIRSUTISM

Occasionally, after a diagnostic evaluation for hirsutism, there is no explanation for the cause of the disorder. By exclusion, this condition is often called **constitutional hirsutism**. Data support the hypothesis that women with **constitutional hirsutism** have greater activity of 5α-reductase and, therefore, more free testosterone than do unaffected women.

Treatment

Treatment of constitutional hirsutism is primarily androgen blockade and mechanical removal of the excess hair. Spironolactone 25 to 100 mg/day is the most commonly used androgen blocker. Spironolactone also inhibits testosterone production by the ovary and reduces 5α-reductase activity. Other androgen blockers include flutamide and cyproterone acetate. The activity of 5α-reductase can also be inhibited directly through the use of drugs such as finasteride (5 mg orally daily). Eflornithine hydrochloride 13.9% is an irreversible inhibitor of L-ornithine decarboxylase, which slows and shrinks hair. This cream has been approved for facial use with satisfactory local effects. Patients taking an androgen receptor or 5α-reductase blocker should be placed on concomitant oral contraceptives because of the teratogenic and demasculinizing effects on a fetus should pregnancy occur. Oral contraceptives may also improve the efficacy of these treatments through the decreased androgen and increased SHBG production effects associated with their use.

IATROGENIC ANDROGEN EXCESS

Some drugs with androgen activity have been implicated in hirsutism and virilization, including danazol and progestin-containing oral contraceptives.

Danazol

Danazol is an attenuated androgen used for the suppression of pelvic endometriosis. It has androgenic properties, and some women develop hirsutism, acne, and deepening of the voice while taking the drug. If these symptoms occur, the value of the danazol should be weighed against the side effects before continuing therapy. Symptoms of voice changes may be irreversible upon discontinuation of treatment. Pregnancy should be ruled out before initiating a course of danazol therapy, because it can produce virilization of the female fetus.

Oral Contraceptives

The progestins in oral contraceptives are impeded androgens. Rarely, a woman taking oral contraceptives develops acne and even hirsutism. If this occurs, another product with a less androgenic progestin should be selected, or the pill should be discontinued. Moreover, evaluation for the coincidental development of late-onset adrenal hyperplasia should be done.

CLINICAL FOLLOW-UP

Physical examination shows a normal female body hair distribution with just a few scant hairs noted around the nipples. Examination of her face shows a few dark hairs on her chin and fine dark hairs over her upper lip. Her family history reveals that this hair pattern is similar to other postmenopausal women in her family. The patient is reassured when she is told that the changes of menopause result in a reduced level of hormones but a relative dominance of androgens.

---

thePoint® Visit http://thePoint.lww.com/activate for an interactive USMLE-style question bank and more!

CHAPTER 41
Menopause

This chapter deals primarily with APGO Educational Topic Area:

TOPIC 47   MENOPAUSE

Students should be able to define and describe the physiologic changes associated with menopause. They should outline a basic approach to evaluation and management of the perimenopausal or menopausal patient. They should identify common presenting signs and symptoms and physical examination findings. They should list factors that influence age of menopause and severity of symptoms. They should be able to counsel women about the menopausal transition including long-term changes.

CLINICAL CASE

A 54-year-old woman comes to see you because she has been having trouble sleeping. She reports that her youngest child recently left for college, and she has just felt "off" recently. She has been irritable with her husband and feels somewhat tired. Her husband complains that her tossing and turning at night keeps him awake. Also her menstrual cycle has been irregular with her last bleeding occurring 4 months ago.

INTRODUCTION

Menopause is the permanent cessation of menses after significant decrease of ovarian estrogen production. This is evidenced by 12 consecutive months with no menstrual bleeding. **Perimenopause** is the period before menopause, that is, the transition from the reproductive to the nonreproductive years during which ovarian estrogen production may fluctuate unpredictably. The time period during which the changes of menopause occur is called the **climacteric**. An increasing proportion of American women are included in these groups, because the female life expectancy has lengthened, and the number of women in this age group is expanding (Fig. 41.1).

MENSTRUATION AND MENOPAUSE

Although male gametes are renewed on a daily basis, female gametes are of a fixed number that progressively diminish throughout a woman's reproductive life. At the time of birth, the female infant has approximately 1 to 2 million oocytes; by puberty, she has approximately 400,000 oocytes remaining. By ages 30 to 35 years, the number of oocytes would have decreased to approximately 100,000. For the remaining reproductive years, the process of oocyte maturation and ovulation becomes increasingly inefficient, with the continued loss of functional oocytes.

A woman ovulates approximately 400 oocytes during her reproductive years. The process of **oocyte selection** is complex. During the reproductive cycle, a cohort of oocytes is stimulated to begin maturation, but only one or two dominant follicles complete the process and are eventually ovulated.

Follicular maturation is induced and stimulated by the pituitary release of the follicle-stimulating hormone (FSH) and luteinizing hormone (LH). FSH binds to its receptors in the follicular membrane of the oocyte and stimulates follicular maturation, providing estradiol (E_2), which is the major estrogen of the reproductive years. LH stimulates the theca luteal cells surrounding the oocyte to produce androgens as well as estrogens and serves as the triggering mechanism to induce ovulation. With advancing reproductive age, the remaining oocytes become increasingly resistant to FSH. Thus, plasma concentrations of FSH begin to increase several years in advance of actual menopause, when the FSH is generally found to be >30 mIU/mL (Table 41.1).

Menopause marks the end of a woman's natural reproductive life. The average age for menopause in the United States is between 50 and 52 years (median 51.5), with 95% of women experiencing this event between 44 and 55 years. The age of menopause is not influenced by the age of menarche, number of ovulations or pregnancies, lactation, or the use of oral contraceptives. Race, socioeconomic status, education, and height also have no effect on the age of menopause. Genetics and lifestyle, however, *can* affect the age of menopause. Undernourished women and smokers, for example, tend to have an earlier menopause, although the effect is slight. Approximately 1% of women undergo menopause before the age of 40 years, which is generally referred to as **primary ovarian insufficiency.** Women spend roughly one-third of their lifespan in menopause.

Contrary to popular belief, the ovaries of postmenopausal women are not quiescent. Under the stimulation of LH, theca cell islands in the ovarian stroma produce hormones, primarily the androgens testosterone and androstenedione. Testosterone appears to be the major product of the

345

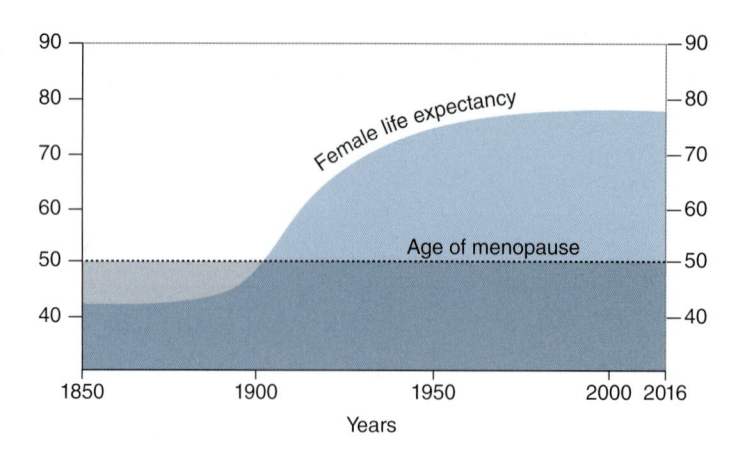

FIGURE 41.1. Age of menopause and female life expectancy.

TABLE 41.1 RELATIVE CHANGES IN FOLLICLE-STIMULATING HORMONE AS A FUNCTION OF LIFE STAGES

Life Stages	FSH (mIU/mL)
Childhood	<4
Prime reproductive years	6–10
Perimenopause	14–24
Menopause	>30

FSH, follicle-stimulating hormone.

postmenopausal ovary. Testosterone concentrations decline after menopause, but remain two times higher in menopausal women with intact ovaries than in those whose ovaries have been removed. **Estrone** (E_1) is the predominant endogenous estrogen in postmenopausal women. It is termed **extragonadal estrogen** because the concentration is directly related to body weight. Androstenedione is converted to E_1, proportionate to the amount of fatty tissue (Table 41.2). Because estrogen promotes endometrial proliferation, obese menopausal women have a higher risk of endometrial hyperplasia and carcinoma.

Conversely, slender menopausal women are at a higher risk for menopausal symptoms.

SYMPTOMS AND SIGNS OF MENOPAUSE

Menopause is a physiologic process that can be associated with symptoms that may affect a woman's quality of life. Decreased estrogen production can result in multiple adverse systemic effects (Fig. 41.2). Many of these symptoms can be ameliorated with hormone therapy (HT). The need for HT should be individualized based on a woman's specific risk factors.

Menstrual Cycle Alterations

Beginning at approximately the age of 40 years, the number of a woman's ovarian follicles diminishes, and subtle changes occur in the frequency and length of menstrual cycles. A woman may note shortening or lengthening of her cycles. The luteal phase of the cycle remains constant at 13 to 14 days, whereas the variation of cycle length is related to a change in the follicular phase. As a woman approaches menopause, the frequency of ovulation decreases from 13 to 14 times per year to 11 to 12 times per year. With advancing reproductive age, ovulation frequency may decrease to three to four times per year.

TABLE 41.2 STEROID HORMONE SERUM CONCENTRATIONS IN PREMENOPAUSAL WOMEN, POSTMENOPAUSAL WOMEN, AND WOMEN AFTER OOPHORECTOMY

Hormone	Premenopausal (Normal Ranges)	Postmenopausal	Postoophorectomy
Testosterone (ng/dL)	325 (200–600)	230	110
Androstenedione (ng/dL)	1,500 (500–3,000)	800–900	800–900
Estrone (pg/mL)	30–200	25–30	30
Estradiol (pg/mL)	35–500	10–15	15–20

Vulva and vagina
  Dyspareunia (atrophic vaginitis)
  Blood tinged discharge (atrophic vaginitis)
  Vulvar pruritus

Urethra, bladder, and pelvic floor
  Urgency, frequency
  Urinary stress incontinence
  Pelvic floor relaxation or prolapse

Skin and mucous membranes
  Dryness or pruritus
  Decreased collagen, increased wrinkles
  Mild hirsutism
  Dry mouth
  Dry hair or alopecia

Hearts and vasculature
  Angina and coronary arterial disease

Bones and joints
  Bone loss (osteoporosis, fractures)
  Joint pain

Breasts
  Mastalgia

Other
  Decreased concentration
  Decreased energy
  Impaired balance
  Mood changes
  Fatigue
  Sleep disturbance
  Vasomotor symptoms (hot flashes, diaphoresis)

FIGURE 41.2. Effects of menopause.

With the change in reproductive cycle length and frequency, there are concomitant changes in the plasma concentration of FSH and LH. More FSH is required to stimulate follicular maturation. Beginning in the late thirties and early forties, the concentration of FSH begins to increase from normal cyclic ranges (6–10 mIU/mL) to perimenopausal levels (14–24 mIU/mL). During this period, women begin to experience sometimes unpleasant symptoms and signs of decreasing estrogen levels. Some women are not symptomatic yet have significant clinical effects such as early osteoporosis. Levels of FSH are 30 mIU/mL or more at menopause.

● HOT FLUSHES AND VASOMOTOR INSTABILITY

Coincident with the change in reproductive cycle length and frequency, **hot flush** is usually the first physical manifestation of decreasing ovarian function and is a symptom of vasomotor instability.

Hot flushes are recurrent, transient episodes of flushing, perspiration, and a sensation ranging from warmth to intense heat on the upper body and face, sometimes followed by chills. When they occur during sleep and are associated with perspiration, they are termed **night sweats**. Occasional hot flushes begin several years before actual menopause. Other conditions that can cause hot flushes include thyroid disease, epilepsy, infection, and use of certain drugs.

The hot flush is the most common symptom of decreased estrogen production and is considered one of the hallmark signs of perimenopause. However, its incidence varies widely. Some U.S. studies have found that about 75% of women experienced hot flushes during the transition from perimenopause to menopause. Outside the United States, rates vary even more widely, from about 10% in Hong Kong to 62% in Australia. Reasons for these differences are unknown. In the United States, prevalence rates also differ among perimenopausal women of racial and ethnic groups, with African Americans most frequently reporting symptoms (45.6%), followed by Hispanic Americans (35.4%), Caucasians (31.2%), Chinese Americans (20.5%), and Japanese Americans (17.6%). More recent studies seem to indicate that differences in body mass index (BMI) would be a more reliable indicator of the incidence of hot flushes.

Hot flushes have a rapid onset and resolution. When a hot flush occurs, a woman experiences a sudden sensation of warmth. The skin of the face and the anterior chest wall becomes flushed for approximately 90 seconds. With resolution of the hot flush, a woman feels cold and diaphoretic. The entire phenomenon lasts less than 3 minutes. The exact cause of hot flushes has not been determined, although it seems that declining 17β-estradiol secretion by the ovarian follicles plays a significant role. As a woman approaches menopause, the frequency and intensity of hot flushes increase. Hot flushes may be disabling during the day and even more so at night when they are a significant cause of clinical sleep disturbance.

When perimenopausal and postmenopausal women receive HT, hot flushes usually resolve in 3 to 6 weeks, though sometimes even more rapidly, depending on the dose administered. If a menopausal woman does not receive HT, hot flushes usually resolve spontaneously within 2 to 3 years, although some women experience them for 10 years or longer.

Hot flushes are not simply an uncomfortable part of the normal perimenopause and menopause. They are associated with significant adverse outcomes, such as hampered job productivity and sleep deprivation.

Sleep Disturbances

Declining E_2 levels induce a change in a woman's sleep cycle so that restful sleep becomes difficult and, for some, impossible. The latent phase of sleep (i.e., the time required to fall asleep) is lengthened, with alterations in rapid eye movement patterns; the actual period of sleep is shortened. Therefore, perimenopausal and postmenopausal women complain of having difficulty falling asleep and of waking up soon after going to sleep. Sleep disturbances are one of the most common and disabling effects of menopause.

Women with marked sleep aberration are understandably often tense and irritable and have difficulty with concentration and interpersonal relationships. With HT, the sleep cycle is improved.

Vaginal Dryness and Genital Tract Atrophy

The vaginal epithelium, cervix, endocervix, endometrium, myometrium, and uroepithelium are estrogen-dependent tissues. With decreasing estrogen production, these tissues become atrophic, resulting in various symptoms. The vaginal epithelium becomes thin and cervical secretions diminish. Women experience vaginal dryness while attempting or having sexual intercourse, leading to diminished sexual enjoyment and dyspareunia. **Atrophic vaginitis** also may present with itching and burning. The thinned epithelium is also more susceptible to becoming irritated by common skin irritants or infected by local flora. This discomfort can be relieved with systemic HT or the topical use of estrogen.

The endometrium also becomes atrophic, sometimes resulting in postmenopausal spotting. The paravaginal tissues that support the bladder and rectum become atrophic. When this is combined with the effects of childbearing, it can result in loss of support for the bladder or and rectum (see Chapter 30). In addition, uterine prolapse is more common in the hypoestrogenic patient. Because of atrophy of the lining of the urinary tract, there may be symptoms of dysuria and urinary frequency, a condition called **atrophic urethritis**. HT can relieve the symptoms of urgency, frequency, and dysuria. Loss of support to the urethrovesical junction may result in stress urinary incontinence; in some cases, pelvic muscle (Kegel) exercises may relieve some of these symptoms.

Mood Changes and Memory Changes

Perimenopausal and postmenopausal women often complain of mood swings. Some women experience memory loss, depression, apathy, and "crying spells." These may be related to menopause, sleep disturbances, or both. The physician should provide counseling and emotional support as well as medical therapy, if indicated. Because there may be a comorbid sleep disorder, such as obstructive sleep apnea and restless legs syndrome (RLS), consultation with a sleep medicine expert for consideration of an overnight sleep study may be appropriate in some cases. Although sex steroid hormone receptors are present in the central nervous system (CNS), there is insufficient evidence about the role of estrogens in CNS function to implicate a direct mechanism.

Skin, Hair, and Nail Changes

Some women notice changes in their hair and nails with the hormonal changes of menopause. Estrogen influences skin thickness. With declining estrogen production, the skin tends to become thin, less elastic, and eventually more susceptible to abrasion and trauma. Estrogen stimulates the production of the sex hormone–binding globulin (SHBG), which binds androgens and estrogens. With declining estrogen production, less SHBG is available, thereby increasing the level of free testosterone. Increased testosterone levels may result in increased facial hair. Moreover, changes in estrogen production affect the rate of hair shedding. Hair from the scalp is normally lost and replaced in an asynchronous way. With changes in estrogen production, hair is shed and replaced in a synchronous way, resulting in the appearance of increased scalp hair loss at a given point in time. Disturbing as physiologic scalp hair loss may be, physicians should reassure patients that the process is self-limiting and requires no therapy. Nails become thin and brittle with estrogen deprivation but are restored to normal over time or with estrogen therapy.

Osteoporosis

Bone demineralization is a natural consequence of aging. Diminishing bone density occurs in both men and women. However, the onset of bone demineralization occurs 15 to 20 years earlier in women than in men because of acceleration after ovarian function ceases. Bone demineralization not only occurs with natural menopause but also has been reported in association with decreased estrogen production in certain groups of young women (such as those with eating disorders or elite athletes with an exercise-associated lower BMI). Risk factors warranting earlier screening for **osteoporosis** are shown in Box 41.1.

Alternatively FRAX® is a tool designed by the World Health Organization to assess fracture risk using a mathematical model that takes into account various factors in the patient's medical history such as BMI, personal medical history, parental history of fracture, and alcohol use, to name just a few. The ACOG recommends screening patients under the age of 65 years for osteoporosis if their FRAX risk of major osteoporotic fracture is 9.3% or greater or if they have one of several risk factors.

BOX 41.1 When to Screen for Bone Density Before Age 65 Years

Bone density should be screened in postmenopausal women younger than 65 years if any of the following risk factors are noted:
- Medical history of a fragility fracture
- Body weight less than 127 lb
- Medical causes of bone loss (medications or diseases)
- Parental medical history of hip fracture
- Current smoker
- Alcoholism
- Rheumatoid arthritis

American College of Obstetricians and Gynecologists. Osteoporosis. Practice Bulletin 129. Washington, DC: American College of Obstetricians and Gynecologists; September, 2012.

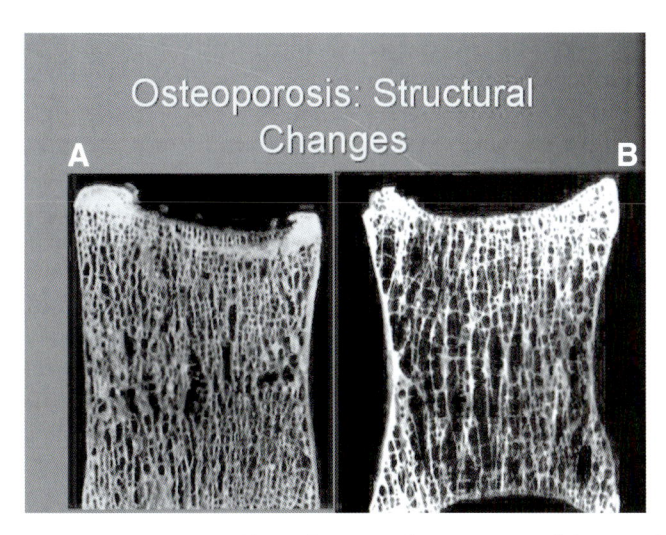

FIGURE 41.3. Structural bone changes with osteoporosis. (A) Normal bone. (B) Osteoporotic trabecular bone. (From Randolph JF, Lobo RA. Menopause. In: *Precis: Reproductive Endocrinology.* 3rd ed. Washington, DC: ACOG; 2007:185. Used with permission from American College of Obstetricians and Gynecologists.)

Estrogen receptors (ERs) are present in osteoblasts, which suggests a permissive and perhaps even an essential role for estrogen in bone formation. Estrogen affects the development of cortical and trabecular bone, although the effect on the latter is more pronounced. Bone density diminishes at the rate of approximately 1% to 2% per year in postmenopausal women, compared with approximately 0.5% per year in perimenopausal women (Fig. 41.3). HT, especially when combined with appropriate calcium supplementation and weight-bearing exercise, can help slow bone loss in menopausal women. Weight-bearing activity such as walking for as little as 30 minutes a day increases the mineral content of older women.

Calcium is beneficial to prevent bone loss; women older than 50 years should meet the Recommended Dietary Allowance of 1,200 mg. Calcium therapy combined with estrogen therapy is more effective than calcium alone. In addition, for those with limited sun exposure and lacking other dietary sources, supplementation with vitamin D should be considered: 600 IU/day from ages 51 to 70 years and 800 IU/day for ages greater than 70 years.

Progressive, linear decrease in bone mineral mass is noted in women who do not receive HT in the first 5 to 10 years following menopause. When HT is initiated before or at the time of menopause, bone density loss is greatly reduced, although this benefit is lost 1 to 2 years after discontinuation. HT begun in a woman 5 or more years after menopause may still have a positive effect on bone density loss. However, osteoporosis is not the primary indication for HT. Several bisphosphonates, such as alendronate, ibandronate, and risedronate, can be used for the management of menopause-associated bone loss. These agents reduce bone resorption through the inhibition of osteoclastic activity (Table 41.3).

Selective estrogen receptor modulators (SERMs) provide another nonhormonal management option. Most estrogenic responses are mediated in the body by one of two receptors, either ERα or ERβ. SERMs are ER ligands that act like estrogens in some tissues but block estrogen action in others. An example is raloxifene, which exhibits ER antagonist activity in the breast but agonist activity in the bone. As with the bisphosphonates, it also lacks the capabilities of mitigating many of the other estrogen deprivation symptoms, such as hot flushes and sleeplessness, and may even exacerbate these symptoms. It is important also to consider the effects of SERMs on the endometrium as they can increase the risk of hyperplasia and endometrial cancer.

Cardiovascular Lipid Changes

With perimenopause, changes occur in the cardiovascular lipid profile. Total cholesterol increases, high-density lipoprotein cholesterol decreases, and low-density lipoprotein cholesterol increases. HT may promote changes in the lipid profile that are favorable to the cardiovascular system. Retrospective case–control studies suggest that estrogens have a cardioprotective effect. However, data from the Women's Health Initiative (WHI) suggest that no such protection exists in placebo-controlled clinical trials, although some have criticized these trials because of various methodological flaws, including the late age of onset of treatment in a large group of the study subjects. Current trials are underway using transdermal estrogen and natural progesterone administered to women in their fifties to better understand whether earlier HT carries the same risk as shown in the

TABLE 41.3 NONHORMONAL REGIMENS FOR OSTEOPOROSIS

Drug	Drug Class	Mechanism of Action
Risedronate	Bisphosphonate	Inhibits osteoclast bone resorption
Ibandronate	Bisphosphonate	Inhibits osteoclast bone resorption
Alendronate	Bisphosphonate	Inhibits osteoclast bone resorption
Calcium carbonate	Natural	Provides substrate for bone remodeling and strengthening
Raloxifene	Selective estrogen receptor modulator, selectively binds estrogen receptors, inhibiting bone resorption and turnover	Inhibits bone resorption and turnover

WHI. At this time, HT should not be offered to patients with the primary goal of protection against heart disease.

● PRIMARY OVARIAN INSUFFICIENCY

The diagnosis of primary ovarian insufficiency applies to the approximately 1% of women who experience menopause before the age of 40 years. The diagnosis should be suspected in a young woman with hot flushes and other symptoms of hypoestrogenism and secondary amenorrhea (e.g., a woman seeking treatment for infertility). The diagnosis is confirmed by laboratory findings of menopausal FSH levels (>30–40 mIU/mL) on two separate occasions. Interestingly, hot flushes are not as common as might be expected in this group of patients. The diagnosis has profound reproductive and emotional implications for most patients, especially if their desires for childbearing have not been fulfilled, as well as metabolic and constitutional implications. There are many causes of premature loss of oocytes and premature menopause; some of the more common causes are discussed here. Given its potential dramatic impact, primary ovarian insufficiency demands a careful workup in order to identify the underlying cause and permit appropriate management.

Genetic Factors

Several factors influence a woman's reproductive lifespan. Genetic information that determines the length of a woman's reproductive life is carried on the distal long arm of the X chromosome. Partial deletion of the long arm of one X chromosome results in primary ovarian insufficiency. Total loss of the long arm of the X chromosome, as seen in Turner syndrome, results in ovarian failure at birth or in early childhood. When suspected, these diagnoses can be established by careful mapping of the X chromosome. Additionally, screening for premutations for the fragile X syndrome should be offered because of its association with primary ovarian insufficiency.

These patients are at risk for having children with mental disabilities. Evaluation for any Y chromosome material should also be performed, because, if identified, oophorectomy should be performed as a result of the risk of cancer in these patients.

Autoimmune Disorders

Some women develop autoantibodies against thyroid, adrenal, and ovarian endocrine tissues. These autoantibodies may cause ovarian failure. These women may need HT for the indications described above; some will spontaneously resume ovarian function.

Smoking

Women who smoke tobacco can undergo ovarian failure some 3 to 5 years earlier than the expected time of menopause. It is established that women who smoke metabolize E_2 primarily to 2-hydroxyestradiol. The 2-hydroxylated estrogens are termed catecholestrogens because of their structural similarity to catecholamines. The catecholestrogens act as antiestrogens and block estrogen action. The effects of smoking should be taken into consideration when counseling women about the menopausal transition.

Alkylating Cancer Chemotherapy

Alkylating cancer chemotherapeutic agents affect the membrane of ovarian follicles and hasten follicular atresia. One of the consequences of cancer chemotherapy in reproductive age women is loss of ovarian function. Young women being treated for malignant neoplasms should be counseled of this possibility and advised that they may be candidates for cryopreservation and other fertility preservation methods.

Hysterectomy

Surgical removal of the uterus (hysterectomy) in reproductive age women is associated with hormonal aspects of menopause some 3 to 5 years earlier than the expected age. The mechanism for this occurrence is unknown. It is likely to be associated with alteration of collateral ovarian blood flow resulting from the surgery.

● MANAGEMENT OF MENOPAUSE

The changes of menopause result from declining 17β-estradiol production by the ovarian follicles. 17β-estradiol and its metabolic byproducts, E_1 and estriol, are used in HT, the objective of which is to diminish the signs and symptoms of menopause.

Estrogen Therapy

Several different estrogen preparations are available through various routes of administration, including oral medications, transdermal preparations, and topical preparations. When administered orally, 17β-estradiol is oxidized in the enterohepatic circulation to E_1. 17β-estradiol remains unaltered when it is administered transdermally, transbuccally, transvaginally, intravenously, or intramuscularly (IM). Unfortunately, IM E_2 administration results in unpredictable fluctuations in plasma concentration. When E_2 is administered across the vaginal epithelium, absorption is poorly controlled, but remains at very low levels when appropriately used. Pharmacologic plasma concentrations of E_2 can result when excessive amounts are used. Transdermal administration of E_2 results in steady, sustained estrogen blood levels and may be a preferable alternative to oral dosing for many patients.

Combined Estrogen and Progestin Therapy

The administration of continuous unopposed estrogens can result in endometrial hyperplasia and an increased risk of endometrial adenocarcinoma. Therefore, it is essential to administer a progestin in conjunction with estrogens in women who have not undergone hysterectomy. Progestins may include any variety of synthetics, such as medroxyprogesterone acetate, norethindrone, or micronized progesterone. To achieve this protective effect, the progestin chosen may be given continuously in low doses or sequentially in higher doses. Sequential dosing is usually administered for 10 or 12 days of each calendar month. Progestins, particularly medroxyprogesterone acetate, may be associated with unacceptable side effects, such as depressive symptoms and weight gain. If estrogen is administered alone because of unacceptable side effects of progestins, then it is imperative to counsel the patient about the need for endometrial surveillance given the increased risk for neoplastic changes.

There are two principal regimens for HT. Continuous estrogen replacement with cyclic progestin administration results in excellent resolution of symptoms and cyclic withdrawal bleeding from the endometrium. One of the difficulties of this method of therapy is that many postmenopausal women do not want a return of cyclic bleeding. As a result, many physicians and patients choose to avoid the problem of cyclic withdrawal bleeding by the daily administration of both an estrogen and a low-dose progestin.

There are a variety of estrogen preparations available. Most perimenopausal and menopausal women respond to one of these preparations, all of which ameliorate acute menopausal symptoms and relieve vaginal atrophy. The administration of progestins for 10 to 12 days of each month converts the proliferative endometrium into a secretory endometrium, brings about endometrial sloughing, and prevents endometrial hyperplasia or cellular atypia. Continuous oral progestin therapy or a levonorgestrel intrauterine device may be used to produce endometrial decidualization and eventually atrophy.

Numerous preparations combining estrogen and progestins are available in both oral and transdermal formulation. Treatment goals include alleviating the patient's symptoms with the smallest dose, producing the least number of side effects. Treatment should be limited and patient expectations and continued symptomatology should be revisited periodically.

CAUTIONS IN HORMONE THERAPY

The results of the WHI in 2002 revealed epidemiologic findings that have modified the contemporary use of HT. This large, multicenter, randomized clinical trial (approximately 17,000 women) studied the effects of HT, dietary modification, and calcium and vitamin D supplementation as related to heart disease, fractures, breast cancer, and colorectal cancer. Although there are features of this study that are not applicable to many younger menopausal patients, the overall results suggested that when compared with placebo, a combination of conjugated equine estrogens and continuous low-dose medroxyprogesterone acetate resulted in an increased risk of heart attack, stroke, thromboembolic disease, and breast cancer, with a reduced risk of colorectal cancer and hip fractures. One arm of the study reviewed the same outcomes in women taking unopposed estrogen and found that these women had no increased risk of cardiac events and a trend toward decrease in breast cancer compared to women on combined therapy.

Some of the data contradicted prior large-scale observational studies, and, therefore, many physicians have changed their practice regarding HT to center more on the relief of short-term symptoms of estrogen deprivation, including hot flushes, sleeplessness, and vaginal atrophy. Although reappraisals of the study have focused on its flaws, current opinion suggests that initiation early in menopause is associated with a good risk/benefit ratio, with preference for the transdermal route. Nonetheless, the current recommendations from numerous organizations, including the American College of Obstetricians and Gynecologists, are that HT should only be used for the short-term relief of menopausal symptoms and should be individually tailored to a woman's need for treatment (Box 41.2). Furthermore, those with a uterus should be provided estrogen along with progestin to reduce the risk of endometrial hyperplasia and cancer.

HT in women with prior history of breast and endometrial cancer requires special consideration. Prospective studies using low-dose HT in women with a prior history of limited lesion breast cancer demonstrate unacceptable risk; HT is not recommended in these patients. Similar studies in women with prior treated limited-lesion, low-risk endometrial cancer have been completed and show no increased risk of recurrence for estrogen users. As with all clinical decisions, a careful risk–benefit analysis should be performed taking into account patient goals.

ALTERNATIVES TO HORMONE THERAPY

Because of the controversy surrounding HT, many women are seeking alternative therapies. When counseling patients, physicians must take a holistic approach. Most women seek relief of the most common symptom of menopause—hot flushes—but as noted earlier, menopause affects women in different ways. As women age, their risk for heart disease begins to rise and, therefore, it is important to advocate heart-healthy and bone-healthy lifestyle changes.

The body of research on alternative therapies is unfortunately fraught with methodologic issues, short-term results, and

---

BOX 41.2 Contraindications to Hormone Therapy

- Undiagnosed abnormal genital bleeding
- Known or suspected estrogen-dependent neoplasia except in appropriately selected patients
- Active deep vein thrombosis, pulmonary embolism, or a history of these conditions
- Active or recent arterial thromboembolic disease (stroke and myocardial infarction)
- Liver dysfunction or liver disease
- Known or suspected pregnancy
- Hypersensitivity to HT preparations

many types of bias. Additionally, the placebo effect on vasomotor symptoms is high. Alternative therapies for the short-term treatment of common symptoms of menopause with mixed results include the following:

- Phytoestrogens
- Acupuncture
- Black cohosh
- Exercise

Therapies showing no convincing benefit include:

- Relaxation techniques
- Chinese herbal medicines
- Evening primrose oil

For each of these, further more definitive studies need to be performed and safety of the therapy should be taken into consideration. Simple environmental and behavioral changes can be used for mild hot flashes such as lowering the temperature of the room, utilizing bedsheets that wick away moisture and heat and avoid triggers.

Most well-controlled studies of the common over-the-counter (OTC) remedies have not shown dramatic, long-term improvements. In addition, many of these OTC botanical supplements are not U.S. Food and Drug Administration regulated. Consequently, there is little quality control. The same can be said for bioidentical hormones. Patients need to be informed that "natural" does not necessarily mean safe. Moreover, many of these products have undesired side effects. Many soy products interact with thyroid medications, and dong quai and red clover potentiate warfarin and other anticoagulants.

One of the most commonly used off-label medications is progesterone. Numerous randomized, placebo-controlled studies have demonstrated its efficacy, usually in the form of depot medroxyprogesterone acetate, in the treatment of hot flushes. Selective serotonin reuptake inhibitors and selective serotonin norepinephrine reuptake inhibitors have also been used with some success. In randomized, double-blind studies, venlafaxine, paroxetine, escitalopram, and fluoxetine were all shown to significantly decrease hot flushes. In addition, both gabapentin and clonidine were found to provide moderate relief of vasomotor symptoms.

Lastly, patients should be advised of the potential relief achieved by lifestyle changes, such as eating a healthy diet that is less than 30% fat and rich in calcium, getting regular exercise, maintaining a healthy weight, avoiding smoking, limiting alcohol and caffeine intake, and getting regular health care. These practices may not only help relieve some menopausal symptoms, but may also help prevent other health problems.

CLINICAL FOLLOW-UP

On physical examination, speculum examination reveals a dry, irritated vaginal mucosa. Given this information, a serum FSH level is obtained and reported back as 34 mIU/mL. The clinical and laboratory findings are consistent with perimenopause. The risks and benefits of appropriate time-limited estrogen therapy are explained to the patient, who elects treatment. At 6 months she remarks on improvement with her problems but her husband reports that she moves her legs about at night and that his sleep is not improved. A sleep medicine physician is consulted, a sleep study is performed, and RLS is diagnosed. With treatment of her RLS, the husband's complaints are gone 6 months later in follow-up.

CHAPTER 42
Infertility

This chapter deals primarily with APGO Educational Topic Area:

TOPIC 48   **INFERTILITY**

Students should be able to define and describe causes of infertility. They should be able to outline a basic approach to the evaluation and initial management of patients with infertility. They should be able to outline the complex psychosocial and ethical issues associated with this diagnosis.

CLINICAL CASE

A 36-year-old G0 comes to see you regarding her concerns about infertility. She reports that she and her husband of 4 years have been trying to achieve pregnancy for the past 14 months without success. She is particularly frustrated because he has fathered children from his previous marriage. They have been timing intercourse using commercial ovulation predictor kits, but she is unsure whether she is using them correctly. She reports regular menses and no history of tubal surgery or tubal disease.

INTRODUCTION

Infertility is the failure of a couple to conceive after 12 months of frequent, unprotected intercourse. Infertility affects approximately 15% of reproductive-age couples in the United States. **Reproductive age** generally encompasses 15 to 44 years, although pregnancy can occur outside of this age range. The probability of achieving a pregnancy in one menstrual cycle is termed **fecundability** and is estimated to be 20% to 25% in healthy young couples. Similarly, **fecundity** is the probability of achieving a live birth in one menstrual cycle. Fecundability and fecundity both decrease over time; in other words, the probability of conceiving in a given menstrual cycle decreases as the duration of time to achieve conception increases (Fig. 42.1). After 12 months of unprotected intercourse, 85% of couples will achieve pregnancy. Of those who have not achieved pregnancy after 12 months without using contraception, approximately 50% of couples will conceive spontaneously within the following 36 months. If a couple does not conceive by this point, then infertility will likely persist without medical intervention.

Infertility is a condition that encompasses a wide spectrum of reversible and irreversible disorders, and many successful treatments are available. Today, greater numbers of men and women are seeking infertility treatment due to increased public awareness of infertility and changes in social acceptance of infertility, improvements in the availability and range of fertility treatments, and improvements in physicians' ability to evaluate and diagnose infertility. Furthermore, many individuals and same-sex couples seek fertility treatments to conceive. Although this chapter discusses infertility from the standpoint of a heterosexual couple, it is recognized that fertility treatments offer the opportunity of parenthood to many nonheterosexual individuals and couples.

Today, 85% of infertile couples who undergo appropriate treatment can expect to have a child. However, fertility treatment can be a difficult experience for an individual or a couple. The inability to conceive or carry a pregnancy can be emotionally stressful, and fertility treatment can be a significant financial burden. The psychological stress associated with infertility must be recognized, and patients should be counseled accordingly.

ETIOLOGY OF INFERTILITY

Successful conception requires a specific series of complex events: (1) ovulation of a competent oocyte, (2) production of competent sperm, (3) juxtaposition of sperm and oocyte in a functional reproductive tract and subsequent fertilization, (4) generation of a viable embryo, (5) transport of the embryo into the uterine cavity, and (6) successful implantation of the embryo into the endometrium (Fig. 42.2). Any defect in one or more of the essential steps in reproduction can result in diminished fertility or infertility. Conditions that affect fertility are divided into three main categories:

1. Female factors (65%)
2. Male factors (20%)
3. Unexplained or other conditions (15%)

EVALUATION OF INFERTILITY

The most common causes of male and female infertility are investigated during the initial evaluation of infertility. It is

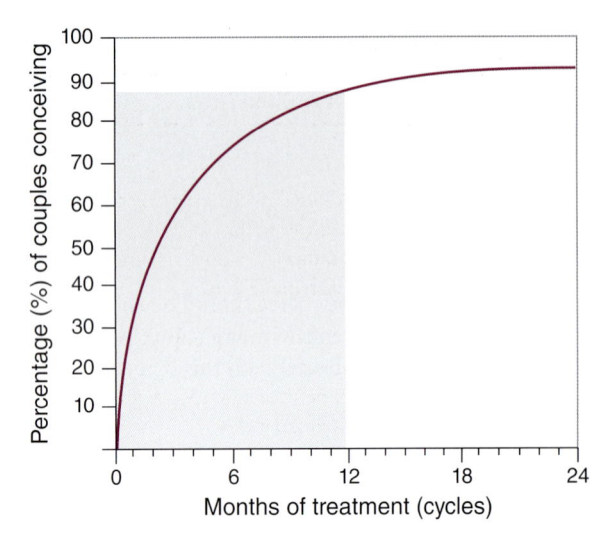

FIGURE 42.1. Conception rates for fertile couples.

important to recognize that more than one factor may be involved in a couple's infertility; thus, comprehensive evaluation is often warranted (Table 42.1). As with any medical condition, a careful history and evaluation should reveal factors that may be involved in a couple's infertility, such as medical disorders, medications, prior surgeries, pelvic infections or pelvic pain, sexual dysfunction, and environmental and lifestyle factors (e.g., diet, exercise, tobacco use, and drug use).

The timing of the initial evaluation depends primarily on the age of the female partner and a couple's risk factors for infertility. Because there is a decline in fecundity with advancing maternal age, women over the age of 35 years may benefit from a preliminary evaluation after only 6 months of attempted conception. The initial assessment and treatment of infertility is commonly provided by an obstetrician–gynecologist. More specialized evaluation and treatment may be performed by a reproductive endocrinologist.

Ovulation

A history of regular, predictable menses strongly suggests ovulatory cycles. Furthermore, many women experience characteristic symptoms associated with ovulation and the production of progesterone: unilateral pelvic discomfort (**mittelschmerz**), fullness and tenderness of the breasts, decreased vaginal secretions, abdominal bloating, slight increase in body weight, and occasional episodes of depression. These changes rarely occur in anovulatory women. Therefore, a history of regular menses with associated cyclic changes may be considered presumptive evidence of ovulation.

Secretion of progesterone by the corpus luteum dominates the luteal phase of the menstrual cycle and persists if conception occurs. Progesterone acts on the endocervix to convert the thin, clear endocervical mucus into a sticky mucoid material. Progesterone also changes the brain's thermoregulatory center set point, resulting in a basal body temperature rise of approximately 0.6°F. In the absence of pregnancy, involution of the corpus luteum is associated with an abrupt decrease in progesterone production, normalization of the basal body temperature, shedding of the endometrium, and the commencement of menstruation.

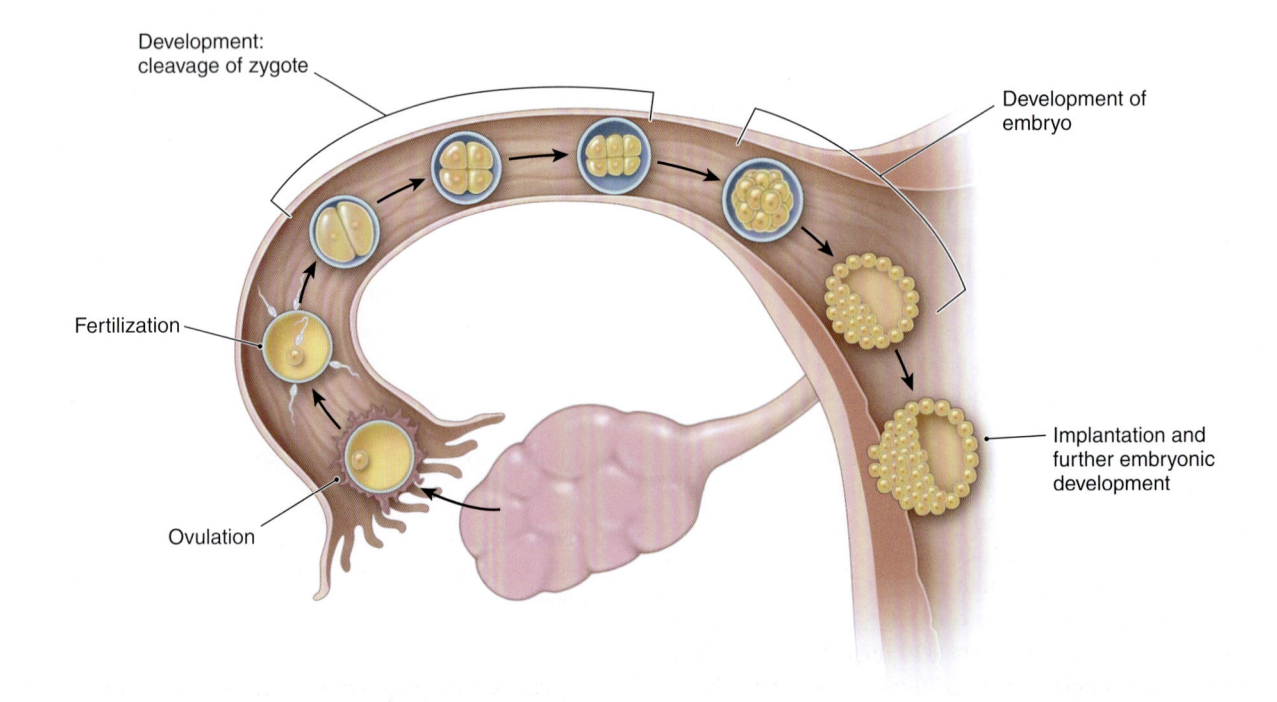

FIGURE 42.2. Steps in successful conception: ovulation, production of viable sperm and fertilization, development of the zygote, early embryonic development, and implantation of the embryo into the endometrium.

TABLE 42.1 TESTS PERFORMED DURING THE EVALUATION OF THE INFERTILE COUPLE

Target of Evaluation	Initial Evaluation	Further Evaluation
Female		
Ovulation	History and physical examination Basal body temperature charting Ovulation predictor kits	Midluteal phase progesterone level Ultrasonography Endometrial biopsy (not routine) Endocrine testing
Uterus	Ultrasonography	Saline infusion sonography Hysterosalpingography Magnetic resonance imaging Hysteroscopy
Fallopian tubes and peritoneum	Hysterosalpingography	Laparoscopy with chromotubation
Male		
Semen	Semen analysis Repeat semen analysis if indicated Postcoital test (not routine)	Genetic evaluation FSH, LH, testosterone level evaluation Prolactin level evaluation Epididymal sperm aspiration Testicular biopsy

FSH, follicle-stimulating hormone; LH, luteinizing hormone.

Ovulation Tests

Two tests provide indirect evidence of ovulation and can help predict the timing of ovulation. **Basal body temperature** measurement reveals a characteristic biphasic temperature curve during most ovulatory cycles (Fig. 42.3). Special thermometers are available for this use. Upon awakening in the morning, the patient must take her temperature immediately before any physical activity. The temperature drops at the time of menses and then rises 2 days after the peak of the luteinizing hormone (LH) surge, coinciding with a rise in peripheral levels of progesterone. Oocyte release occurs 1 day before the first temperature elevation, and the temperature remains elevated for up to 14 days. This test for ovulation is readily available, although it is cumbersome to use; it can retrospectively identify ovulation and the optimal time for intercourse, but it can be difficult to interpret. **Urine LH kits** are also used to prospectively assess the presence and timing of ovulation based on increased excretion of LH in the urine. Ovulation occurs approximately 24 hours after urinary evidence of the LH surge. However, due to the pulsatile nature of LH release, an LH surge can be missed if the test is performed only once daily.

Other diagnostic tests assess ovulation using **serum progesterone** levels and the **endometrial response** to progesterone. A midluteal phase serum progesterone level can be used to retrospectively assess ovulation. A value above 3 ng/mL implies ovulation; however, values between 6 and 25 ng/mL may occur in a normal ovulatory cycle. Due to the pulsatile nature of hormone secretion, a single low progesterone assessment should be repeated. Another diagnostic procedure is the **luteal phase endometrial biopsy**. The identification of secretory endometrium consistent with the day of the menstrual cycle confirms the presence of progesterone; hence, ovulation is implied. However, this procedure is invasive, and histologic assessment of the endometrium does not reliably differentiate infertile and fertile women and may interrupt an early pregnancy. Therefore,

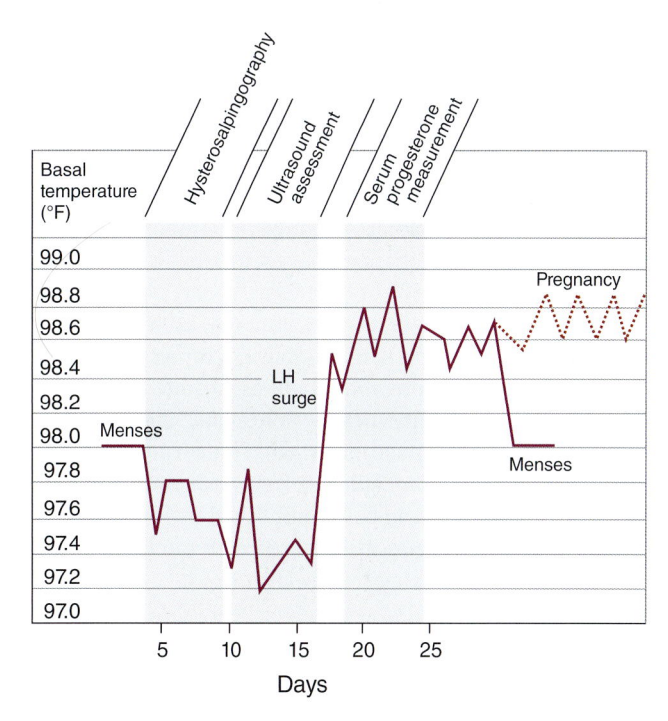

FIGURE 42.3. Biphasic basal body temperature pattern that occurs with an ovulatory cycle. HSG, hysterosalpingography; LH, luteinizing hormone.

the endometrial biopsy is no longer performed to assess ovulation or the endometrium.

Ovulatory Dysfunction

If **oligo-ovulation** (sporadic and unpredictable ovulation) or **anovulation** (absence of ovulation) is established, usually based on clinical and laboratory data, further testing is indicated to determine the underlying cause. A common cause of ovulatory dysfunction in reproductive-age women is **polycystic ovary syndrome (PCOS)**; other causes include thyroid disorders and hyperprolactinemia. Women with PCOS often present with oligomenorrhea and signs of hyperandrogenism such as hirsutism, acne, and weight gain (see Chapter 40).

Some infertile women present with **amenorrhea**, and this usually signifies anovulation. Important causes of amenorrhea include pregnancy (a pregnancy test should always be given), hypothalamic dysfunction (usually stress related), ovarian failure, and obstruction of the reproductive tract. Laboratory testing for ovulatory dysfunction may include assessment of serum levels of human chorionic gonadotropin (hCG), thyroid-stimulating hormone, prolactin, total testosterone, dehydroepiandrosterone sulfate, follicle-stimulating hormone (FSH), LH, and estradiol. Treatment of the etiology of ovulatory dysfunction may lead to resumption of ovulation and improved fertility.

Anatomic Factors

The pelvic anatomy should be assessed as a part of the infertility evaluation. Abnormalities of the uterus, fallopian tubes, and peritoneum can all play a role in infertility.

Uterus

Uterine abnormalities are commonly not sufficient to cause infertility; these disorders are usually associated with pregnancy loss. However, assessment of the uterus is particularly important if there is a history that causes concern, such as abnormal bleeding, pregnancy loss, preterm delivery, or previous uterine surgery. Potential uterine abnormalities include leiomyomas, endometrial polyps, intrauterine adhesions, and congenital anomalies (such as a septate, bicornuate, unicornuate, or didelphic uterus), as shown in Figure 42.4. Assessment of the uterus and endometrial cavity can be accomplished with several imaging techniques; sometimes, a combination of modalities is necessary to best assess pelvic anatomy (Box 42.1).

Fallopian Tubes and Peritoneum

The fallopian tubes are dynamic structures that are essential for ovum, sperm, and embryo transport and fertilization. At ovulation, the fimbriated end of the fallopian tube picks up the oocyte from the site of ovulation or from the pelvic cul-de-sac. The oocyte is transported to the ampullary portion of the fallopian tube where fertilization occurs (see Fig. 42.2). Subsequently, a zygote and then an embryo are formed. At 5 days following fertilization, the embryo enters the endometrial cavity, where implantation into the secretory endometrium occurs, followed by further embryo growth and development.

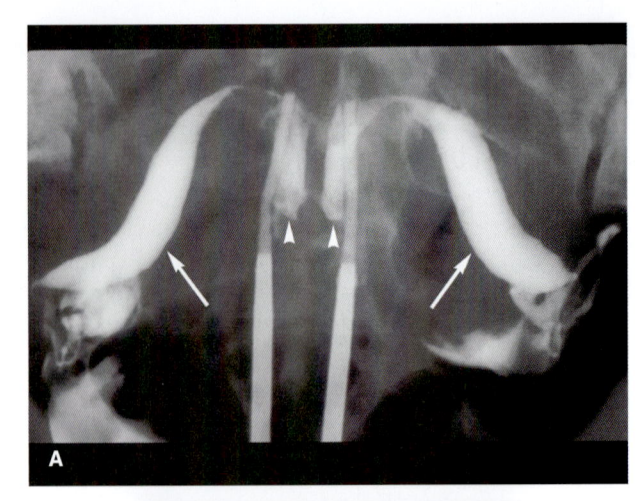

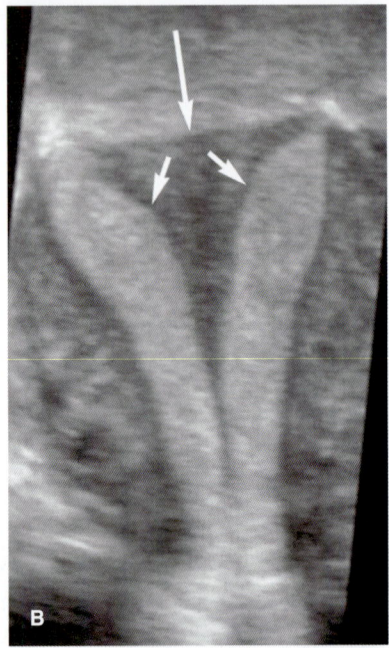

FIGURE 42.4. Uterine abnormalities. **(A)** X-ray hysterosalpingogram confirms a didelphic uterus, with paired contrast-filled cervical canals (*arrowheads*) and anteverted uterine cavities (*arrows*). **(B)** Three-dimensional sonogram indicating a septate uterus. The endometrium is separated into two components (*short arrows*) and the uterine fundus (*long arrow*) has a smooth external contour. Courtesy of Dr. Beryl Benacerraf. (From Doubilet PM, Benson CB. *Atlas of Ultrasound in Obstetrics and Gynecology*. Philadelphia, PA: Lippincott Williams & Wilkins; 2003:291.)

The fallopian tubes and pelvis can be evaluated with **HSG** or laparoscopy.

Hysterosalpingogram

There are several important characteristics of a normal HSG (Fig. 42.5). The uterine cavity should be smooth and symmetrical; indentations or irregularities of the cavity suggest the presence of leiomyomas, endometrial polyps, or intrauterine adhesions. The proximal two-thirds of the fallopian tube should be thin, approximately 1 mm in thickness. The distal third comprises the ampulla and should appear dilated in comparison to

Chapter 42: Infertility 357

> **BOX 42.1 Procedures Used in the Evaluation of Female Infertility**
>
> - **Transvaginal Ultrasonography:** Provides assessment of the cervix, uterus, and ovaries.
> - **3D Transvaginal Ultrasonography:** Provides reconstructed coronal views of the uterus, allowing better visualization of uterine abnormalities.
> - **Saline Infusion Sonography:** Provides assessment of the endometrial cavity, specifically presence or absence of intrauterine lesions and distortion of endometrial cavity shape
> - **Hysterosalpingography (HSG):** Provides information about the uterine cavity shape and fallopian tube patency.
> - **Magnetic Resonance Imaging:** Provides information about uterine abnormalities, including fibroids.
> - **Hysteroscopy:** Provides in vivo assessment and treatment of intrauterine abnormalities identified by imaging studies, such as removal of small leiomyomata, polyps, and adhesions.
> - **Laparoscopy:** Provides in vivo assessment and treatment of pelvic abnormalities, including endometriosis. Chromopertubation (infusion of dye into the fallopian tubes) can also be performed to assess tubal patency.

the proximal portion of the tube. Free spill of dye from the fimbria into the pelvis is appreciated as the cul-de-sac and other structures such as bowel are outlined by the accumulating dye. Failure to observe dispersion of dye through a fallopian tube or throughout the pelvis suggests the possibility of pelvic adhesions that restrict normal fallopian tube mobility. Examples of abnormal HSGs are shown in Figure 42.6.

Pelvic Adhesions

Pelvic adhesions that affect the fallopian tubes or peritoneum may occur because of pelvic infection (e.g., pelvic inflammatory disease and appendicitis), endometriosis, or abdominal or pelvic surgery, particularly tubal surgery. The sequelae of any of these processes or events can include fallopian tube scarring and obstruction. Pelvic infections are usually associated with sexually transmitted infections that cause acute salpingitis; commonly implicated organisms are *Chlamydia trachomatis* and *Neisseria gonorrhoeae* (see Chapter 29). Endometriosis occurs with higher frequency in infertile women compared with fertile women and can cause scarring and distortion of the fallopian tubes and other pelvic organs (see Chapter 31).

Hysteroscopy and Laparoscopy

The HSG detects approximately 70% of anatomic abnormalities of the genital tract. When there are abnormalities, further diagnostic evaluation and treatment can be performed

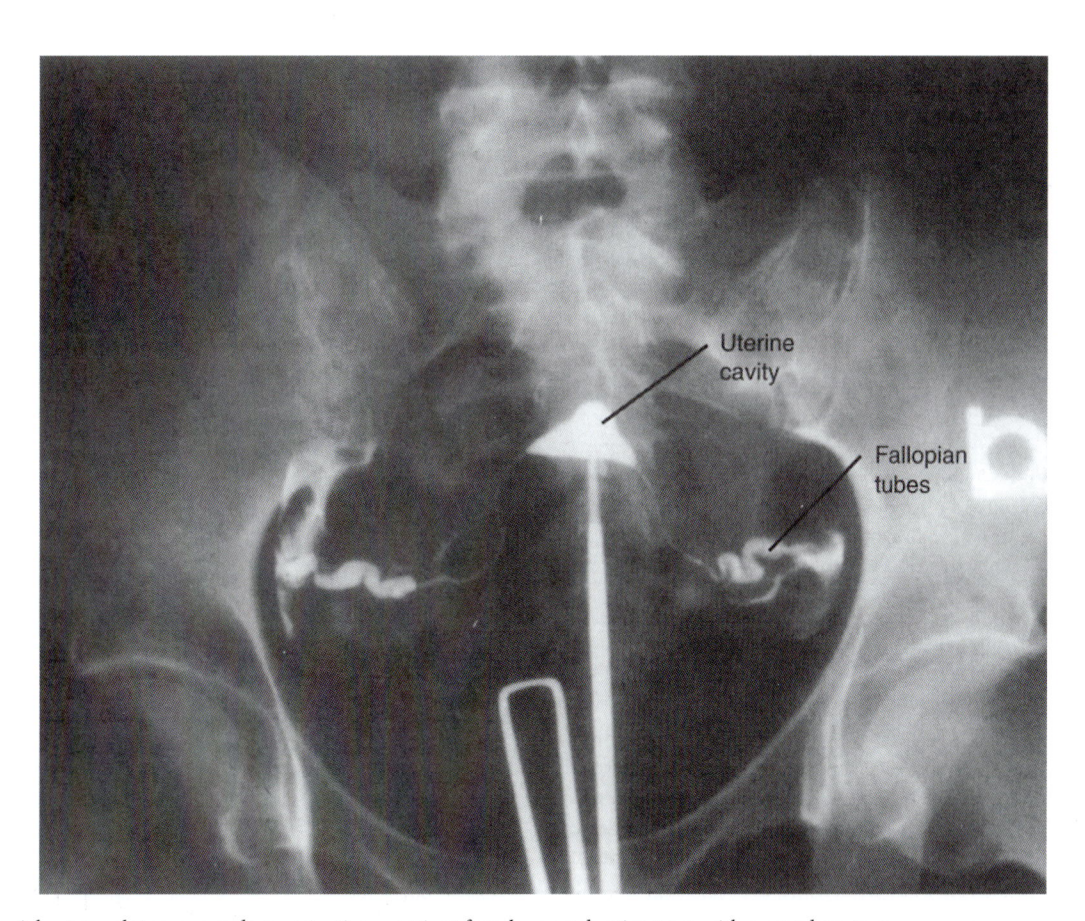

FIGURE 42.5. A hysterosalpingogram demonstrating a patient female reproductive tract with normal anatomy.

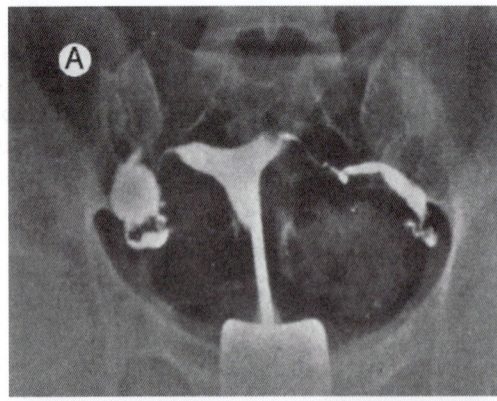

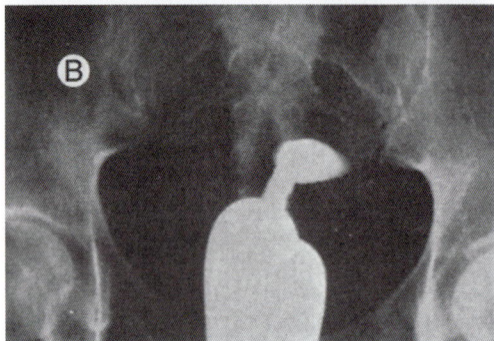

FIGURE 42.6. Abnormal hysterosalpingograms. **(A)** Bilateral hydrosalpinges (dilated fallopian tubes) with distal obstruction at the fimbriated ends; no free spill of dye seen. **(B)** Bilateral proximal tubal occlusion; uterus overdistended with radiopaque dye.

with **hysteroscopy** and **laparoscopy**. Hysteroscopy evaluates the endometrium and the architecture of the uterine cavity. Laparoscopy assesses pelvic structures, including the uterus, ovaries, and fallopian tubes as well as the pelvic peritoneum. During laparoscopy, **chromopertubation** should be performed. Similar to HSG, a catheter is placed in the uterus, and dye is injected into the uterus. Tubal patency and function is confirmed if dye is seen at fimbria bilaterally. Laparoscopy also allows the diagnosis and treatment of any pelvic abnormalities, such as adhesions and endometriosis.

● MALE INFERTILITY

Because male infertility is common, it is important to also perform a **semen analysis** when evaluating an infertile couple.

Semen Analysis

The semen specimen is usually obtained by masturbation after 2 to 3 days of abstinence; frequent ejaculation may lower the sperm concentration. It is important to collect the entire ejaculate, because the first part contains the greatest density of sperm. Analysis of the specimen should be performed within 1 hour of ejaculation (see Table 42.1). The standard semen analysis evaluates the quantity and quality of seminal fluid, sperm concentration, and sperm motility and morphology. Normal semen measurements have been established by the World Health Organization (Table 42.2). A normal semen analysis excludes a male cause for infertility in more than 90% of heterosexual couples. Certain abnormalities identified by semen analysis are associated with specific etiologies of male infertility (Table 42.3). Sperm function can be further evaluated with specialized diagnostic tests, but these tests are not routinely used.

TABLE 42.2 REFERENCE VALUES FOR SEMEN ANALYSIS

Element	Reference Value
Ejaculate volume	>1.5 mL
Sperm concentration	>15 million/mL
Motility	>40%
Rapid progressive motility	>32%
Normal morphology	>4%

Cooper TG, Noonan E, von Eckardstein S, et al. World Health Organization Reference Values for Human Semen Characteristics. *Hum Reprod Update.* 2010;16(3):231–245.

TABLE 42.3 CAUSES OF ABNORMAL SEMEN

Finding	Cause
Low semen volume	Ejaculatory dysfunction Retrograde ejaculation Hypogonadism Poor collection technique
Acidic semen	Ejaculatory duct obstruction Congenital absence of the vas deferens and/or seminal vesicles
Azoospermia or oligospermia	Genetic disorders Endocrine disorders Varicocele Cryptorchidism Infections Exposure to toxins, radiation, medications Genital tract obstruction Idiopathic
Decreased motility (asthenospermia)	Prolonged abstinence Immunologic factors: antisperm antibodies Partial genital tract obstruction Infection Sperm structural defects Idiopathic
Abnormal morphology (teratospermia)	Varicocele Genetic disorder Cryptorchidism Infections Exposure to toxins, radiation, medications Idiopathic

An alternative assessment, the postcoital test, originally used to assess the viability of sperm contained in ovulatory cervical mucus is now considered of limited diagnostic and therapeutic usefulness. Furthermore, conventional fertility treatments, such as **intrauterine insemination** (IUI) and **in vitro fertilization** (IVF), bypass any abnormalities of the cervix or cervical mucus.

Causes of Male Infertility

If the results of the semen analysis are abnormal, the test should be repeated in 1 to 2 weeks. Persistent abnormalities in the semen necessitate further investigation. The male partner should be evaluated by a urologist or reproductive endocrinologist who specializes in male infertility. Occasionally, male infertility may be the presenting sign of a serious medical condition, such as testicular cancer or a pituitary tumor. Etiologies of male infertility include congenital, acquired, and systemic disorders that can be grouped into the following categories: hypothalamic–pituitary disease that causes gonadal dysfunction (1%–2%), testicular disease (30%–40%), post-testicular defects that cause disorders of sperm transport or ejaculation (10%–20%), and unexplained infertility (40%–50%).

Spermatogenesis

Abnormalities in spermatogenesis are a major cause of male infertility. Unlike oocytes, which undergo development in a cyclic fashion, sperm are being produced constantly by the testes. As sperm develop within the germinal epithelium of the testis, they are released into the epididymis where maturation occurs before ejaculation. Sperm production and development take approximately 70 days. Therefore, abnormal results of the semen analysis may reflect events that occurred more than 2 months before the specimen collection. Alternatively, a minimum of 70 days is required to observe changes in sperm production following initiation of any therapy.

Endocrinology

Further evaluation of the infertile male includes endocrine testing. Endocrine evaluation is appropriate for individuals with abnormal sperm concentrations or signs of androgen deficiency. Serum testosterone, FSH, and LH levels will identify primary hypogonadism (low testosterone, or elevated FSH and LH) or secondary hypogonadism (low testosterone, FSH, and LH). A low LH level in the presence of **oligospermia** (sperm concentration <5 million/mL) and a normal testosterone level may indicate exogenous steroid use. A serum **prolactin** level should be assessed in men with low testosterone levels.

Genetics

Genetic abnormalities may affect sperm production or transport. **Genetic testing** is indicated in men with **azoospermia** (no sperm) and severe oligospermia. The most common abnormalities identified include gene mutations in the cystic fibrosis transmembrane conductance regulator (CFTR), somatic and sex chromosome abnormalities, and microdeletions of the Y chromosome. Men with mutations in one or both copies of the *CFTR* gene often exhibit congenital bilateral absence of the vas deferens or other obstructive defects but have no pulmonary symptoms. A karyotype may reveal abnormalities, such as Klinefelter syndrome (47 XXY) or chromosome inversions and translocations. Special testing must be performed to search for Y chromosome microdeletions because they are not detected by routine karyotype analysis; these microdeletions are associated with altered testicular development and spermatogenesis. If a genetic condition is identified, genetic counseling is strongly recommended prior to conception.

Advanced paternal age has been shown to be associated with increased rates of spontaneous autosomal-dominant mutations, with risk progressively increasing with increasing age; however, currently there are no standardized protocols in place to screen for these. There are also data to suggest increased miscarriage rates and pregnancy loss rates with paternal age over 40 years.

Diagnostic Procedures

Men with azoospermia can be further evaluated by two diagnostic procedures. If an obstructive process is suspected (obstructive azoospermia), then sperm should accumulate just before the obstruction. For example, men with congenital absence of the vas deferens or those who underwent a vasectomy have a swollen epididymis where constant production of sperm results in a small collection. **Percutaneous epididymal sperm aspiration** and **microsurgical epididymal sperm aspiration** procedures can retrieve motile, healthy sperm. If no obstruction is present (nonobstructive azoospermia) and a testicular abnormality is suspected, a testicular biopsy may identify a few sperm present in the seminiferous tubules. With either procedure, small numbers of sperm are obtained compared with a normal ejaculated specimen. These retrieved sperm are used to fertilize a single oocyte obtained from the female partner via IVF, a technology called **intracytoplasmic sperm injection** (ICSI).

UNEXPLAINED INFERTILITY

For some couples, comprehensive evaluation of both partners does not identify an etiology for their infertility. Specifically, test results identify a normal semen analysis, evidence of ovulation, a normal uterine cavity, and patient fallopian tubes. Approximately 15% of infertile couples are considered to have unexplained infertility. This diagnosis usually signifies the presence of one or more mild abnormalities in the highly orchestrated sequence of events that result in successful conception. These abnormalities may lie below the level of detection of current tests. These couples have a low rate of spontaneous conception, approximately 1% to 3% each month; this rate is influenced by the age of the female partner and the duration of infertility. If laparoscopy is performed on the female partner, subtle abnormalities such as pelvic adhesions and mild endometriosis may be identified and treated. However, it is reasonable to proceed with medical treatment of infertility without performing laparoscopy.

TREATMENT

A couple's infertility may be related to one or several abnormalities in one or both partners. Numerous medical, surgical, and **assisted reproductive technology** (**ART**) therapies are available for treating the infertile couple. For couples with unexplained infertility, empiric treatment may address one or more mild abnormalities. These couples, as well as the majority of infertile couples, tend to proceed through fertility treatment in a stepwise fashion, starting with conservative interventions and then with more aggressive treatments such as ovarian stimulation, inseminations, and eventually proceeding to IVF (explained later).

Surgical procedures are indicated in certain circumstances. If a woman presents with pelvic pain and infertility, laparoscopy may be used to identify and treat the cause of her pelvic pain as well as evaluate pelvic anatomy from a fertility standpoint. If an obstructed fallopian tube is identified with HSG, it may be possible to correct the obstruction surgically. For these operations to be successful, the endosalpinx must be healthy. If the tubal damage is significant enough to impair gamete transport, then an ART such as IVF may be necessary. When indicated, abnormalities of the uterine cavity, such as submucosal leiomyomas, endometrial polyps, intrauterine adhesions, and a septum, can be surgically corrected with a hysteroscopic procedure.

Ovarian Stimulation

Ovulation induction is indicated in women with anovulation or oligo-ovulation. However, any identified condition associated with ovulatory disorders should be addressed before initiating ovulation induction therapy. Such conditions include thyroid disorders, hyperprolactinemia, PCOS, and high levels of stress (including psychological stress, intense exercise, and eating disorders) causing hypothalamic dysfunction.

Clomiphene
The most commonly used medication for ovulation induction is **clomiphene citrate**. *However, letrozole, an aromatase inhibitor, should be considered as an alternative first-line therapy.*

Clomiphene is a selective estrogen receptor modulator that competitively inhibits estrogen binding to the estrogen receptors at the hypothalamus and pituitary. The antiestrogen effects of clomiphene induce gonadotropin release from the pituitary, which stimulates follicle development in the ovaries. Clomiphene is administered daily for 5 days in the follicular phase of the menstrual cycle, starting between cycle days 3 and 5. If ovulation does not occur, the dose is increased for the subsequent month. Women with ovulatory disorders associated with oligomenorrhea may not have regular menses and may require a progesterone-induced menses to start their clomiphene cycle. When used in women who are already ovulatory, clomiphene may stimulate development of several mature follicles.

With clomiphene, ovulation can occur between 5 and 12 days after the last pill, and it can be monitored in several ways. Urine LH kits can be used each day starting on cycle day 10; when ovulation occurs, exposure to sperm through intercourse or IUI should occur. Transvaginal ultrasound performed on cycle day 11 or 12 may identify a developing follicle. When ultrasound is used and a mature follicle is identified (average diameter > 18 mm), ovulation can be triggered by administering a subcutaneous injection of hCG. The exogenous hCG effectively simulates the LH surge and ovulation occurs; this practice enables the proper timing of intercourse or insemination. Some couples prefer not to monitor ovulation and have regular midcycle intercourse. In this situation, a serum progesterone level on cycle day 21 may provide evidence of ovulation. The use of clomiphene is associated with a 10% risk of multiple gestations, the majority of which are twin gestations, and a small risk of ovarian hyperstimulation and cyst formation.

Aromatase inhibitors work by selective inhibition of the terminal step in estrogen production. Aromatase inhibitors, compared to clomiphene, in recent trials are associated with an increased ovulation rate and increased live-birth rate in patients with PCOS. Some studies have shown a trend toward lower multifetal pregnancies as well.

Controlled Ovarian Hyperstimulation
Alternatively, exogenous gonadotropins can be given to stimulate follicular development. The use of gonadotropins is commonly referred to as **controlled ovarian hyperstimulation** (**COH**). This therapy aims to achieve monofollicular ovulation in anovulatory women (particularly those who do not respond to clomiphene) and ovulation of several mature follicles in other infertile women. Available preparations include purified human menopausal gonadotropins, FSH and LH extracted from the urine of postmenopausal women, and recombinant human FSH. The dose of medication is tailored to a woman's age, body weight, infertility diagnosis, and response to previous fertility treatments. These medications are more potent than clomiphene and require frequent monitoring of follicle growth that usually includes transvaginal ultrasonography and serum estradiol measurements. When at least one mature follicle is identified (average follicle diameter of 18 mm and serum estradiol concentration >200 pg/mL), hCG is administered to trigger ovulation. Timed inseminations are commonly performed within 12 to 36 hours from hCG administration. The risks of this therapy include **ovarian hyperstimulation syndrome**, which can require intensive therapy, a 25% incidence of multiple gestations, and an increased risk of ectopic pregnancy.

Intrauterine Insemination

Before performing IUI, an ejaculated semen specimen is washed to remove prostaglandins, bacteria, and proteins. The sperm is then suspended in a small amount of medium. To perform IUI, a speculum is inserted into the vagina, the specimen is placed in a thin flexible catheter, and the catheter is advanced through the cervix into the uterine cavity where the specimen is deposited (Fig. 42.7). A total motile sperm count (concentration multiplied by motility) of at least 1 million must be present, as pregnancy is rarely achieved with lower counts. In couples with

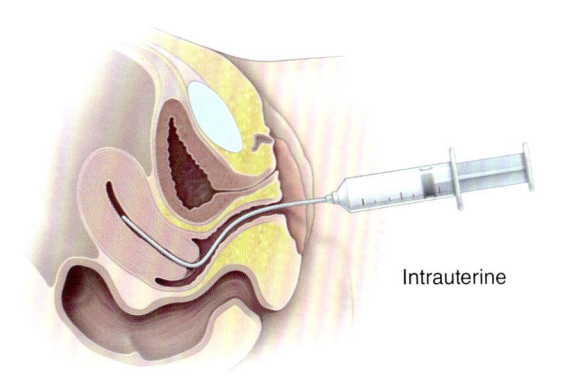

FIGURE 42.7. Intrauterine insemination technique.

infertility, and particularly in those with mild male infertility, pregnancy rates are increased with IUI. However, more severe male infertility may necessitate the use of ART to achieve pregnancy. If the male partner is azoospermic and no sperms are identified during testicular biopsy, or if a woman does not have a male partner, IUI with an anonymous donor sperm is an available alternative.

Assisted Reproductive Technologies

All fertility procedures that involve manipulation of gametes, zygotes, or embryos to achieve conception comprise the ARTs. In the United States, IVF accounts for more than 99% of all ART procedures. The process of IVF involves ovarian stimulation to produce multiple follicles, retrieval of the oocytes from the ovaries, oocyte fertilization in vitro in the laboratory, embryo incubation in the laboratory, and transfer of embryos into a woman's uterus through the cervix. The required medications for IVF include gonadotropins to stimulate follicle development, a gonadotropin-releasing hormone analogue (agonist or antagonist) to prevent premature ovulation during follicle development, and hCG to initiate the final maturation of oocytes prior to their retrieval. As with COH, the IVF process necessitates careful monitoring of ovarian response with transvaginal ultrasonography and serum estradiol measurements. Oocyte retrieval is performed by passing a needle through the vaginal apex under ultrasound guidance to aspirate the fluid from the mature follicles. Oocytes are contained within this fluid and are sent to the lab to ready them for fertilization.

Depending on the etiology of infertility, fertilization can be achieved "naturally," by placing tens of thousands of sperm together with a single oocyte, or with ICSI (Fig. 42.8). Embryos are evaluated for development and quality, and an appropriate number are transferred to the uterus to achieve pregnancy, with the goal of avoiding higher order multifetal pregnancies. Therefore, IVF provides the tools necessary to bypass the normal mechanisms of gamete transport, fertilization, and embryo transport. After oocyte retrieval, daily progesterone supplementation is necessary to insure the appropriate secretory changes in the endometrium and to support the potential pregnancy; if conception occurs, supplementation is continued until at least 10 weeks of gestation.

Indications for IVF include absent or blocked fallopian tubes, tubal sterilization, failed surgery to achieve tubal patency, severe pelvic adhesions, severe endometriosis, poor ovarian response to stimulation, oligo-ovulation, severe male factor infertility, unexplained infertility, and failed treatment with less aggressive therapies. Success rates with IVF depend on the etiology of infertility and the age of the female partner. The chance of conception with one IVF cycle depends on the number and quality of embryos transferred and can be as high as 40% to 50%, with a 30% rate of multiple gestations and at least a 15% rate of spontaneous abortion. In certain situations, embryo quality and

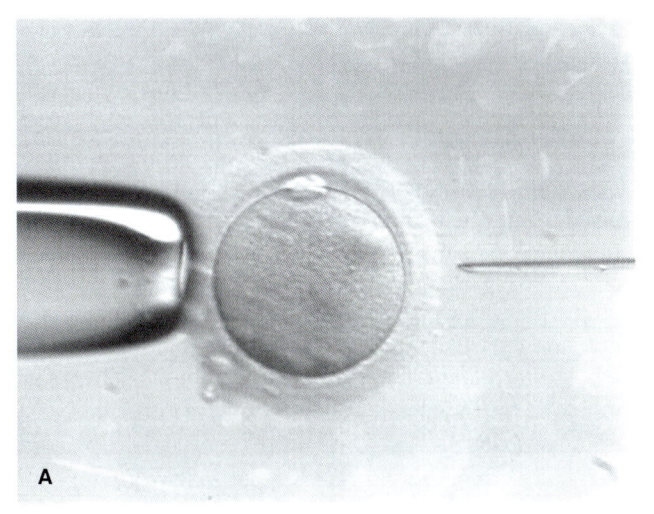

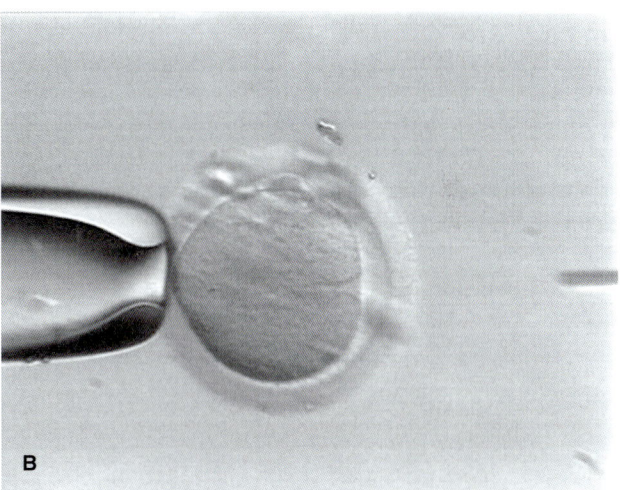

FIGURE 42.8. Intracytoplasmic sperm injection. **(A)** An oocyte is being held by a holding pipette. The injection pipette contains a single sperm. **(B)** The injection pipette has penetrated the zona pellucida and plasma membrane of the oocyte, and the sperm has been microinjected into the oocyte. (Courtesy of James H. Liu, MD. From Fritz MA, Dodson WC, Meldrum D, Johnson JV. Infertility. In: *Precis, An Update in Obstetrics and Gynecology: Reproductive Endocrinology.* 3rd ed. Washington, DC: American College of Obstetricians and Gynecologists; 2007:161.)

number and, thus, chance of conception can be improved using donor gametes.

● COUNSELING

A team approach is frequently helpful in ensuring that patients receive an adequate workup and appropriate counseling. Counseling of patients who are treated with ART should include information regarding the risk of multiple gestation, ethical issues surrounding multifetal pregnancy reduction, the stress associated with undergoing ART, and adoption. Clinicians should also be familiar with any state laws regarding infertility services and treatment and insurance coverage since the cost of these treatments is very high and most often coverage is limited or not at all by third-party payers.

CLINICAL FOLLOW-UP

Because the couple has excellent health care coverage, they agree to undergo a comprehensive workup, which demonstrates a normal day 21 progesterone, normal hysterosalpingogram, and a normal semen analysis. When given the option of expectant management or clomiphene ovulation induction with IUI, they opt for the latter and achieve pregnancy in 3 months. They ultimately deliver a healthy baby girl at term.

thePoint® Visit http://thePoint.lww.com/activate for an interactive USMLE-style question bank and more!

CHAPTER 43
Premenstrual Syndrome and Premenstrual Dysphoric Disorder

This chapter deals primarily with APGO Educational Topic Area:

TOPIC 49 PREMENSTRUAL SYNDROME AND PREMENSTRUAL DYSPHORIC DISORDER

Students should be able to list diagnostic criteria and appropriate treatments for premenstrual syndrome and premenstrual dysphoric disorder, attuned to differences between the two.

CLINICAL CASE

A 32-year-old patient comes to you because her friends have noticed that recently she has become very moody and irritable, particularly before her menstrual period. They have told her they think she has premenstrual syndrome. She reports that, additionally, she is having trouble concentrating, feels anxious, and has trouble sleeping.

INTRODUCTION

Premenstrual syndrome (PMS) is a group of physical, mood-related, and behavioral changes that occur in a regular, cyclic relationship to the luteal phase of the menstrual cycle and that interfere with some aspect of the patient's life. These symptoms occur in most cycles, resolving usually with onset of menses but certainly by cessation of menses. This cyclic symptom complex varies both in severity and in the degree of disruption of the patient's work, home, and/or leisure life. The *Diagnostic and Statistical Manual of Mental Disorders*, 5th edition (DSM-5) lists the diagnostic criteria for **premenstrual dysphoric disorder (PMDD)** as a specific set of at least 5 of 11 possible symptoms, with at least 1 core symptom—specifically, depressed mood, anxiety or tension, irritability, or decreased interest in activities (anhedonia). These symptoms occur regularly during the luteal phase of the menstrual cycle.

The pathophysiology of both entities is not well elucidated. Neither condition should be confused with **molimina**, normal cyclic symptoms associated with ovulation, which do not interfere with the patient's daily routine.

INCIDENCE

Premenstrual symptoms occur in approximately 75% to 85% of women. PMS that causes significant disruption of daily life occurs in approximately 5% to 10% of women. PMDD, rigorously diagnosed as outlined in the DSM-5, affects only 3% to 5% of women. PMS and PMDD can begin with menarche but can also present later in life, even in a woman's forties, although this is often a reflection of the hesitancy of women to seek medical help for their symptoms. The expression or symptom dominance of these disorders differs depending on ethnicity and culture. There is some evidence that the incidence of PMDD varies across cultures as well, with high rates in Mediterranean cultures and the Middle East and low rates in Asia. Twin studies also demonstrate concordance, implying a genetic contribution to the development of these disorders.

SYMPTOMS

More than 200 symptoms have been attributed to PMS. Each patient presents with her own constellation of symptoms, thus making specific symptoms less important than the cyclic occurrence of the symptoms. Somatic symptoms that are most common include abdominal bloating and fatigue. Other symptoms include breast swelling and pain (**mastodynia**), headache, acne, digestive upset, dizziness, sensitivity to external stimuli, and hot flushes. The most common behavioral symptom is emotional lability. Other behavioral symptoms include irritability, depressed mood, anxiety, hostility, tearfulness, increased appetite, difficulty concentrating, and changes in libido. Box 43.1 lists the diagnostic criteria for PMS. Box 43.2 presents the diagnostic criteria for PMDD as described in the DSM-5. The criteria for the diagnosis of PMDD are more rigorous than those of PMS and emphasize the existence of mood-related symptoms. PMS can be diagnosed on the basis of either mood or physical symptoms.

Etiology

Many theories have been proposed to explain PMS, including altered levels of estrogen, progesterone, endorphins, catecholamines, vitamins, and minerals, but none provides a single,

> **BOX 43.1 Diagnostic Criteria for Premenstrual Syndrome**
>
> 1. PMS can be diagnosed if the patient reports at least one of the following affective and somatic symptoms during the 5 days before menses in each of three menstrual cycles:
>   **Affective symptoms**
>   - Depression
>   - Angry outbursts
>   - Irritability
>   - Anxiety
>   - Confusion
>   - Social withdrawal
>
>   **Somatic symptoms**
>   - Breast tenderness
>   - Abdominal bloating
>   - Headache
>   - Swelling of extremities
>
> 2. These symptoms are relieved within 4 days of the onset of menses, without recurrence until at least cycle day 13. The symptoms are present in the absence of any pharmacologic therapy, hormone ingestion, or drug or alcohol use. The symptoms occur reproducibly during two cycles of prospective recording. The patient suffers from identifiable dysfunction in social or economic performance.
>
> Adapted with permission from Mortola JF, Girton L, Yen SS. Depressive episodes in premenstrual syndrome. Am J Obstet Gynecol. 1989;161 (1 pt 1):1682–1687.

unified explanation that accounts for all the variations that are seen. No compelling variations in any of these substances have been found in women who have symptoms compared with women without symptoms, with the exception of some preliminary studies on serotonin. Although it has been proposed that a low luteal-phase progesterone level is the cause of what is now recognized PMDD, measurement of serum progesterone values and clinical results of progesterone supplementation have not supported this theory.

Currently, the data support a theory of **serotoninergic dysregulation** as the basis for **PMDD**. Normal cyclic hormonal fluctuations can trigger an abnormal serotonin response. Monoamine oxidase reduces serotonin availability, progesterone potentiates monoamine oxidase, and estrogen potentiates monoamine oxidase inhibitors. Thus, the availability of serotonin is decreased in the progesterone-dominant luteal phase. However, the interaction must be more complex, because replacement of progesterone alone does not ameliorate symptoms. Absolute levels of progesterone have not been found to be different in women with PMDD and those without, and monoamine oxidase inhibitors do not improve symptoms in these patients. More recent data implicate γ-aminobutyric acid as an important factor in decreasing levels of allopregnanolone, a progesterone metabolite.

Diagnosis

Virtually any condition that results in mood or physical changes in any cyclic fashion may be included in the differential diagnosis of PMS (Box 43.3). Studies have shown that a patient's recall of symptoms and timing of symptoms is often biased and thus inaccurate, because of widespread societal expectations and cultural prominence of "the PMS." The majority of patients who present for treatment of PMS do not actually demonstrate symptoms restricted to the luteal phase; thus, the diagnosis of PMS and PMDD should be rigorously established using the criteria outlined.

The physician must remain open minded at the outset, and not prematurely exclude the primary problem. In the differential diagnosis, the physician should consider medical problems, psychiatric disorders, and premenstrual exacerbations of medical and/or psychiatric conditions. Perimenopause can also present with similar symptoms (see Chapter 41).

Menstrual Diary

Because the etiology of PMS and PMDD is not clear, no definitive physical examination or laboratory markers are available to aid in diagnosis. At present, the definitive diagnosis of PMS and PMDD hinges on documentation of the relationship of the patient's symptoms to the luteal phase. Prospective documentation of symptoms can be accomplished using a **menstrual diary** in two or more consecutive menstrual cycles. The patient is asked to monitor her symptoms and the pattern of menstrual bleeding for two or more cycles. For PMS, she needs only to have one of the listed symptoms but must have a symptom-free interval. For PMDD, the patient is asked to also monitor the severity of symptoms. She must demonstrate 5 of the listed 11 symptoms (see Box 43.2), one of which must be a core symptom. She must also demonstrate a symptom-free follicular phase. If her symptoms persist during the follicular phase but are less severe, luteal phase worsening of a different disorder (sometimes called **entrainment**) should be considered.

Many physical and psychiatric disorders are known to worsen in the luteal phase, including irritable bowel syndrome and MDD. It is important to distinguish these disorders from PMDD. It is particularly important to distinguish MDD and PMDD because of the risk of suicide in patients with MDD. A variety of diagnostic tools exist to assist patients with keeping their menstrual diaries. Figure 43.1 shows one such tool called "Daily Record of Severity of Problems."

Diagnostic Tests

Patients with PMDD should be evaluated to rule out specific pathology, although it is also important to understand that no specific physical findings are diagnostic of PMDD. It is reasonable to perform a complete blood count and evaluate the thyroid-stimulating hormone level, because thyroid disease and anemia are quite common in young menstruating women; however, there is no evidence that anemia and thyroid disease occur more frequently in patients who present for treatment of PMS or PMDD.

BOX 43.2 Diagnostic Criteria for Premenstrual Dysphoric Disorder

A. In the majority of menstrual cycles, at least five symptoms must be present in the final week before onset of menses, start to *improve* within a few days after the onset of menses, and become *minimal* or absent in the week postmenses.
B. One (or more) of the following symptoms must be present:
   1. Marked affective lability (e.g., mood swings, feeling suddenly sad or tearful, or increased sensitivity to rejection)
   2. Marked irritability or anger or increased interpersonal conflicts
   3. Marked depressed mood, feelings of hopelessness, or self-deprecating thoughts
   4. Marked anxiety, tension, and/or feelings of being keyed up or on edge
C. One (or more) of the following symptoms must additionally be present, to reach a total of *five* symptoms when combined with symptoms from Criterion B above.
   1. Decreased interest in usual activities (e.g., work, school, friends, hobbies)
   2. Subjective difficulty in concentration
   3. Lethargy, easy fatigability, or marked lack of energy
   4. Marked change in appetite; overeating; and/or specific food cravings
   5. Hypersomnia or insomnia
   6. A sense of being overwhelmed or out of control
   7. Physical symptoms such as breast tenderness or swelling, headaches, joint or muscle pain, a sensation of "bloating," or weight gain

Note: The symptoms in Criteria A to C must have been met for most menstrual cycles that occurred in the preceding year.

D. The symptoms are associated with clinically significant distress or interfere with work, school, usual social activities, or relationships with others (e.g., avoidance of social activities; decreased productivity and efficiency at work, school, or home).
E. The disturbance is not merely an exacerbation of the symptoms of another disorder, such as major depressive disorder (MDD), panic disorder, persistent depressive disorder (dysthymia), or a personal disorder (although it may co-occur with any of these disorders).
F. Criterion A should be confirmed by prospective daily ratings during at least two consecutive symptomatic cycles. (*Note:* The diagnosis may be made provisionally prior to this confirmation.)
G. The symptoms are not attributable to the physiologic effects of a substance (e.g., a drug of abuse, a medication, other treatment) or other medical condition (e.g., hyperthyroidism).

Reprinted with permission from American Psychiatric Association. *Diagnostic and Statistical Manual of Mental Disorders,* Fifth Edition. Arlington, VA, American Psychiatric Association; 2013.

TREATMENT

The prospective charting of symptoms not only documents the cyclic or noncyclic nature of the patient's symptoms but also allows her to play a key role in the diagnostic and management team. This will allow her to regain some control of her symptoms. For some women, providing a diagnostic label helps relieve the fear that they are "going crazy." A patient's symptoms may become more bearable as she gains insight. The symptom calendar is usually continued during the treatment phase to monitor the effectiveness of treatment and to suggest the need for further focused therapy.

Nonpharmacologic Treatment

Diet recommendations emphasize eating fresh rather than processed foods. The patient is encouraged to eat more fruits and vegetables and minimize the intake of refined sugars and fats. Minimizing salt intake may help with bloating, and eliminating caffeine and alcohol from the diet can reduce nervousness and anxiety. None of these therapies have shown statistically significant improvements in PMS and PMDD, but they are reasonable, benign, and a good part of general health improvement. In some studies, these interventions have demonstrated trends toward improvement. Clearly, they yield low risks and are generally healthful behaviors.

Lifestyle interventions that have demonstrated significant improvement in symptoms include aerobic exercise and calcium carbonate and magnesium supplementation. Aerobic exercise, as opposed to static (e.g., weightlifting) exercise, has been found to be helpful in some patients, possibly by increasing endogenous production of endorphins. Calcium decreases water retention, food cravings, pain, and negative affect compared with placebo.

Other interventions have been studied but demonstrate conflicting results. These include vitamins E and D and chaste tree berry extract as well as relaxation therapy, cognitive therapy, and light therapy. Many of these therapies have no untoward side effects and can be considered for certain patients. Studies have shown that vitamin B_6 supplementation has limited clinical

BOX 43.3 Differential Diagnosis of Premenstrual Syndrome

Allergy
Breast disorders (fibrocystic change)
Chronic fatigue states
Anemia
Chronic cytomegalovirus infection
Lyme disease
Connective tissue disease (lupus erythematosus)
Drug and substance abuse
Endocrinologic disorders
- Adrenal disorders (Cushing syndrome and hypoadrenalism)
- Adrenocorticotropic hormone–mediated disorders
- Hyperandrogenism
- Hyperprolactinemia
- Panhypopituitarism
- Pheochromocytoma
- Thyroid disorders (hypothyroidism and hyperthyroidism)

Family, marital, and social stress
- Physical or sexual abuse

Gastrointestinal conditions
Inflammatory bowel disease
- Crohn disease
- Ulcerative colitis

Irritable bowel syndrome
Gynecologic disorders
- Dysmenorrhea
- Endometriosis
- Pelvic inflammatory disease
- Perimenopause
- Uterine leiomyomata

Idiopathic edema
Neurologic disorders
- Migraine
- Seizure disorders

Psychiatric and psychological disorders
- Anxiety neurosis
- Bulimia
- Personality disorders
- Psychosis
- Somatoform disorders
- Unipolar and bipolar affective disorders

From Smith RP. *Gynecology in Primary Care*. Baltimore, MD: Lippincott Williams & Wilkins; 1996:434.

benefit. Patients should be cautioned that dosages in excess of 100 mg/day may cause medical harm, including peripheral neuropathy. Studies of evening primrose oil demonstrate no benefit. Alternative therapies include meditation, aromatherapy, reflexology, acupuncture, acupressure, and yoga. Further research is warranted in these areas.

Pharmacologic Treatment

In addition to lifestyle changes, behavioral therapies, and dietary supplementation, some pharmacologic agents have been shown to provide symptomatic relief. Nonsteroidal anti-inflammatory agents have been found in controlled trials to be useful in PMS patients with dysmenorrhea, breast pain, and leg edema but not useful in treating other aspects of PMS. This effect is possibly related to prostaglandin production in various sites in the body. Spironolactone decreases bloating but does not relieve other symptoms.

Ovulation Suppression

Because the underlying mechanism appears to be normal hormone fluctuations triggering an abnormal serotonin response, it would seem that medications to induce anovulation *should* be beneficial in the treatment of PMS/PMDD; however, ovulation suppression does not seem to help patients with PMDD. The research on PMS/PMDD has been fraught with multiple challenges because the strict criteria for diagnosis of PMS/PMDD have only relatively recently been established and standardized. Many previous studies suffered from poor methodology, and the placebo effect (30%–70%) in patients with PMS/PMDD is significant. Because symptoms are associated with ovulatory cycles, suppressing ovulation is beneficial for some patients with PMS and can be accomplished by using oral contraceptives. Oral contraceptives are a logical first choice for patients who also require contraception. Some patients, however, find that their symptoms worsen when taking oral contraceptives.

Selective Serotonin Reuptake Inhibitors

The medical treatment of PMDD differs from that of PMS. In patients who have been diagnosed with PMDD using strict criteria, the gold standard of treatment is the selective serotonin reuptake inhibitors (SSRIs). Though many medications have been studied, only four are U.S. Food and Drug Administration approved for the treatment of PMDD: fluoxetine, sertraline, controlled-release paroxetine, and drospirenone/ethinyl estradiol. In a Cochrane Database Review, 15 randomized placebo-controlled trials demonstrated benefit with SSRIs. The combination of drospirenone and ethinyl estradiol is the only oral contraceptive regimen that has demonstrated benefit and is the newest therapeutic choice for the treatment of PMDD. SSRIs are effective when dosed continuously (daily dosage) or dosed intermittently (taken only during the luteal phase [14 days prior to the onset of menses]). Patients often report improvement with their first cycle of use, lending credence to the idea that the pathophysiology of PMDD is different from that of MDD, in which treatment can take weeks to demonstrate improvement. Side effects of SSRIs include gastrointestinal upset, insomnia, sexual dysfunction, weight gain, anxiety, hot flushes, and nervousness.

Other Treatments

The use of danazol and gonadotropin-releasing hormone (GnRH) agonists has been demonstrated to be beneficial in short-term

DAILY RECORD OF SEVERITY OF PROBLEMS

Please print and use as many sheets as you need for at least two FULL months of ratings.

Name or Initials _____
Month/Year _____

Each evening note the degree to which you experienced each of the problems listed below. Put an "x" in the box which corresponds to the severity: 1–not at all, 2–minimal, 3–mild, 4–moderate, 5–severe, 6–extreme.

Enter day (Monday="M", Thursday="R", etc) >
Note spotting by entering "S" >
Note menses by entering "M" >
Begin rating on correct calendar day >

1. Felt depressed, sad, "down,", or "blue" or felt hopeless; or felt worthless or guilty
2. Felt anxious, tense, "keyed up" or "on edge"
3. Had mood swings (i.e., suddenly feeling sad or tearful) or was sensitive to rejection or feelings were easily hurt
4. Felt angry, or irritable
5. Had less interest in usual activities (work, school, friends, hobbies)
6. Had difficulty concentrating
7. Felt lethargic, tired, or fatigued; or had lack of energy
8. Had increased appetite or overate; or had cravings for specific foods
9. Slept more, took naps, found it hard to get up when intended; or had trouble getting to sleep or staying asleep
10. Felt overwhelmed or unable to cope; or felt out of control
11. Had breast tenderness, breast swelling, bloated sensation, weight gain, headache, joint or muscle pain, or other physical symptoms
12. At work, school, home, or in daily routine, at least one of the problems noted above caused reduction of productivity or inefficiency
13. At least one of the problems noted above caused avoidance of or less participation in hobbies or social activities
14. At least one of the problems noted above interfered with relationships with others

FIGURE 43.1. Daily Record of Severity of Problems. © 1977 Jean Endicott, PhD, and Wilma Harrison, MD.

studies, but long-term effects of such drugs for PMDD have not been fully evaluated, and these medications are associated with significant, often prohibitive, side effects. The use of either constitutes a "medical oophorectomy" and may be used as a trial before surgical oophorectomy is undertaken. Oophorectomy should be used only for those severely affected patients who meet strict diagnostic criteria for PMDD and who do not respond to any potentially effective therapy other than GnRH agonists.

CLINICAL FOLLOW-UP

After filling out 2 months worth of prospective daily ratings, the data demonstrate that she meets the criteria for PMDD and does *not* meet criteria for MDD. She starts taking an SSRI and feels better within a month. She plans to continue this for at least a couple of years after which point she will reassess with her physician.

---

thePoint®   Visit http://thePoint.lww.com/activate for an interactive USMLE-style question bank and more!

VI Gynecologic Oncology and Uterine Leiomyoma

CHAPTER 44
Cell Biology and Principles of Cancer Therapy

Students should be able to understand the fundamentals of cell biology and relate them to the behavior of malignant cells and their response to chemotherapy, radiation, and other novel approaches to cancer treatment.

CLINICAL CASE

A 60-year-old patient has just completed her ovarian cancer debulking surgery and returns for postoperative care and consultation regarding chemotherapy. She has questions regarding the side effects of the treatment.

INTRODUCTION

Treatment of cancers involving the breast and genital organs may involve surgery, chemotherapy, radiation therapy, or hormone therapy, used alone or in combination. The specific treatment plan depends on the type of cancer, the stage of the cancer, and the characteristics of the individual patient. Individualizing treatment is an important aspect of cancer therapy.

CELL CYCLE AND CANCER THERAPY

Knowledge of the cell cycle is important in understanding cancer therapies. The ideal cancer treatment would be a drug that targets only cancer cells with no effect on healthy tissues. In order to optimally target only cancerous tissue, it is imperative to understand not only how normal cells function but also how cancer cells differ from normal cells.

Many treatments are based on the fact that cancer cells are constantly dividing, making them more vulnerable to agents that interfere with cell division.

The cell cycle consists of four phases in addition to a resting state (Fig. 44.1). During the **G_1 phase** (**postmitotic phase**), RNA and protein synthesis, cell growth, and DNA repair take place. Once these processes are complete, the cell enters the **S phase** (**synthesis phase**), during which the DNA is completely replicated. The **G_2 phase** is a period of additional synthesis of RNA, protein, and specialized DNA. Cell division occurs during the **M phase** (**mitosis**). After mitosis, cells can again enter the G_1 phase, or can "drop out" of the cell cycle and enter a **resting phase** (G_0). Cells in G0 do not engage in the synthetic activities characteristic of the cell cycle and are not vulnerable to therapies aimed at actively growing and dividing cells. The **growth fraction** is the proportion of cells in a tumor that are actively involved in cell division (i.e., not in the G_0 phase). The growth fraction of tumors decreases as they enlarge, because vascular supply and oxygen levels are decreased. Surgical removal of tumor tissue (cytoreductive debulking surgery) can result in G0 cells reentering the cell cycle, thereby making them more vulnerable to chemotherapy and radiation therapy.

The **generation time** is the length of the cell cycle, from one M phase to the next M phase. For a given cell type, the lengths of the S and M phases are relatively constant, whereas G_2 and, especially, G_1 vary. The variable length of G_1 can be explained by cells entering the resting phase (G_0) for a period and then reentering the cycle. The length of G_1 has a profound effect on the cell's susceptibility to treatment.

Chemotherapeutic agents and radiation kill cancer cells by first-order kinetics. This means that each dose kills a constant fraction of tumor cells, instead of a constant number. The resulting clinical implication is that several intermittent doses are more likely to be curative than a single large dose.

CHEMOTHERAPY

Chemotherapeutic agents can be (1) **cell cycle (phase) nonspecific**, which means that they can kill in all phases of the cell cycle and are useful in tumors with a low growth index, or (2) **cell cycle (phase) specific**, which means that they kill in a specific

369

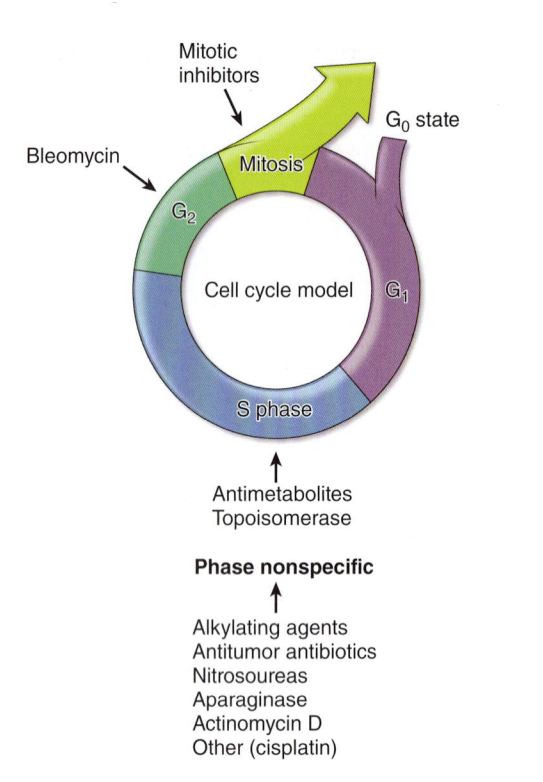

FIGURE 44.1. Actions of antineoplastic agents within the cell cycle.

phase of the cell cycle and are most useful in tumors that have a large proportion of actively dividing cells. Figure 44.1 illustrates common drugs and their sites of action within the cell cycle.

Several classes of **antineoplastic drugs** are available (Table 44.1). **Alkylating agents** and **alkylating-like agents** bind and cross-link DNA, interfering with DNA replication and, ultimately, with RNA transcription. Dividing cells, especially those in the late G_1 and S phases, are most sensitive to the effects of these drugs; however, these drugs are considered phase nonspecific (i.e., they are effective in all phases of the cell cycle). The major side effect of the alkylating agents is myelosuppression. The alkylating-like agents behave similarly and include the platinum-based agents cisplatin and carboplatin.

Antitumor antibiotics inhibit DNA-directed RNA synthesis and are also involved in the formation of free radicals, causing strand breakage. They are phase nonspecific. Their general side effects are similar to those of the alkylating agents; however, each drug has its own toxicity.

Antimetabolites are structural analogues of normal molecules necessary for cell function. They competitively interfere with the enzymes involved with normal synthesis of nucleic acids and, therefore, are most active during the S phase of cell division. They may cause bone marrow suppression or gastrointestinal (GI) mucositis when given in a bolus.

Mitotic inhibitors interfere with the M phase of cell division by preventing the assembly of microtubules. They may cause bone marrow suppression or an anaphylactoid reaction.

Topoisomerase inhibitors result in cell death by inhibiting topoisomerase I (TOPO-I) and topoiseomerase II (TOPO-II), enzymes required for DNA replication. In a normally replicating cell, TOPO-I induces reversible single-strand breaks in the DNA. TOPO-I inhibitors combine with the DNA and TOPO-I and prevent repair of the breaks in the single strand of DNA, resulting in cellular death.

ENDOCRINE THERAPY

Hormonal agents are frequently used in gynecologic cancer treatment because these cancers contain estrogen, progesterone, and other endocrine receptors. These therapies are not specifically aimed at killing cancer cells but control disease via biochemical pathways. They are commonly used along with other therapies.

TABLE 44.1 CLASSES OF CHEMOTHERAPEUTIC DRUGS

Class	Mechanism of Action	Primary Toxicities	Representative Drugs
Alkylating agents	Bind and cross-link DNA interstrand, intrastrand, or to proteins; prevent replication and transcription	Hemorrhagic cystitis, alopecia, nephrotoxicity	Cyclophosphamide, ifosfamide, melphalan
Alkylating-like agents	Cross-link DNA strands (interstrand)	Nephrotoxicity, neurotoxicity, myelosuppression	Cisplatin, carboplatin, doxorubicin
Antibiotics	Interfere with DNA replication through free radical formation and intercalation between bases	Variable	Bleomycin, actinomycin D
Antimetabolites	Block enzymes required for DNA synthesis	Gastrointestinal, myelosuppression, dermatologic, hepatotoxicity	Methotrexate, 5-fluorouracil
Mitotic inhibitors	Inhibit microtubule assembly	Myelosuppression	Vincristine, vinblastine, paclitaxel
Topoisomerase inhibitors	Inhibit topoisomerase, resulting in DNA strand breaks	Myelosuppression, alopecia, gastrointestinal	Etoposide, topotecan

Toxicity of Chemotherapy

Antineoplastic drugs are toxic because they act on normal as well as cancer cells. Table 44.2 describes the major applications and side effects of antineoplastic agents. Rapidly dividing cell types of the erythroid, myeloid, and megakaryocytic lineages are most sensitive to damage by common neoplastic drugs. Anemia, granulocytopenia (neutropenia), and thrombocytopenia are predictable side effects. Patients with anemia will often experience incapacitating lethargy. Patients with neutropenia are at high risk for fatal sepsis, and those with sustained thrombocytopenia are at risk for spontaneous GI or acute intracranial hemorrhage. Prophylactic antibiotics are administered to patients with febrile neutropenia or in neutropenic patients to prevent serious infection. Platelet transfusions can be used to decrease the risk of hemorrhage.

Combination Chemotherapy

The use of single agents is limited by development of drug resistance and toxicity. **Combination chemotherapy** is used to counteract these limitations. Several strategies can be used to select drugs for combination chemotherapy. In **sequential blockade**, the drugs block sequential enzymes in a single biochemical pathway. In **concurrent blockade**, the drugs attack parallel biochemical pathways leading to the same end product. Complementary inhibition interferes with different steps in the synthesis of DNA, RNA, or protein.

The interactions between drugs used in combination are defined as **synergistic** (result in improved antitumor activity or decreased toxicity, compared with when each agent is used alone), **additive** (result in enhanced antitumor activity equal to the sum of the antitumor activities resulting from using the individual agents separately), or **antagonistic** (result in less antitumor activity than if each individual agent is used alone). Drugs used in combinations should (1) be effective when used singly; (2) have different mechanisms of action; and (3) be additive or, preferably, synergistic in action.

Chemotherapy Regimens

Chemotherapy is administered in various regimens. **Adjuvant** chemotherapy is usually a set course of combination chemotherapy that is given in a high dose to patients who have no evidence of residual cancer after radiotherapy or surgery. The purpose is to eliminate any residual cancer cells, typically with the intent to cure disease. **Neoadjuvant** chemotherapy aims to eradicate micrometastases or reduce inoperable disease to prepare patients for surgery and/or radiotherapy. **Induction** chemotherapy is usually a combination chemotherapy given in a high dose to cause a remission. **Maintenance** chemotherapy (consolidation chemotherapy) is a long-term and low-dose regimen that is given to a patient in remission to maintain the remission by inhibiting the growth of remaining cancer cells.

Endocrine therapy with **selective estrogen receptor modulators** (**SERMs**) acts in estrogen-sensitive breast tumors to block the interaction of estrogen with estrogen receptors (ERs). The therapeutic importance of cellular ERs has been well established in breast cancers. ER-positive tumors are responsive to endocrine therapy. Normally, estrogen enters cells and binds to ERs in the cytoplasm. The complex is translocated to the nucleus, where it binds to acceptor sites on chromosomes, resulting in activation of RNA and protein synthesis. SERMs act as competitive inhibitors of estrogen binding; the SERM–ER complex binds to chromosomes but does not activate cell metabolism. The subsequent decrease in cellular activity and cell division results in reduced tumor growth.

Additionally, SERMs are used to prevent cancer recurrence. The two SERMs most frequently prescribed in the United States are tamoxifen and raloxifene. Although relatively nontoxic, some SERMs increase the risk of endometrial cancer and uterine sarcomas as well as benign endometrial pathology.

Aromatase inhibitors (**AIs**), such as anastrozole and letrozole, which suppress intratumor and plasma estrogen levels, are being used in postmenopausal patients for the treatment of advanced breast cancer that has progressed beyond tamoxifen therapy. In addition, they are being used as an adjuvant therapy, often sequentially with tamoxifen, to prevent breast cancer recurrence. AIs have been associated with bone loss secondary to the induced hypoestrogenic state.

Progestational agents have been found to be useful in the treatment of early-stage endometrial cancer when surgery is not feasible, unsafe, or not desired. Progestational therapy is also useful for some patients with recurrent disease. The most common progestational agents used are medroxyprogesterone, megestrol, and the levonorgestrel intrauterine device.

Research is ongoing to search for other hormonal agents effective for the treatment or prevention of hormonally related neoplasms. Other agents that have demonstrated efficacy in cases of recurrent disease include goserelin (synthetic hormone) and arzoxifene (SERM).

RADIATION THERAPY

Ionizing radiation causes the production of free hydrogen ions and hydroxyl (•OH) radicals. With sufficient oxygen, hydrogen peroxide (H_2O_2) is formed, which disrupts the structure of DNA and, eventually, the cell's ability to divide. As with chemotherapy, killing is by first-order kinetics. Because dividing cells are more sensitive to radiation damage and because not all cells in a given tumor are dividing at any one time, fractionated doses of radiation are more likely to be effective than a single dose. Providing multiple lower doses of radiation also reduces the deleterious effects on normal tissues.

The basis of fractionated dosage comes from the **"four Rs" of radiobiology**:

1. **Repair of sublethal injury**: When a dose is divided, the number of normal cells that survive is greater than if the dose were given at one time (higher total amounts of radiation can be tolerated in fractionated doses as opposed to single dose).
2. **Repopulation**: Reactivation of stem cells occurs when radiation is stopped; thus, regenerative capacity depends on the number of available stem cells.
3. **Reoxygenation:** Cells are more vulnerable to radiation damage with oxygen present; as tumor cells are killed, surviving

TABLE 44.2 MAJOR APPLICATION AND SIDE EFFECTS OF CHEMOTHERAPEUTIC AGENTS

Drug	Application	Off-Label Use	Dose-Limiting Toxicity	Other Toxicities
Paclitaxel (mitotic inhibitor)	Ovarian cancer	Cervical cancer (advanced) Endometrial cancer (advanced)	Myelosuppression (neutropenia) Peripheral neuropathy	Alopecia Myalgias/arthralgias GI toxicity Hypersensitivity reaction
Carboplatin (alkylating-like agent)	Ovarian cancer	Cervical cancer (recurrent, metastatic) Endometrial cancer	Myelosuppression (thrombocytopenia)	Nephrotoxicity Ototoxicity GI toxicity Alopecia Hypersensitivity reaction
Cisplatin (alkylating-like agent)	Ovarian cancer	Cervical cancer Endometrial cancer Germ cell tumors	Nephrotoxicity	Neurotoxicity GI toxicity Hypersensitivity reaction
Bleomycin (antibiotic)	Nongynecologic cancers	Germ cell tumors	Pulmonary fibrosis	Dermatologic (mucositis, hyperpigmentation)
Topotecan (topoisomerase inhibitor)	Ovarian cancer (metastatic) Cervical cancer (resistant, recurrent)	Ovarian cancer	Myelosuppression (neutropenia)	Alopecia GI toxicity
Liposomal doxorubicin	Ovarian cancer (metastatic)	Endometrial cancer Leiomyosarcoma	Myelosuppression, cardiac toxicity	Palmar-plantar erythrodysesthesia GI toxicity (stomatitis, N&V)
Gemcitabine hydrochloride (antimetabolite)	Ovarian cancer	Cervical cancer (recurrent, persistent) Leiomyosarcoma	Neutropenia	Hepatotoxicity Nephrotoxicity Hemolytic uremic syndrome
Etoposide (topoisomerase inhibitor)	Nongynecologic cancers	Ovarian cancer Gestational trophoblastic neoplasia	Myelosuppression (neutropenia)	Alopecia GI toxicity Acute MI Acute leukemia
Ifosfamide (alkylating agent)	Nongynecologic cancer	Cervical cancer (recurrent, metastatic) Ovarian cancer	Hemorrhagic cystitis	Nephrotoxicity GI toxicity Alopecia Mild leukopenia
Methotrexate (antimetabolite)	Gestational trophoblastic neoplasia Molar pregnancies		Myelosuppression (all cell lines)	Hepatotoxicity Nephrotoxicity Dermatologic (photosensitivity, rashes, vasculitis)
Dactinomycin/actinomycin D (antibiotic)	Endometrial cancer Gestational trophoblastic neoplasia	Ovarian (germ cell) cancer	Myelosuppression (all cell lines)	GI toxicity (N&V, mucositis) Alopecia Extravasation necrosis
Cyclophosphamide (alkylating agent)	Gestational trophoblastic neoplasia		Myelosuppression	Hemorrhagic cystitis Alopecia SIADH
Vincristine (plant alkaloid)	Gestational trophoblastic neoplasia		Myelosuppression	Alopecia GI toxicity Myalgias Peripheral neuropathy

GI, gastrointestinal; MI, myocardial infarction; N&V, nausea and vomiting; SIADH, syndrome of inappropriate secretion of antidiuretic hormone.

tumor cells are brought into contact with capillaries, making them radiosensitive.

4. **Redistribution in the cell cycle**: Because tumor cells are in various phases of the cell cycle, fractionated doses make it more likely that a given cell is irradiated when it is most vulnerable.

The **radiation absorbed dose** (**rad**) has been used as a measure of the amount of energy absorbed per unit mass of tissue. A standard measure of absorbed dose is the *Gray*, which is defined as 1 J/kg; 1 Gray is equal to 100 rad. Radiation is delivered in two general ways: external irradiation (teletherapy) and local irradiation (brachytherapy). **Teletherapy** depends on the use of high-energy (>1 million eV) beams; it spares the skin and delivers less toxic radiation to the bone. Tolerance for external radiation depends on the vulnerability of surrounding normal tissues. Teletherapy is usually used to shrink tumors before localized radiation. **Brachytherapy** depends on the inverse square law: the dose of radiation at a given point is inversely proportional to the square of the distance from the radiation source. To put the radioactive material at the closest possible distance, brachytherapy uses encapsulated sources of ionizing radiation implanted directly into tissues (interstitial) or placed in natural body cavities (intracavitary). **Intracavitary devices** can be placed within the uterus, cervix, or vagina, and then loaded with radioactive sources in the form of either low-dose radiotherapy (cesium-137) or high-dose radiotherapy (iridium-192 and cobalt-60). This method protects health personnel from radiation exposure. A new method of treating early breast cancer involves high-dose rate brachytherapy inserted by a balloon catheter into the cavity created by lumpectomy. **Interstitial implants** use isotopes (iridium-192 and iodine-125) formulated as wires or seeds. These implants are usually temporary, but permanent seed implants are being investigated.

New strategies are being developed for radiation therapy. For example, **intraoperative** therapy is being used for previously irradiated patients with recurrent disease who would require unacceptably high dosages of external radiation.

Complications

Complications associated with radiation therapy can be acute or late (chronic). **Acute reactions** affect rapidly dividing tissues, such as epithelia (skin, GI mucosa, bone marrow, and reproductive cells). Manifestations are cessation of mitotic activity, cellular swelling, tissue edema, and tissue necrosis. Early problems associated with irradiation of gynecologic cancers include enteritis, acute cystitis, vulvitis, proctosigmoiditis, topical skin desquamation, and, occasionally, bone marrow depression. **Chronic complications** occur months to years after completion of radiation therapy. These include obliteration of small blood vessels or thickening of the vessel wall, fibrosis, and reductions in epithelial and parenchymal cell populations. Chronic proctitis, hemorrhagic cystitis, formation of ureterovaginal or vesicovaginal fistula, rectal or sigmoid stenosis, and bowel obstructions as well as GI fistulae may result.

NOVEL CHEMOTHERAPEUTIC AGENTS

The next horizon for cancer treatment is molecularly targeted agents, cancer vaccines, and gene therapy. Several drugs are currently available that target specific molecules or proteins in cancer cells. For example, trastuzumab is a DNA-derived monoclonal antibody to the human epidermal growth factor receptor 2 protein (HER-2). Treatment with trastuzumab is currently indicated in patients with metastatic breast cancer whose tumors overexpress HER-2. Some ovarian, cervical, and endometrial tumors express the HER-2/*neu* receptor; therefore, investigation is currently ongoing regarding the usefulness of this agent in gynecologic tumors. Additionally, bevacizumab is a monoclonal antibody designed to target the vascular endothelial growth factor protein and inhibit angiogenesis in tumors. It is currently approved for treatment of a variety of tumors, including cervical and epithelial ovarian cancer.

Tumor vaccines are also currently being investigated for the treatment of ovarian cancer. The underlying principle behind these therapeutic vaccines is to inoculate the patient with a modified cancer cell line in an attempt to stimulate the patient's immune system to recognize and eliminate the tumor. Inactivated virus strains have also been studied as a vector for the vaccines in hopes of creating higher immunogenicity. Currently, the response to this type of therapy has been modest, but studies are ongoing.

Because a large proportion of gynecologic cancers result from the loss of genetic function through DNA mutations, investigational therapies have also focused on genetic manipulation of the tumors, or **gene therapy**. For instance, because half of ovarian cancers exhibit deleterious mutations in the *p53* gene, research has focused on delivering a normal *p53* gene product to the tumor using a variety of viral vectors. The hope is that the wild-type gene product would then be expressed by the tumor, and the growth would then be inhibited. So far, response has been minimal, but investigation continues.

The potential benefits of these novel therapeutic concepts are manifold, whether considered as primary or adjunct therapy. Work in this area is in the experimental stage, but eliminating cancer cells with minimal toxicity remains the goal of cancer therapeutics.

CLINICAL FOLLOW-UP

As the physician, you explain the toxic effects of chemotherapy to the patient including a change in her blood cell counts causing her increased risk of infection, changes in her kidney functioning, loss of hair, changes in hearing, and gastrointestinal symptoms as well as aches and pains. She is now prepared to undergo chemotherapy with a better understanding of what she might expect.

CHAPTER 45
Gestational Trophoblastic Neoplasia

This chapter deals primarily with APGO Educational Topic Area:

TOPIC 50 GESTATIONAL TROPHOBLASTIC NEOPLASIA

Students should be able to outline a basic approach to diagnosis, management, and follow-up of patients with gestational trophoblastic neoplasia (GTN). They should identify risk factors, common presenting signs and symptoms, and physical examination findings. They should be able to contrast molar pregnancy and malignant GTN.

CLINICAL CASE

A 27-year-old G1 presents to you with vaginal bleeding. She is 8 weeks pregnant based on her last menstrual period. She states that she is also having severe nausea and vomiting. You perform an ultrasound, which demonstrates a snowstorm pattern and no fetus in the uterus.

INTRODUCTION

GTN is a rare variation of pregnancy of unknown etiology and usually presents as a benign disease called **hydatidiform mole** (**molar pregnancy**). GTN is a clinical spectrum that includes all neoplasms that derive from abnormal placental (trophoblastic) proliferation. There are two varieties of molar pregnancies, complete mole (no fetus) and incomplete mole (fetal parts in addition to molar degeneration). **Persistent or malignant disease** will develop in approximately 20% of patients with molar pregnancy. Persistent or malignant GTN is responsive to chemotherapy.

Key clinical features of GTN include (1) clinical presentation as pregnancy; (2) reliable means of diagnosis by pathognomonic ultrasound findings; and (3) a specific tumor marker, **human chorionic gonadotropin** (**hCG**). Persistent GTN may occur with any pregnancy, although it most commonly follows molar pregnancy.

EPIDEMIOLOGY

The incidence of molar pregnancy varies among different national and ethnic groups. The incidence in the United States is approximately 1 in 1,500 pregnancies. The risk of GTN is increased in women over age 35 years and under age 20 years, although the incidence is higher in women in between these age ranges because pregnancy is more common at these ages. Complete moles are associated with low dietary carotene consumption and vitamin A deficiency. Both complete and partial moles are associated with a history of infertility and spontaneous abortion.

HYDATIDIFORM MOLE

A hydatidiform mole includes abnormal proliferation of the syncytiotrophoblast and replacement of normal placental trophoblastic tissue by **hydropic placental villi**. **Complete moles** do not have identifiable embryonic or fetal structures. **Partial moles** are characterized by focal trophoblastic proliferation, degeneration of the placenta, and identifiable fetal or embryonic structures.

The genetic constitutions of the two types of molar pregnancy are different (Table 45.1). Complete moles have chromosomes entirely of paternal origin as the result of the fertilization of a blighted ovum by a haploid sperm that reduplicates or, rarely, fertilization of a blighted ovum with two sperm. The karyotype of a complete mole is usually 46XX. The fetus of a partial mole is usually a triploid. This consists of one haploid set of maternal chromosomes and two haploid sets of paternal chromosomes, the consequence of dispermic fertilization of a normal ovum. Complete moles are more common than partial moles and are more likely to undergo malignant transformation.

Clinical Presentation

Patients with molar pregnancy have findings consistent with a confirmed pregnancy as well as uterine size and date discrepancy, exaggerated subjective symptoms of pregnancy, and painless second-trimester bleeding. With the increased early prevalence of first-trimester ultrasound, moles are now frequently diagnosed in the first trimester of pregnancy before symptoms are present. Abnormal bleeding is the most characteristic presenting symptom which prompts evaluation for threatened abortion. Lack of fetal heart tones detected at the first

TABLE 45.1 FEATURES OF PARTIAL AND COMPLETE HYDATIDIFORM MOLES

Feature	Partial Mole	Complete Mole
Karyotype	69XXX or 69XXY	45XX or 46XY
Pathology		
Fetus	Often present	Absent
Amnion, fetal red blood cells	Usually present	Absent
Villous edema	Variable, focal	Diffuse
Trophoblastic proliferation	Focal, slight to moderate	Diffuse, slight to severe
Clinical presentation		
Diagnosis	Missed abortion	Molar gestation
Uterine size	Small or appropriate for gestational age	50% larger for gestational age
Theca lutein cysts	Rare	>25% depending on diagnostic modality
Medical complications	Rare	Becoming rare with early diagnosis
Postmolar invasion and malignancy	5%	15% and 4%, respectively

From *ACOG Practice Bulletin #53*. Washington, DC: American College of Obstetricians and Gynecologists; June 2004 (reaffirmed 2016).

obstetric appointment can also prompt evaluation (depending on the estimated gestational age). Ultrasound imaging confirms the diagnosis of molar pregnancy by its characteristic "**snowstorm**" appearance and absence of fetal parts (complete mole) as shown in Figure 45.1. In cases of partial mole, ultrasonography reveals an abnormally formed fetus (Fig. 45.2). Quantitative hCG levels are excessively elevated for gestational age, and the uterus is usually larger than expected.

Molar pregnancies may present with other signs and symptoms, including severe nausea and vomiting; marked gestational hypertension; proteinuria; and, rarely, clinical hyperthyroidism. Most of these findings can be attributed to the high levels of hCG produced by the abnormal pregnancy. Rarely, patients experience tachycardia and shortness of breath, arising from intense hemodynamic changes associated with acute hypertensive crisis. In these patients, physical examination reveals not only the date and size discrepancy of the uterine fundus and absent fetal heart tones but also changes associated with developing severe hypertension such as hyperreflexia. Bimanual pelvic examination may reveal large adnexal masses (**theca lutein cysts**; see Chapter 50), which represent marked enlargement of the ovaries secondary to hCG stimulation.

With earlier diagnosis, the medical complications of molar pregnancy are becoming less common. In any woman who presents with findings suggestive of severe hypertension prior to 20 weeks in pregnancy, a molar pregnancy should be immediately suspected.

Twin pregnancies with a normal fetus coexisting with a complete or partial mole are exceedingly rare. Women with these pregnancies should be treated in a tertiary hospital center with specialized care. Medical complications in molar twin gestations rarely allow these pregnancies to reach term. These pregnancies also have a higher risk of persistent metastatic or nonmetastatic GTN.

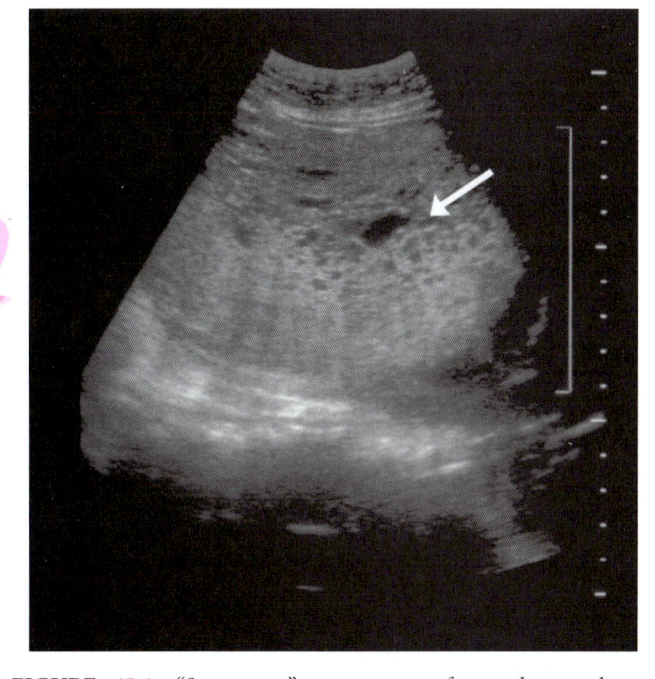

FIGURE 45.1. "Snowstorm" appearance of complete mole on ultrasound examination. The arrow points to intrauterine tissue. (From Soper JT. Gestational trophoblastic disease. *Obstet Gynecol.* 2006;108(1):178.)

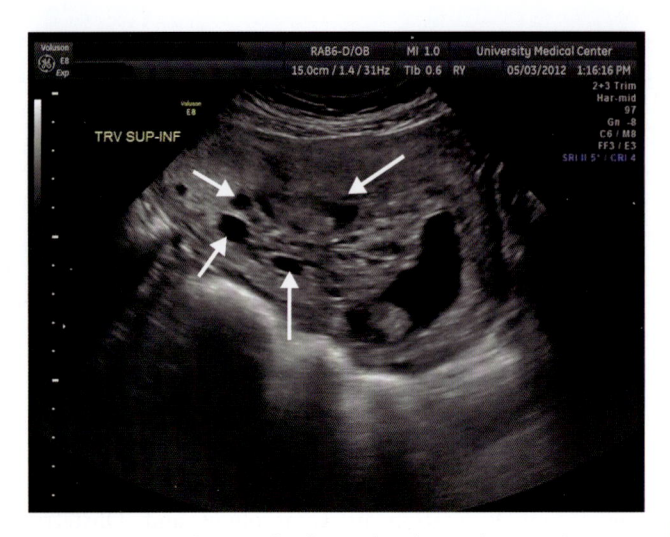

FIGURE 45.2. Hydropic villi of partial mole on ultrasound examination. *Arrows point* to variable and focal villous edema. (Courtesy of Eric Blackwell, M.D.)

BOX 45.1 Classification of Gestational Trophoblastic Neoplasia

Hydatidiform mole (primary nonmalignant nonmetastatic disease)
- Complete mole
- Partial mole

Malignant GTN
- Persistent nonmetastatic GTN
- Metastatic GTN
  - Good-prognosis metastatic disease
  - Poor-prognosis metastatic disease

Placental site tumors (malignant, usually nonmetastatic)

BOX 45.2 Preoperative Evaluation of Molar Pregnancy

1. Baseline quantitative hCG level
2. Baseline chest X-ray to check for metastatic disease
3. Complete blood count
4. Blood type with type and screen
5. Clotting function studies
6. Other appropriate tests if clinical evidence of hyperthyroidism and/or gestational hypertension

---

Whereas both partial and complete molar pregnancies present as abnormal pregnancies, partial mole most often presents as a missed abortion. Vaginal bleeding is less common in partial molar pregnancy than in complete molar pregnancy. Uterine growth is less than expected for the gestational age in partial molar pregnancy. Ultrasound reveals molar degeneration of the placenta and a grossly abnormal fetus or embryo. Medical complications, theca lutein cysts, and subsequent malignancies are rare (see Table 45.1).

Treatment

In most cases of molar pregnancy, the definitive treatment is prompt evacuation of the uterine contents. Uterine evacuation is done most often by dilation of the cervix and suction curettage followed by gentle sharp curettage. Because the evacuation of larger moles is sometimes associated with uterine atony and excessive blood loss, appropriate preparations should be made for uterotonic administration and blood transfusion, if needed. In rare cases of a late presenting partial molar pregnancy, there may be an additional need for larger grasping instruments to remove the abnormal fetus. In general, the larger the uterus, the greater the risk of pulmonary complications associated with trophoblastic emboli, fluid overload, and anemia.

This is particularly true in patients with associated severe gestational hypertension, who may experience concomitant hemoconcentration and alteration in vascular hemodynamics (see the section on preeclampsia in Chapter 22). Hysterectomy or induction of labor with prostaglandins is not usually recommended, because of the increased risk of blood loss and other sequelae. The bilaterally enlarged multicystic ovaries (theca lutein cysts) resulting from follicular stimulation by high levels of circulating hCG do not represent malignant changes. The theca lutein cysts invariably regress within a few months of evacuation and, therefore, do not require surgical removal.

Patients who have no interest in further childbearing or have other indications for hysterectomy may be treated by hysterectomy with ovarian preservation. Despite removal of the entire primary neoplasm, the risk of persistent GTN is 3% to 5%.

Postevacuation Management

Because of the predisposition for recurrence, patients should be monitored closely for 6 to 12 months after the evacuation of a molar pregnancy. Rh-negative patients should be given Rh immunoglobulin. Follow-up consists of periodic physical examination to check for vaginal metastasis and appropriate involution of pelvic structures. Quantitative hCG levels should be checked within 48 hours following evacuation, every 1 to 2 weeks while elevated, and at 1 to 2 months thereafter. Quantitative hCG levels that rise or reach a plateau are an indication of persistent disease and the need for further treatment after a new pregnancy has been ruled out. During the first year, the patient should be provided with a reliable contraceptive method to prevent an intercurrent pregnancy. Multiple studies have proven the safety of oral contraceptive use after a molar pregnancy. The benefits certainly outweigh any risks. The risk of recurrence after 1 year of remission is 1%. The risk of recurrence with subsequent pregnancies is 1% to 2%. There is no increase in congenital anomalies or complications in future pregnancies.

MALIGNANT GESTATIONAL TROPHOBLASTIC NEOPLASIA

Postmolar or **persistent GTN** is often diagnosed when hCG levels do not fall appropriately after a molar pregnancy but can also occur after a normal pregnancy. This disease can be localized or widespread (metastatic). An **invasive mole**, a localized form, is histologically identical to a complete mole. It invades the myometrium without any intervening endometrial stroma seen on histologic sample. Occasionally, it may be diagnosed on curettage at the time of initial molar evacuation.

Although invasive moles are histologically identical to antecedent molar pregnancies while invading the myometrium, **choriocarcinomas** are a malignant transformation of trophoblastic tissue. Instead of hydropic chorionic villi, the tumor has a red, granular appearance on cut section and consists of intermingled syncytiotrophoblastic and cytotrophoblastic elements with many abnormal cellular forms. Clinically, choriocarcinomas are characterized by rapid myometrial and uterine vessel invasion and systemic metastases resulting from hematogenous embolization. Lung, vagina, central nervous system, kidney, and liver are common metastatic locations. Choriocarcinoma may follow a molar pregnancy, normal-term pregnancy, abortion, or ectopic pregnancy. In the United States, choriocarcinoma is associated with approximately 1 in 20,000–40,000 pregnancies, approximately half of those after term pregnancies.

Treatment

Early identification and treatment are important. Abnormal bleeding for more than 6 weeks after any pregnancy should be evaluated with hCG testing to exclude a new pregnancy or GTN. Failure of quantitative hCG levels to regress after treatment of a molar pregnancy suggests that further treatment is needed. Identified metastatic sites should not be biopsied to avoid bleeding complications. Most GTN, including malignant forms, are highly sensitive to chemotherapy, which often results in a cure, allowing for future reproduction.

Nonmetastatic persistent GTN is completely treated by single-agent chemotherapy. Single-agent chemotherapy is either **methotrexate** or **actinomycin D**. The prognosis for metastatic GTN is more complex, divided into *good* and *poor* prognostic categories (Table 45.2). The World Health Organization has developed a prognostic scoring system for GTN that includes a number of epidemiologic and laboratory findings; this system was later combined into the International Federation of Gynecology and Obstetrics (FIGO) staging system (Table 45.3). A FIGO score of 7 or above classifies metastatic GTN as high risk, requiring multiagent chemotherapy.

The combination chemotherapeutic regimen with the highest success rate is called **EMACO**, which stands for **e**toposide, **m**ethotrexate, **a**ctinomycin D, **c**yclophosphamide, and vincristine (**O**ncovin). Adjunctive radiotherapy is sometimes performed with patients who have brain or liver metastasis. Surgery may be necessary to control hemorrhage, remove chemotherapy-resistant disease, and treat other complications to stabilize high-risk patients during intensive chemotherapy. The 5-year survival rate for nonmetastatic and good-prognosis disease approaches 100%. The 5-year survival rate for poor-prognosis metastatic disease is 80%.

TABLE 45.2 CLINICAL CLASSIFICATION SYSTEM FOR MALIGNANT GESTATIONAL TROPHOBLASTIC DISEASE

Category	Criteria
Nonmetastatic gestational trophoblastic disease	No evidence of metastases; not assigned to prognostic category
Metastatic gestational trophoblastic disease	Any extrauterine metastasis
Good prognosis	No risk factors: 1. Short interval from antecedent pregnancy <4 months 2. Pretherapy human chorionic gonadotropin (hCG) level < 40,000 mIU/mL 3. No brain or liver metastases 4. No antecedent term pregnancy 5. No prior chemotherapy
Poor prognosis	Any risk factor: 1. ≥4 months since last pregnancy 2. Pretherapy hCG level 40,000 mIU/mL 3. Brain or liver metastases 4. Antecedent term pregnancy 5. Prior chemotherapy

From the American College of Obstetricians and Gynecologists. Diagnosis and treatment of gestational trophoblastic disease. *ACOG Practice Bulletin No. 53.* Washington, DC: American College of Obstetricians and Gynecologists; 2004;103:1365–1377. Used with permission.

TABLE 45.3 REVISED (2010) FIGO SCORING SYSTEM FOR GESTATIONAL TROPHOBLASTIC NEOPLASIA

Finding	FIGO Score[a]			
	0	1	2	4
Age (years)	<40	≥40		
Antecedent pregnancy	Hydatidiform mole	Abortion	Term pregnancy	
Interval from last pregnancy (months)	<4	4–6	7–12	>12
Pretreatment hCG level	1,000	1,000–10,000	>10,000–100,000	>100,000
Largest tumor size including uterus (cm)	3	3–4	≥5	
Site of metastases	Lung	Spleen, kidney	Gastrointestinal tract	Brain, liver
Number of metastases	0	1–4	5–8	>8
Previous failed chemotherapy			Single drug	Two or more drugs

FIGO, International Federation of Gynecology and Obstetrics; hCG, human chorionic gonadotropin.
[a] The total score for a patient is obtained by adding the individual scores for each prognostic factor. Total score: 0–6, low risk; ≥7, high risk.
International Federation of Gynecology and Obstetrics. Modified WHO Prognostic Scoring System as Adapted by FIGO. Accessed at http://www.cancer.gov/cancertopics/pdq/treatment/gestationaltrophoblastic/HealthProfessional/page3, August 8, 2016.

Placental Site Tumors

Placental site tumor is a rare form of trophoblastic disease. The tumor is composed of monomorphic populations of intermediate cytotrophoblastic cells that are locally invasive at the site of placental implantation. The tumor only secretes small amounts of hCG and can be better followed by human placental lactogen levels. Another rare variant of placental site tumor is epithelioid trophoblastic tumor. It often presents in advanced stages.

CLINICAL FOLLOW-UP

You diagnose her with a complete mole and plan a dilation and curettage. You have uterotonics on hand. She recovers well from this procedure and sees you regularly for quantitative beta human chorionic gonadotropin levels for a full 12 months. One year later, you clear her, and she conceives again in 18 months. She is carefully monitored throughout the pregnancy and ultimately delivers a healthy baby at term.

CHAPTER 46
Vulvar and Vaginal Disease and Neoplasia

This chapter deals primarily with APGO Educational Topic Area:

TOPIC 51 VULVAR NEOPLASMS

Students should be able to identify the risk factors for vulvar neoplasms and list indications for vulvar biopsy.

CLINICAL CASE

A 51-year-old patient comes to see you secondary to vulvar itching. She reports that it has been going on for about 5 months and she has tried over-the-counter vaginal preparations for yeast, but these have not helped. She even went to an urgent care clinic and obtained a prescription for metronidazole for bacterial vaginosis, but that too did not help. On examination, you notice some erythema with a keyhole lesion on the perineal body.

INTRODUCTION

Evaluation of vulvar symptoms and examination of patients for vulvar disease and neoplasia constitute a significant part of health care for women. The major symptoms of vulvar disease are pruritus, burning, nonspecific irritation, and/or appreciation of a mass. The vulvar region is particularly sensitive to irritants, more so than other regions of the body. It has been suggested that the layer overlying the vulva—the stratum corneum—may be less of a barrier to irritants, thereby making the vulva more susceptible to irritations and contributing to the "itch–scratch" cycle. Noninflammatory vulvar pathology is found in women of all ages but is especially significant in perimenopausal and postmenopausal women because of concern regarding the possibility of vulvar neoplasia.

Diagnostic aids for the assessment of noninflammatory conditions are relatively limited in number and include careful history, inspection, and biopsy. Because vulvar lesions are often difficult to diagnose, use of vulvar biopsy is central to good care. **Punch biopsies** of vulvar abnormalities are most helpful to determine if cancer is present or to histologically determine the specific cause of a perceived abnormality of the vulva. Cytologic evaluation of the vulva is of limited value, insofar as the vulvar skin is keratinized and epithelium shedding does not occur as readily as that of the cervix. **Colposcopy** is useful for evaluating known vulvar atypia and intraepithelial neoplasia. However, colposcopic evaluation of the vulva for human papillomavirus (HPV) with acetic acid can be limited by the degree of keratinization.

This chapter provides discussions of a range of vulvar pathologic conditions, including non-neoplastic dermatoses, localized vulvodynia (formerly known as *vestibulitis*), benign vulvar mass lesions, vulvar intraepithelial neoplasia (VIN), and vulvar cancer. Benign vaginal masses and vaginal neoplasia are also discussed. Inflammatory conditions of the vulva are discussed in Chapter 28.

BENIGN VULVAR DISEASE

In the past, the classification of benign, noninfectious vulvar disease used descriptive terminology based on gross clinical morphologic appearance such as *leukoplakia*, *kraurosis vulvae*, and *hyperplastic vulvitis*. Currently, these diseases are classified into three categories: *squamous cell hyperplasia*, *lichen sclerosus*, and *other dermatoses*.

In 2006, the International Society for the Study of Vulvar Disease (ISSVD) constructed a new classification using **histologic morphology** based on consensus among gynecologists, dermatologists, and pathologists involved in the care of women with vulvar disease. Common ISSVD classifications are outlined in Table 46.1. In 2011, the ISSVD developed guidelines for clinical terminology and diagnosis.

Lichen Sclerosus

Lichen sclerosus has confused clinicians and pathologists because of inconsistent terminology and its frequent association with other types of vulvar pathology, including those of the acanthotic variety. As with the other disorders, chronic vulvar pruritus occurs in most patients. Typically, the vulva is diffusely involved, with very thin, whitish epithelial areas, termed "onion skin" epithelium (Fig. 46.1A).

TABLE 46.1 2006 INTERNATIONAL SOCIETY FOR THE STUDY OF VULVAR DISEASE CLASSIFICATION OF VULVAR DERMATOSES: MOST COMMON PATHOLOGIC SUBSETS AND THEIR CLINICAL CORRELATES

Histologic Pattern	Characteristic	Clinical Correlate
Lichenoid	Band-like lymphocytic infiltration of the upper dermis and epidermal basal layer damage	Lichen sclerosus Lichen planus
Dermal homogenization/sclerosis	Partial or complete obliteration of collagen bundle boundaries with "hyalinized/glassy" dermis	Lichen sclerosus
Acanthotic (formerly squamous cell hyperplasia)	Hyperkeratosis—increased number of epithelial cells leading to epidermal thickening or hyperplasia	Lichen simplex chronicus Primary (idiopathic) Secondary (superimposed on lichen sclerosis/planus) Psoriasis
Spongiotic	Intercellular edema within the epidermis with widening of the intercellular space	Irritant dermatitis Atopic dermatitis Allergic contact dermatitis

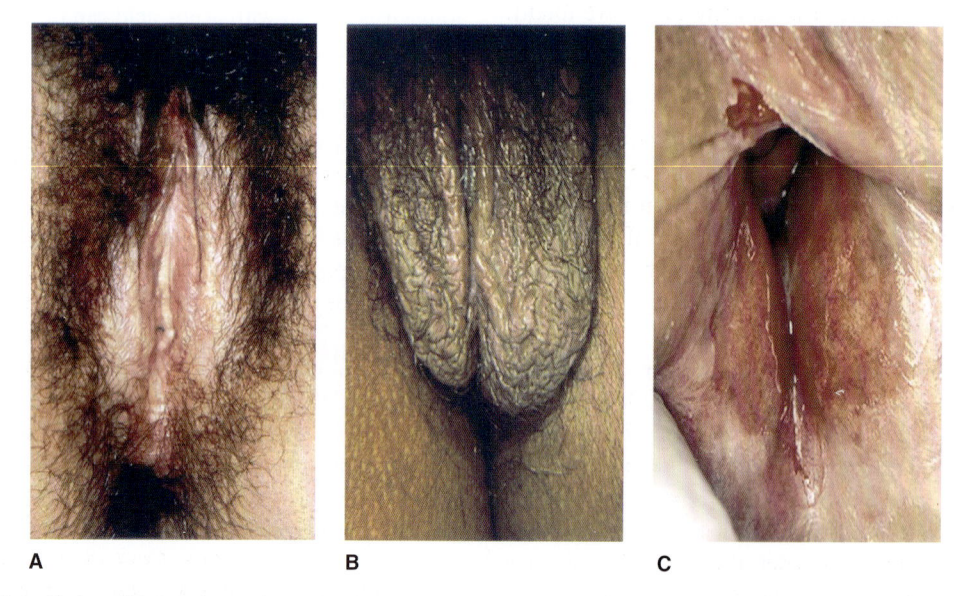

FIGURE 46.1. The three "lichens." (A) Lichen sclerosus. (B) Lichen simplex chronicus. (C) Lichen planus. (Used with permission from Foster DC. Vulvar disease. *Obstet Gynecol.* 2002;100(1):149.)

The epithelium has been termed "cigarette paper" skin and described as "parchment-like." Most patients have involvement on both sides of the vulva, with the most common sites being the labia majora, labia minora, the clitoral and periclitoral epithelium, and the perineal body. The lesion may extend to include a perianal "halo" of atrophic, whitish epithelium, forming a figure-8 or keyhole configuration with the vulvar changes. In severe cases, many normal anatomic landmarks are lost, including obliteration of the labial and periclitoral architecture, sometimes resulting in fusion of the normal labial and periclitoral folds, as well as severe stenosis of the vaginal introitus. Some patients have areas of cracked skin, which are prone to bleeding with minimal trauma. Patients with these severe anatomic changes complain of difficulty in having normal coital function.

The etiology of lichen sclerosus is unknown, but a familial association has been noted, as well as associations with disorders of the immune system, including thyroid disorders and class II human leukocyte antigens. However, the response to topical steroids further indicates the underlying inflammatory process and the role of prostaglandins and leukotrienes in the hallmark symptom of pruritus. Histologic evaluation for confirmation of lichen sclerosis is often necessary and useful because it allows specific therapy. The histologic features of the lichenoid pattern include a band of chronic inflammatory cells, consisting mostly of lymphocytes, in the upper dermis with a zone of homogeneous, pink-staining, collagenous-like material beneath the epidermis due to cell death. The rete pegs, normally projectile in appearance, are flattened. The obliteration of boundaries between collagen bundles gives the dermis a "hyalinized" or "glassy" appearance. This dermal homogenization/sclerosis pattern is virtually pathognomonic.

In 27% to 35% of patients, there are associated areas of acanthosis characterized by **hyperkeratosis**—an increase in the number of epithelial cells (keratinocytes) with flattening of the rete pegs. These areas may be mixed throughout or adjacent to the typically lichenoid areas. In patients with this mixed pattern, both components need to be treated to effect resolution of symptoms. Patients in whom a large acanthotic component has been histologically confirmed should be treated initially with well-penetrating corticosteroid creams. With improvement of these areas (usually 2–3 weeks), therapy can then be directed to the lichenoid component.

Treatment for lichen sclerosis includes the use of topical high-dose steroid (clobetasol) preparations in an effort to ameliorate symptoms. The lesion is unlikely to resolve totally. Intermittent treatment or maintenance therapy may be needed indefinitely.

Lichen sclerosus is associated with an increased risk of developing squamous cell cancer (SCC) of the vulva. It has been estimated that this risk is in the 4% range. Due to the frequent coexistence with acanthosis, the condition needs to be followed carefully and repeat biopsy performed if lesions are therapeutically resistant because acanthosis can be a harbinger of SCC.

Lichen Simplex Chronicus

In contrast to many dermatologic conditions that may be described as "rashes that itch," **lichen simplex chronicus** can be described as *"an itch that rashes."* Most patients develop this disorder secondary to an irritant dermatitis, which progresses to lichen simplex chronicus as a result of the effects of chronic mechanical irritation from scratching and rubbing an already irritated area. The mechanical irritation contributes to epidermal thickening or hyperplasia and inflammatory cell infiltrate, which, in turn, leads to heightened sensitivity that triggers more mechanical irritation.

Accordingly, the history of these patients is one of progressive vulvar pruritus and/or burning, which is temporarily relieved by scratching or rubbing with a washcloth or some similar material. Etiologic factors for the original pruritic symptoms are often unknown, but may include sources of skin irritation from the environment (laundry detergents, fabric softeners, scented hygienic preparations applied topically, perspiration, bubble bath, scented pads and panty liners) or other preexisting skin conditions. These potential sources of symptoms must be investigated. Any domestic or hygienic irritants must be removed, in combination with treatment, to break the cycle described.

On clinical inspection, the skin of the labia majora, labia minora, and perineal body often shows diffusely reddened areas with occasional hyperplastic or hyperpigmented plaques of red to reddish brown (see Fig. 46.1B). Occasionally, areas of linear hyperplasia are also seen, which show the effect of grossly hyperkeratotic ridges of epidermis. Biopsy of patients who have these characteristic findings is usually not warranted.

Empiric treatment to include antipruritic medications such as diphenhydramine hydrochloride (Benadryl) or hydroxyzine hydrochloride (Atarax) that inhibit nighttime, unconscious scratching, combined with a mild to moderate topical steroid cream applied to the vulva, usually provides relief. A steroid cream, such as hydrocortisone (1–2%), or for patients with significant areas of obvious hyperkeratosis, a moderate strength steroid cream such as triamcinolone acetonide or betamethasone valerate may be used. If significant relief is not obtained within 3 months, diagnostic vulvar biopsy is warranted.

The prognosis for this disorder is excellent when the offending irritating agents are removed and a topical steroid preparation is used appropriately. In most patients, these measures cure the problem and eliminate future recurrences.

Lichen Planus

Lichen planus is a rare inflammatory skin condition that can be generalized or isolated to the vulva and vagina. In the latter situation, it usually presents as a desquamative lesion of the vagina; occasionally, patients develop lesions on the vulva near the inner aspects of the labia minora and vulvar vestibule. Patients may have areas of whitish, lacy bands (Wickham striae) of keratosis near the reddish ulcerated-like lesions characteristic of the disease (see Fig. 46.1C). Typically, complaints include chronic vulvar burning and/or pruritus, insertional dyspareunia, and a profuse vaginal discharge.

Because of the patchiness of this lesion and the concern raised by atypical appearance of the lesions, biopsy may be warranted to confirm the diagnosis in some patients. In lichen planus, the biopsy shows no atypia. Examination of the vaginal discharge in these patients frequently reveals large numbers of acute inflammatory cells without significant numbers of bacteria. Histologically, the epithelium is thinned, and there is a loss of the rete ridges with a lymphocytic infiltrate just beneath, associated with basal cell liquefaction necrosis.

Treatment for lichen planus includes lifestyle modification to optimize treatment response to topical steroid preparations similar to those used for lichen simplex chronicus. Additional treatment options include systemic steroids, tacrolimus, methotrexate, and other medications. Patients should be counseled that lichen planus is a chronic condition and goals of treatment are realistically control of symptoms and not cure.

Psoriasis

Psoriasis can involve vulvar skin as part of a generalized dermatologic process. It is a dermatologic disorder with a multifactorial pattern of inheritance. With approximately 2% of the general population suffering from psoriasis, the physician should be alert to its prevalence and the likelihood of vulvar manifestation, because it may appear during menarche, pregnancy, and menopause.

The lesions are typically slightly raised round or ovoid patches with a silver scale appearance atop an erythematous base. Vulvar lesions most often measure approximately 1 × 1 to 1 × 2 cm. Though pruritus is usually minimal, these silvery lesions will reveal punctate bleeding areas if removed (Auspitz sign). The diagnosis is generally known because of psoriasis found elsewhere on the body, obviating the need for vulvar biopsy to confirm the diagnosis. Histologically, a prominent **acanthotic pattern** is seen, with distinct dermal papillae that are clubbed and chronic inflammatory cells between them.

Treatment often occurs in conjunction with consultation by a dermatologist. Like lesions elsewhere, vulvar lesions usually respond to topical coal tar preparations, followed by exposure to ultraviolet light as well as corticosteroid medications, either topically or by intralesional injection. However, coal tar preparations are extremely irritating to the vagina and labial mucous membranes and should not be used in these areas. With very severe disease, systemic therapy may need to be implemented. Emollients to keep the skin moist help reduce itching. Other therapies include topical vitamin D analogues, retinoids, and calcineurin inhibitors. Because vulvar application of some of the photoactivated preparations can be somewhat awkward, topical steroids are most effective, using compounds such as betamethasone valerate 0.1%.

Dermatitis

Vulvar dermatitis falls into two main categories: **eczema** and **seborrheic dermatitis**. Eczema can be further subdivided into **exogenous** and **endogenous forms**. **Irritant** and **allergic contact dermatitis** are forms of exogenous eczema. They are usually reactions to potential irritants or allergens found in soaps, laundry detergents, textiles, and feminine hygiene products. Careful history can be helpful in identifying the offending agent and in preventing recurrences. **Atopic dermatitis** is a form of endogenous eczema that often affects multiple sites, including the flexural surfaces of the elbows and knees, retroauricular area, and scalp. The lesions associated with these three forms of dermatitis can appear similarly as symmetric eczematous lesions, with underlying erythema. Histology alone will not distinguish these three types of dermatitis. They all exhibit a **spongiotic pattern** characterized by intercellular edema within the epidermis, causing widening of the space between the cells. Therefore, these entities must often be distinguished clinically.

Although **seborrheic dermatitis** is a common problem, isolated vulvar seborrheic dermatitis is rare. It involves a chronic inflammation of the sebaceous glands, but the exact cause is unknown. The diagnosis is usually made in patients complaining of vulvar pruritus who are known to have seborrheic dermatitis in the scalp or other hair-bearing areas of the body. The lesion may mimic other entities, such as psoriasis or lichen simplex chronicus. The lesions are pale red to a yellowish pink and may be covered by an oily-appearing, scaly crust. Because this area of the body remains continually moist, occasional exudative lesions include raw "weeping" patches, caused by skin maceration, which are exacerbated by the patient's scratching. As with psoriasis, vulvar biopsy is usually not needed when the diagnosis is made in conjunction with known seborrheic dermatitis in other hair-bearing areas. The histologic features of seborrheic dermatitis are a combination of those seen in the acanthotic and spongiotic patterns.

Treatment for vulvar dermatitis involves removing the offending agent and careful perineal hygiene including wearing nonocclusive clothing, gentle water-based cleansers, gentle drying after cleaning and toileting, and use of emollients to keep moisture in and irritants out. Topical corticosteroid lotions or creams containing a mixture of an agent that penetrates well, such as betamethasone valerate, in conjunction with crotamiton, can be used for symptom control. As with lichen simplex chronicus, the use of antipruritic agents as a bedtime dose in the first 10 days to 2 weeks of treatment frequently helps break the sleep–scratch cycle and allows the lesions to heal. Table 46.2 summarizes the clinical characteristics of the common vulvar dermatoses.

Localized Vulvodynia

Localized vulvodynia is a condition of unknown etiology. It involves the acute and chronic inflammation of the vestibular glands, which lie just inside the vaginal introitus near the hymenal ring. The involved glands may be circumferential to include areas near the urethra, but this condition most commonly involves posterolateral vestibular glands between the 4 and 8 o'clock positions (Fig. 46.2). The diagnosis should be suspected in all patients who present with new-onset insertional dyspareunia. Patients with this condition frequently complain of progressive insertional dyspareunia to the point where they are unable to have intercourse. The history may go on for a few weeks but most typically involves progressive worsening over the course of 3 or 4 months. Patients also complain of pain on tampon insertion; on sitting; and, at times, during washing or bathing the perineal area. Sexual history should be carefully reviewed.

Physical examination is helpful to making the diagnosis. Because the vestibular glands lie between the folds of the hymenal ring and the medial aspect of the vulvar vestibule, diagnosis is frequently missed when inspection of the perineum does not include these areas. After carefully inspecting the proper anatomic area by applying gentle traction to the vestibule, a light touch with a moistened cotton applicator recreates the pain exactly and allows for quantification of the pain. In addition, the regions affected are most often evident as small, reddened, patchy areas. Using a speculum is not recommended during this examination because it causes too much patient discomfort.

Because the etiology of localized vulvodynia is unknown, treatments vary and range from changing or eliminating environmental factors, temporary sexual abstinence, and application

TABLE 46.2 CLINICAL CHARACTERISTICS OF THE COMMON VULVAR DERMATOSES

Disorder	Lesion	Hallmarks
Lichen sclerosis	Atrophic, thin, whitish epithelium with frequent perianal halo or "keyhole" distribution	"Cigarette paper," parchment-like skin, halo or loss of elasticity
Lichen planus	White lacy network (Wickham striae) with flat-topped lilac papules and plaques	Erosive vaginitis with demarcated edges
Lichen simplex chronicus	Lichenified, hyperplastic plaques of red to reddish brown	Symmetric with variable pigmentation
Psoriasis	Annular pink plaques with silvery scale that bleed if removed (Auspitz sign)	Elbows, knees, scalp also often affected
Dermatitis irritant, allergic, or atopic	Eczematous lesions with underlying erythema	Symmetric with extension into areas of irritant or allergen contact
Seborrheic	Pale red to yellowish pink plaques, often oily appearing, scaly crust	Other hair-bearing areas often affected—scalp and chest; also back and face

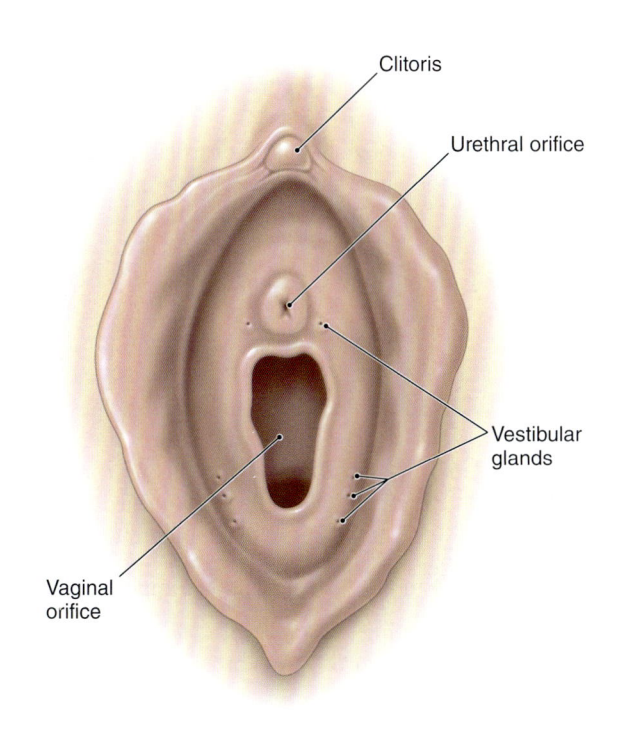

FIGURE 46.2. Vestibular glands.

of cortisone ointments and topical lidocaine (jelly) to more radical treatments such as surgical excision of the vestibular glands. A combination of treatment modalities may be necessary. Treatment must be individualized, based on the severity of patient symptoms and the disability.

Some patients may benefit from low-dose tricyclic medication (amitriptyline and desipramine) or fluoxetine to help break the cycle of pain. Other limited reports suggest the use of calcium citrate to change the urine composition by removing oxalic acid crystals or consumption of a low-oxalate diet. Those advocating changing the urine chemistry cite evidence to suggest that oxalic acid crystals are particularly irritating when precipitated in the urine of patients with high urinary oxalic acid composition. Other modalities include biofeedback, physical therapy with electrical stimulation, and intralesional injections with triamcinolone and bupivacaine. Pudendal nerve block and botulinum toxin may also help.

Vulvar Lesions

Sebaceous or **inclusion cysts** are caused by inflammatory blockage of the sebaceous gland ducts and are small, smooth, nodular masses, usually arising from the inner surfaces of the labia minora and majora, that contain cheesy, sebaceous material. They may be easily excised if their size or position is troublesome.

The round ligament inserts into the labium majus, carrying an investment of peritoneum. On occasion, peritoneal fluid may accumulate therein, causing a **cyst of the canal of Nuck**, or **hydrocele**. If such cysts reach symptomatic size, excision is usually required. **Fibromas (fibromyomas)** arise from the connective tissue and smooth muscle elements of vulva and vagina and are usually small and asymptomatic. Sarcomatous change is extremely uncommon, although edema and degenerative changes may make such lesions suspicious for malignancy. Treatment is surgical excision when the lesions are symptomatic or with concerns about malignancy. **Lipomas** appear much like fibromas, are rare, and are also treated by excision if symptomatic. **Hidradenitis suppurativa** is a chronic skin condition involving follicles in areas with a high density of sweat glands, including the groin, axillae, and perineal and inner thigh regions. The clinical presentation can range from a few indurated, occluded follicles to a more serious confluence, leading to scarring, draining, and fistula formation. Effective medical treatments include antibiotics, anti-inflammatories, and even antiandrogens, particularly in women. More serious disease requires surgical management in the form of incision and drainage or even excision of the glands of the affected area. **Hidradenoma** is a rare lesion arising from the sweat glands of the vulva. It is almost always benign, is usually found on the inner surface of the labia majora, and is treated with excision. It is not related to hidradenitis suppurativa. **Nevi** are benign, usually asymptomatic, pigmented lesions whose importance is that they must be distinguished from malignant melanoma, 3% to 4% of which occur on the external genitalia in females. Biopsy of pigmented vulvar lesions may be warranted, depending on clinical suspicion.

VULVAR INTRAEPITHELIAL NEOPLASIA

Much like the vulvar dermatoses, the classification and terminology of **VIN** has undergone multiple revisions and reclassifications over the years. The currently accepted terminology is the Lower Anogenital Squamous Tract Terminology classification, which is espoused by the American College of Obstetricians and Gynecologists, the American Society for Colposcopy and Cervical Pathology (ASCCP), and the World Health Organization (WHO) (see Table 46.3).

Low-Grade Squamous Intraepithelial Lesion of the Vulva

Low-grade squamous intraepithelial lesion of the vulva (vulvar LSIL) is a low-grade lesion that demonstrates minimal to mild squamous atypia limited to the lower epidermis. Vulvar LSIL is either a non-neoplastic, reactive atypia or an effect of an HPV infection. Vulvar LSIL occurs most often in **condylomata acuminata**. Lesions that are condylomatous in origin do not have the features of attenuated maturation, pleomorphism, and atypical mitotic figures that are found in other forms of VIN.

The features of vulvar LSIL are uncommon histologic findings, and there is little evidence that vulvar LSIL is a cancer precursor. Previously this was classified as VIN I, but in 2004, the ISSVD abolished the term *VIN 1* from their classification system. The diagnosis of vulvar LSIL must be made by biopsy, and treatment is the same as for condyloma.

High-Grade Squamous Intraepithelial Lesion of the Vulva

High-grade squamous intraepithelial lesions of the vulva (vulvar HSIL) are high-grade, HPV-related lesions distinguished only by the degree of abnormality. They represent true neoplasia with a high predilection for progression to severe intraepithelial lesions and, eventually, carcinoma, if left untreated. Almost 60% of women with vulvar HSIL or vaginal intraepithelial neoplasia (VAIN) vaginal HSIL will also have cervical HSIL lesions. Furthermore, 10% of women with cervical HSIL will have either vulvar HSIL or vaginal HSIL.

Smoking or second-hand smoke is a common social history finding in patients with vulvar HSIL. Presenting complaints include vulvar pruritus, chronic irritation, and a development of raised mass lesions. Normally, the lesions are localized, fairly well-isolated, and raised above the normal epithelial surface to include a slightly rough texture. They are usually found along the posterior, hairless area of vulva and in the perineal body but can occur anywhere on the vulva. The color changes in these lesions range from white, hyperplastic areas to reddened or dusky, patch-like involvement, depending on whether associated hyperkeratosis is present. Figure 46.3 illustrates the variation in appearance of vulvar HSIL.

In patients without obvious raised or isolated lesions, careful inspection of the vulva is warranted, using a colposcope. Applying a 3% to 5% solution of acetic acid to the vulva using soaked gauze pads for 2 to 5 minutes often accentuates the white lesions and may also help in revealing abnormal vascular patterns. These areas must be selectively biopsied in multiple sites to thoroughly investigate the type of vulvar HSIL and reliably exclude invasive carcinoma. Vulvar HSIL, previously called VIN usual type, is subdivided into three histologic subtypes—warty, basaloid, and mixed—depending on the features present. They all have atypical mitotic figures and nuclear pleomorphism, with loss of normal differentiation in the lower one-third to one-half of the epithelial layer. Full thickness loss of maturation indicates lesions that are at least severely dysplastic, including areas that may represent true carcinoma in situ (CIS).

The goal in treating vulvar HSIL is to quickly and completely remove all involved areas of skin. These lesions can

TABLE 46.3 GRADING SYSTEMS FOR VULVAR INTRAEPITHELIAL LESIONS

2003 WHO	Clinical, "Bethesda-like"	2004 ISSVD	2015 ISSVD similar to LAST
VIN 1 (mild dysplasia)	Low-grade VIN	Term abolished	Low-grade SIL of the vulva (includes flat condyloma, HPV effect)
VIN 2 (moderate dysplasia)	High-grade VIN	VIN, usual type a. VIN, warty b. VIN, basaloid c. VIN, mixed	High-grade SIL of the vulva (includes VIN)
VIN 3 (severe dysplasia, CIS)			
VIN 3, simplex type (CIS)		VIN, differentiated type	VIN, differentiated type

CIS, carcinoma in situ; ISSVD, International Society for the Study of Vulvar Disease; WHO, World Health Organization; VIN, vulvar intraepithelial neoplasia; LAST, Lower Anogenital Squamous Tract Terminology.

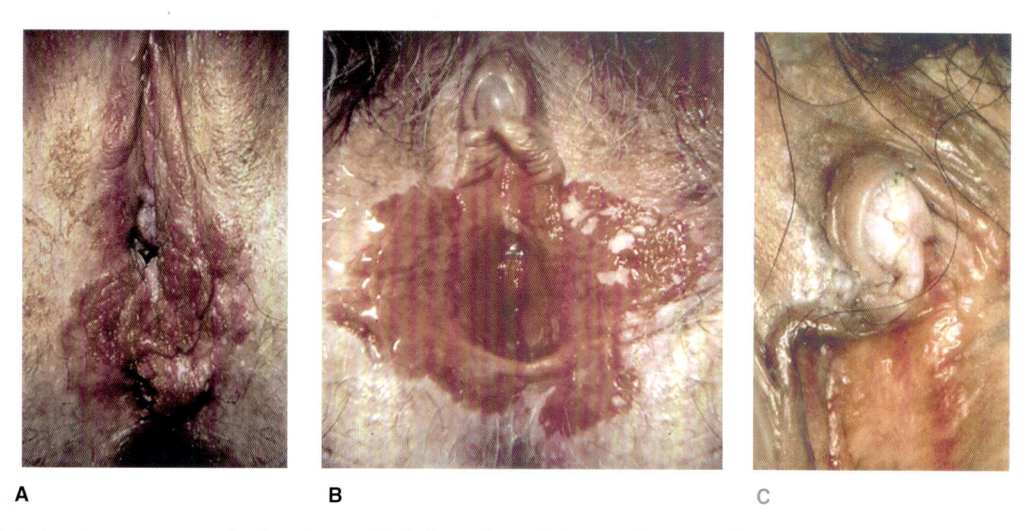

FIGURE 46.3. Variation in appearance of vulvar intraepithelial neoplasia. (A) Large, hypertrophic, pigmented lesion; (B) associated with erosive lichen planus; and (C) isolated to the clitoris. (Used with permission from Foster DC. Vulvar disease. *Obstet Gynecol.* 2002;100(1):157.)

be removed after appropriate biopsies confirm the absence of invasive cancer. Removal options include wide local excision or laser ablation. A variety of nonsurgical treatments for patients with vulvar HSIL have been reported, including phototherapy, corticosteroids, 5-fluorouracil (5-FU), and imidazoquinolones (particularly imiquimod). Results to date are mixed. 5-FU is poorly tolerated, although it has acceptable response rates; imidazoquinolones have been shown to be effective. Careful evaluation to exclude invasive disease is of paramount importance, insofar as VIN, usual type, is seen adjacent to 30% of SCCs of the vulva.

VIN, Differentiated Type

The less common simplex type of VIN (CIS) in the WHO system is now called **VIN, differentiated type** by the ISSVD (see Table 46.3). The lesion is either a hyperkeratotic plaque, warty papule, or an ulcer, seen primarily in older women. It is often associated with keratinizing SCCs or lichen sclerosus and is not HPV related. It is thought that VIN, differentiated type is underdiagnosed due to a relatively short intraepithelial phase before progression to invasive carcinoma. Clinical awareness of this entity and its features as different from vulvar HSIL would help improve diagnosis before cancer has supervened. Biopsy is mandatory, and the mainstay of treatment is excision.

PAGET DISEASE

Paget disease is characterized by extensive intraepithelial disease whose gross appearance is described as a fiery, red background mottled with whitish hyperkeratotic areas. The histology of these lesions is similar to that of the breast lesions, with large, pale cells of apocrine origin below the surface epithelium (Fig. 46.4). Although not common, Paget disease of the vulva may be associated with adenocarcinoma in or around the

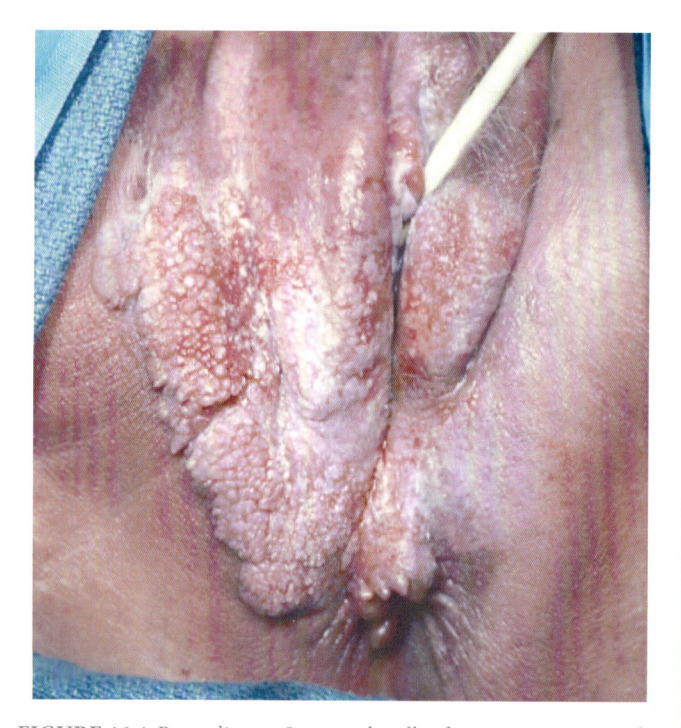

FIGURE 46.4. Paget disease. Large, pale cells of apocrine origin involving the surface epithelium. (Used with permission from Berek JS. *Berek and Novak's Gynecology.* 15th ed. Philadelphia: Lippincott Williams & Wilkins; 2011.)

lesion. As many as 20 to 30% of women with Paget disease have other associated but noncontiguous cancers, such as breast, gastrointestinal, genitourinary, and workup for these should be considered. Similarly, patients with Paget disease of the vulva have a higher incidence of underlying internal carcinoma, particularly of the colon and breast.

The treatment for vulvar Paget disease is wide local excision or simple vulvectomy, depending on the amount of involvement. Recurrences are more common with this disorder than with VIN, necessitating wider margins when local excision or vulvectomy is performed.

VULVAR CANCER

Vulvar carcinoma accounts for approximately 5% of all gynecologic malignancies. Approximately 90% of these carcinomas are SCCs. The second most common variety is melanoma, which accounts for 2% of all vulvar carcinomas, followed by sarcoma. Less common types include basal cell carcinoma and adenocarcinoma.

The typical clinical profile of vulvar carcinoma includes women in their postmenopausal years, most commonly between 70 and 80 years. However, about 20% of these cancers are discovered in women younger than 50 years. Vulvar pruritus is the most common presenting complaint. In addition, patients may notice a red or white ulcerative or exophytic lesion arising most commonly on the posterior two-thirds of either labium majus. An exophytic ulcerative lesion need not be present, further underscoring the need for thorough biopsy in patients of the age group who complain of vulvar symptoms. Patients in this older age group may be reluctant to consult their physicians about these signs and symptoms, which can result in a delay in treatment.

Although a specific cause for vulvar cancer is not known, progression has been shown from prior intraepithelial lesions, including those that are associated with certain types of HPV. Smokers have a high preponderance in this population of patients.

Natural History

SCC of the vulva generally remains localized for long periods of time and then spreads in a predictable fashion to the regional lymph nodes, including those of the inguinal and femoral chain. Lesions 2 cm wide and 0.5 cm deep have an increased chance of nodal metastases. The overall incidence of lymph node metastasis is approximately 30%. Lesions arising in the anterior one-third of the vulva may spread to the deep pelvic nodes, bypassing regional inguinal and femoral lymphatics.

Evaluation

The staging classification for vulvar cancer was revised by the Federation of Gynecology and Obstetrics in 2009 (Table 46.4). Prior to 1988, vulvar cancers were staged clinically. However, noted discrepancies in regard to predicting nodal metastasis led to a change from clinical to surgical staging. This staging convention uses the analysis of the removed vulvar tumor and microscopic assessment of the regional lymph nodes as its basis.

Treatment

Although the mainstay for the treatment of invasive vulvar cancer is surgical, many advances have been made to help individualize care in an effort to reduce the amount of radical surgery, without compromising survival. Accordingly, not all patients should undergo radical vulvectomy with bilateral nodal dissections. Other approaches include the following:

- Conservative vulvar operations for unifocal lesions
- Elimination of routine pelvic lymphadenectomy
- Avoidance of groin dissection in unilateral lesions less than 1 mm deep
- Elimination of contralateral groin dissection in unilateral lesions 1 cm from the midline with negative ipsilateral nodes
- Separate groin incisions for patients with indicated bilateral groin dissection
- Postoperative radiation therapy to decrease groin recurrence in patients with two or more positive groin nodes.

Concomitant use of radiation and chemotherapy (5-FU plus cisplatin or mitomycin or cisplatin alone) is gaining favor for the treatment of vulvar cancers that require radiation therapy.

TABLE 46.4 INTERNATIONAL FEDERATION OF GYNECOLOGY AND OBSTETRICS 2009 STAGING OF VULVAR CANCER

Stage	Definition
0	
I	Tumor confined to the vulva and/or perineum, 2 cm or less in greatest dimension; no nodal metastasis
IA	Stromal invasion no greater than 1.0 mm^a
IB	Stromal invasion greater than 1.0 mm^a
II	Tumor confined to adjacent areas (1/3 lower urethra, 1/3 lower vagina, anus); no nodal metastasis
III	Tumor of any size with regional (inguinal or femoral) node metastasis
IIIA	(i) One node metastasis 5 mm or greater (ii) One to two node metastasis(es) less than 5 mm
IIIB	(i) Two or more node metastases 5 mm or greater (ii) Three or more node metastases less than 5 mm
IIIC	Nodal involvement with extracapsular spread
IV	Tumor with regional (2/3 upper urethra, 2/3 upper vagina) or distant involvement
IVA	Tumor invades any of the following: 2/3 upper urethra, 2/3 upper vagina, bladder mucosa, and rectal mucosa, or is fixed to bone (i) No fixed or ulcerated regional (inguinal or femoral) lymph nodes (ii) Fixed or ulcerated regional (inguinal or femoral) lymph nodes
IVB	Any distant metastasis including pelvic lymph nodes

^{a}The depth of invasion is defined as the measurement of the tumor from the epithelial–stromal junction of the adjacent most superficial dermal papilla to the deepest point of invasion.

Treatment with chemotherapy in cases of recurrent vulvar cancer has only limited value.

Prognosis

The corrected 5-year survival rate for all vulvar carcinoma is approximately 70%. Five-year survival rates for SCC are 60% to 80% for stage I and II disease. Survival rates for patients with stage III disease are 45%, and those with stage IV have rates of 15%.

Other Types of Vulvar Cancer

Melanoma

Melanoma is the most common non-SCC of the vulva. Vulvar melanoma usually presents with a raised, irritated, pruritic, pigmented lesion. Most commonly, melanotic lesions are located on the labia minora or the clitoris. Melanoma accounts for approximately 6% of all vulvar malignancies, and, when suspected, wide local excision is necessary for diagnosis and staging. Survival approaches 100% when the lesions are confined to the intrapapillary ridges, decreasing rapidly as involvement includes the papillary dermis; reticular dermis; and, finally, subcutaneous tissues. In the latter instance, survival is generally 20% because of substantial incidence of nodal involvement. Because early diagnosis and treatment by wide excision are so crucial, it is important to recognize that irritated, pigmented, vulvar lesions mandate the excisional biopsy for definitive treatment.

Carcinoma of the Bartholin Gland

Carcinoma of the Bartholin gland is uncommon (1%–2% of all vulvar carcinomas). Malignancies that arise from the Bartholin gland include adenocarcinomas, SCCs, adenosquamous carcinomas, and adenoid cystic and transitional cell carcinomas. These arise mainly as a result of changes occurring within the different histologic areas of the gland and ducts leading from it. Bartholin carcinoma on average occurs in women over age 60 years; however, any new solid Bartholin mass in a woman over age 40 years should be excised. Treatment of diagnosed Bartholin cancers is radical vulvectomy and bilateral lymphadenectomy. Recurrence is disappointingly common, and a 5-year overall survival rate of 85% is noted.

VAGINAL DISEASE

Vaginal disease can be classified into three broad categories: *benign*, *precancerous*, and *cancerous*. There are important differences in the management and prognosis of these conditions. Vaginal neoplasias are rare and usually occur secondary to cervical or vulvar cancers that have spread to the vagina from the primary site.

Benign Vaginal Masses

Gartner duct cysts arise from vestigial remnants of the Wolffian or mesonephric system that course along the outer anterior aspect of the vaginal canal. These cystic structures are usually small and asymptomatic, but, on occasion, they may be larger and symptomatic so that excision is required.

Inclusion cysts are usually seen on the posterior lower vaginal surface, resulting from imperfect approximation of childbirth lacerations or episiotomy. They are lined with stratified squamous epithelium, their content is usually cheesy, and they may be excised if symptomatic.

Vaginal Intraepithelial Neoplasia

VAIN can be classified into three types:

- VAIN 1 involves the basal epithelial layers
- VAIN 2 involves up to two-thirds of the vaginal epithelium
- VAIN 3 involves more than two-thirds of the vaginal epithelium (including CIS).

VAIN is most commonly located in the upper third of the vagina, a finding that may be partially related to its association with the more common cervical neoplasias. It is estimated that one-half to two-thirds of all patients with VAIN have had cervical or vulvar neoplasia.

In 2012, the College of American Pathologists and the ASCCP proposed these three categories of VAIN be consolidated into two categories: low-grade squamous intraepithelial lesion (LSIL) which includes VAIN 1 and high-grade squamous intraepithelial lesion (HSIL) which includes VAIN 2 and 3. Patients with VAIN 1 can be monitored and typically will not require therapy. Many of these patients have HPV infection and atrophic change of the vagina. Topical estrogen therapy may be useful in some women. VAIN 2 and 3 should be treated.

VAIN 3 appears to occur more commonly in the third decade of life onward, although its exact incidence is unknown. Approximately 1% to 2% of patients who undergo hysterectomy for cervical intraepithelial neoplasia (CIN) 3 and many patients who undergo radiation therapy for other gynecologic malignancy ultimately develop VAIN 3. Vaginal Pap tests should be performed for a period of time in patients who have a hysterectomy for the treatment of CIN, particularly CIN 2 and 3. The importance of VAIN 3 is its potential for progression to invasive vaginal carcinoma, as the lesions themselves are usually asymptomatic and have no intrinsic morbidity.

VAIN 3 must be differentiated from other causes of red, ulcerated, or white hyperplastic lesions of the vagina such as herpes, traumatic lesions, hyperkeratosis associated with chronic irritation (e.g., from a poorly fitting diaphragm), and adenosis. Inspection and palpation of the vagina are the mainstay of diagnosis, but, unfortunately, this is often done in a cursory fashion during the routine pelvic examination. Pap tests of the vaginal epithelium can disclose findings that are useful in the diagnosis, although colposcopy with directed biopsy is the definitive method of diagnosis, just as it is with CIN.

The goals of treatment of VAIN 3 are ablation of the intraepithelial lesion while preserving vaginal depth, caliber, and sexual function. Laser ablation, local excision, intracavitary radiation, and chemical treatment with 5-FU cream are all used for limited lesions; total or partial vaginectomy with application of a split thickness skin graft is usually reserved for failure of the previously described treatments. The treatment chosen is dependent on the severity of disease, side-effect profile of treatments, certainty of exclusion of carcinoma, patient's health and associated surgical risks, and patient's sexual functioning. Cure rates of 80% to 95% may be expected.

Vaginal Cancer

Invasive vaginal cancer accounts for approximately 1% to 3% of gynecologic malignancies. SCC makes up approximately 80% to 90% of these malignancies, which occur primarily in women 55 years or older. The majority of the remainder of vaginal carcinomas consists of adenocarcinoma of the vagina, vaginal melanoma, and sarcoma. Small cell cancer, lymphoma, and carcinoid cancers together make up 1% of primary vaginal cancers.

The staging of vaginal carcinoma is nonsurgical (Table 46.5). Surgery, radiation, and neoadjuvant chemotherapy are potential treatments. The patient's sexual functioning and exact anatomic location need to be considered. Radiation would not be appropriate for cancers in close proximity to radiation-sensitive tissues. Some anatomic locations would preclude achieving an appropriate margin of resection; thus, surgery would not be appropriate. The overall 5-year survival rate for SCC of the vagina is approximately 42%, and for clear cell adenocarcinoma of the vagina, 78%, with stage I and II patients having the best prognosis. Melanoma is treated with radical surgery; radiation therapy is used as an alternative or adjunct therapy for specific clinical situations.

Sarcoma botryoides (or, *embryonal rhabdomyosarcoma*) is a rare tumor that presents as a mass of grape-like polyps protruding from the introitus of pediatric age patients. It arises from the undifferentiated mesenchyme of the lamina propria of the anterior vaginal wall. Bloody discharge is an associated symptom in

TABLE 46.5 INTERNATIONAL FEDERATION OF GYNECOLOGY AND OBSTETRICS 2009 STAGING OF CARCINOMA OF THE VAGINA

Stage	Definition
I	Carcinoma limited to the vaginal wall
II	Carcinoma involving subvaginal tissue but not extending to the pelvic wall
III	Carcinoma extending to the pelvic wall
IV	Carcinoma extending beyond the true pelvis or has involved the mucosa of the bladder or rectum; bullous edema as such does not permit a case to be allotted to stage IV
IVA	Tumor invades bladder and/or rectal mucosa and/or direct extension beyond the true pelvis
IVB	Spread to distant organs

these tumors. The tumor spreads locally, although it may have distant hematogeneous metastases. Combination chemotherapy administered prior to surgery appears to be effective, resulting in a marked reduction in tumor size. This permits more conservative surgery than was performed in the past, preserving as much bowel and bladder function as possible.

CLINICAL FOLLOW-UP

You perform a vulvar biopsy, which shows lichen sclerosus. You treat her with high-potency steroids for 3 months. At that time, her symptoms have improved and her vulvar examination appears more normal.

CHAPTER 47

Cervical Neoplasia and Carcinoma

This chapter deals primarily with APGO Educational Topic Area:

TOPIC 52 CERVICAL DISEASE AND NEOPLASIA

Students should be able to outline appropriate screening for cervical neoplasia as well as management of patients with abnormal screening. They should be able to discuss pathogenesis of cervical cancer and to identify risk factors, common presenting signs and symptoms, and physical examination findings.

CLINICAL CASE

A 27-year-old comes to see you because her cervical cytology smear shows atypical cells. Her primary care physician stated that she would need a procedure and that this could signify cervical cancer. She is clearly concerned.

INTRODUCTION

Although the incidence and mortality from cervical cancer have decreased substantially in the past several decades among women in the United States, cervical cancer remains the third most common gynecologic cancer. In countries where cytologic screening is not widely available, cervical cancer remains common. Worldwide, it is the fourth most common cancer among women (after breast, colon, and lung cancer) and the most common cause of mortality from gynecologic malignancy, accounting for more than 250,000 deaths per year.

Cervical cancer can be thought of as a preventable cancer. It is preceded by an identifiable precursor lesion (**cervical intraepithelial neoplasia [CIN]**) that may (but not always) progress to invasive cancer. CIN can be easily detected by an inexpensive and noninvasive screening test (cervical cytology test) that may be augmented with supplemental tests such as human papillomavirus (HPV) DNA typing and a follow-up diagnostic procedure (colposcopy). CIN is treatable with simple and effective therapies, including cryotherapy, laser ablation, loop electrosurgical excision procedure (LEEP), and cold knife cone biopsy, all of which have high cure rates. It is also one of only a few cancers for which a vaccine exists that may have a significant impact in reducing an individual's risk.

CERVICAL INTRAEPITHELIAL NEOPLASIA

Etiology

Cervical cancer and CIN are caused by HPV. Of the approximately 170 types of HPV, about 30 infect the anogenital tract. Approximately 15 of these types (16, 18, 31, 33, 35, 39, 45, 51, 52, 56, 58, 59, 68, 73, and 82) are associated with cancer and are known as **high-risk HPV types**. The majority of cervical cancers are caused by HPV 16 and 18. Low-risk HPV types are not associated with cancer. However, low-risk types 6 and 11 are associated with **genital warts** (**condylomata acuminata**) and with low-grade squamous intraepithelial lesions (LSILs).

HPV infects the cells of the cervix. The size and shape of the cervix change depending on age, hormonal status, and number of children (parity). The upper part of the cervix that opens into the endometrial cavity is called the **internal os**; the lower part that opens into the vagina is called the **external os**. The exterior portion of the cervical canal is called the **ectocervix**, and the interior cervical canal is called the **endocervical canal**. The walls of the endocervical canal contain numerous folds and plicae.

The histology of the cervix is complex (Fig. 47.1A, B). Overlying the fibrous stroma of the cervix is the cervical epithelium, a meshwork of cells. The epithelium is of two types: columnar (glandular) and stratified nonkeratinizing squamous epithelia. The columnar epithelium consists of a single layer of mucus-secreting cells that are arranged into deep folds or crypts. The area where the two types of epithelia meet is called the **squamocolumnar junction** (**SCJ**). The SCJ is clinically important, because it is the site where more than 90% of cervical neoplasias arise. During childhood, the SCJ is located just inside the external os. Under the influence of hormones and the acidification of the vaginal environment during puberty, subcolumnar cells undergo metaplasia, a process of transformation. The metaplasia of these cells causes the SCJ to "roll out," or evert, from its prepubertal position inside the external os to a position on the enlarged cervical surface. Columnar epithelium is also rolled onto the cervical surface, where it is exposed to vaginal secretions, irritants, and a changing hormonal milieu. The area between the original SCJ (on ectocervix) and the active SCJ (variable throughout reproductive life) is called the

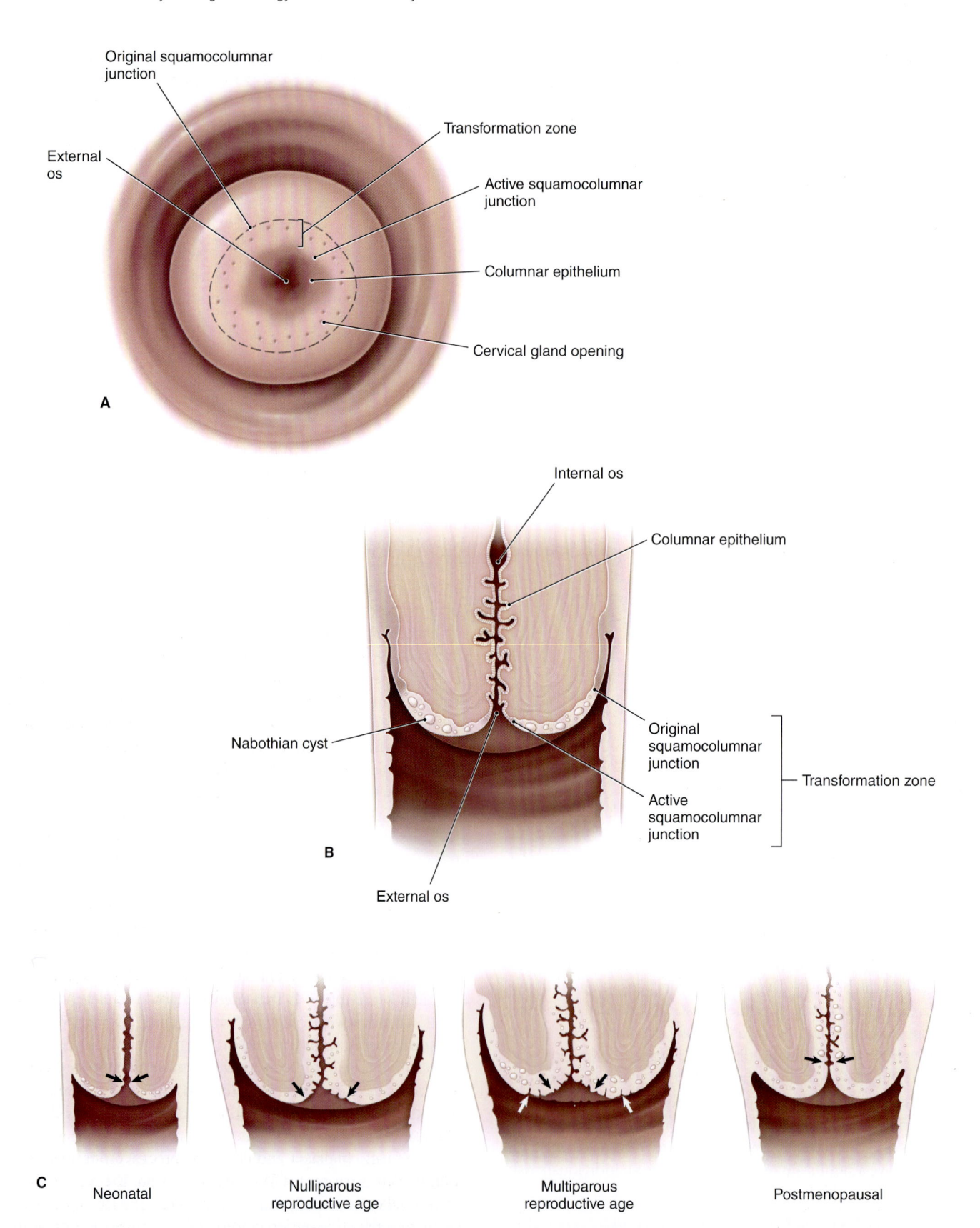

FIGURE 47.1. Anatomy of the cervix. (A) The cervix and the transformation zone. (B) Anterior view of the cervix and exocervix. (C) Different locations of the transformation zone and the squamocolumnar junction during a woman's lifetime. The *arrows* mark the active transformation zone. (Based on Berek JS. *Berek and Novak's Gynecology.* 15th ed. Philadelphia: Lippincott Williams & Wilkins; 2011.)

transformation zone (TZ). As metaplasia continues, the metaplastic epithelium covers and eventually becomes indistinguishable from the original squamous epithelium. Glands within the columnar epithelium may become trapped during this metaplastic activity by squamous epithelium, causing **Nabothian cysts**. These cysts are not considered pathologic but are a normal consequence of the dynamic histology of the cervix.

The metaplastic cells within the TZ represent the newest and least mature cells in the cervix, and it is thought that they are the most vulnerable to oncogenic change. The rate of metaplasia is highest during adolescence and early pregnancy. During perimenopause, the new SCJ recedes upward into the endocervical canal, often out of direct visual contact (see Fig. 47.1C).

HPV infection of cervical cells may or may not result in neoplastic change. Most HPV infections are transient, indicating that the host's immune system is able to eradicate the virus before it can cause neoplastic changes in cervical cells. It is likely that several as-yet unidentified host or environmental factors act as cofactors. If the HPV DNA is not integrated into the host genome, encapsulated virions are produced that are expressed histologically as "koilocytes," cells with shrunken or withered-appearing nuclei surrounded by perinuclear clearing. If HPV DNA is integrated into the host DNA, the expression of the cell's regulatory genes may be altered, leading to the transformation of the cells into intraepithelial lesions or cancer.

Risk Factors

Several factors have been identified that may increase the risk of cervical neoplasia (Box 47.1). A higher incidence of HPV infection and progression of intraepithelial neoplasia is seen in immunosuppressed patients, including those infected with human immunodeficiency virus as well as those who are organ transplant recipients, who have chronic renal failure or a history of Hodgkin lymphoma, or who have undergone immunosuppressive therapy for other reasons. Another factor is cigarette smoking. The risk of cervical cancer is 3.5 times greater among smokers than among nonsmokers. Carcinogens from cigarette smoke have been found in high concentrations in the cervical mucus of smokers, suggesting a plausible biologic explanation for this association. First intercourse at a young age may increase a woman's risk of cervical neoplasia because of the high rate of metaplasia that occurs in the TZ during adolescence and a higher proportion of new or immature cervical cells in this region. However, age of onset of screening is not affected by age of first intercourse and remains age 21.

Persistent HPV infection increases the risk of persistent or progressive cervical dysplasia. HPV 16 infection is more likely to be persistent than infections caused by other oncogenic HPV types. Individuals may possess a genetic susceptibility to cervical cancer, but the relative risks are small.

Classification

The goal of all cervical cancer classification systems is to establish management guidelines that decrease the likelihood of progression of precursor lesions to more advanced lesions. The 2001 Bethesda System is the most widely used system in the United States for reporting and classifying cervical cytologic studies. Established in 1988 and updated in 1991, 2001, and 2014, the Bethesda Classification outlines the various possible results of the cervical cytology test, specifies accepted methodologies of reporting the cervical cytology results, and provides for interpretation of findings. This categorization allows for defined management options regarding the initial results of the cervical cytology test (Box 47.2). Additionally, the Lower Anogenital Tract Squamous Terminology consensus conference uses terminology similar to Bethesda and can help provide some clarity around more equivocal pathologic findings. Details about how the cervical cytology test is performed are found in Chapter 1. Guidelines for cervical cancer screening are found in Chapter 2.

The classification used by the Bethesda system divides epithelial lesions into two categories: *squamous lesions* and *glandular lesions*. In both categories, lesions are either precancerous or cancerous. Squamous precursor lesions are described as **ASCs**, **LSILs**, or **HSILs**, whereas cancerous lesions are termed **invasive squamous carcinoma**. ASC is further divided into **ASC-US** and **ASC-H**. Precancerous glandular lesions are classified as **atypical glandular cells (AGCs)**; **atypical, favor neoplastic**; and **endocervical AIS**. Cancerous glandular lesions are classified as **adenocarcinoma**. AGC is also classified as *endocervical*, *endometrial*, or *NOS*.

Before the intraepithelial lesion terminology was created, the term **cervical intraepithelial neoplasia** was used, and lesions were graded as **CIN 1**, **CIN 2**, or **CIN 3**. The CIN classification system replaced an even earlier classification scheme that used the term **dysplasia** and classified precancerous lesions as *mild*, *moderate*, or *severe*. With each revision, the terminology for cervical cancer results has become more precise and reflects the current scientific understanding of the progression of cervical cancer. The CIN terminology, however, is still used with the current Bethesda terminology. LSIL encompasses HPV infection, mild dysplasia, or CIN 1. HSIL encompasses CIN 2 and CIN 3. CIN 3 is also designated CIS (Table 47.1).

BOX 47.1 Risk Factors for Cervical Neoplasia

- More than one sexual partner or a male sexual partner who has had sex with more than one person
- First intercourse at an early age (younger than 18 years)
- Male sexual partner who has had a sexual partner with cervical cancer
- Smoking
- Human immunodeficiency virus infection
- Organ (especially kidney) transplant
- Sexually transmitted disease infection
- Diethylstilbestrol exposure
- History of cervical cancer or high-grade squamous intraepithelial lesions
- Infrequent or absent cervical cytology screening tests

BOX 47.2 The 2014 Bethesda System

Specimen Type
- Indicate conventional smear (cervical cytology smear) vs. liquid based vs. other

Specimen Adequacy
- Satisfactory for evaluation (*describe the presence or absence of endocervical/TZ component and any other quality indicators, e.g., partially obscuring blood and inflammation*)
- Unsatisfactory for evaluation (*specify reason*)
  ▸ Specimen rejected/not processed (*specify reason*)
  ▸ Specimen processed and examined, but unsatisfactory for evaluation of epithelial abnormality because of (*specify reason*)

General Categorization (*optional*)
- Negative for intraepithelial lesion or malignancy
- Epithelial cell abnormality: See Interpretation/Result (*specify* squamous *or* glandular *as appropriate*)
- Other: See Interpretation/Result (*e.g., endometrial cells in a woman 40 years of age*)

Interpretation/Result

Negative for Intraepithelial Lesion or Malignancy

Organisms
- *Trichomonas vaginalis*
- Fungal organisms morphologically consistent with *Candida* spp.
- Shift in flora suggestive of bacterial vaginosis
- Bacteria morphologically consistent with *Actinomyces* spp.
- Cellular changes consistent with Herpes simplex virus

Other Non-neoplastic Findings (Optional to Report; List Not Inclusive)
- Reactive cellular changes associated with
  ▸ inflammation (includes typical repair)
  ▸ radiation
  ▸ intrauterine contraceptive device
- Glandular cell status posthysterectomy
- Atrophy

Other
- Endometrial cells (*in a woman ≥45 years of age*) (Specify if *"negative for squamous intraepithelial lesion"*)

Epithelial Cell Abnormalities

Squamous Cell
- Atypical squamous cells (ASCs)
  ▸ of undetermined significance (ASC-US)
  ▸ cannot exclude HSIL (ASC-H)
- LSIL encompassing: HPV/mild dysplasia/CIN 1
- High-grade squamous intraepithelial lesion (HSIL) encompassing: moderate and severe dysplasia, carcinoma in situ (CIS)/CIN 2 and CIN 3
  ▸ with features suspicious for invasion (*if invasion is suspected*)
- Squamous cell carcinoma (SCC)

Glandular Cell
- Atypical
  ▸ endocervical cells
  ▸ endometrial cells
  ▸ glandular cells
- Atypical
  ▸ endocervical cells, favor neoplastic
  ▸ glandular cells, favor neoplastic
- Endocervical adenocarcinoma in situ (AIS)
- Adenocarcinoma
  ▸ endocervical
  ▸ endometrial
  ▸ extrauterine
  ▸ not otherwise specified (NOS)
- Other Malignant Neoplasms: (specify)

Adjunctive Testing
- Computer-Assisted Interpretation of Cervical Cytology

Educational Notes and Suggestions (*Optional*)
- Suggestions should be concise and consistent with clinical follow-up guidelines published by professional organizations (references to relevant publications may be included).

Modified from The 2014 Bethesda System: Terminology for Reporting Results of Cervical Cytology. *Journal of the American Medical Association* (2002;287:2114-2119).

Despite decades of study, the natural history of cervical intraepithelial lesions is still not completely understood. The once widely held concept that low-grade lesions are necessary precursors to the high-grade lesions that, in turn, may progress to invasive cancer has been questioned as the sole pathogenesis. It has been observed, for example, that many women present with CIN 2 or CIN 3 without prior CIN 1 lesions. Although multiple longitudinal studies have attempted to document the rates of "progression" and "regression" of CIN, results of these studies must be interpreted with caution due to varying methods of diagnostic criteria, populations, and duration of follow-up.

Evaluation of Abnormal Cervical Cytology Test Results

An abnormal cervical cytologic finding from a cervical cytology test should be followed by visual inspection of the vagina and a bimanual examination. The first objective is to exclude

TABLE 47.1 COMPARISON OF CERVICAL CYTOLOGY DESCRIPTIVE CONVENTIONS

CIN system	Normal	Inflammatory	CIN I	or	CIN II	CIN III	Suggestive of cancer
Bethesda 2001	Negative for intraepithelial lesion or malignancy	ASC-US / ASC-H	LSIL		HSIL		Squamous cell carcinoma
Histology	Basal cells	WBCs	Basement membrane				Invasive cervical cancer

the presence of invasive carcinoma. Once this has been accomplished, the objectives are to determine the grade and distribution of the intraepithelial lesion. Options for evaluation include repeat cytology, high-risk HPV testing, colposcopy with directed biopsies (see Chapter 34), and endocervical assessment.

Colposcopy and Endocervical Curettage

Colposcopy with directed biopsy has been the standard of care for disease detection and remains the technique of choice for treatment decisions. A **colposcope** is a binocular stereomicroscope with variable magnification (usually 7× to 15×) and a light source with a green filter to aid in the identification of abnormal-appearing blood vessels that may be associated with intraepithelial neoplasia. With colposcopy, areas with changes consistent with dysplasia are identified, allowing directed biopsy (i.e., biopsy of the area where dysplasia is most likely). Colposcopic criteria, such as white epithelium, abnormal vascular patterns, and punctate lesions help identify such areas (Fig. 47.2). To facilitate the examination, the cervix is washed with a 3% to 4% acetic acid solution, which dehydrates cells, causing those with large nuclei (i.e., those undergoing metaplasia, dysplasia, or HPV infection) to appear white. Lesions usually appear with relatively discrete borders near the SCJ within 10 to 90 seconds of acetic acid application. Tissue samples for biopsy can be collected; the number of samples obtained will vary depending on the number and severity of abnormal areas found. Visualization of the entire SCJ is required for a colposcopy to be considered satisfactory. If the SCJ is not visualized in its entirety, or if the margins of abnormal areas are not seen in their entirety, the colposcopic assessment is termed unsatisfactory, and other evaluations such as cervical conization and **endocervical curettage (ECC)** are indicated. In this procedure,

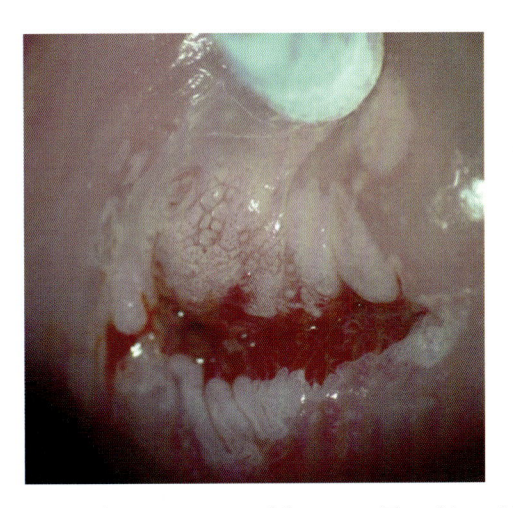

FIGURE 47.2. Colposcopic image of the cervix. The white epithelium and coarse mosaic pattern of the underlying capillaries in this colpophotograph are suggestive of cervical intraepithelial neoplasia. (Case Studies in Colposcopy Case #53—March 2007. Kevin J. Mitchell, MD, Chair, with pathology courtesy of Mary Chacho MD, Department of Pathology, Danbury Hospital, Danbury, CT, 2006–08 Section on the Cervix. Downloaded on 7-21-08 from http://www.asccp.org/edu/case_studies.shtml#. (From Berek, J.S. (2007). Berek & Novak's Gynecology, 14th edition. Philadelphia, PA: Lippincott Williams & Wilkins.))

a small curette is used to collect cells from the endocervical canal. An endocervical brush can be used to retrieve additional cells dislodged in the curette specimen. This endocervical sample is obtained so that potential disease farther inside the cervical canal, which is not visualized by the colposcope, may be detected. The cervical biopsies and ECC are then submitted separately for pathologic assessment.

Human Papillomavirus DNA Testing

Testing for the presence of high-risk HPV DNA is now being used as an adjunct screening tool for cervical neoplasia in women older than 30 years. It is also used as a triage tool for women with cervical cytology test results reported as ASC-US and in the management of nonadolescent women with LSIL. HPV DNA can identify women whose cervical cytology test results are caused by other, non–HPV-associated phenomena, such as infection, thus preventing unnecessary colposcopic evaluations. Because HPV is more prevalent in younger women and the rate of CIN 2 and CIN 3 increases with age, HPV DNA testing is more useful as a triage tool in older women. HPV DNA testing is also used in the initial workup of women with AGC.

Management Guidelines for Cervical Epithelial Cell Abnormalities

The American Society for Colposcopy and Cervical Pathology issues guidelines and protocols for the appropriate management of women with cervical cytologic or histologic abnormalities. The most recent updates to these recommendations occurred in 2012 and were published shortly thereafter. These guidelines, including practice algorithms, are available at http://www.asccp.org/asccp-guidelines. The following sections summarize these guidelines.

Low-Grade Squamous Intraepithelial Lesions and Atypical Squamous Cells of Undetermined Significance

A patient with an ASC-US result should either undergo reflex HPV DNA testing (on the liquid-based sample already collected) or repeat cytology with cotesting, HPV testing done at the same time, at 12 months following the abnormal cervical cytology test result. The rationale for HPV DNA testing is that a negative result obviates the need for colposcopy; patients with ASC-US who are negative for high-risk HPV DNA need repeat cotesting in 3 years. Women who screen positive for HPV DNA with ASC-US results on cervical cytology should be managed in the same way as women with LSIL, with no HPV results or positive HPV result—both groups should be referred for a colposcopic evaluation. Patients with ASC-US results, who were originally not tested for HPV and have another ASC-US (or worse) at the 12th-month repeat cytology screening, should be referred for colposcopy; if repeat cytology in 12 months is negative, then the patient may resume routine screening (Fig. 47.3).

About 3% of cervical cytology test results are reproducibly classified as LSIL. Colposcopy is recommended for LSIL with no HPV test, LSIL with positive HPV, and ASCUS with positive HPV as earlier. Management and follow-up are the same following colposcopy for these women. If the patient has LSIL and a negative HPV test, then she can be monitored closely in the form of repeat cotesting in 12 months. If this repeat cotesting is negative, then she can have her next cotesting in 3 years (Fig. 47.4).

Management protocols differ for younger women (ages 21–24 years) and pregnant women. ASC and LSIL are more common in younger women, and the likelihood of spontaneous regression is higher. Because HPV DNA positivity is also higher in this population, using HPV DNA screening as a triage method is not useful. Young women (21–24 years) with LSIL or ASC-US with no HPV result may be managed with repeat cytologic testing at

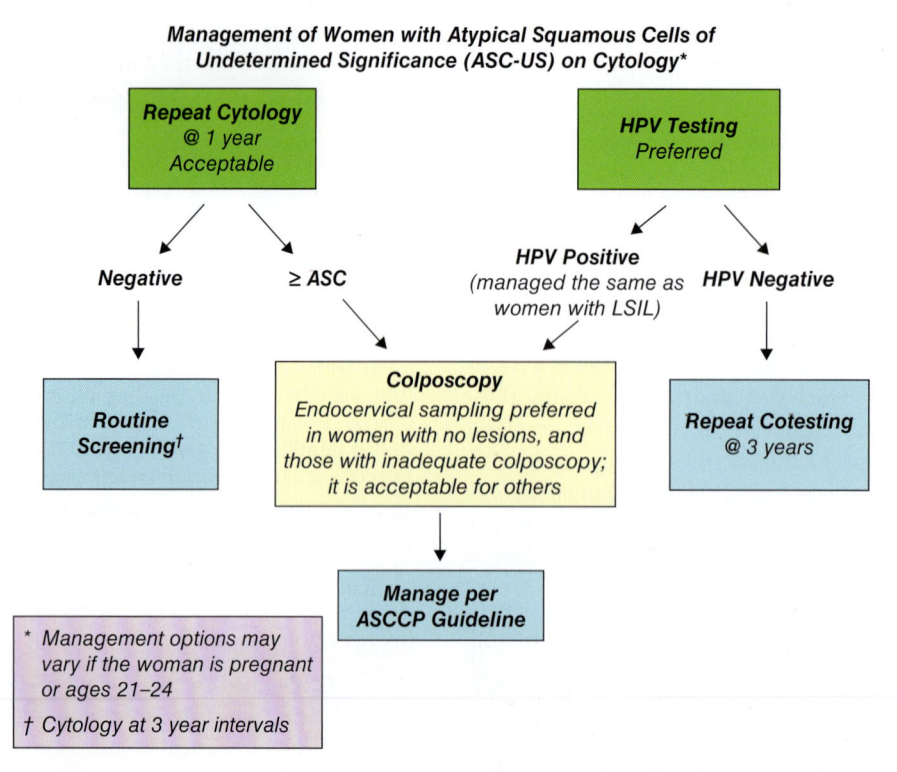

FIGURE 47.3. Management of women with atypical squamous cells of undetermined significance (ASCCP). ASC, atypical squamous cells; HPV, human papillomavirus; LSIL, low-grade squamous intraepithelial lesion. (Reprinted from *The Journal of Lower Genital Tract Disease* Volume 17, Number 5, with the permission of ASCCP © American Society for Colposcopy and Cervical Pathology 2013. No reproductions of the Work, in whole or in part, may be made without the prior written consent of ASCCP.)

**Management of Women Ages 21–24 Years with either
Atypical Squamous Cells of Undetermined Significance (ASC-US) or
Low-grade Squamous Intraepithelial Lesion (LSIL)**

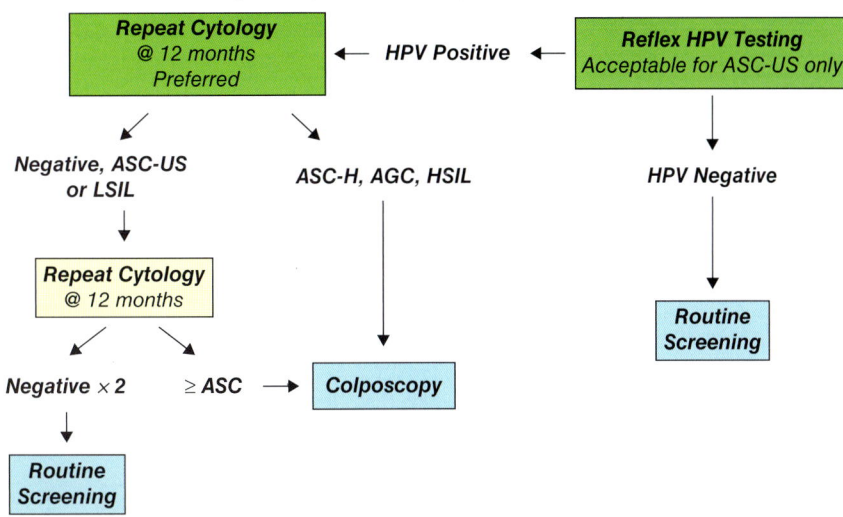

```
                Repeat Cytology                          Reflex HPV Testing
                  @ 12 months       ← HPV Positive ←    Acceptable for ASC-US only
                   Preferred
                   ↙       ↘                                       ↓
          Negative, ASC-US   ASC-H, AGC, HSIL                 HPV Negative
            or LSIL                                                 ↓
                ↓                                              Routine
          Repeat Cytology                                      Screening
           @ 12 months
            ↙       ↘
       Negative × 2   ≥ ASC  →  Colposcopy
            ↓
         Routine
         Screening
```

FIGURE 47.4. Management of women ages 21 to 24 years with either atypical squamous cells of undetermined significance (ASC-US) or low-grade squamous intraepithelial lesion (LSIL). AGC, atypical glandular cell; ASC, atypical squamous cells; HPV, human papillomavirus; HSIL, high-grade squamous epithelial lesion. (Reprinted from *The Journal of Lower Genital Tract Disease* Volume 17, Number 5, with the permission of ASCCP © American Society for Colposcopy and Cervical Pathology 2013. No reproductions of the Work, in whole or in part, may be made without the prior written consent of ASCCP.)

12 months. Those whose repeat cytology results show HSILs are referred for colposcopy; otherwise, they can have a repeat cervical cytology in another 12 months (Fig 47.5). Pregnant women with LSIL should not undergo ECC and should not have more than one colposcopy during pregnancy. Performing colposcopic biopsy during pregnancy should be reserved for situations when there is strong clinical suspicion of cancer. The cervix should be carefully inspected colposcopically to examine for suspicious lesions. Colposcopic examination for evaluation can also be deferred until at least 6 weeks following delivery.

Earlier guidelines for postmenopausal women with LSIL cervical cytology test results offered repeat cytologic screening after treatment with vaginal estrogen cream as a triage option, insofar as atrophy of the vaginal mucosa may contribute to the abnormal test result. However, current guidelines recommend that postmenopausal women with LSIL and ASC-US test results be managed in the same way as the general population. At the age of 65 years, screening should be discontinued in any woman with adequate history of normal cervical screening results and no history of CIN 2 or higher.

High-Grade Squamous Intraepithelial Lesions and Atypical Squamous Cells—Cannot Exclude High-Grade Squamous Intraepithelial Lesion

In the United States, approximately 0.5% of all cervical cytology test results are reported as HSIL. The rate of HSIL decreases with age. CIN 2 or CIN 3 is identified in 84% to 97% of women with HSIL cervical cytology results, and invasive cancer is identified in 2%. Because the rate of CIN 2 or CIN 3 is so high in adults with HSIL cytologic findings, immediate treatment with LEEP (see below) is an acceptable management approach. The other management approach is colposcopic examination, followed by appropriate treatment and follow-up (see Fig. 47.6). ASC-H is evaluated by colposcopy because, like HSIL, it carries a higher risk of underlying CIN 2 to CIN 3 lesions. Further management depends upon results of colposcopy and presence of CIN 2 or CIN 3 (Figs. 47.7).

Atypical Glandular Cells and Other Glandular Abnormalities

Glandular cell abnormalities comprise 0.4% of epithelial cell abnormalities. The risk associated with AGC is dramatically higher than that seen with ASC. The risk associated with glandular abnormalities increases as the description in the Bethesda classification system advances from AGC-NOS to AGC, favor neoplasia and, finally, to AIS. Women with AGC of any type except for atypical endometrial cells should undergo colposcopic evaluation, HPV DNA testing, and ECC. If a woman is 35 years or older or is at risk for endometrial neoplasia (i.e., she has unexplained vaginal bleeding or conditions suggesting chronic anovulation), endometrial sampling should also be performed. Women with atypical endometrial cells should have an endometrial biopsy and ECC (Fig 47.8).

Knowledge of HPV status in women with AGC who do not have CIN 2 or CIN 3 or glandular neoplasia allows expedited triage. These women should have cotesting at 12 months. Women with a positive HPV test or an abnormal cervical cytology test result should be referred to colposcopy; women who have negative results on both tests can have repeating cotesting after another 12 months or 24 months from the original cervical cytology.

Treatment

Both excisional and ablative techniques are used to treat CIN. The underlying concept in the treatment of CIN is that excision or ablation of the precursor lesion prevents progression to carcinoma.

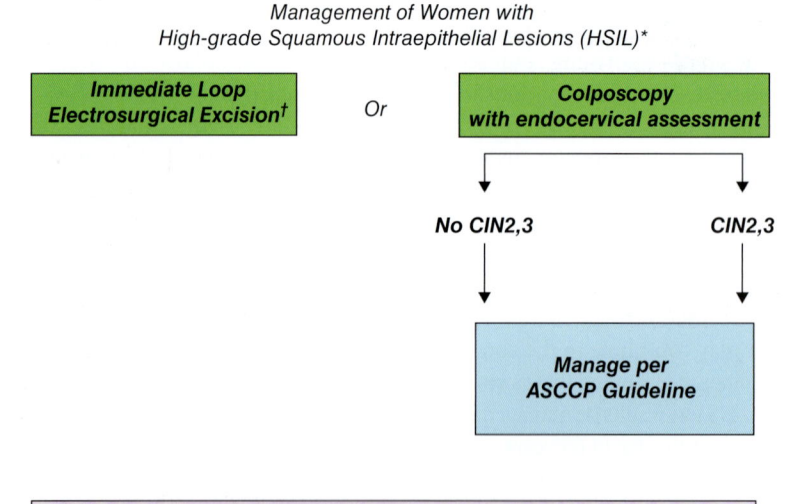

FIGURE 47.5. Management of women with LSIL (ASCCP). ASC, atypical squamous cells; CIN, cervical intraepithelial neoplasia; HPV, human papillomavirus. (Reprinted from *The Journal of Lower Genital Tract Disease* Volume 17, Number 5, with the permission of ASCCP © American Society for Colposcopy and Cervical Pathology 2013. No reproductions of the Work, in whole or in part, may be made without the prior written consent of ASCCP.)

FIGURE 47.6. Management of women with HSIL (ASCCP). CIN, cervical intraepithelial neoplasia. (Reprinted from *The Journal of Lower Genital Tract Disease* Volume 17, Number 5, with the permission of ASCCP © American Society for Colposcopy and Cervical Pathology 2013. No reproductions of the Work, in whole or in part, may be made without the prior written consent of ASCCP.)

Ablative Methods

Ablative methods destroy the affected cervical tissue and include cryotherapy, laser ablation, electrofulguration, and cold coagulation, all of which are outpatient procedures that can be performed with regional anesthesia. Ablative methods should be used only with an adequate colposcopy and appropriate correlation between cervical cytology test results and colposcopically directed biopsy.

Laser therapy is now only rarely performed in the United States. **Cryotherapy** is a commonly used outpatient method used

Management of Women with Atypical Squamous Cells: Cannot Exclude High-grade SIL (ASC-H)*

```
         Colposcopy
      Regardless of HPV status
       /              \
   No CIN2,3        CIN2,3
       ↓               ↓
   Manage per       Manage per
   ASCCP Guideline  ASCCP Guideline
```

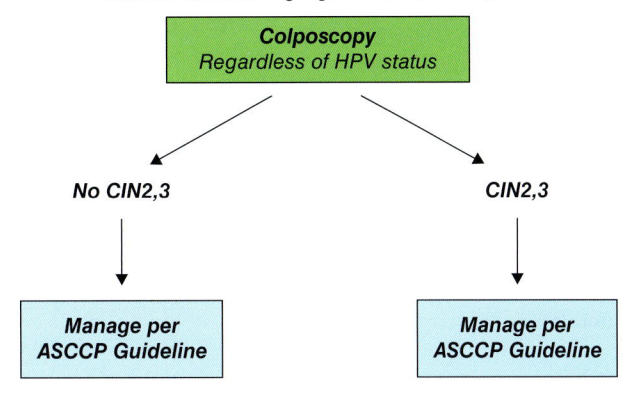

*Management options may vary if the woman is pregnant or ages 21–24 years.

FIGURE 47.7. Management of women with ASC-H. HPV, human papillomavirus; ASC, atypical squamous cells; CIN, cervical intraepithelial neoplasia. (Reprinted from *The Journal of Lower Genital Tract Disease* Volume 17, Number 5, with the permission of ASCCP © American Society for Colposcopy and Cervical Pathology 2013. No reproductions of the Work, in whole or in part, may be made without the prior written consent of ASCCP.)

Initial Workup of Women with Atypical Glandular Cells (AGC)

```
All Subcategories                    Atypical Endometrial Cells
(except atypical endometrial cells)          ↓
        ↓                            Endometrial and
Colposcopy with endocervical         Endocervical Sampling
sampling and                                 ↓
Endometrial Sampling                 No Endometrial Pathology
(if ≥ 35 yrs or at risk for                  ↓
endometrial neoplasia*)              Colposcopy
```

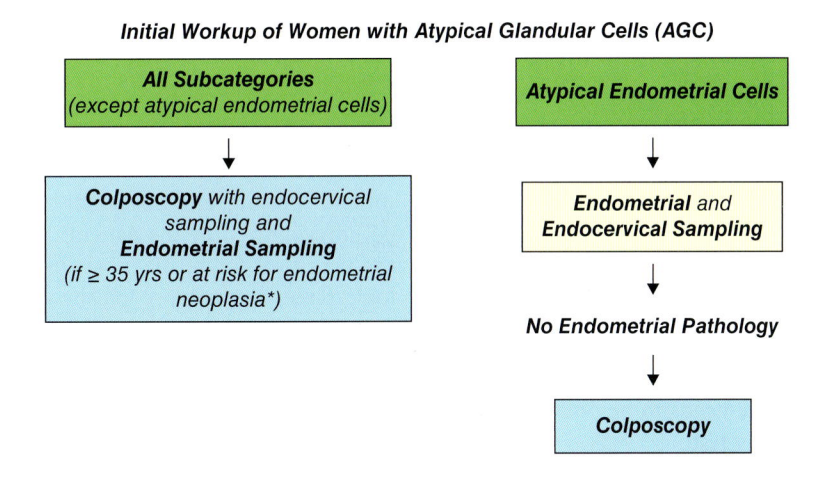

*Includes unexplained vaginal bleeding or conditions suggesting chronic anovulation

FIGURE 47.8. Initial workup of women with AGC. (Reprinted from *The Journal of Lower Genital Tract Disease* Volume 17, Number 5, with the permission of ASCCP © American Society for Colposcopy and Cervical Pathology 2013. No reproductions of the Work, in whole or in part, may be made without the prior written consent of ASCCP.)

to treat persistent CIN 1. The procedure involves covering the SCJ and all identified lesions with a stainless steel probe, which is then supercooled with liquid nitrogen or compressed gas (carbon dioxide or nitrous oxide). The size and shape of the probe depend on the size and shape of the cervix and the lesion to be treated. The most common technique involves a 3-minute freeze followed by a 5-minute thaw, with a repeat 3-minute freeze. The thaw period between the two freezing episodes allows the damaged tissue from the first freeze to become edematous and swell with intracellular fluid. With the second freeze, the edematous cellular architecture is refrozen and extends the damaged area slightly deeper into the tissue. Healing after cryotherapy may take up to 4 or 5 weeks, because the damaged tissue slowly sloughs and is replaced by new cervical epithelium. This process is associated with profuse watery discharge often mixed with necrotic cellular debris. The healing process is complete within 2 months. A follow-up cervical cytology test is usually performed 12 weeks following the freezing to ascertain the effectiveness of the procedure. The cure rate for CIN 1 using this technique approaches 90% to 95%.

Excisional Methods

Excisional methods remove the affected tissue and provide a specimen for pathologic evaluation. These methods include cold knife conization (CKC), LEEP (also called *large loop excision of the transformation zone* [*LLETZ*]), laser conization, and electrosurgical needle conization. These procedures are performed under regional or general anesthesia. A cone-shaped specimen is removed from the cervix, which encompasses the SCJ, all identified lesions on the ectocervix, and a portion of the endocervical canal, the extent of which depends on whether the ECC was positive or negative. Because LEEP uses electrosurgical energy, thermal damage may occur at the margins of the specimen, obscuring the histology. Thermal damage is usually not considered a problem in the evaluation of squamous epithelial abnormalities, but it may be a substantial issue in the evaluation of glandular epithelial lesions, where abnormal cells in the bottom of glandular crypts may be altered. In cases of glandular abnormalities, CKC may be more appropriate.

If the margins of the biopsy are not free of disease, the patient should have either repeat conization or close follow-up because of the possibility that disease remains. If the margins are positive for a high-grade epithelial lesion or CIS, the most appropriate treatment may be hysterectomy, if the patient has no desire for future childbearing. If the patient wants to preserve her fertility, colposcopy with ECC and HPV DNA testing is an acceptable management protocol.

Excisional procedures are also indicated when an ECC is positive as well as in the following situations:

- Unsatisfactory colposcopy: If the SCJ is not visualized in its entirety or if the margins of abnormal areas are not seen in their entirety during colposcopy, the colposcopic assessment is termed unsatisfactory and other evaluation such as cervical conization or ECC is indicated.
- If a substantial discrepancy is seen between the screening cervical cytology and the histologic data from biopsy and ECC (i.e., the biopsy does not explain the source of the abnormal cervical cytology test). In this situation, which occurs in approximately 10% of colposcopies with directed biopsies and ECC, more tissue needs to be obtained by an excisional procedure for further testing.

CKC, LEEP, and LLETZ are associated with an increased risk of second-trimester pregnancy loss secondary to cervical incompetence, preterm labor, preterm premature rupture of membranes, and cervical stenosis. Both types of excisional procedures are also associated with the usual risks of any surgery (bleeding, infection, and anesthetic risks).

Follow-Up

After treatment for noninvasive epithelial cell abnormalities, specifically, CIN 2 or CIN 3, either by ablation or excision, a period of follow-up cotesting (cervical cytology with HPV testing) at 12 months and 24 months after the treatment is recommended. If this follow-up testing is normal, repeat cotest is performed 3 years after treatment and then patients can return to routine testing for at least 20 years. If any of the follow-up testing is abnormal, then colposcopy with endocervical evaluation is performed. The importance of follow-up should be stressed to the patient, because of the greater risk of recurrent abnormalities.

CERVICAL CARCINOMA

Between 1950 and 1992, the death rate from cervical cancer declined by 74%. The main reason for this steep decrease is the increasing use of cervical cytology cancer screening. The death rate continues to decline by approximately 4% per year. Despite the progress made in early detection and treatment, approximately 11,000 new cases of invasive cervical carcinoma are diagnosed annually, with 3,870 deaths.

The average age at diagnosis for invasive cervical cancer is approximately 50 years, although the disease may occur in the very young as well as the very old patient. In studies following patients with advanced CIN, this precursor lesion precedes invasive carcinoma by approximately 10 years. In some patients, however, this time of progression may be considerably less. The etiology of cervical cancer is HPV in more than 90% of the cases. The two major histologic types of invasive cervical carcinomas are SCCs and adenocarcinomas. SCCs comprise 80% of cases, and adenocarcinoma or adenosquamous carcinoma comprise approximately 15%. The remaining cases are made up of various rare histologies that behave differently from SCC and adenocarcinoma.

Clinical Evaluation

The signs and symptoms of early cervical carcinoma are variable and nonspecific, including watery vaginal discharge, intermittent spotting, and postcoital bleeding. Often the symptoms go unrecognized by the patient. Because of the accessibility of the cervix, accurate diagnosis often can be made with cytologic screening, colposcopically directed biopsy, or biopsy of a gross or palpable lesion. In cases of suspected microinvasion and early-stage cervical carcinoma, conization of the cervix is indicated to evaluate the possibility of invasion or to define the depth and extent of microinvasion. CKC provides the most accurate evaluation of the margins.

Staging is based on the International Federation of Gynecology and Obstetrics staging classification (Table 47.2). This classification is based both on the histologic assessment of the tumor sample and on physical and laboratory examination to ascertain the extent of disease. It is useful because of the predictable manner in which cervical carcinoma spreads by direct invasion and by lymphatic metastasis (Fig. 47.9). Careful clinical examination should be performed on all patients. Examinations should be conducted by experienced examiners and may be performed under anesthesia. Pretreatment evaluation of women with cervical carcinoma often can be helpful if provided by an obstetrician–gynecologist with advanced surgical training, experience, and demonstrated competence, such as a gynecologic oncologist. Various optional examinations, such as ultrasonography, computed tomography, magnetic resonance imaging, lymphangiography, laparoscopy, and fine-needle aspiration, are valuable for treatment planning and to help define the extent of tumor growth, especially in patients with locally advanced disease (i.e., stage IIb or more advanced). Surgical findings provide extremely accurate information about

TABLE 47.2 INTERNATIONAL FEDERATION OF GYNECOLOGY AND OBSTETRICS STAGING OF CERVICAL CANCER

Stage	Description
Stage I: The carcinoma is strictly confined to the cervix (extension to the corpus would be disregarded)	
Ia	Invasive carcinoma which can be diagnosed only by microscopy, with deepest invasion ≤5 mm and largest extension ≥7 mm
Ia1	Measured stromal invasion of ≤3.0 mm in depth and extension of ≤7.0 mm
Ia2	Measured stromal invasion of >3.0 mm and not >5.0 mm with an extension of not >7.0 mm
Ib	Clinically visible lesions limited to the cervix uteri or preclinical cancers greater than stage IA[a]
Ib1	Clinically visible lesion ≤4.0 cm in greatest dimension
Ib2	Clinically visible lesion >4.0 cm in greatest dimension
Stage II: Cervical carcinoma invades beyond the uterus, but not to the pelvic wall or to the lower third of the vagina	
IIa	Without parametrial invasion
IIa1	Clinically visible lesion ≤4.0 cm in greatest dimension
IIa2	Clinically visible lesion >4 cm in greatest dimension
IIb	With obvious parametrial invasion
Stage III: The tumor extends to the pelvic wall and/or involves lower third of the vagina and/or causes hydronephrosis or nonfunctioning kidney[b]	
IIIa	Tumor involves lower third of the vagina, with no extension to the pelvic wall
IIIb	Extension to the pelvic wall and/or hydronephrosis or nonfunctioning kidney
Stage IV: The carcinoma has extended beyond the true pelvis or has involved (biopsy proven) the mucosa of the bladder or rectum. A bullous edema, as such, does not permit a case to be allotted to Stage IV	
IVa	Spread of the growth to adjacent organs
IVb	Spread to distant organs

[a] All macroscopically visible lesions—even with superficial invasion—are allotted to stage IB carcinomas. Invasion is limited to a measured stromal invasion with a maximal depth of 5.00 mm and a horizontal extension of not >7.00 mm. Depth of invasion should not be >5.00 mm taken from the base of the epithelium of the original tissue—superficial or glandular. The depth of invasion should always be reported in mm, even in those cases with "early (minimal) stromal invasion" (~1 mm). The involvement of vascular/lymphatic spaces should not change the stage allotment.
[b] On rectal examination, there is no cancer-free space between the tumor and the pelvic wall. All cases with hydronephrosis or nonfunctioning kidney are included, unless they are known to be due to another cause.
Modified from FIGO COMMITTEE ON GYNECOLOGIC ONCOLOGY. Revised FIGO Staging for Carcinoma of the Vulva, Cervix, and Endometrium. Originally published in *Int J Gynecol Obstet*. 2009;105:103–104.

the extent of disease and will guide treatment plans but will not change the results of clinical staging. Cervical cancer is considered a clinically staged entity.

Management

The clinician should be familiar with the options for treating women with both early and advanced cervical cancer and should facilitate referrals for this treatment. Surgery or radiation therapy may be options for treatment, depending on the stage and size of the lesion:

- Patients with squamous cell cancers and those with adenocarcinomas should be managed similarly, except for those with microinvasive disease. Criteria for microinvasive adenocarcinomas have not been established.
- For stage Ia1, microinvasive squamous carcinoma of the cervix, treatment with conization of the cervix or simple extrafascial hysterectomy may be considered.
- Stage Ia2, invasive squamous carcinoma of the cervix, should be treated with radical hysterectomy with lymph node dissection or radiation therapy, depending on clinical circumstances.
- Stage Ib1 should be distinguished from stage Ib2 carcinoma of the cervix, because the distinction predicts nodal involvement and overall survival and may, therefore, affect treatment and outcome.
- For bulky stage Ib and selected IIa carcinomas of the cervix, either radical hysterectomy and lymph node dissection or

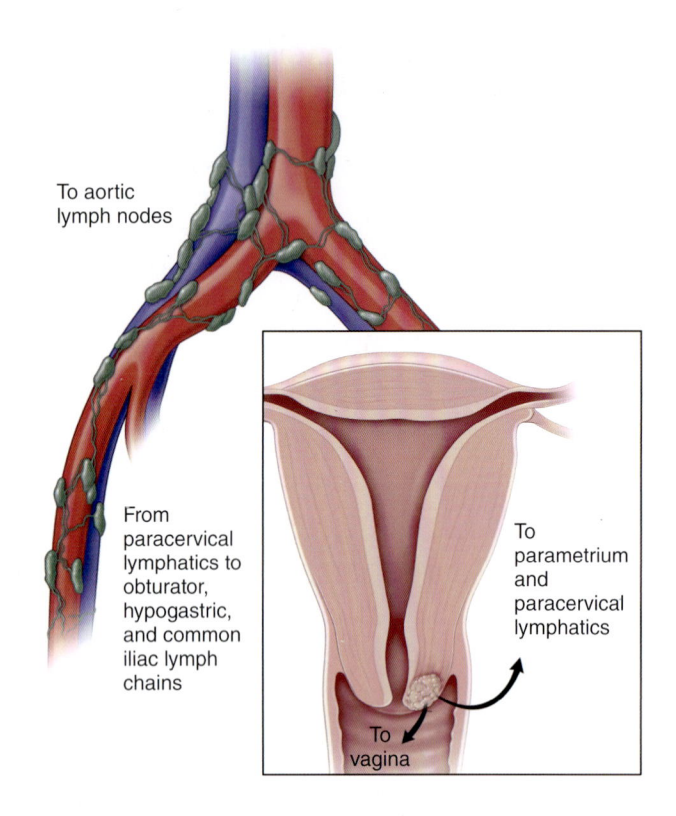

FIGURE 47.9. Spread patterns of cervical carcinoma.

radiation therapy with cisplatin-based chemotherapy should be considered. Adjuvant radiation therapy may be required in those treated surgically, based on pathologic risk factors, especially in those with stage Ib2 carcinoma.
- Stage IIb and greater should be treated with external beam and brachytherapy radiation and concurrent cisplatin-based chemotherapy.

Brachytherapy delivers radiation close to the affected organ or structure. Both high- and low-dose brachytherapy are used to treat cervical cancer. The brachytherapy radiation is delivered using special apparatuses known as *tandem and ovoid devices* placed through the cervix into the uterus and at the apices of the vagina. The external beam radiation is applied primarily along the paths of lymphatic extension of cervical carcinoma in the pelvis.

The structures close to the cervix, such as the bladder and distal colon, tolerate radiation relatively well. Radiation therapy doses are calculated by individual patient needs to maximize radiation to the tumor sites and potential spread areas, while minimizing the amount of radiation to adjacent uninvolved tissues. Complications of radiation therapy include radiation cystitis and proctitis, which are usually relatively easy to manage. Other more unusual complications include intestinal or vaginal fistulae, small bowel obstruction, and difficult-to-manage hemorrhagic proctitis or cystitis. Tissue damage and fibrosis incurred by radiation therapy progress over many years, and these effects may complicate long-term management.

Following treatment for cervical carcinoma, patients should be monitored regularly, for example, with follow-up examinations every 4 months for the first 2 years and visits every 6 months subsequently to year 5, followed by cervical cytology annually to perpetuity and chest x-rays annually for up to 5 years. The 5-year survival rates for cervical cancer are listed in Table 47.3.

Treatment for recurrent disease is associated with poor cure rates. Most chemotherapeutic protocols have only limited usefulness and are reserved for palliative efforts. Likewise, specific "spot" radiation to areas of recurrence also provides only limited benefit. Occasional patients with central recurrence (i.e., recurrence of disease in the upper vagina or the residual cervix and uterus in radiation patients) may benefit from ultraradical surgery with partial or total pelvic exenteration. These candidates are few, but when properly selected, may benefit from this aggressive therapy.

PREVENTION

Preventive approaches to cervical cancer include sexual abstinence, vaccination with the HPV vaccine, the use of barrier protection with or without spermicides, and regular gynecologic examination and cytologic screening with treatment of precancerous lesions according to established protocols. It is estimated that gynecologic examination and cervical cytology administered according to current guidelines may reduce cancer incidence and mortality by 40%. Limiting the number of sexual partners also may decrease the risk of sexually transmitted diseases, including HPV.

The HPV vaccine prevents transmission and acquisition of type-specific HPV through sexual and nonsexual contact. Currently, there are three vaccines on the market (bivalent, quadrivalent, and 9-valent). One is active against oncogenic

TABLE 47.3 FIVE-YEAR SURVIVAL RATES FOR CERVICAL CANCER

Stage	5-Year Survival Rate (%)
0	93
IA	93
IB	80
IIA	63
IIB	58
IIIA	35
IIIB	32
IVA	16
IVB	15

American Cancer Society. (2010). Retrieved from https://www.cancer.org/cancer/cervical-cancer/detection-diagnosis-staging/survival.html.

> **BOX 47.3** Current Guidelines for Administration of the Human Papillomavirus Vaccine
>
> - Currently, there are at least three vaccines which are approved by the Food and Drug Administration for preventing HPV infection. They differ in the number of serotypes covered.
> - The HPV vaccine is given as two or three separate doses depending on age of first dose. If the first dose is administered before age 15, then only two doses are required, 6 to 12 months apart. If, for some reason, the second doses are administered less than 5 months apart, then a third dose is required.
> - If the first dose is administered at the age of 15 or older, then three doses are required. The second dose should be given 1 to 2 months after the first dose, and the third dose given 6 months after the first dose.
> - It is recommended as a routine vaccination for boys and girls aged 11 to 12 years. However, it can be given as young as 9 years.
> - Previous exposure to HPV is not a contraindication to vaccination. Testing for HPV is currently not recommended before vaccination.
> - The vaccine is not recommended for pregnant women, but is safe for women who are breastfeeding.
> - Current cervical cytology screening recommendations remain unchanged and should be followed regardless of vaccination status.
>
> Used with permission from the American College of Obstetricians and Gynecologists. Human Papillomavirus Vaccination. ACOG Committee Opinion 704, Washington, DC: American College of Obstetricians and Gynecologists, June 2017;129:e173–8.

HPV types 16 and 18 only, one is active against HPV 5 types 16, 18, as well as two types that cause genital warts, HPV types 6 and 11. The other vaccine is active against oncogenic HPV types 16 and 18, with some possible protection against seven other genotypes including 45 and 31. These vaccines contain virus-like particles that consist of the main structural HPV-L1 protein but lack the viral genetic material and, thus, are noninfectious. These vaccines stimulate the production of immunoglobulin G–type-specific antibodies to prevent acquisition of type-specific HPV in the genital and vulvar areas. The quadrivalent vaccine has been shown to prevent 91% of new and 100% of persistent infections.

Currently, HPV vaccines are indicated only for prophylaxis (Box 47.3). However, it is anticipated that the guidelines for their use will continue to change regarding age group, sex, and therapeutic indications. The development of new vaccines may also broaden the horizon for HPV treatment.

CLINICAL FOLLOW-UP

You explain that a colposcopy is a diagnostic procedure that will provide more information. On colposcopic examination, you see the full TZ and notice a small acetowhite area at the 3:00 position, which you biopsy. The biopsy results demonstrate no evidence of dysplasia or cancer. You relay this information to the patient and make a plan for future follow-up with cervical cytology.

CHAPTER 48

Uterine Leiomyoma and Neoplasia

This chapter deals primarily with APGO Educational Topic Area:

TOPIC 53 **UTERINE LEIOMYOMAS**

Students should be able to outline a basic approach to patients with uterine leiomyoma, including diagnosis and the range of management options. They should identify prevalence, common presenting signs and symptoms, and physical examination findings.

CLINICAL CASE

A 46-year-old G2P2002 comes to see you because she feels a lump in the lower part of her abdomen. She states that it does not cause her any pain, but she has noticed an increase in the number of times she needs to urinate and estimates she urinates 10 times a day and 2 to 3 times each night. She denies any irregular bleeding and reports normal menstrual periods.

INTRODUCTION

Uterine leiomyomata (also called **fibroids** and **myomas**) represent localized proliferation of smooth muscle cells surrounded by a pseudocapsule of compressed muscle fibers. The highest prevalence occurs during the fifth decade of a woman's life, when they may be present in one in four white women and one in two African American women. Studies in which careful pathologic examination of the uterus is carried out suggest that the prevalence may be as high as 80%. Uterine fibroids vary in size, from microscopic to large multinodular tumors that literally fill the patient's abdomen. Leiomyomata are the most common indication for hysterectomy, accounting for approximately 30% of this operation. Additionally, they account for a large number of more conservative operations, including myomectomy, uterine curettage, operative hysteroscopy, and uterine artery embolization (UAE).

Leiomyomata are classified into subgroups based on their anatomic relationship to the layers of the uterus. The three most common types are **intramural** (in the muscular wall of the uterus), **subserosal** (just beneath the uterine serosa), and **submucosal** (just beneath the endometrium). A subset of the subserosal category is the **pedunculated leiomyoma**, which remains connected to the uterus by a stalk. Most leiomyomata initially develop from within the myometrium as intramural leiomyomata. About 5% of uterine myomas originate from the cervix. Rarely, leiomyomata may occur without evidence of a uterine origin in places such as the broad ligament and peritoneal cavity. Leiomyomata are considered hormonally responsive, benign tumors, because estrogen may induce their rapid growth in high-estrogen states, such as pregnancy. In contrast, menopause generally causes cessation of tumor growth and even some atrophy. Estrogen may work by stimulating the production of progesterone receptors in the myometrium. In turn, progesterone binding to these sites stimulates the production of several growth factors, causing the growth of myomas. Although exact mechanisms are unknown, chromosomal translocations/deletions, peptide growth factor, and epidermal growth factor are implicated as potential pathogenic factors of leiomyomata. Sensitive DNA studies suggest that each myoma arises from a single smooth muscle cell and that, in many cases, the smooth muscle cell is vascular in origin.

The uterine smooth muscle may also develop a rare cancer, such as **leiomyosarcoma**. These are not thought to represent "degeneration" of a fibroid, but, rather, a new neoplasm. Uterine malignancy is more typical in postmenopausal patients who present with rapidly enlarging uterine masses, postmenopausal bleeding, unusual vaginal discharge, and pelvic pain. An enlarging uterine mass in a postmenopausal patient should be evaluated with considerably more concern for malignancy than one found in a younger woman. These heterologous, mixed tumors contain other sarcomatous tissue elements not necessarily found only in the uterus (see Chapter 49).

SYMPTOMS

Bleeding is the most common presenting symptom in uterine fibroids; many fibroids are found incidentally. Although the kind of abnormal bleeding may vary, the most common presentation includes the development of progressively heavier menstrual flow that lasts longer than the normal duration (**menorrhagia**, defined as menstrual blood loss of >80 mL). This bleeding may result from significant distortion of the endometrial cavity by the underlying tumor. Three generally accepted but unproven mechanisms for increased bleeding include the following:

1. Alteration of normal myometrial contractile function in the small artery and arteriolar blood supply underlying the endometrium
2. Inability of the overlying endometrium to respond to the normal estrogen/progesterone menstrual phases, which contributes to incomplete sloughing of the endometrium
3. Pressure necrosis of the overlying endometrial bed, which exposes vascular surfaces that bleed in excess of that normally found with endometrial sloughing.

Characteristically, the best example of leiomyoma contributing to this bleeding pattern is the so-called **submucous leiomyoma**. In this variant, most of the distortion created by the smooth muscle tumor projects toward the endometrial cavity, rather than toward the serosal surface of the uterus. Enlarging intramural fibroids likewise may contribute to excessive bleeding if they become large enough to significantly distort the endometrial cavity.

Blood loss from this type of menstrual bleeding may be heavy enough to contribute to chronic **iron-deficiency anemia** and, rarely, to profound acute blood loss. The occurrence of isolated submucous (subendometrial) leiomyomata is unusual. Commonly, these are found in association with other types of leiomyomata (Fig. 48.1).

Another common symptom is a progressive increase in "pelvic pressure." This may be a sense of progressive pelvic fullness, "something pressing down," or the sensation of a pelvic mass. Most commonly, this is caused by slowly enlarging myomas, which, on occasion, may attain a massive size. These leiomyomata are most easily palpated on bimanual or abdominal examination and contribute to a characteristic "lumpy-bumpy,"

or cobblestone, sensation when multiple myomas are present. Occasionally, these large myomas present as a large asymptomatic pelvic or even abdominopelvic mass. Such large leiomyomata may cause an uncommon but significant clinical problem: pressure on the ureters as they traverse the pelvic brim leading to **hydroureter** (dilation of the ureter) and possibly **hydronephrosis** (dilation of the renal pelvis and calyces). These conditions can also occur if fibroids lower within the pelvis grow laterally between the leaves of the broad ligament. Occasionally, large fibroids can cause urinary symptoms or problems with defecation.

Another presentation is the onset of **secondary dysmenorrhea**. Other pain symptoms, although rare, may be the result of rapid enlargement of a leiomyoma. This can result in areas of tissue necrosis or areas of subnecrotic vascular ischemia, which contribute to alteration in myometrial response to prostaglandins similar to the mechanism described for primary dysmenorrhea. Occasionally, torsion of a pedunculated myoma can occur, resulting in acute pain. Dull, intermittent, low midline cramping (labor-like) pain is the clinical presentation when a submucous (subendometrial) myoma becomes pedunculated and progressively prolapses through the internal os of the cervix.

DIAGNOSIS

The diagnosis of fibroids is usually based on physical examination or imaging studies. Often the diagnosis is incidental to pathologic assessment of a uterine specimen removed for other indications. On abdominopelvic examination, uterine leiomyomata usually present as a large, midline, irregular-contoured mobile pelvic mass with a characteristic "hard feel" or solid quality. The degree of enlargement is usually stated in terms ("weeks size") that are used to estimate equivalent gestational size.

The fibroid uterus is described separately from any adnexal disease, although, on occasion, a pedunculated myoma may be difficult to distinguish from a solid adnexal mass. Pelvic ultrasound may be used for confirmation of uterine myomas. There may be areas of acoustic "shadowing" amid otherwise normal myometrial patterns, and there may be a distorted endometrial stripe. Often, a round mass is identified within the myometrium. Occasionally, cystic components may be seen as hypoechogenic areas and are consistent in appearance with myomas undergoing degeneration. Adnexal structures, including the ovaries, are usually identifiable separately from these masses.

Computerized axial tomography and magnetic resonance imaging (MRI) may be useful in evaluating extremely large myomas when ultrasonography may not characterize a large myoma well. Hysteroscopy, hysterosalpingography, and saline infusion ultrasonography are the best techniques for identifying intrauterine lesions such as submucosal myomata and polyps. An indirect appreciation for uterine enlargement may be gained by uterine sounding, which may be done as part of an endometrial biopsy. If a patient has irregular uterine bleeding and endometrial carcinoma is a consideration, endometrial sampling is useful to evaluate for this possibility, independent of the presence of myomas.

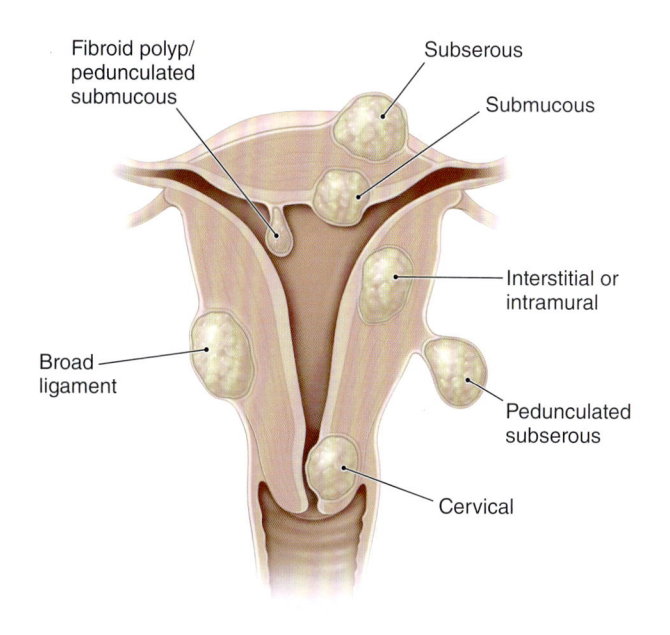

FIGURE 48.1. Common types of leiomyomata.

Hysteroscopy may be used to evaluate the enlarged uterus by directly visualizing the endometrial cavity. The increased size of the cavity can be documented, and submucous fibroids can be visualized and removed. Although the efficacy of hysteroscopic resection (removal) of submucous myomas has been documented, long-term follow-up suggests that up to 20% of patients require additional treatment during the subsequent 10 years.

Surgical evaluation may be required when physical examination and ultrasound cannot differentiate whether the patient has a leiomyomata or other potentially more serious disease such as adnexal neoplasia. Laparoscopic resection of subserosal or intramural myoma has gained in popularity, although the long-term benefit of this procedure has not been well established.

TREATMENT

Treatment is generally first directed toward the symptoms caused by the myomas. If this approach fails (or there are other indications present), surgical or other extirpative procedures may be considered.

For example, if a patient presents with menstrual aberrations that are attributable to the myomas, specifically bleeding that is not heavy enough to cause her significant hygiene or lifestyle problems and that is not contributing to iron-deficiency anemia, reassurance and observation may be all that are necessary. Further uterine growth may be assessed by repeat pelvic examinations or serial pelvic ultrasonography.

Medical Treatment

An attempt may be made to minimize uterine bleeding by using intermittent **progestin supplementation** and/or prostaglandin synthetase inhibitors, which decrease the amount of secondary dysmenorrhea and amount of menstrual flow. Iron supplementation should be considered if the patient is anemic. If significant endometrial cavity distortion is caused by intramural or submucous myomas, hormonal supplementation may be ineffective. If effective, this conservative approach can potentially be used until the time of menopause. Progestin can be delivered in the form of oral contraceptives, the levonorgestrel intrauterine system, progestin injections, or pills. Nonsteroidal anti-inflammatory drugs and, more recently, antifibrinolytic agents, such as tranexamic acid, have been used to treat menorrhagia, with mixed results in patients with fibroids.

Pharmacologic inhibition of estrogen secretion has been used to treat fibroids. This is particularly applicable in the perimenopausal years when women are more likely anovulatory, with relatively more endogenous estrogen. Pharmacologic removal of the ovarian estrogen source can be achieved by suppression of the hypothalamic–pituitary–ovarian axis through the use of **gonadotropin-releasing hormone agonists**, which can reduce fibroid size by as much as 40% to 60%. This treatment is commonly used before a planned hysterectomy to reduce blood loss as well as the difficulty of the procedure. It can also be used as a temporizing medical therapy until natural menopause occurs.

Therapy is generally limited to 6 months of drug treatment secondary to the risk of clinically significant bone loss during this hypoestrogenic state. Therapy can be extended beyond 6 months if hormonal add-back therapy is used concurrently to decrease the rate of bone loss. More recently, aromatase inhibitors have been used, but this treatment is not well studied.

In patients with an adequate endogenous estrogen source, this treatment does not permanently reduce the size of uterine myomas, because withdrawal of the medication predictably results in regrowth of the myomas. Although less successful, other pharmacologic agents such as **danazol** have historically also been used as medical treatment for myomas by reducing endogenous production of ovarian estrogen. It is important to address the multiple side effects associated with danazol with patients prior to use.

Surgical Treatment

Of the surgical options available, **myomectomy** is warranted in patients who desire to retain childbearing potential or whose fertility is compromised by the myomas, creating significant intracavitary distortion. Indications for a myomectomy include a rapidly enlarging pelvic mass, symptoms unrelieved with medical management, and enlargement of an asymptomatic myoma to the point of causing hydronephrosis. Contraindications to myomectomy include current pregnancy, advanced adnexal disease, malignancy, and the situation in which enucleation of the myomas would completely compromise the function of the uterus. Potential complications of myomectomy include excessive intraoperative blood loss; postoperative hemorrhage, infection, and pelvic adhesions; and even the need for emergency hysterectomy. Within 20 years of a myomectomy procedure, one in four women has a hysterectomy, the majority for recurrent symptomatic leiomyomas.

Although **hysterectomy** is commonly performed for uterine myomas, it should be considered as definitive treatment only in symptomatic women who have completed childbearing. Indications should be specific and well documented. Depending on the size of the fibroids and the skill of the surgeon, both myomectomy and hysterectomy can be performed using minimally invasive techniques. The ultimate decision whether to perform a hysterectomy should include an assessment of the patient's future reproductive plans as well as careful assessment of clinical factors, including the amount and timing of bleeding, the degree of enlargement of the tumors, and the associated disability for the individual patient. Asymptomatic uterine myomas alone do not necessarily warrant hysterectomy. Large asymptomatic myomas should be monitored for symptoms and size clinically.

Other Therapies

Other therapeutic modalities have been introduced, including **myolysis** (via direct procedures or by the delivery of external radio- or ultrasonic energy) and **UAE**. The safety and efficacy of UAE have been studied to the point that it is now considered a viable alternative to hysterectomy and myomectomy for selected patients. The procedure involves selective uterine artery catheterization with embolization using polyvinyl alcohol particles, which creates acute infarction of the target myomas. For maximal efficacy, bilateral uterine artery cannulation and embolization are necessary. In assessing outcomes data, the three most common symptoms of myomas—bleeding, pressure, and pain—are ameliorated in over 85% of patients. Acute postembolization pain and fever that requires hospitalization occur in approximately 10% to 15% of patients. Other complications include delayed infection and/or passage of necrotic fibroids through the cervix up to 30 days after the procedure. Occasionally, these complications necessitate hysterectomy. Although successful pregnancies have been reported after selective embolization, UAE is currently not recommended as a procedure to consider in patients who desire future childbearing.

MRI-guided focused ultrasound surgery is a new approach used to treat myomata. A focused ultrasound unit delivers sufficient ultrasound energy to a targeted point to raise the temperature to approximately 70°C. This results in coagulative necrosis and a decrease in myoma size. Treatment is associated with minimal pain and appears to improve self-reported bleeding patterns and quality of life. Multiple treatments are typically needed.

EFFECT OF LEIOMYOMATA IN PREGNANCY

Although leiomyomata may be associated with infertility, patients with leiomyoma do become pregnant. Pregnancy with small leiomyomata is usually unremarkable, with a normal antepartum course, labor, and delivery. However, women with multiple myomas or large myomas may have significantly increased rates of preterm labor, fetal growth abnormalities, malpresentation, pelvic pain, abnormal labor, cesarean delivery, and postpartum hemorrhage. Myomas may sometimes cause pain, because they can outgrow their blood supply during pregnancy, resulting in **red**, or **carneous**, **degeneration**.

Bed rest and strong analgesics are usually sufficient as treatment, although, on occasion, myomectomy may be needed. The risk of abortion or preterm labor following myomectomy during pregnancy is relatively high, so prophylactic β-adrenergic tocolytics are frequently used. Myomectomy during pregnancy should be limited to myomas with a discrete pedicle that can be clamped and easily ligated. Myomas should otherwise not be removed during the time of delivery, because bleeding may be profuse, resulting in hysterectomy. Vaginal birth after myomectomy is controversial and must be decided on a case-by-case basis. Generally, if removal of the myoma requires entry into the endometrial cavity, cesarean delivery is recommended because there is a theoretical risk of uterine rupture during a subsequent pregnancy, even at times remote from labor. Rarely, myomas are located below the fetus, in the lower uterine segment or cervix, causing a soft tissue dystocia, leading to a need for cesarean birth.

CLINICAL FOLLOW-UP

You do a physical examination and note the lump she describes. You order an ultrasound, and it demonstrates a single 7-cm fibroid over the lower anterior portion of her uterus. You counsel her about the options, and, together, you formulate a plan for myomectomy, which she undergoes without complication. Two months after surgery, her urinary patterns are back to normal.

thePoint® Visit http://thePoint.lww.com/activate for an interactive USMLE-style question bank and more!

CHAPTER 49
Cancer of the Uterine Corpus

This chapter deals primarily with APGO Educational Topic Area:

TOPIC 54 ENDOMETRIAL HYPERPLASIA AND CARCINOMA

Students should be able to outline a basic approach to the causes and diagnosis of endometrial hyperplasia or cancer, particularly in the postmenopausal patient who presents with bleeding. They should identify risk factors, common presenting signs and symptoms, and physical examination findings.

CLINICAL CASE

A 42-year-old patient comes to see you because of irregular bleeding. She reports that she has had regular menstrual cycles until 3 months ago, when she started noticing that she was having two "periods" a month. She denies any light-headedness, pain, bloating, or fever.

INTRODUCTION

Approximately 2% to 3% of women will develop uterine cancer during their lifetime. Ninety-seven percent of all uterine cancers arise from the glands of the endometrium and are known as **endometrial carcinomas**. The remaining 3% of uterine cancers arise from mesenchymal uterine components and are classified as **sarcomas**.

Endometrial carcinoma is the most common genital tract malignancy and the fourth most common cancer after breast, lung, and colorectal carcinoma. In 2013, over 50,000 new cases were diagnosed, resulting in over 8,000 deaths. Fortunately, patients with this disease usually present early in the disease course with some form of abnormal uterine bleeding (AUB), particularly postmenopausal bleeding. With early diagnosis, survival rates are excellent.

ENDOMETRIAL HYPERPLASIA

Endometrial hyperplasia is the most common precursor to endometrial adenocarcinoma. In 2015, the World Health Organization simplified the classification system of endometrial hyperplasia. Previously it was based on four types of simple and complex hyperplasia, with or without **atypia** (Table 49.1). Now there are only two types: hyperplasia without atypia and atypical hyperplasia.

Types

Hyperplasia without Atypia
Simple hyperplasia is the least significant form of endometrial hyperplasia and is not commonly associated with progression to endometrial carcinoma. In this type of hyperplasia, both glandular elements and stromal cell elements proliferate excessively. Histologically, glands vary markedly in size, from small to cystically enlarged (the hallmark of this hyperplasia). Cystic glandular hyperplasia should not be confused with a normal postmenopausal variant—cystic involution of the endometrium—which is histologically not a hyperplastic condition.

Complex hyperplasia represents an abnormal proliferation of primarily glandular elements without concomitant proliferation of stromal elements. This increased gland-to-stroma ratio gives the endometrium a "crowded" picture, frequently with glands appearing almost back-to-back. As the severity of the hyperplasia increases, the glands become more crowded and more structurally bizarre. It is thought that complex hyperplasia represents a true intraepithelial neoplastic process, and it is occasionally found coexisting with areas of endometrial adenocarcinoma.

Atypical Hyperplasia and Endometrioid Intraepithelial Neoplasia
Hyperplasia characterized by significant numbers of glandular elements that exhibit cytological atypia and disordered maturation (loss of cellular polarity, nuclear enlargement with increased nucleus-to-cytoplasm ratio, dense chromatin, and prominent nucleoli) is considered a precursor lesion to endometrial carcinoma (Fig. 49.1).

Pathophysiology and Risk Factors

The primary process central to the development of endometrial hyperplasia (and most endometrial cancer) is overgrowth

TABLE 49.1 WORLD HEALTH ORGANIZATION'S CLASSIFICATION OF ENDOMETRIAL HYPERPLASIA

New Term	Synonyms	Genetic Changes	Coexistent Invasive Endometrial Carcinoma	Progression to Invasive Carcinoma
Hyperplasia without atypia	Benign endometrial hyperplasia; simple nonatypical endometrial hyperplasia; complex nonatypical endometrial hyperplasia; simple endometrial hyperplasia without atypia; complex endometrial hyperplasia without atypia	Low level of somatic mutations in scattered glands with morphology on HE staining showing no changes	<1%	RR: 1.01–1.03
Atypical hyperplasia/endometrioid intraepithelial neoplasia	Complex atypical endometrial hyperplasia; simple atypical endometrial hyperplasia; endometrial intraepithelial neoplasia (EIN)	Many of the genetic changes typical for endometrioid endometrial cancer are present, including: microsatellite instability; PAX2 inactivation; mutation of PTEN, KRAS, and CTNNB1 (β-catenin)	25–33% 59%	RR: 14–45

Source: Emons, G., Beckmann, M.W., Schimdt, D., & Mallmann, P. and the Uterus Commission of the Gynecologic Oncology Working Group. (2015). New WHO classification of endometrial hyperplasias. *Geburtshilfe Frauenheilkd.* 2015 Feb; 75(2): 135–136. Retrieved from https://www.ncbi.nlm.nih.gov/pmc/articles/PMC4361167/table/TB877-1/ doi: 10.1055/s-0034-1396256

of the endometrium in response to excess unopposed estrogen. Sources of estrogen may be **endogenous** (ovarian; peripheral conversion of androgenic precursors) or **exogenous** (Box 49.1). Endometrial proliferation represents a normal part of the menstrual cycle and occurs during the follicular, or estrogen-dominant, phase of the cycle. With continued estrogen stimulation through either endogenous mechanisms or exogenous administration, simple endometrial proliferation will become endometrial hyperplasia. Research suggests that this transformation may be time and dose dependent. When proliferation becomes hyperplasia is not clear, although studies showing sequential change suggest it requires 6 months or longer of stimulation without progesterone opposition. The risk factors for hyperplasia and endometrial cancer are identical (Table 49.2). The risk of progression to cancer with the various forms of hyperplasia is detailed in Table 49.1. In one study, more than 42% of women with endometrial atypia had invasive endometrial cancer demonstrated when hysterectomy was performed within 3 months.

Patient History

AUB is the hallmark symptom of both endometrial hyperplasia and cancer. Further evaluation to rule out underlying carcinoma is warranted in two general scenarios: (1) any patient with AUB over age 45 years and (2) a woman with AUB ≤45 years in the presence of additional risk factors (family history of breast, colon, or gynecologic cancer; obesity; prior endometrial hyperplasia; chronic anovulation; tamoxifen use; or estrogen therapy).

Evaluation

Endometrial Evaluation

Histologic evaluation of a sample of the endometrium establishes the diagnosis of endometrial hyperplasia or carcinoma. **Endometrial biopsy** is most easily accomplished by any number of different atraumatic aspiration devices used in the office. The diagnostic accuracy of office endometrial biopsy is 90% to 98%, compared with dilation and curettage (D&C) or hysterectomy.

Routine cervical cytology is not reliable in diagnosing endometrial hyperplasia or cancer, because only 30% to 40% of patients with endometrial carcinoma have abnormal cervical cytology results. On the other hand, endometrial carcinoma must be considered, and endometrial sampling obtained, when atypical endometrial cells or atypical glandular cells of undetermined significance are found by cervical cytology.

The most common indication for endometrial sampling is abnormal bleeding. After ruling out pregnancy in premenopausal women, an adequate tissue sample can be obtained with relatively little discomfort. Further management is usually dictated by the results of the biopsy specimen. **D&C** with **hysteroscopy** and directed endometrial biopsy may be undertaken when outpatient sampling is not possible (e.g., because of a stenotic cervical os or a patient who cannot tolerate the outpatient procedure) or when the outpatient sampling has been nondiagnostic. Repeat endometrial evaluation should be considered in a patient who has normal results but recurrent bleeding.

Sometimes the office endometrial biopsy will be reported as having "insufficient tissue for diagnosis." In a postmenopausal woman who is not taking hormone therapy, this result is compatible with the normal atrophic condition of the endometrium.

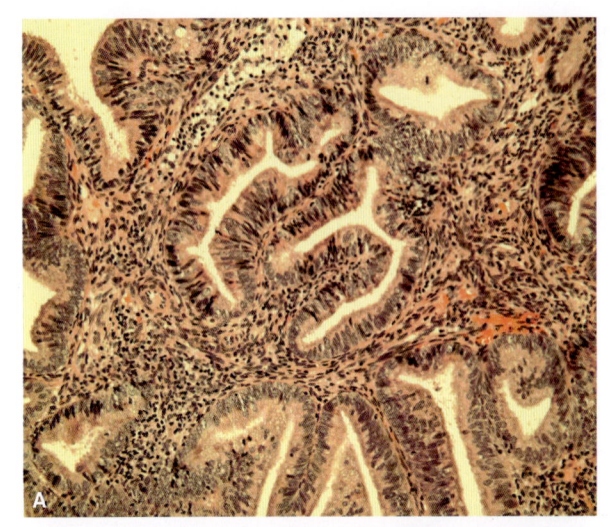

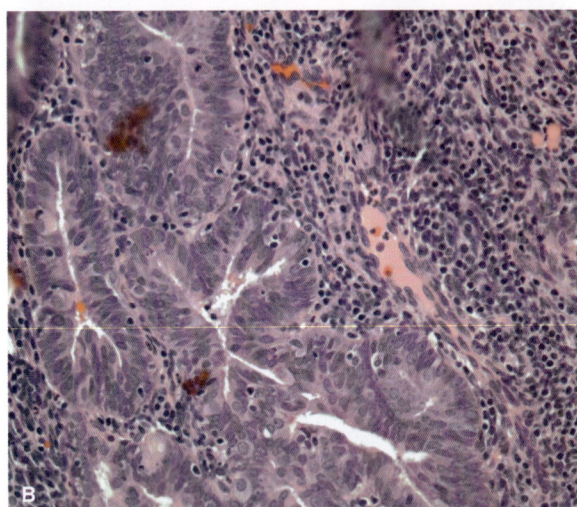

FIGURE 49.1. Complex hyperplasia with severe nuclear atypia of endometrium. (A) The proliferative endometrial glands reveal considerable crowding and papillary infoldings. The endometrial stroma, although markedly diminished, can still be recognized between the glands. (B) Higher magnification demonstrates disorderly nuclear arrangement and nuclear enlargement and irregularity. Some contain small nucleoli. (Provided by Gordana Stevanovic, MD, and Jianyu Rao, MD, Department of Pathology, UCLA; Berek JS. *Berek & Novak's Gynecology.* 14th ed. Philadelphia, PA: Lippincott Williams & Wilkins; 2007:1347, Fig. 33.1.)

In other cases, the clinical suspicion of a possible hyperplastic endometrial process may be high enough to warrant hysteroscopic evaluation with directed sampling, which allows more complete evaluation of the endometrium as well as direct visualization of polyps, myomas, and structural abnormalities (Fig. 49.2).

Ultrasound

Transvaginal ultrasound (with or without the instillation of fluid for contrast, sonohysterography) may be used as an adjunct means of evaluation for endometrial hyperplasia as well as for polyps, myomas, and structural abnormalities of the uterus. An endometrial thickness of >4 mm in a postmenopausal patient, a polypoid mass, or fluid collection is considered an indication for further evaluation and obtaining histologic samples via sonohysterography, hysteroscopy, or endometrial biopsy (Fig. 49.3). It is also useful in patients who have multiple medical problems, to help determine if the risks of endometrial sampling are less than the risk of not sampling. Multiple meta-analyses have demonstrated that the probability of endometrial cancer, though not zero, is low, approximately 1%, with an endometrial stripe thickness of 4 mm or less. The value of measuring the endometrial

---

BOX 49.1 Estrogen Sources

Endogenous
- Glandular
  - Estradiol (ovary)
  - Estrone (ovary)
- Peripheral
  - Estrone (fat, conversion of androstenedione)
- Tumor
  - Granulosa cell of ovary (an uncommon tumor and source)

Exogenous
- Conjugated estrogen (mostly estrone)
- Lyophilized estradiol
- Cutaneous patches
- Vaginal creams

TABLE 49.2 RISK FACTORS FOR ENDOMETRIAL HYPERPLASIA AND CANCER

Factors Influencing Risk	Estimated Relative Risk
Long-term use of high dosages of menopausal estrogens	10–20
Residency in North America or Northern Europe	3–18
High cumulative doses of tamoxifen	3–7
Stein-Leventhal disease or estrogen-producing tumors	>5
Obesity	2–5
Nulliparity	3
Older age	2–3
History of infertility	2–3
Late age of natural menopause	2–3
Early age of menarche	1.5–2

Adapted from the American College of Obstetricians and Gynecologists. *Management of Uterine Cancer.* ACOG Practice Bulletin # 65. Washington, DC: American College of Obstetricians and Gynecologists; 2005:2. Reaffirmed 2011.

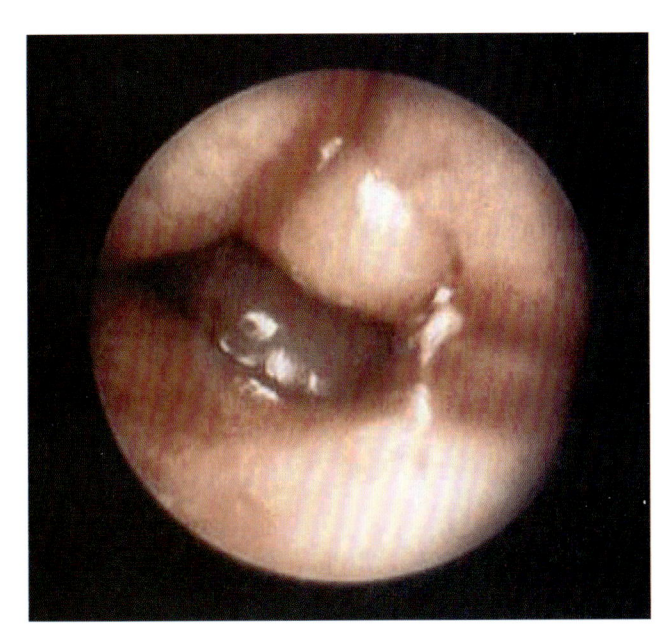

FIGURE 49.2. Diffuse hyperplasia as seen by hysteroscopy. The thickened walls of the uterus are closely opposed. (Baggish MS, Valle RF, Guedj H. *Hysteroscopy: Visual Perspectives of Uterine Anatomy, Physiology & Pathology.* 3rd ed. Philadelphia, PA: Lippincott Williams & Wilkins; 2007:233, figure 18.19.)

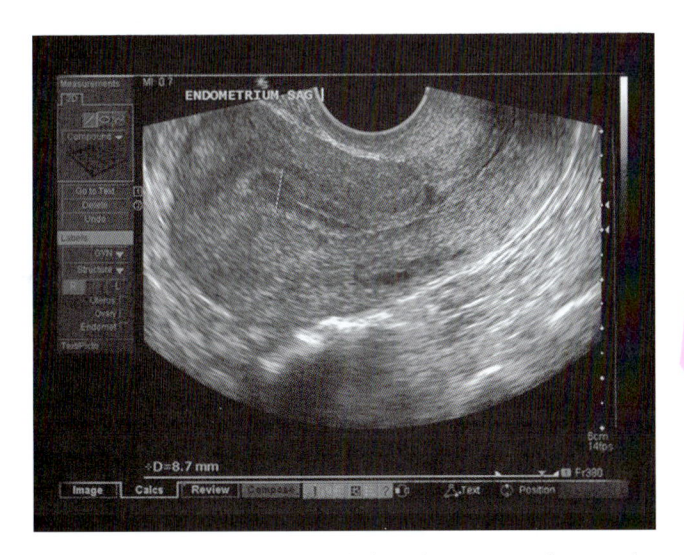

FIGURE 49.3. Endometrial stripe (calipers) as seen on ultrasound.

stripe in a premenopausal woman is less significant, given day-to-day variations throughout the menstrual cycle.

Management

The primary goals of treating endometrial hyperplasia are to reduce the risk of malignant transformation and to control the presenting symptoms.

In women with breast cancer treated with tamoxifen, the optimal manner of monitoring the endometrium is unclear. Tamoxifen acts as a weak estrogen and is associated with increased risk of endometrial hyperplasia and carcinoma. Most agree that unless the patient has been identified to be at high risk for endometrial cancer, a routine ultrasonography and endometrial biopsy in asymptomatic women are not necessary. Endometrial abnormalities should be excluded in the presence of new symptoms, such as bloody vaginal discharge, spotting, and AUB.

Medical Therapy

Synthetic progesterones or other progestins are central in the medical treatment of endometrial hyperplasia. They act through a number of pathways. First, they work to alter the enzymatic pathways, which eventually convert endogenous estradiol to weaker estrogens. Second, they decrease the number of estrogen receptors in the endometrial glandular cells, rendering them less susceptible to exogenous stimulation. Finally, the stimulation of progesterone receptors results in thinning of the endometrium and stromal decidualization. With time, this results in a decrease in endometrial glandular proliferation, which renders the endometrium atrophic.

In cases of hyperplasia without atypia, medical therapy is utilized first. The mean duration of progression from endometrial hyperplasia to carcinoma in those that do progress is relatively long: perhaps 10 years for those without atypia and 4 years for those with atypia. The most common treatment regimen is cyclic medroxyprogesterone acetate, which is administered for 10 to 14 days each month for at least 3 to 6 months. Continuous or daily administration is another alternative and may aid with compliance in patients who have an irregular cycle length. A levonorgestrel intrauterine device may also be placed for continuous progestin treatment and to improve compliance.

Beyond Medical Therapy

Many view hyperplasia with atypia as a continuum with endometrial cancer. Hence, aggressive therapy for these patients is warranted, given the increased likelihood of progression to endometrial cancer. After initial diagnosis, D&C is indicated to better sample the endometrium and exclude the possibility of a coexistent endometrial cancer. In young women who desire future fertility, long-term, high-dose progestin therapy with megestrol acetate may be used in an attempt to avoid a hysterectomy. As an alternative to oral therapy, the levonorgestrel intrauterine contraceptive has been reported to have response rates ranging from 58% to 100%. Definitive therapy by hysterectomy is recommended after a patient has completed childbearing. Patients who are treated medically for atypical hyperplasia should also be followed with periodic endometrial sampling (every 3 months after therapy), so treatment response can be monitored.

ENDOMETRIAL POLYPS

Most endometrial polyps represent focal, accentuated, benign hyperplastic processes. Their histologic architecture is characteristic and may commonly be found in association with other types of endometrial hyperplasia or even carcinoma. Polyps occur most frequently in perimenopausal or immediately postmenopausal women, when ovarian function is characterized by persistent estrogen production due to chronic anovulation. *The most common presenting symptom is abnormal bleeding.*

Small polyps may often be incidentally found as part of endometrial sampling or curettage done for evaluating AUB. Rarely, a large polyp may begin to protrude through the cervical canal. Such cases present with bleeding irregularities, and low, dull, midline pain, as the cervix is slowly dilated and effaced. In these cases, surgical removal is necessary to reduce the amount of bleeding and to prevent infection developing within the exposed endometrial surface. Less than 5% of polyps show malignant change. When they do, however, they may represent any endometrial histologic variant. Polyps in postmenopausal women or women taking tamoxifen are more likely to be associated with endometrial carcinoma than those found in reproductive-age women.

ENDOMETRIAL CANCER

Endometrial carcinoma is typically a disease of postmenopausal women. Between 5% and 10% of postmenopausal women with bleeding have endometrial cancer, with risk increasing with age beyond menopause. A majority of cases are diagnosed while in stage I (72%). Despite recognition at early stages, endometrial

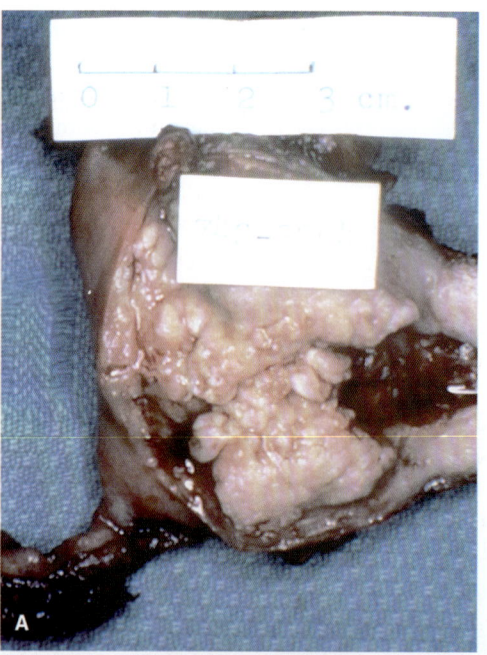

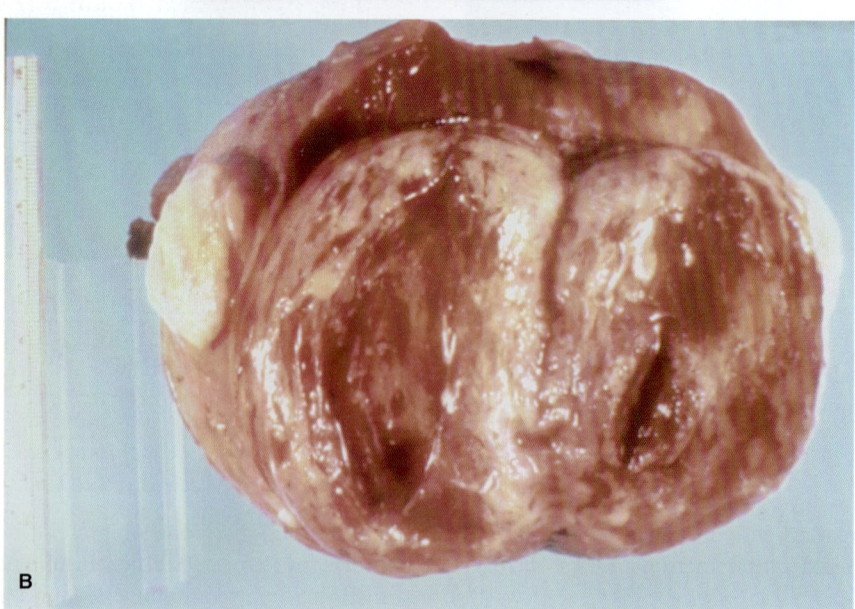

FIGURE 49.4. Types of endometrial tumors. (A) Endometrial adenocarcinoma. This polypoid exophytic tumor has invaded the outer third of the myometrium. (B) Serous carcinoma of the endometrium. The tumor is a polypoid mass arising in an atrophic uterus. Extensive myometrial lymphatic spread and involvement of the ovary are evident. (From Berek JS, Hacker NF. *Berek & Hacker's Practical Gynecologic Oncology.* 4th ed. Philadelphia: Lippincott Williams & Wilkins; 2009.)

TABLE 49.3 HISTOLOGIC TYPES OF ENDOMETRIAL CARCINOMA

Histologic Type	Histologic subtype	Discussion	Percentage
Type 1: Endometrioid	Endometrioid, endometrioid with squamous differentiation, villoglandular, secretory endometrioid	Composed of glands that resemble normal endometrial glands but that contain more solid areas, less glandular formation, and more cytologic atypia as they become less well differentiated, can exist mixed with other histologic types of tissue including squamous and villoglandular tissues	80%
Type II: Non-Endometriod	Serous, clear cell, mucinous, squamous, transitional cell, menonephric, undifferentiated	Represents many different histologic patterns, some resembling other tissue, some (clear cell) very aggressive	20%

cancer is the eighth leading site of cancer-related mortality among women in the United States.

Most primary endometrial carcinomas are **adenocarcinomas** (Fig. 49.4). Because squamous epithelium may coexist with the glandular elements in an adenocarcinoma, descriptive terms that include the squamous element may be used. In cases where the squamous element is benign and makes up less than 10% of the histologic picture, the term **adenoacanthoma** is used. Uncommonly, the squamous element may appear malignant on histologic assessment and is then referred to as **adenosquamous carcinoma**. Other descriptions, such as **clear cell carcinoma** and **papillary serous adenocarcinoma**, may be applied, depending on the histologic architecture. All of these carcinomas are considered under the general category of adenocarcinoma of the endometrium and are treated in a similar manner.

Pathogenesis and Risk Factors

Two kinds of endometrial carcinoma have been identified. Type I endometrial carcinoma is "**estrogen dependent**" and accounts for approximately 90% of cases. It is most commonly caused by an excess of estrogen unopposed by progestins. These cancers tend to have low-grade nuclear atypia, endometrioid cell types, and an overall favorable prognosis. The second type, type II or "**estrogen-independent**" endometrial carcinoma, occurs spontaneously, characteristically in thin, older postmenopausal women without unopposed estrogen excess, arising in an atrophic endometrium rather than a hyperplastic one. These cancers tend to be less differentiated, with a poorer prognosis. Estrogen-independent cancer is less common than the estrogen-dependent cancer. Unusual histologic subtypes, including papillary serous adenocarcinoma and clear cell adenocarcinoma of the endometrium, tend to be more aggressive than the more common adenocarcinoma (Table 49.3).

Endometrial carcinoma usually spreads throughout the endometrial cavity first and then begins to invade the myometrium; endocervical canal; and, eventually, the lymphatics. Hematogenous spread occurs with endometrial carcinoma more readily than in cervical cancer or ovarian cancer. Invasion of adnexal structures may occur through lymphatics or direct implantation through the fallopian tubes. After extrauterine spread to the peritoneal cavity, cancer cells may spread widely in a fashion similar to that of ovarian cancer.

As mentioned earlier, the risk factors for developing endometrial cancer are identical to those for endometrial hyperplasia (see Table 49.2).

Diagnosis

Endometrial sampling, prompted by vaginal bleeding, most frequently establishes the diagnosis of endometrial cancer. Vaginal bleeding or discharge is the only presenting complaint in 80% to 90% of women with endometrial carcinoma. In some, often older patients, cervical stenosis may sequester the blood in the uterus, with the presentation being hematometra or pyometra and a purulent vaginal discharge. In more advanced disease, pelvic discomfort or an associated sensation of pressure caused by uterine enlargement or extrauterine disease spread may accompany the complaint of vaginal bleeding or even be the presenting complaint. Between 5% and 20% of women found to have endometrial carcinoma are asymptomatic.

Special consideration should be given to the patient who presents with **postmenopausal bleeding** (i.e., bleeding that occurs after 12 months of amenorrhea in a patient who has been diagnosed as menopausal). In this group of patients, it is mandatory to assess the endometrium histologically because the risk of endometrial carcinoma is approximately 10% to 15%, although other causes are more common (Table 49.4). Other gynecologic assessments should also be made, including careful physical and pelvic examination, as well as screening cervical cytology. Preoperative measurement of the CA-125 level may be appropriate, because it is frequently elevated in women with advanced-stage disease. Elevated levels of CA-125 may assist in predicting treatment response or in posttreatment surveillance.

Prognostic Factors

The current International Federation of Gynecology and Obstetrics (FIGO) staging of endometrial cancer (adopted in 2009) lists three grades of endometrial carcinoma:

TABLE 49.4 CAUSES OF POSTMENOPAUSAL UTERINE BLEEDING

Cause	Frequency (%)
Atrophy of the endometrium	31
Endometrial cancer	7
Endometrial polyps	38
Endometrial hyperplasia	2
Other	22

Source: Data from Goodman, A. (2017). Postmenopausal uterine bleeding. UpToDate. Retrieved from https://www.uptodate.com/contents/postmenopausal-uterine-bleeding?source=search_result&search=postmenopausal%20bleeding&selectedTitle=1~75

- G1 is well-differentiated adenomatous carcinoma (less than 5% of the tumor shows a solid growth pattern).
- G2 is moderately differentiated adenomatous carcinoma with partly solid areas (6%–50% of the tumor shows a solid growth pattern).
- G3 is poorly differentiated or undifferentiated (greater than 50% of the tumor shows a solid growth pattern).

Most patients with endometrial carcinoma have G1 or G2 lesions by this classification, with 15% to 20% having undifferentiated or poorly differentiated G3 lesions.

The FIGO staging system incorporates elements correlated with prognosis and risk of recurrent disease—histologic grade, nuclear grade, depth of myometrial invasion, cervical glandular or stromal invasion, vaginal and adnexal metastasis, cytology status, disease in the pelvic and/or periaortic lymph nodes, and presence of distant metastases (Table 49.5). The single most important prognostic factor for endometrial carcinoma is **histologic grade**. Histologically, poorly differentiated or undifferentiated tumors are associated with a considerably poorer prognosis because of the likelihood of extrauterine spread through adjacent lymphatic and peritoneal fluid. **Depth of myometrial invasion** is the second most important prognostic factor. Survival rates vary widely, depending on the grade of tumor and depth of penetration into the myometrium. A patient with a G1 tumor that does not invade the myometrium has a 95% 5-year survival rate, whereas a patient with a poorly differentiated (G3) tumor with deep myometrial invasion may have a 5-year survival rate of only 20%.

Treatment

Hysterectomy is the primary treatment of endometrial cancer. The addition of complete surgical staging, which includes bilateral salpingo-oophorectomy, lymph node dissection, and peritoneal washing, is not only therapeutic but also associated with improved survival. Complete surgical staging includes pelvic washings, bilateral pelvic and periaortic lymphadenectomy, and complete resection of all disease. Sampling of the common iliac nodes, regardless of depth of penetration or histologic grade, may provide further information about the histologic grade and depth of invasion. Palpation of lymph nodes is equally inaccurate and should not be used as a substitute for surgical resection of nodal tissue for histopathology.

Exceptions to the need for surgical staging include young or perimenopausal women with G1 endometrioid adenocarcinoma associated with atypical endometrial hyperplasia and women at increased risk for mortality secondary to comorbidities. Women in the former group who desire to maintain their fertility may be treated with high-dose progestin monitored by serial endometrial sampling. Women in the latter group may be treated with vaginal hysterectomy. In ultra-high–risk surgical patients, therapeutic radiation may be used as primary treatment, although results are suboptimal.

TABLE 49.5 INTERNATIONAL FEDERATION OF GYNECOLOGY AND OBSTETRICS SURGICAL STAGING SYSTEM FOR ENDOMETRIAL CANCER

Stage	Description
Stage I: Tumor confined to the corpus uteri[a]	
IA[a]	No or less than half myometrial invasion
IB[a]	Invasion equal to or more than half of the myometrium
Stage II: Tumor invades cervical stroma, but does not extend beyond the uterus[a,b]	
Stage III: Local and/or regional spread of the tumor[a]	
IIIA[a]	Tumor invades the serosa of the corpus uteri and/or adnexa[c]
IIIB[a]	Vaginal and/or parametrial involvement[c]
IIIC[a]	Metastases to pelvic and/or para-aortic lymph nodes[c]
IIIC1[a]	Positive pelvic nodes
IIIC2[a]	Positive para-aortic lymph nodes with or without positive pelvic lymph nodes
Stage IV: Tumor invades bladder and/or bowel mucosa, and/or distant metastases[a]	
IVA[a]	Tumor invasion of bladder and/or bowel mucosa
IVB[a]	Distant metastases

[a] Either G1, G2, or G3.
[b] Endocervical glandular involvement only should be considered as Stage I and no longer as Stage II.
[c] Positive cytology has to be reported separately without changing the stage.
Modified from Figo Committee on Gynecologic Oncology. Revised FIGO Staging for Cancer of the Vulva, Cervix, and Endometrium. *Int J Gynecol Obstet,* 2009;105:3–4.

Postoperative radiation therapy should be tailored to known metastatic disease or used in cases of recurrence. In patients with surgical stage I disease, radiation therapy may reduce the risk of recurrence, but does not improve the survival. For women with positive lymph nodes (stage IIIc), radiation therapy is critical in improving survival rates. Women with intraperitoneal disease are treated with surgery, followed by systemic chemotherapy or radiation therapy or both.

Recurrent Endometrial Carcinoma

Postoperative surveillance for women who have not received radiation therapy involves speculum and rectovaginal examinations every 3 to 4 months for 2 to 3 years, and then twice a year to detect pelvic recurrent disease, particularly in the vagina. Women who have received radiation therapy have a decreased risk of vaginal recurrence as well as fewer therapeutic options to treat recurrence. Therefore, these women benefit less from frequent surveillance with cytology screening and pelvic examinations for the detection of recurrent disease.

Recurrent endometrial carcinoma occurs in about 25% of patients treated for early disease, one-half of those within 2 years, increasing to three-fourths of those within 3 to 4 years. In general, those with recurrent vaginal disease have a better prognosis than those with pelvic recurrence, who, in turn, fare better than those with distant metastatic disease (lung, abdomen, lymph nodes, liver, brain, and bone).

Recurrent estrogen-dependent or progestin-dependent cancer may respond to high-dose **progestin** therapy. A major advantage of high-dose progestin therapy is its minimal complication rate. Systemic chemotherapy may produce occasional favorable short-term results, but long-term remissions with these therapies are rare.

Hormone Therapy after Treatment for Endometrial Carcinoma

The use of **estrogen therapy** in patients previously treated for endometrial carcinoma has long been considered contraindicated because of the concern that estrogen might activate occult metastatic disease. For women with a history of endometrial carcinoma, hormone therapy can potentially be used for the same indications as for any other woman, except that the selection of appropriate candidates for estrogen treatment should be based on prognostic indicators, and the patient must be willing to assume the risk. Cautious individualized assessment of risks and benefits should, therefore, be made on a case-by-case basis.

UTERINE SARCOMA

Uterine sarcomas represent an unusual gynecologic malignancy, accounting for approximately 3% of cancers involving the body of the uterus, and only about 0.1% of all myomas. Progressive uterine enlargement occurring in the postmenopausal years should not be assumed to be the result of simple uterine leiomyomata, because appreciable endogenous ovarian estrogen secretion is absent, thereby minimizing the potential for growth of benign myomas. Even postmenopausal women on low-dose hormone therapy are not at risk for stimulation of uterine enlargement. When progressive growth is present in postmenopausal women, uterine sarcoma should be strongly considered. Other symptoms of uterine sarcoma include postmenopausal bleeding, unusual pelvic pain coupled with uterine enlargement, and an increase in unusual vaginal discharge. Surgical removal is the method of most reliable diagnosis. Accordingly, hysterectomy is usually indicated in patients with documented and, especially, progressive uterine enlargement (Fig. 49.5).

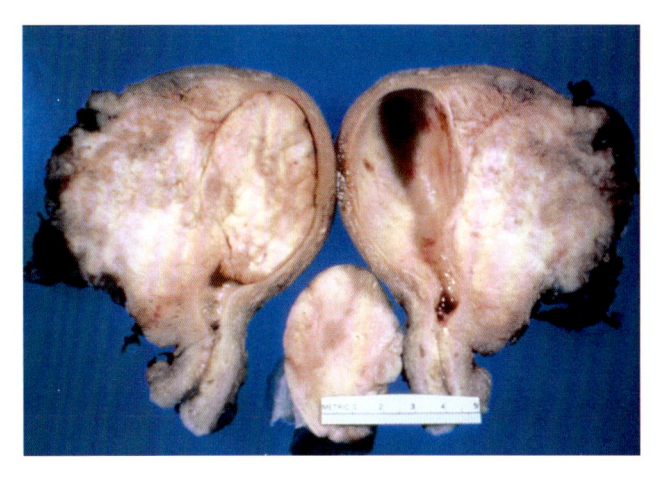

FIGURE 49.5. Uterine sarcoma. This hysterectomy specimen shows a large, partially necrotic polypoid mass filling the endometrial cavity and extensively invading the uterine wall. (From Berek JS, Hacker NF. *Berek & Hacker's Practical Gynecologic Oncology.* 4th ed. Philadelphia: Lippincott Williams & Wilkins; 2009.)

Sarcomas originate from the myometrium or the stromal components of the endometrium. There are many types of uterine sarcoma. They are histologically divided into *nonepithelial type* and *mixed epithelial–nonepithelial type*. Nonepithelial-type uterine sarcomas include **endometrial stromal sarcoma**, **undifferentiated endometrial sarcoma**, **leiomyosarcoma**, and **mixed endometrial stromal and smooth muscle tumors**. Mixed epithelial–nonepithelial tumors include **adenosarcomas**, which contain a benign epithelial component and a malignant stromal element.

The virulence of uterine sarcomas is directly related to the number of mitotic figures and degree of cellular atypia as defined histologically. These tumors are very aggressive and are more likely to spread hematogenously than endometrial adenocarcinoma. When uterine sarcoma is suspected, patients should undergo a tumor survey to assess for distant metastatic disease. At the time of hysterectomy, it is necessary to thoroughly explore the abdomen and sample commonly affected node chains, including the iliac and periaortic areas. The staging for uterine sarcoma is surgical and identical to that for endometrial adenocarcinoma.

Unfortunately, the 5-year survival of patients with a uterine sarcoma is worse than those with similar stage endometrial carcinoma. Survival ranges from 29% to 76%. Radiation and chemotherapy provide little survival advantage as adjuvant therapy to hysterectomy but can decrease recurrence rate. Adjuvant therapy in the form of hormonal antagonists and analogues, such as aromatase inhibitors, progestins, and gonadotropin-releasing hormone agonists, have demonstrated similar results.

CLINICAL FOLLOW-UP

You perform an endometrial biopsy, which demonstrates simple hyperplasia without atypia. You explain that this represents abnormal cells with a heightened potential for endometrial cancer. She opts for progesterone treatment, which she continues for 1 year. Follow-up biopsies of the endometrium are normal.

---

thePoint®   Visit **http://thePoint.lww.com/activate** for an interactive USMLE-style question bank and more!

CHAPTER 50
Ovarian and Adnexal Disease

This chapter deals primarily with APGO Educational Topic Area:

TOPIC 55 OVARIAN NEOPLASMS

Students should be able to outline a basic approach to patients with ovarian abnormalities. They should identify risk factors, common presenting signs and symptoms, and physical examination findings. They should be able to distinguish physiologic cysts, benign neoplasms, and malignant neoplasms as well as the basic three histological types of ovarian neoplasms.

CLINICAL CASE

A 26-year-old patient comes to see you because of increasing girth in her abdomen. She reports that she has been trying to lose weight and feels she has been successful except in her abdominal area. Other than this planned weight loss, she denies any other symptoms. On physical examination, the abdomen is soft and nontender, but you feel an unusual amount of fluctuance. A computed tomography (CT) of the abdomen demonstrates a 22-cm fluid-filled mass.

INTRODUCTION

The area between the lateral pelvic wall and the cornu of the uterus is called the **adnexal space**. The structures in this space are called the adnexa and include the ovaries, fallopian tubes, upper portion of the broad ligament and mesosalpinx, and remnants of the embryonic Müllerian duct. Of these, the organs most commonly affected by disease processes are the ovaries and fallopian tubes.

DIFFERENTIAL DIAGNOSIS

Because the adnexal space is located near urinary and gastrointestinal (GI) organs, disorders of these organs may cause symptoms in the pelvic area that need to be distinguished from gynecologic disorders. The most common urologic disorders are upper and lower **urinary tract infection**, and the less common are **renal and ureteral calculi**. Even rarer are anatomic abnormalities such as a **ptotic kidney**, which may present as a solid pelvic mass. An isolated pelvic kidney may likewise present as an asymptomatic, solid, cul-de-sac mass. Acute **appendicitis** should be considered in the differential diagnosis of acute right lower-quadrant pain and tenderness. Less commonly, symptoms in the right adnexa may be related to intrinsic **inflammatory bowel disease** involving the ileocecal junction. Left-sided bowel disease involving the rectosigmoid is seen more often in older patients, as in acute or chronic diverticular disease. Because of the age of these patients and the proximity of the left ovary to the sigmoid, **sigmoid diverticular disease** is included in the differential diagnosis of a left-sided adnexal mass. Finally, left-sided pelvic pain or a mass may be related to **rectosigmoid carcinoma**. Midline disease can sometimes be related to a process involving a Meckel diverticulum or a sacral tumor. An adnexal mass can of course originate from the Fallopian tube, including hydrosalpinx and ectopic pregnancy.

EVALUATION OF OVARIAN DISEASE

A thorough pelvic examination is essential for evaluation of the ovary. Symptoms that may arise from physiologic and pathologic processes of the ovary must be correlated with physical examination findings. Also, because some ovarian conditions are asymptomatic, incidental physical examination findings may be the only information available when an evaluation begins. Interpretation of examination findings requires knowledge of the physical characteristics of the ovary during the stages of the life cycle. In the **premenarchal age group**, the ovary should not be palpable. If it is, a pathologic condition is presumed, and further evaluation is necessary.

In the **reproductive-age group**, the normal ovary is not always palpable depending on patient body mass index, history of abdominal surgery with associated scarring, size and orientation of uterus, and other factors. Other important considerations include ovarian size, shape, consistency (firm or cystic), and mobility. In reproductive-age women taking ovulation-inhibiting contraceptives, the ovaries are palpable less frequently and are smaller and more symmetric than in women who are not using these types of contraceptives.

In postmenopausal women, the ovaries are less responsive to gonadotropin secretion; therefore, their surface follicular activity diminishes over time, becoming nonpalpable in most women within 3 years of the onset of natural menopause.

Perimenopausal women are more likely to have residual functional cysts. In general, palpable ovarian enlargement in postmenopausal women should be assessed more critically than in a younger woman, because the incidence of ovarian malignant neoplasm is increased in this age group.

A significant portion of all ovarian masses in postmenopausal women are malignant, whereas in reproductive-age women less than 10% of ovarian tumors are malignant. This risk was considered so great in the past that any ovarian enlargement in a postmenopausal woman was an indication for surgical investigation, the so-called *palpable postmenopausal ovary syndrome*. With the advent of more sensitive pelvic imaging techniques to assist in diagnosis, routine removal of minimally enlarged postmenopausal ovaries is no longer recommended.

Pelvic ultrasound is the primary component of evaluation. Simple, unilocular cysts less than 10 cm in diameter confirmed by transvaginal ultrasonography are almost universally benign and may safely be followed without intervention regardless of age; however, patients should be made aware of possible complications such as ovarian torsion or cyst rupture.

Biomarkers may also be helpful. CA-125 is a serum marker that is sometimes used to help distinguish benign from malignant pelvic masses. Any CA-125 elevation in a postmenopausal woman with a pelvic mass is highly suspicious, but not diagnostic, for cancer. There are currently serum tumor marker panels that are Food and Drug Administration (FDA) approved to assess the risk of ovarian cancer in women with adnexal masses.

Finally, algorithms have been developed based on mathematical modeling to help us determine the risk of ovarian cancer using results from the previously mentioned evaluative tools. These include International Ovarian Tumor Analysis that uses ultrasound features and patient characters to determine risk.

FUNCTIONAL OVARIAN CYSTS

Functional ovarian cysts are not neoplasms but, rather, anatomic variations that arise as a result of normal ovarian function. They may present as an asymptomatic adnexal mass or become symptomatic, requiring evaluation and, possibly, treatment.

Follicular Cyst

When an ovarian follicle fails to rupture during follicular maturation, ovulation does not occur, and a **follicular cyst** may develop. This process, by definition, involves a lengthening of the follicular phase of the cycle, with resultant transient secondary amenorrhea. Follicular cysts are lined by normal granulosa cells, and the fluid contained in them is rich in estrogen.

A follicular cyst becomes clinically significant if it is large enough to cause pain or if it persists beyond one menstrual interval. For poorly understood reasons, the granulosa cells lining the follicular cyst persist through the time when ovulation should have occurred and continue to enlarge through the second half of the cycle. A cyst may enlarge beyond 5 cm and continue to fill with follicular fluid from the thickened granulosa cell layer. Symptoms associated with a follicular cyst may include mild to moderate unilateral lower abdominal pain and alteration of the menstrual interval. The latter may be the result of both failed subsequent ovulation and bleeding stimulated by the large amount of estradiol produced in the follicle. This hormonal environment, along with the lack of ovulation, overstimulates the endometrium and causes irregular bleeding. Pelvic examination findings may include unilateral tenderness with a palpable, mobile, and cystic adnexal mass.

Pelvic ultrasonography can be used as an adjunct to physical examination and is often warranted in reproductive-age patients who have cysts larger than 5 cm in diameter. A benign tumor tends to appear as a unilocular simple cyst without any of the following solid components: thick septations, soft tissue elements, evidence of internal or external excrescences, and papillations (Fig. 50.1).

Most follicular cysts spontaneously resolve within 6 weeks. If a contraceptive is given to suppress gonadotropin stimulation of the cyst, it does not shrink the existing cyst, but, instead, may suppress the development of a new cyst and permit resolution of the existing problem. If the presumed functional cyst persists despite expectant management, another type of cyst or neoplasm should be suspected and further evaluated by imaging studies and/or surgery.

On occasion, rupture of a follicular cyst may cause acute pelvic pain. Because release of follicular fluid into the peritoneum produces only transient symptoms, surgical intervention is rarely necessary, and analgesics may be prescribed for short-term, symptomatic relief.

Corpus Luteum Cysts

A **corpus luteum cyst** is the other common type of functional ovarian cyst, designated a cyst rather than simply a corpus

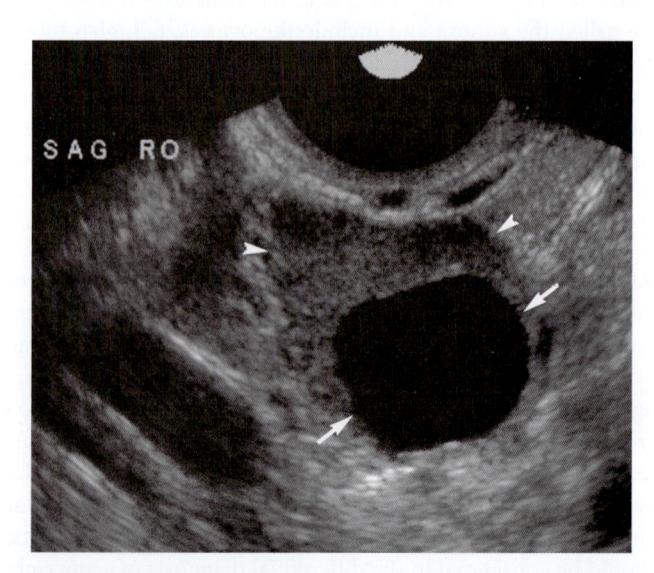

FIGURE 50.1. Sagittal ultrasonographic view of an ovarian cyst (*arrows*). Normal ovarian tissue (*arrowheads*) is seen around a portion of the cyst. (From Doubilet PM, Benson CB. *Atlas of Ultrasound in Obstetrics and Gynecology.* Philadelphia, PA: Lippincott Williams & Wilkins; 2003:304.)

luteum when its diameter exceeds approximately 3 cm. It is related to the postovulatory (i.e., progesterone-dominant) phase of the menstrual cycle. Two variations of corpus luteum cysts are encountered. The first is a slightly enlarged corpus luteum, which may continue to produce progesterone for longer than the usual 14 days. Menstruation is delayed from a few days to several weeks, although it usually occurs within 2 weeks of the missed period. Persistent corpus luteum cysts are often associated with ipsilateral dull lower-quadrant pain. This pain and occasionally a missed menstrual period are the most common complaints associated with persistent corpus luteum cysts. Pelvic examination usually discloses an enlarged, tender, cystic, or solid adnexal mass. Because of the triad of missed menstrual period, unilateral lower-quadrant pain, and adnexal enlargement, ectopic pregnancy is often considered in the differential diagnosis. A negative pregnancy test eliminates this possibility, whereas a positive pregnancy test mandates further evaluation regarding the location of the pregnancy. Patients with recurrent persistent corpus luteum cysts may benefit from cyclic oral contraceptive therapy.

A second, less common type of corpus luteum cyst is the rapidly enlarging **luteal-phase cyst** into which there is spontaneous hemorrhage. Sometimes called the **corpus hemorrhagicum**, this hemorrhagic corpus luteum cyst may rupture late in the luteal phase. A typical patient would be one not using oral contraceptives, with regular periods, who presents with acute pain late in the luteal phase. Some patients present with evidence of hemoperitoneum as well as hypovolemia and require surgical resection of the bleeding cyst. In others, the acute pain and blood loss are self-limited. These patients may be managed with mild analgesics and reassurance. Patients at risk for repetitive hemorrhagic corpus luteum cysts include those who are taking anticoagulation medication and those who have a clotting disorder. This clinical presentation may be the genesis of a coagulopathy investigation.

Theca Lutein Cyst

The third type of functional cyst is the least common, the **theca lutein cyst**, which is associated with pregnancy. Usually bilateral, they are most common in multiple gestations, trophoblastic disease, and ovulation induction with clomiphene and human menopausal gonadotropin/human chorionic gonadotropin (hCG). They may not only become large and multicystic but also regress spontaneously in most cases without intervention.

BENIGN OVARIAN NEOPLASMS

Although most ovarian enlargements in the reproductive-age group are functional cysts, about 25% prove to be **nonfunctional ovarian neoplasms**. In the reproductive-age group, 90% of these neoplasms are benign, whereas the risk of malignancy rises to approximately 25% when postmenopausal patients are also included. Thus, ovarian masses in older patients and in reproductive-age patients that show no response to expectant management are of special concern. Unfortunately, unless the mass is particularly large or becomes symptomatic, these masses may remain undetected. Ovarian neoplasms are usually categorized by the cell type of origin:

- **Epithelial cell tumors**, the largest class of ovarian neoplasm
- **Germ cell tumors**, the most common ovarian neoplasm in reproductive-age women, the benign cystic teratoma or dermoid
- **Stromal cell tumors**, some of the rarer types
- The classification of ovarian tumors by cell line of origin is presented in Box 50.1.

Benign Epithelial Cell Neoplasms

The exact cell source for the development of **epithelial cell tumors** of the ovary is unclear; however, the cells are characteristic of typical glandular epithelial cells. Evidence exists to suggest that these cells are derived from mesothelial cells lining the peritoneal cavity. Because the Müllerian duct–derived tissue becomes the female genital tract by differentiation of the mesothelium from the gonadal ridge, it is hypothesized that these tissues are also capable of differentiating into glandular tissue. The more common epithelial tumors of the ovary are grouped into serous, mucinous, and endometrioid neoplasms, as shown in Box 50.2.

The most common epithelial cell neoplasm is **serous cystadenoma** (Fig. 50.2). Seventy percent of serous tumors are benign; approximately 10% have intraepithelial cellular characteristics, which suggest that they are of **low malignant potential**, and the

---

BOX 50.1 **Histologic Classification of All Ovarian Neoplasms**

From Coelomic Epithelium (epithelial)
- Serous
- Mucinous
- Endometrioid
- Brenner

From Gonadal Stroma
- Granulosa theca
- Sertoli-Leydig (arrhenoblastoma)
- Lipid cell fibroma

From Germ Cell
- Dysgerminoma
- Teratoma
- Endodermal sinus (yolk sac)
- Choriocarcinoma

Miscellaneous Cell Line Sources
- Lymphoma
- Sarcoma
- Metastatic
  - Colorectal
  - Breast
  - Endometrial

BOX 50.2 Histologic Classification of the Common Epithelial Tumors of the Ovary

Serous Tumors
- Serous cystadenomas
- Serous cystadenomas with proliferating activity of the epithelial cells and nuclear abnormalities but with no infiltrative destructive growth (low potential malignancy)
- Serous cystadenocarcinoma

Mucinous Tumors
- Mucinous cystadenomas
- Mucinous cystadenomas with proliferating activity of the epithelial cells and nuclear abnormalities but with no infiltrative destructive growth (low potential malignancy)
- Mucinous cystadenocarcinoma

Endometrioid Tumors (similar to adenocarcinomas in the endometrium)
- Endometrioid benign cysts
- Endometrioid tumors with proliferating activity of the epithelial cells and nuclear abnormalities but with no infiltrative destructive growth (low potential malignancy)

Other
- Brenner tumor (transitional cell)
- Carcinosarcoma
- Undifferentiated carcinoma

---

remaining 20% are frankly malignant by both histologic criteria and clinical behavior.

Treatment of serous tumors is surgical, because of the relatively high rate of malignancy. In the younger patient with smaller tumors, ovarian cystectomy may be attempted to minimize the amount of ovarian tissue removed. For large, unilateral serous tumors in young patients, unilateral oophorectomy with preservation of the contralateral ovary is indicated to maintain fertility.

In patients past reproductive age, bilateral oophorectomy along with hysterectomy may be indicated, not only because of the chance of future malignancy but also because of the increased risk of a coexistent serous tumor in the contralateral ovary.

The **mucinous cystadenoma** is the second most common epithelial cell tumor of the ovary. The malignancy rate of 15% is lower than that for serous tumors. These cystic tumors can become quite large, sometimes filling the entire pelvis and extending into the abdominal cavity (Fig. 50.3). Ultrasound assessment will often reveal multilocular septations. Surgery is the treatment of choice.

A third type of benign epithelial neoplasm is **endometrioid tumor**. Most benign endometrioid tumors take the form of endometriomas, which are cysts lined by well-differentiated, endometrial-like glandular tissue. For further discussion of this neoplasm, see Section "Malignant Ovarian Neoplasms" later in the chapter.

Brenner cell tumor is an uncommon benign epithelial cell tumor of the ovary. This tumor is usually described as a solid ovarian tumor because of the large amount of stroma and fibrotic tissue that surrounds the epithelial cells. It is more common in older women, and occasionally occurs in association with mucinous tumors of the ovary. When discovered as an isolated tumor of the ovary, it is relatively small compared with the large size often attained by the serous and especially by the mucinous cystadenomas. It is rarely malignant.

Benign Germ Cell Neoplasms

Germ cell tumors are derived from the primary germ cells. They arise in the ovary and may contain relatively differentiated structures, such as the hair and bone. The most common tumor found in women of all ages is **benign cystic teratoma**, also called a **dermoid cyst** or **dermoid** (Fig. 50.4). Eighty percent occur during the reproductive years, with a median age of occurrence of 30 years. In children and adolescents, mature cystic teratomas account for about one-half of benign ovarian neoplasms. Dermoids may contain differentiated tissue from all three embryonic germ layers (i.e., ectoderm, mesoderm, and endoderm). The most common elements found are of ectodermal origin, primarily squamous cell tissue such as skin appendages (e.g., sweat, sebaceous glands) with associated hair follicles

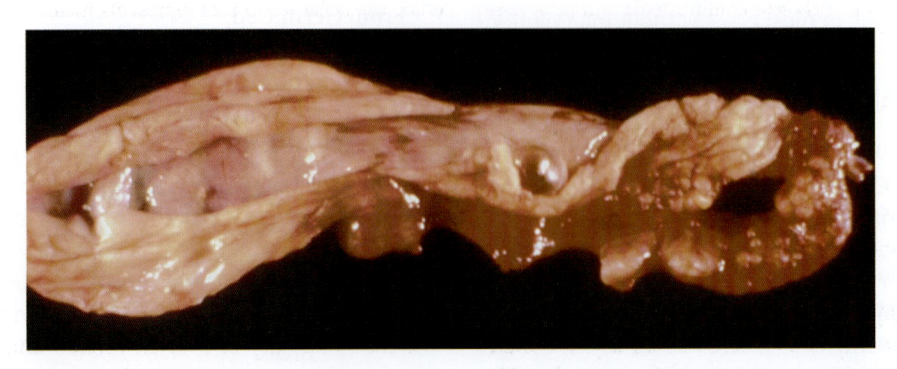

FIGURE 50.2. Serous cystadenoma of the ovary. This unilocular cyst has a smooth lining, microscopically resembling the fallopian tube epithelium. (From Berek JS, Hacker NF. *Berek & Hacker's Practical Gynecologic Oncology*. 4th ed. Philadelphia: Lippincott Williams & Wilkins; 2000.)

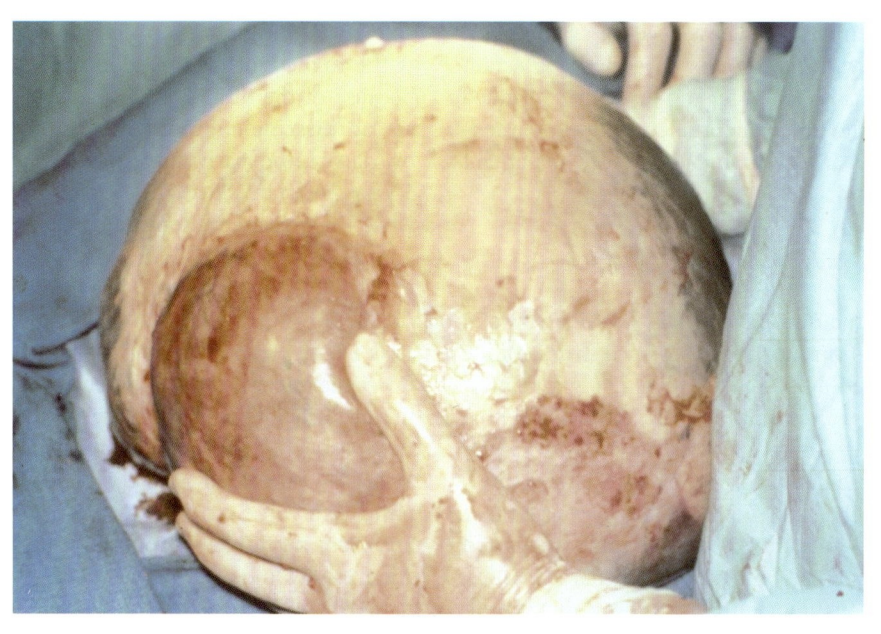

FIGURE 50.3. Mucinous cystadenoma. This cyst is extremely large and fills the entire pelvic cavity. (From Berek JS, Hacker NF. *Berek & Hacker's Practical Gynecologic Oncology.* 4th ed. Philadelphia: Lippincott Williams & Wilkins; 2000.)

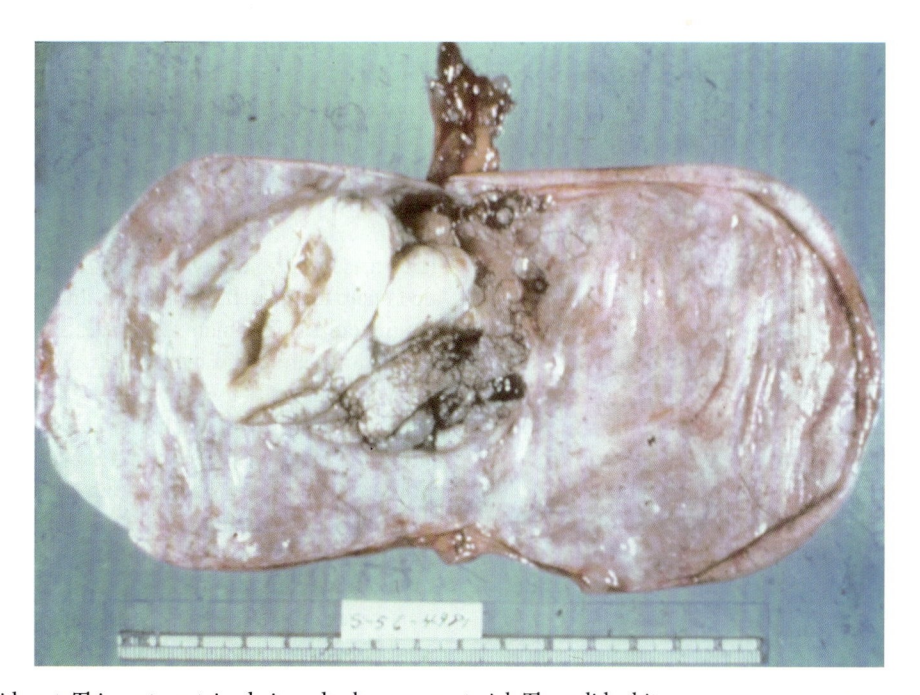

FIGURE 50.4. Dermoid cyst. This cyst contains hair and sebaceous material. The solid white area represents mature cartilage. (From Berek JS, Hacker NF. *Berek & Hacker's Practical Gynecologic Oncology.* 4th ed. Philadelphia: Lippincott Williams & Wilkins; 2000.)

and sebum. It is because of this predominance of dermoid derivatives that the term "dermoid" is used. Other constituents of dermoids include central nervous system tissue, cartilage, bone, teeth, and intestinal glandular elements, most of which are found in well-differentiated form. One unusual variant is *struma ovarii*, in which functioning thyroid tissue is found.

A dermoid is frequently encountered as an asymptomatic, unilateral adnexal mass that is mobile and nontender. This tumor often has a high fat content that makes it more readily identified by CT evaluation, as well as giving it a more buoyant tendency in the pelvis, resulting in a relatively high rate of ovarian torsion (15%) in comparison with other types of neoplasms.

Treatment of dermoids depends on size, patient symptoms, surgical risk, and suspicion of malignancy. The rate of malignancy is low, but surgical removal should be considered because of the possibility of ovarian torsion and rupture, resulting in intense chemical peritonitis due to the sebaceous contents and the subsequent surgical emergency. Between 10% and 20% of these cysts are bilateral, underscoring the need for examination of the contralateral ovary at the time of surgery. If expectant management is chosen, then close follow-up with continued ultrasound monitoring should be undertaken, with close attention to increase in size or development of more malignant appearing radiologic characteristics.

Benign Stromal Cell Neoplasms

Stromal cell tumors of the ovary are usually considered solid tumors and are derived from specialized sex cord stroma of the developing gonad. These tumors may develop along a primarily female cell type into **granulosa theca cell tumors**, or into a primarily male gonadal type of tissue, known as **Sertoli-Leydig cell tumors**. Both of these tumors are referred to as "functioning tumors" because of their hormone production. Granulosa theca cell tumors primarily produce estrogenic components and may be manifest in patients through feminizing characteristics, whereas Sertoli-Leydig cell tumors produce androgenic components, which may contribute to hirsutism or virilization. These neoplasms occur with approximately equal frequency in all age groups, including pediatric patients. When the granulosa cell tumor occurs in the pediatric age group, it may contribute to signs and symptoms of precocious puberty, including precocious thelarche and vaginal bleeding. Vaginal bleeding may also occur when this tumor develops in the postmenopausal years. Both granulosa cell tumor and the Sertoli-Leydig cell tumor have malignant potential, as discussed later.

The **ovarian fibroma** is the result of collagen production by spindle cells. These tumors account for 4% of ovarian tumors and are most common during middle age. It is unlike other stromal cell tumors in that it does not secrete sex steroids. It is usually a small, solid tumor with a smooth surface and is occasionally clinically misleading because ascites are present. The combination of benign ovarian fibroma coupled with ascites and right pleural effusion has historically been referred to as **Meigs syndrome**.

Key Points

The following are the key points that can be made regarding benign ovarian neoplasms:

- They are more common than malignant tumors of the ovary in all age groups.
- The risk of malignant transformation increases with increasing age.
- Surgical treatment should be considered if there is high potential for malignancy or torsion.
- Preoperative assessment with pelvic imaging techniques such as ultrasound is necessary.
- Surgical treatment may be conservative for benign tumors, especially if future reproduction is desired.

● MALIGNANT OVARIAN NEOPLASMS

Ovarian cancer is the fifth most common cause of cancer death in women in the United States (following, in order, lung, breast, colorectal, and pancreatic). The mortality rate of this disease is the highest of all the gynecologic malignancies, primarily because of the difficulty in detecting the disease before widespread dissemination. Of the estimated 22,400 new cases of ovarian cancer yearly, approximately 50% to 65% will die within 5 years. About 65% to 70% are diagnosed at an advanced state when the 5-year survival rate is approximately 20%.

Clinical Presentation

Risk Factors and Early Symptoms

Ovarian cancer presents most commonly in the fifth and sixth decades of life. The incidence of ovarian cancer in Western European countries and in the United States is higher, with a five- to sevenfold greater incidence than the age-matched populations in East Asia. In the United States, White women are 250% more likely to develop ovarian cancer than African American women.

Symptoms of ovarian cancer are often confused with benign conditions or interpreted as part of the aging process, with the final diagnosis often delayed. The most common symptoms are abdominal bloating or distension, abdominal or pelvic pain, decreased energy or lethargy, early satiety, and urinary urgency. Usually these symptoms occurred more frequently and were more severe than in patients without cancer. Because no clinically applicable screening test is available, approximately two-thirds of patients with ovarian cancer have advanced disease at the time of diagnosis.

The risk of a woman developing ovarian cancer during her lifetime is approximately 1 in 70. The risk increases with age until approximately 70 years. In addition to age, the epidemiologic factors associated with development of ovarian cancer include nulliparity, primary infertility, and endometriosis. Approximately 8% to 13% of cases of ovarian cancer are caused by inherited mutations in the cancer susceptibility genes *BRCA1* and *BRCA2*. The risk of ovarian cancer through age 70 years for women with Lynch syndrome is estimated to be 5% to 10%, compared with approximately 1% in the general population.

Long-term suppression of ovulation may protect against the development of ovarian cancer, at least for epithelial cell tumors. It has been suggested that the so-called *incessant ovulation* may predispose to neoplastic transformation of the epithelial cell surfaces of the ovary. Five years of cumulative suppression of ovulation through the use of oral contraceptives appears to decrease the lifetime risk of ovarian cancer by one-half. No evidence exists to implicate the use of postmenopausal hormone therapy in the development of ovarian cancer.

Pathogenesis and Diagnosis

Malignant ovarian epithelial cell tumors spread primarily by direct extension within the peritoneal cavity as a result of direct cell sloughing from the ovarian surface. This process explains the widespread peritoneal dissemination at the time of diagnosis, even with relatively small primary ovarian lesions. Although epithelial cell ovarian cancers also spread by lymphatic and bloodborne routes, their direct extension into the virtually unlimited space of the peritoneal cavity is the primary basis for their late clinical presentation.

Currently, it appears that the best way to detect early ovarian cancer is for both the patient and her clinician to be aware of early warning signs (Box 50.3). These signs should not be ignored in postmenopausal women (median age at diagnosis is 63 years).

The early diagnosis of ovarian cancer in the symptomatic patient is made even more difficult by the lack of effective screening tests. Neither pelvic ultrasound nor CA-125 should be routinely used to screen for ovarian cancer. CA-125 should be used primarily to follow response to therapy and evaluate for recurrent disease. CA-125 can also be used to evaluate the presence of ovarian cancer in selected cases:

- In premenopausal women with symptoms, a CA-125 measurement has not been shown to be useful in most circumstances, because elevated levels of CA-125 are associated with a variety of common benign conditions, including uterine leiomyomata, pelvic inflammatory disease, endometriosis, adenomyosis, pregnancy, and even menstruation. Nongynecologic conditions associated with elevated CA-125 include cirrhosis, pleural effusion, and peritoneal effusion.
- In postmenopausal women with a pelvic mass, a CA-125 measurement may be helpful in predicting a higher likelihood of a malignant tumor than a benign tumor. However, a normal CA-125 measurement alone does not rule out ovarian cancer, because up to 50% of early-stage cancers and 20% to 25% of advanced cancers are associated with normal values.

Histologic Classification and Staging

The cell type of origin, similar to their benign counterparts, is used to categorize malignant ovarian neoplasms: **malignant epithelial cell tumors**, which are the most common type; **malignant germ cell tumors**; and **malignant stromal cell tumors** (see Box 50.1). Most ovarian tumors have a histologically similar but benign counterpart (i.e., serous cystadenoma is the benign counterpart of serous cystadenocarcinoma). The relationship between a benign ovarian neoplasm and its malignant counterpart is clinically important: If a benign ovarian neoplasm is found in a patient, removal of both ovaries is considered, because there is a possibility of future malignant transformation in the remaining ovary1. The decision regarding removal of one or both ovaries, however, must be individualized based on age, type of tumor, desire for future fertility, genetic predisposition for malignancy, and the patient's concern regarding future risks.

The staging of ovarian carcinoma is based on the extent of spread of tumor and histologic evaluation of the tumor. The International Federation of Gynecology and Obstetrics classification of ovarian cancer is presented in Table 50.1.

Borderline Ovarian Tumors

Approximately 10% of seemingly benign epithelial cell tumors may contain histologic evidence of intraepithelial neoplasia, commonly referred to as borderline malignancies, or "tumors of low malignant potential" as shown in Fig. 50.5. These tumors generally remain confined to the ovary, are more common in premenopausal women (ages 30–50 years), and have good prognoses. About 20% of such tumors show spread beyond the ovary. They require carefully individualized therapy following the initial surgical resection of the primary tumor. If frozen section pathology demonstrates borderline histology, unilateral oophorectomy with a staging procedure and follow-up is appropriate, assuming the woman wishes to retain ovarian function and/or fertility and understands the risks of such conservative management.

Epithelial Cell Ovarian Carcinoma

Approximately 90% of all ovarian malignancies are of the epithelial cell type, derived from mesothelial cells. The ovary contains these cells as part of an ovarian capsule just overlying the actual stroma of the ovary. When these mesothelial cell elements are situated over developing follicles, they go through metaplastic transformation whenever ovulation occurs. Repeated ovulation is, therefore, associated with the histologic change in these cells derived from coelomic epithelium.

Malignant epithelial serous tumors (serous cystadenocarcinoma) are the most common malignant epithelial cell tumors. Approximately 50% of these cancers are thought to be derived from their benign precursors (serous cystadenoma), and as many as 30% of these tumors are bilateral at the time of clinical presentation. They are typically multiloculated and often have external excrescences on an otherwise smooth capsular surface. Calcified, laminated structures, **psammoma bodies**, are found in more than one-half of serous carcinomas.

Another epithelial cell variant that contains cells reminiscent of endocervical glandular mucous-secreting cells is the **malignant mucinous epithelial tumor (mucinous cystadenocarcinoma)**. They make up approximately one-third of all epithelial tumors, the majority of which are benign or of low malignant potential; only 5% are cancerous. These tumors have a lower rate of bilaterality and can be among the largest of ovarian tumors, often measuring more than 20 cm. They may be associated with

---

BOX 50.3 Early Warning Signs of Ovarian Cancer

- Increase in abdominal size
- Abdominal bloating
- Fatigue
- Abdominal pain
- Indigestion
- Inability to eat normally
- Urinary frequency
- Constipation
- Back pain
- Urinary incontinence of recent onset
- Unexplained weight loss

TABLE 50.1 INTERNATIONAL FEDERATION OF GYNECOLOGY AND OBSTETRICS STAGING FOR PRIMARY CARCINOMA OF THE OVARY

Stage	Description
Stage I:	Growth limited to the ovaries
IA	Growth limited to one ovary; pelvic washings contain no malignant cells; no tumor on the external surface; capsule intact
IB	Growth limited to both ovaries; pelvic washings contain no malignant cells; no tumor on the external surface; capsule intact
IC	Tumor limited to one or both ovaries
1C1	Tumor limited to one or both ovaries with surgical spill
1C2	Tumor limited to one or both ovaries with tumor on surface of one or both ovaries or with capsule ruptured
1C3	Tumor limited to one or both ovaries with pelvic washings or ascites containing malignant cells
Stage II:	Growth involving one or both ovaries with pelvic extension or primary peritoneal cancer
IIA	Extension and/or metastases to the uterus and/or tubes
IIB	Extension to other pelvic tissues
Stage III:	Tumor involving one or both ovaries with peritoneal implants outside the pelvis and/or positive retroperitoneal nodes
IIIA1	Tumor involving one or both ovaries with positive retroperitoneal lymph nodes only
IIIA2	Tumor involving one or both ovaries with microscopic metastasis outside of pelvis with or without positive retroperitoneal lymph nodes
IIIB	Tumor of one or both ovaries with histologically confirmed implants outside of pelvis with or without positive retroperitoneal lymph nodes; none exceeding 2 cm wide; extension to hepatic/splenic capsules
IIIC	Tumor of one or both ovaries with histologically confirmed implants outside of pelvis and positive retroperitoneal lymph nodes > 2 cm wide with or without positive retroperitoneal nodes; extension to hepatic/splenic capsules
Stage IV:	Growth involving one or both ovaries with distant metastasis, not peritoneal metastasis
IVA	Growth involving one or both ovaries with distant metastasis and pleural effusion containing malignant cells
IVB	Growth involving one or both ovaries with distant metastasis; with metastasis to liver, spleen, or other extra-abdominal organs

Modified Prat J; FIGO Committee on Gynecologic Oncology. Staging classification for cancer of the ovary, fallopian tube, and peritoneum. *Int J Gynecol Obstet.* 2014;124:1-5.

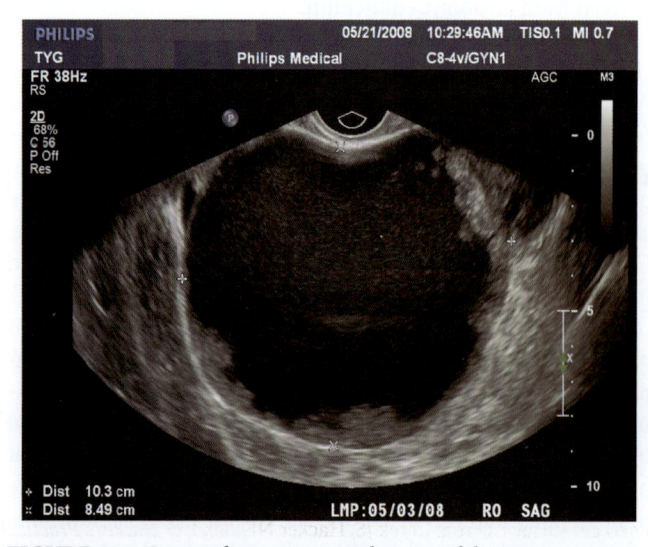

FIGURE 50.5. Low malignant potential tumor of the ovary.

widespread peritoneal extension with thick, mucinous ascites, termed **pseudomyxomatous peritonei**.

Hereditary Epithelial Ovarian Cancer

Although most epithelial carcinomas occur sporadically, a small percentage (5%–10%) occurs in familial or hereditary patterns involving first- or second-degree relatives with a history of epithelial ovarian cancer. Having a first-degree relative (i.e., mother, sister, and daughter) with an epithelial carcinoma confers a 5% lifetime risk for ovarian cancer, whereas having two first-degree relatives increases this risk to 20% to 30%. Such hereditary ovarian cancers generally present in patients at a younger age than nonhereditary tumors.

Women with **breast/ovarian familial cancer syndrome**, a combination of epithelial ovarian and breast cancers in first- and second-degree family members, are at two to three times the risk of these cancers as the general population. Women with this syndrome have an increased risk of bilaterality of breast cancer and developing ovarian tumors at a younger age. This syndrome has been associated with the *BRCA1 or BRCA2* gene mutations, which are inherited in an autosomal-dominant fashion. Women with these gene mutations have a cumulative lifetime risk of 50% to 85% for breast cancer and 15% to 45% for ovarian cancer. Women of Ashkenazi Jewish ancestry have a 1 in 40 chance of carrying this gene, a 10-fold risk over the general population.

Lynch syndrome occurs in families with first- and second-degree members with combinations of colon, ovarian, endometrial, and breast cancers. Women in families with this syndrome may have a threefold or more increased risk of ovarian cancer over the general population, with those cancers occurring at a younger age. Women in families with these syndromes should have more frequent screening tests and may benefit from risk-reducing salpingo-oophorectomy.

Endometrioid Tumors

Most **endometrioid tumors** are malignant. These tumors contain histologic features similar to those of endometrial carcinoma and are commonly found in association with endometriosis or are coincident with endometrial cancer of the uterus.

Other Epithelial Cell Ovarian Carcinomas

Of the remaining epithelial cell carcinomas of the ovary, clear cell carcinomas are thought to arise from mesonephric elements, and Brenner tumors are thought to arise rarely from their benign counterpart. Brenner tumors may occur in the same ovary that contains mucinous cystadenoma; the reason for this is unclear.

Germ Cell Tumors

Germ cell tumors are the most common ovarian cancers in women younger than 20 years. Germ cell tumors may be functional, producing hCG or α-fetoprotein (AFP), both of which can be used as tumor markers. The most common germ cell malignancies are dysgerminoma and immature teratoma. Other tumors are recognized as mixed germ cell tumors, endodermal sinus tumors, and embryonal tumors. Improved chemotherapeutic and radiation protocols have resulted in greatly improved 5-year survival rates.

Dysgerminomas are usually unilateral and are the most common type of germ cell tumor seen in patients with gonadal dysgenesis (Fig. 50.6). These tumors often arise in benign counterparts, called the *gonadoblastoma*. The tumors are particularly radiosensitive and chemosensitive.

Because of the young age of patients with dysgerminomas, removing only the involved ovary while preserving the uterus and contralateral tube and ovary may be considered if the tumor is less than approximately 10 cm and if no evidence of extraovarian spread is found. Unlike the epithelial cell tumors, these malignancies are more likely to spread by lymphatic channels, and, therefore, the pelvic and periaortic lymph nodes must be sampled at the time of surgery. If disease has spread outside the ovaries, conventional hysterectomy and bilateral salpingo-oophorectomy are necessary, usually followed by cisplatin-based chemotherapy that is used in combination with bleomycin and etoposide. The prognosis of these tumors is generally excellent. The overall 5-year survival rate for patients with dysgerminoma is 90% to 95% when the disease is limited to one ovary.

Immature teratomas are the malignant counterpart of benign cystic teratomas (dermoids). These tumors are the second most common germ cell cancer and are most often found in women younger than age 25 years. They are usually unilateral, although, on occasion, a benign counterpart may be found in the contralateral ovary. Because these tumors are rapidly growing, they may produce painful symptomatology relatively early, due to hemorrhage and necrosis. The disease is, therefore, diagnosed

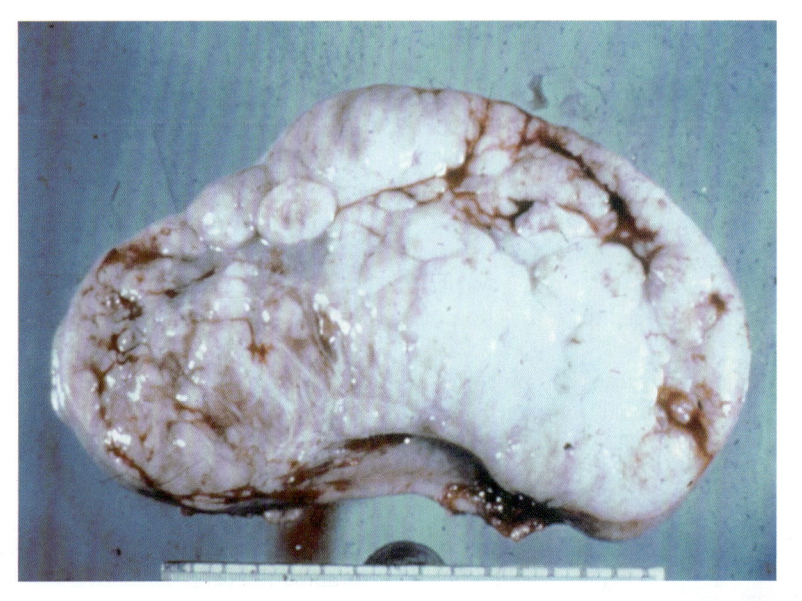

FIGURE 50.6. Dysgerminoma. This solid tumor has a gray, fleshy, and lobulated cut surface. (From Berek JS, Hacker NF. *Berek & Hacker's Practical Gynecologic Oncology.* 4th ed. Philadelphia: Lippincott Williams & Wilkins; 2009.)

when it is limited to one ovary in two-thirds of patients. As with dysgerminoma, if an immature teratoma is limited to one ovary, unilateral oophorectomy is sufficient. Treatment with chemotherapeutic agents provides a good prognosis.

Rare Germ Cell Tumors

Endodermal sinus tumors and **embryonal cell carcinomas** are uncommon malignant ovarian tumors that have had a remarkable improvement in cure rate. Previously, these tumors were almost uniformly fatal. New chemotherapeutic protocols have resulted in an overall 5-year survival rate of more than 70%. These tumors typically occur in childhood and adolescence, with the primary treatment being surgical resection of the involved ovary followed by combination chemotherapy. The endodermal sinus tumor produces AFP, whereas the embryonal cell carcinoma produces both AFP and β-hCG.

Gonadal Stromal Cell Tumors

The gonadal stromal cell tumors make up an unusual group of tumors characterized by hormone production; hence, these tumors are called **functioning tumors**. They can be both benign and malignant though malignant forms are more rare. The hormonal output from these tumors is usually in the form of female or male sex steroids or, on occasion, adrenal steroid hormones.

The **granulosa cell tumor** is the most common in this group. These tumors occur in all ages, although, in older patients, they are more likely to be benign. Granulosa cell tumors may secrete large amounts of estrogen, which, in some older women, may cause endometrial hyperplasia or endometrial carcinoma. Thus, endometrial sampling is especially important when ovarian tumors such as the granulosa tumor are estrogen producing. Surgical treatment should include removal of the uterus and both ovaries in postmenopausal women as well as in women of reproductive age who no longer wish to remain fertile. In a young woman with the lesion limited to one ovary with an intact capsule, unilateral oophorectomy with careful surgical staging may be adequate. This tumor may demonstrate recurrences up to 10 years later. This is especially true with large tumors, which have a 20% to 30% chance of late recurrence.

Sertoli-Leydig cell tumors (arrhenoblastoma) are the rare, testosterone-secreting counterparts to granulosa cell tumors. They usually occur in older patients and should be suspected in the differential diagnosis of perimenopausal or postmenopausal patients with hirsutism or virilization and an adnexal mass. Treatment for these tumors is similar to that for other ovarian malignancies in this age group and is based on extirpation of uterus and ovaries.

Other stromal cell tumors include **fibromas** and **thecomas**, which rarely demonstrate malignant potential, and their malignant counterparts, the **fibrosarcoma** and **malignant thecoma**.

Other Ovarian Cancers

Rarely, the ovary may be the site of initial manifestation of lymphoma. These tumors are usually found in association with lymphoma elsewhere, although cases have been reported of primary ovarian lymphoma. Once diagnosed, their management is similar to that of lymphoma of other origin. **Malignant mesodermal sarcomas** (**carcinosarcomas**), another rare type of ovarian tumor, usually show aggressive behavior and are diagnosed at late stages. The survival rate is poor, and the clinical experience with these tumors is limited.

Cancer Metastatic to the Ovary

Classically, the term **Krukenberg tumor** describes an ovarian tumor that is metastatic from other sites such as the GI tract and breast. Between 5% and 10% of women thought to have a primary ovarian malignancy ultimately will receive the diagnosis of a nongenital tract malignancy. Most of these tumors are characterized as infiltrative, mucinous carcinoma of predominantly **signet-ring cell type**. They are often bilateral and associated with widespread metastatic disease. On occasion, these tumors are associated with abnormal uterine bleeding or virilization, leading to the supposition that some may produce estrogens or androgens. Breast cancer metastatic to the ovary is common, with autopsy data suggesting ovarian metastasis in one-quarter of cases.

In approximately 10% of patients with cancer metastatic to the ovary, an extraovarian primary site cannot be demonstrated. In this regard, it is important to consider ovarian preservation versus prophylactic oophorectomy at the time of hysterectomy in patients who have a strong family history (i.e., first-degree relatives) of epithelial ovarian cancer, primary GI tract cancer, or breast cancer. In patients previously treated for breast or GI cancer, consideration should be given to the incidental removal of the ovaries at the time of hysterectomy, because these patients have a high predilection for the development of ovarian cancer. The prognosis for most patients with carcinoma metastatic to the ovary is generally poor.

FALLOPIAN TUBE DISEASE

Normal fallopian tubes cannot be palpated and are usually not considered in the differential diagnosis of adnexal disease in the asymptomatic patient. Common problems involving the fallopian tubes include ectopic pregnancy, salpingitis, hydrosalpinx, tubo-ovarian abscess, and endometriosis. These conditions are discussed in other chapters.

Benign Disease of the Fallopian Tube and Mesosalpinx

Paraovarian cysts develop in the mesosalpinx from vestigial Wolffian duct structures, tubal epithelium, and peritoneum inclusions. These are differentiated from paratubal cysts, which are found near the fimbriated end of the fallopian tube, are common, and are called **hydatid cysts of Morgagni**. Both are usually small and symptomatic, although, rarely, they can reach large proportions.

Carcinoma of the Fallopian Tube

Primary fallopian tube carcinoma is usually an adenocarcinoma, although other cell types, including adenosquamous carcinoma and sarcoma, are rarely reported. About two-thirds of patients with this rare gynecologic cancer (1% of gynecologic cancers) are postmenopausal. Grossly, these tumors are often rather large, resembling a hydrosalpinx, and unilateral. Microscopically, most appear like typical papillary serous cystadenocarcinomas of the ovary. The symptoms of this tumor are so minimal that the tumor is often advanced before a problem is recognized. The most common complaint associated with fallopian tube carcinoma is postmenopausal bleeding, followed by abnormal vaginal discharge. Profuse serosanguineous discharge, called **hydrotubae profluens**, is sometimes considered diagnostic of this tumor; however, other findings are watery vaginal discharge, pain, and pelvic mass.

Staging is surgical, similar to that for ovarian carcinoma (Table 50.2). Progression is similar to that of ovarian carcinoma, with intraperitoneal metastases and ascites. Because the fallopian tubes are richly permeated with lymphatic channels, periaortic and pelvic lymph node spread often occurs. Seventy percent of fallopian tube cancers present as stage I or II disease. The overall 5-year survival rate is 35% to 45%, with stage I having the most favorable rate. Too few data are available to ascertain whether adjunctive therapy is useful, and this management must be made on a case-by-case basis; however, initial management with staging and debulking is the same as for ovarian cancer treatment.

Carcinoma Metastatic to the Fallopian Tube

Carcinoma metastatic to the fallopian tube, coming mainly from the uterus and ovary, is far more common than the primary fallopian tube carcinoma. Other rare tumors of the fallopian tube include malignant mixed Müllerian tumors, primary choriocarcinoma, fibroma, and adenomatoid tumors.

TABLE 50.2 INTERNATIONAL FEDERATION OF GYNECOLOGY AND OBSTETRICS STAGING FOR PRIMARY TUBAL CARCINOMA

Stage	Description
Stage I: Growth limited to the Fallopian tubes	
IA	Growth limited to one tube; pelvic washings contain no malignant cells; no tumor on the external surface; capsule intact
IB	Growth limited to both tubes; pelvic washings contain no malignant cells; no tumor on the external surface; capsule intact
IC	Tumor limited to one or both tubes
1C1	Tumor limited to one or both tubes with surgical spill
1C2	Tumor limited to one or both tubes with tumor on surface of one or both tubes or with capsule ruptured
1C3	Tumor limited to one or both tubes with pelvic washings or ascites containing malignant cells
Stage II: Growth involving one or both tubes with pelvic extension or primary peritoneal cancer	
IIA	Extension and/or metastases to the uterus and/or ovaries
IIB	Extension to other pelvic tissues
Stage III: Tumor involving one or both tubes with peritoneal implants outside the pelvis and/or positive retroperitoneal nodes	
IIIA1	Tumor involving one or both tubes with positive retroperitoneal lymph nodes only
IIIA2	Tumor involving one or both tubes with microscopic metastasis outside of pelvis with or without positive retroperitoneal lymph nodes
IIIB	Tumor of one or both tubes with histologically confirmed implants outside of pelvis with or without positive retroperitoneal lymph nodes; none exceeding 2 cm wide; extension to hepatic/splenic capsules
IIIC	Tumor of one or both tubes with histologically confirmed implants outside of pelvis and positive retroperitoneal lymph nodes > 2 cm wide with or without positive retroperitoneal nodes; extension to hepatic/splenic capsules
Stage IV: Growth involving one or both tubes with distant metastasis, not peritoneal metastasis	
IVA	Growth involving one or both tubes with distant metastasis and pleural effusion containing malignant cells
IVB	Growth involving one or both tubes with distant metastasis; with metastasis to liver, spleen, or other extra-abdominal organs

Modified from Prat J; FIGO Committee on Gynecologic Oncology. Staging classification for cancer of the ovary, fallopian tube, and peritoneum. *Int J Gynecol Obstet.* 2014;124:1–5.

MANAGEMENT OF OVARIAN AND FALLOPIAN TUBE CANCERS

Primary surgical therapy is indicated in most of the ovarian malignancies, using the principle of **cytoreductive surgery**, or **"tumor debulking."** The rationale for cytoreductive surgery is that adjunctive radiation therapy and chemotherapy are more effective when all tumor masses are reduced to less than 1 cm in size (see Chapter 44). Because direct peritoneal seeding is the primary method of intraperitoneal spread, multiple adjacent structures commonly contain tumor, resulting in cytoreductive procedures that are often extensive. Each procedure includes the following:

1. Peritoneal cytology is obtained on entering the abdomen to assess microscopic spread of tumor. Gross ascites is aspirated and submitted for cytologic analysis or, if no ascites are found, saline irrigation is used to "wash" the peritoneal cavity in an attempt to find microscopic disease.
2. Inspection and palpation of the entire peritoneal cavity are performed to determine the extent of disease. This involves palpation of the pelvis, paracolic gutters, omentum, and upper abdomen, including the liver, spleen, and undersurface of the diaphragm.
3. Partial omentectomy is usually performed for histologic examination of the omental tissue, whether or not tumor involvement is grossly evident.
4. Sampling of the pelvic and periaortic lymph nodes is performed. Without gross disease, biopsies are obtained from the anterior and posterior cul-de-sac, right and left pelvic sidewalls, right and left pericolic gutters, and diaphragm.

Because most ovarian cancer presents at an advanced stage, adjunctive treatment using chemotherapy is usually necessary. First-line chemotherapy is with **paclitaxel** (**Taxol**) combined with **carboplatin** or **cisplatin**.

With recurrence of disease, other chemotherapeutic agents may be used, including ifosfamide, doxorubicin, topotecan, gemcitabine, etoposide, vinorelbine, docetaxel, pemetrexed, bevacizumab, cyclophosphamide, leucovorin-modulated 5-fluorouracil, and tamoxifen. **Radiation therapy** has only a limited role in the management of ovarian cancer. **Follow-up** consists of clinical history and examination, various imaging studies (ultrasound and/or CT), and in epithelial cell tumors, the use of serum tumor markers such as CA-125.

CLINICAL FOLLOW-UP

You perform an exploratory laparotomy with pelvic washings and planned excision of the tumor. It appears to originate from the ovary and is filled with 13 L of fluid. Pathology on the specimen reveals a serous cystadenoma. The patient is pleased that her abdomen is no longer so rotund and recovers well from surgery.

Appendix A
The American College of Obstetricians and Gynecologists Well-Woman Recommendations by Age Group

Annual assessments provide an excellent opportunity to counsel patients about preventive care and to provide or refer for recommended services. These assessments should include screening, evaluation and counseling, and immunizations based on age and risk factors. The interval for individual services varies. These recommendations, based on age and risk factors, serve as a framework for care that may be provided by a single physician or a team of health care professionals. The scope of services provided by obstetrician–gynecologists in the ambulatory setting will vary from practice to practice. The recommendations should serve as a guide for the obstetrician–gynecologist and others providing health care for women and should be adapted as necessary to meet patients' needs.

This information should not be construed as dictating an exclusive course of treatment or procedure to be followed.

Note: Because immunization recommendations change frequently, we direct readers to the CDC website to obtain the latest information: https://www.cdc.gov/vaccines/index.html

Ages 13–18

Screening	Laboratory and Other Tests	Evaluation and Counseling
History	*Periodic*	*Sexuality*

Screening

History
- ☐ Reason for visit
- ☐ Health status: medical/surgical, menstrual, reproductive health
- ☐ Family medical history
- ☐ Dietary/nutrition assessment
- ☐ Physical activity
- ☐ Use of medications, including complementary and alternative medicine
- ☐ Tobacco, alcohol, other drug use
- ☐ Emotional, physical, and sexual abuse
- ☐ Sexual practices (including vaginal, anal, and oral sex; sexual orientation, number of partners; contraceptive use; exchange sex for drugs or money)

Physical Examination
- ☐ Height
- ☐ Weight
- ☐ Body mass index (BMI)
- ☐ Blood pressure
- ☐ Secondary sexual characteristics (Tanner staging)
- ☐ Pelvic examination (when indicated by the medical history)
- ☐ Abdominal examination
- ☐ Additional physical examinations as clinically appropriate

For more information, see *Guidelines for Adolescent Health Care.*

Laboratory and Other Tests

Periodic
- ☐ Chlamydia and gonorrhea testing (if female is 24 years and younger and sexually active)
- ☐ HIV testing (if sexually active)—*Physicians should be aware of and follow their states' HIV screening requirements. Visit the Centers for Disease Control and Prevention for more information.*

High-Risk Groups
- ☐ Colorectal cancer screening—*Only for those with a family history of familial adenomatous polyposis or 8 years after the start of pancolitis.*
- ☐ Diabetes testing
- ☐ Genetic testing/counseling
- ☐ Hemoglobin level assessment
- ☐ Hepatitis B virus testing
- ☐ Hepatitis C virus testing (not sexually active)
- ☐ HIV testing
- ☐ Lipid profile assessment
- ☐ Sexually transmitted infection testing
- ☐ Tuberculosis skin testing

Evaluation and Counseling

Sexuality
- ☐ Development
- ☐ High-risk sexual behaviors (number of partners, exchange sex for drugs or money)
- ☐ Preventing unwanted/unintended pregnancy
- ☐ Postponing sexual involvement
- ☐ Contraceptive options, including emergency contraception, and LARC
- ☐ Sexually transmitted infections—barrier protection
- ☐ Internet/phone safety

Fitness and Nutrition
- ☐ Physical activity
- ☐ Dietary/nutrition (including eating disorders and obesity)
- ☐ Multivitamin with folic acid
- ☐ Calcium intake

Psychosocial Evaluation
- ☐ Suicide: depressive symptoms
- ☐ Interpersonal/family relationships
- ☐ Sexual orientation and gender identity
- ☐ Personal goal development
- ☐ Behavioral/learning disorders
- ☐ Emotional, physical, and sexual abuse by family or partner
- ☐ School experience
- ☐ Peer relationships
- ☐ Acquaintance rape prevention
- ☐ Bullying

Cardiovascular Risk Factors
- ☐ Family history
- ☐ Hypertension
- ☐ Dyslipidemia
- ☐ Obesity
- ☐ Diabetes mellitus
- ☐ Personal history of preeclampsia, gestational diabetes, or pregnancy-induced hypertension

Health/Risk Assessment
- ☐ Hygiene (including dental), fluoride supplementation
- ☐ Injury prevention
- ☐ Exercise and sports safety
- ☐ Weapons, including firearms
- ☐ Hearing
- ☐ Occupational hazards
- ☐ Recreational hazards
- ☐ Safe driving practices (seat belt use, no distracted driving, or driving while under the influence of substances)
- ☐ Helmet use
- ☐ Skin exposure to ultraviolet rays
- ☐ Tobacco, alcohol, other drug use
- ☐ Piercing and tattooing

Ages 19–39

Screening	Laboratory and Other Tests	Evaluation and Counseling
History	*Periodic*	*Sexuality and Reproductive Planning*
☐ Reason for visit	☐ Cervical cytology:	☐ Contraceptive options for prevention of unwanted pregnancy, including emergency contraception
☐ Health status: medical/surgical, menstrual, reproductive health	Age 21–29 years: Screen every 3 years with cytology alone	☐ Discussion of a reproductive health plan
☐ Family medical history	Age 30 years and older:	☐ High-risk behaviors
☐ Dietary/nutrition assessment	Preferred–Co-test with cytology and HPV testing every 5 years;	☐ Preconception and genetic counseling
☐ Physical activity	Option–Screen with cytology alone every 3 years	☐ Sexual function
☐ Use of complementary and alternative medicine	Age 25 years and older: the FDA-approved primary HPV screening test can be considered as an alternative to current cytology-based cervical cancer screening methods.	☐ Sexually transmitted infections—barrier protection
☐ Tobacco, alcohol, other drug use	☐ Chlamydia and gonorrhea testing (if female is 24 years and younger and sexually active)	*Fitness and Nutrition*
☐ Abuse/neglect		☐ Physical activity
☐ Sexual practices (including vaginal, anal, and oral sex; sexual orientation, number of partners; contraceptive use; exchange sex for drugs or money)	☐ Genetic testing/counseling (screening for spinal muscular atrophy, cystic fibrosis carrier, and assessment for risk of a hemoglobinopathy should be offered to all women who are considering pregnancy)	☐ Dietary/nutrition assessment (including eating disorders and obesity)
		☐ Folic acid supplementation
		☐ Calcium intake
☐ Urinary and fecal incontinence	☐ HIV testing—*Physicians should be aware of and follow their states' HIV screening requirements. Visit the Centers for Disease Control and Prevention for more information.*	*Psychosocial Evaluation*
Physical Examination		☐ Interpersonal/family relationships
☐ Height		☐ Intimate partner violence
☐ Weight	*High-Risk Groups*	☐ Acquaintance rape prevention
☐ Body mass index (BMI)	☐ Bone mineral density screening	☐ Work satisfaction
☐ Blood pressure	☐ Colorectal cancer screening	☐ Lifestyle/stress
☐ Neck: adenopathy, thyroid	☐ Diabetes testing	☐ Sleep disorders
☐ Breasts (Offer 1–3 year screening for women ages 25–39 years)	☐ Genetic testing/counseling (fragile X syndrome, Tay–Sachs disease)	*Cardiovascular Risk Factors*
☐ Abdomen	☐ Hemoglobin level assessment	☐ Family history
☐ Pelvic examination: ages 19–20 years when indicated by the medical history; age 21 or older, periodic pelvic examination	☐ Hepatitis C virus testing	☐ Hypertension
	☐ Lipid profile assessment	☐ Dyslipidemia
	☐ Mammography	☐ Obesity
	☐ Sexually transmitted infection testing	☐ Diabetes mellitus
☐ Additional physical examinations as clinically appropriate	☐ Thyroid-stimulating hormone testing	☐ Personal history of preeclampsia, gestational diabetes, or pregnancy-induced hypertension
	☐ Tuberculosis skin testing	☐ Lifestyle
		Health/Risk Assessment
		☐ Breast self-awareness (may include breast self-examination)
		☐ Chemoprophylaxis for breast cancer (for high-risk women aged 35 years or older)
		☐ Hygiene (including dental)
		☐ Injury prevention
		Exercise and sports involvement
		Firearms
		Hearing
		Occupational hazards
		Recreational hazards
		Safe driving practices (seat belt use, no distracted driving or driving while under the influence of substances)
		☐ Skin exposure to ultraviolet rays
		☐ Suicide: depressive symptoms
		☐ Tobacco, alcohol, other drug use

(Continued)

Ages 40–64

Screening	Laboratory and Other Tests	Evaluation and Counseling
History	*Periodic*	*Sexuality (Preconception and genetic counseling is appropriate for certain women in this age group.)*
☐ Reason for visit ☐ Health status: medical/surgical, menstrual, reproductive health ☐ Family medical history ☐ Dietary/nutrition assessment ☐ Physical activity ☐ Use of complementary and alternative medicine ☐ Tobacco, alcohol, other drug use ☐ Pelvic prolapse ☐ Menopausal symptoms ☐ Abuse/neglect ☐ Sexual practices (including vaginal, anal, and oral sex; sexual orientation, number of partners, contraceptive use; exchange sex for drugs or money) ☐ Urinary and fecal incontinence *Physical Examination* ☐ Height ☐ Weight ☐ Body mass index (BMI) ☐ Blood pressure ☐ Neck: adenopathy, thyroid ☐ Breasts (Offer every 1–3 years for women aged 25–39 years; May be offered annually for women 40 years and older) ☐ Abdomen ☐ Pelvic examination ☐ Additional physical examinations as clinically appropriate	☐ Colorectal cancer screening:* Beginning at age 50 years [for most women] [*Beginning at age 45 for African American women] ☐ Diabetes testing—beginning at age 45 years (If tests are normal, repeat testing carried out at a minimum of 3-year intervals is reasonable.) ☐ Genetic testing/counseling (screening for spinal muscular atrophy, cystic fibrosis carrier, and assessment for risk of hemoglobinopathy should be offered to all women who are considering pregnancy) ☐ Hepatitis C virus testing—one-time testing for persons born from 1945 through 1965 and unaware of their infection status ☐ HIV testing—Physicians should be aware of and follow their states' HIV screening requirements. Visit the Centers for Disease Control and Prevention for more information. ☐ Lipid profile assessment—every 5 years beginning at age 45 years ☐ Mammography - Annual or biennial; Offer starting at 40; Initiate at ages 40–49 years after counseling, if patient desires; Recommend no later than age 50 if patient has not already initiated. *High-Risk Groups* ☐ Bone mineral density screening ☐ Colorectal cancer screening ☐ Diabetes testing ☐ Genetic testing/counseling (fragile X syndrome, Tay-Sachs disease) ☐ Hemoglobin level assessment ☐ Lipid profile assessment ☐ Sexually transmitted infection testing ☐ Thyroid-stimulating hormone testing ☐ Tuberculosis skin testing	☐ High-risk behaviors ☐ Contraceptive options for prevention of unwanted pregnancy, including emergency contraception ☐ Sexual function ☐ Sexually transmitted infections—barrier protection *Fitness and Nutrition* ☐ Physical activity ☐ Dietary/nutrition assessment (including eating disorders and obesity) ☐ Folic acid supplementation ☐ Calcium intake *Psychosocial Evaluation* ☐ Family relationships ☐ Intimate partner violence ☐ Work satisfaction ☐ Lifestyle/stress ☐ Sleep disorders ☐ Advance directives *Cardiovascular Risk Factors* ☐ Family history ☐ Hypertension ☐ Dyslipidemia ☐ Obesity ☐ Diabetes mellitus ☐ Personal history of preeclampsia, gestational diabetes, or pregnancy-induced hypertension ☐ Lifestyle *Health/Risk Assessment* ☐ Aspirin prophylaxis to reduce the risk of stroke (ages 55–79 years)* ☐ Breast self-awareness (may include breast self-examination) ☐ Chemoprophylaxis for breast cancer (for high-risk women) ☐ Hormone therapy ☐ Hygiene (including dental) ☐ Injury prevention ☐ Exercise and sports involvement ☐ Firearms ☐ Hearing ☐ Occupational hazards ☐ Recreational hazards ☐ Safe driving practices (seat belt use, no distracted driving or driving while under the influence of substances) ☐ Sun exposure ☐ Suicide: depressive symptoms ☐ Tobacco, alcohol, other drug use *The recommendation for aspirin prophylaxis must weigh the benefits of stroke prevention against the harm of gastrointestinal bleeding. Visit the U.S. Preventive Services Task Force for more information.*

Ages 65 Years and Older

Screening	Laboratory and Other Tests	Evaluation and Counseling
History	*Colorectal Cancer Screening*	*Sexuality*
☐ Reason for visit	☐ Aged 76–85 years: screening should be made on an individual basis, taking into account the patient's overall health and prior screening history.	☐ Sexual function
☐ Health status: medical/surgical, menstrual, reproductive health		☐ Sexual behaviors
☐ Family medical history		☐ Sexually transmitted infections—barrier protection
☐ Dietary/nutrition assessment	*Periodic*	*Fitness and Nutrition*
☐ Physical activity	☐ Bone mineral density screening (*In the absence of new risk factors, screen no more frequently than every 2 years.*)	☐ Physical activity
☐ Pelvic prolapse	☐ Cervical cytology:	☐ Dietary/nutrition assessment (including eating disorders and obesity)
☐ Menopausal symptoms	Age 65: Preferred-Co-test with cytology and HPV testing every 5 years; Option–Screen with cytology alone every 3 years.	☐ Calcium intake
☐ Use of complementary and alternative medicine	Age 66 years and older: Discontinue in women with evidence of adequate negative prior screening test results and no history of CIN 2 or higher. Adequate negative prior screening test results are defined as three consecutive negative cytology results or two consecutive negative cotest results within the previous 10 years, with the most recent test performed within the past 5 years.	*Psychosocial Evaluation*
☐ Tobacco, alcohol, other drug use, and concurrent medication use		☐ Neglect/abuse
☐ Abuse/neglect		☐ Intimate partner violence
☐ Sexual practices (including vaginal, anal, and oral sex; sexual orientation; number of partners; contraceptive use; exchange sex for drugs or money)		☐ Lifestyle/stress
		☐ Depression/sleep disorders
		☐ Family relationships
	☐ Other methods include:	☐ Advance directives
☐ Urinary and fecal incontinence	1. Fecal occult blood testing or fecal immunochemical test, annual patient-collected (each method requires two or three samples of stool collected by the patient at home and returned for analysis. A single stool sample obtained by digital rectal examination is not adequate for the detection of colorectal cancer.)	*Cardiovascular Risk Factors*
Physical Examination		☐ Hypertension
☐ Height		☐ Dyslipidemia
☐ Weight		☐ Obesity
☐ Body mass index (BMI)		☐ Diabetes mellitus
☐ Blood pressure	2. Flexible sigmoidoscopy every 5 years	☐ Personal history of preeclampsia, gestational diabetes, or pregnancy-induced hypertension
☐ Neck: adenopathy, thyroid	3. Double contrast barium enema every 5 years	☐ Sedentary lifestyle
☐ Breasts (Offer annually)	4. Computed tomography colonography every 5 years	*Health/Risk Assessment*
☐ Abdomen	5. Stool DNA	☐ Aspirin prophylaxis (for women aged 79 years or younger)*
☐ Pelvic examination (*When a woman's age or other health issues are such that she would not choose to intervene on conditions detected during the routine examination, it is reasonable to discontinue pelvic exams.*)	☐ Diabetes testing (every 3 years)	☐ Breast self-awareness (may include breast self-examination)
	☐ Hepatitis C virus testing (one-time testing for persons born from 1945 through 1965 and unaware of their infection status)	☐ Chemoprophylaxis for breast cancer (for high-risk women)
	☐ Lipid profile assessment (every 5 years)	☐ Hearing
☐ Additional physical examinations as clinically appropriate	☐ Mammography (annual or biennial; begin no later than 50 if patient has not already initiated; decision to discontinue after 75 should be based on a shared decision-making process that includes a discussion of the woman's health status and longevity)	☐ Hormone therapy
		☐ Hygiene (including dental)
		☐ Injury prevention
		Exercise and sports involvement
		Firearms
		Occupational hazards
		Prevention of falls
		Recreational hazards
	☐ Thyroid-stimulating hormone testing (every 5 years)	Safe driving practices (seat belt use, no distracted driving or driving while under the influence of substances)
	☐ Urinalysis	☐ Skin exposure to ultraviolet rays
	The College supports stopping routine screening at age 75 years.	☐ Suicide: depressive symptoms
	High-Risk Groups	☐ Tobacco, alcohol, other drug use
	☐ Hemoglobin level assessment	☐ Visual acuity/glaucoma
	☐ Human immunodeficiency virus (HIV) testing	*The recommendation for aspirin prophylaxis must weigh the benefits of stroke prevention against the harm of gastrointestinal bleeding. Visit the U.S. Preventive Services Task Force for more information.*
	☐ Sexually transmitted infection testing	
	☐ Thyroid-stimulating hormone testing	
	☐ Tuberculosis skin testing	

Appendix B

The American College of Obstetricians and Gynecologists Antepartum Record and Postpartum Form

The American College of Obstetricians and Gynecologists
WOMEN'S HEALTH CARE PHYSICIANS

Patient Addressograph

Date: — —   ID #: _____

ANTEPARTUM RECORD

Hospital of Delivery: _____

Name: _____
  LAST   FIRST   MIDDLE

Newborn Care Provider:	Referred By:
Primary Care Provider/Group:	Address:
Final EDD:	
Birth Date: Age: Race: Marital Status: S M W D Sep	Address:
	Zip: Phone: (1) (2)
Occupation: Education: (Last Grade Completed)	E-Mail:
Language: Ethnicity:	Insurance Carrier/Medicaid #:
Partner: Phone:	Policy #:
Father Of Baby: Phone:	Emergency Contact: Phone:

Total Preg:	Full Term:	Premature:	Ab, Induced:	Ab, Spontaneous:	Ectopics:	Multiple Births:	Living:

Menstrual History

Lmp ☐ Definite ☐ Approximate (Month Known)   Duration: Q _____ Days   Frequency: Q _____ Days   Menarche: _____ (Age Onset)
     ☐ Unknown   ☐ Normal Amount/Duration   Prior Menses: _____ Date   Contraception ☐ Yes ☐ No   Hcg + ___/___/___
     ☐ Final: _____   at conception

Past Pregnancies (Last Five)

Date Month/Year	GA Weeks	Length Of Labor	Birth Weight	Sex M/F	Type Of Delivery	Anes	Place Of Delivery	Breastfeeding Duration	Lactation Consult Needed Yes/No	Comments/Complications

Medical History

	P*	F*	Detail Positive Remarks Include Date & Treatment		P*	F*	Detail Positive Remarks Include Date & Treatment
A. Drug/Latex Allergies/Reactions				17. Dermatologic Disorders			
B. Allergies (Food, Seasonal, Environmental)				18. Operations/Hospitalizations (Year & Reason)			
1. Neurologic/Epilepsy				19. Gyn Surgery (Year & Reason)			
2. Thyroid Dysfunction				20. Anesthetic Complications			
3. Breast Disease/Breast Surgery				21. History Of Blood Transfusions			
4. Pulmonary (TB, Asthma)				22. Infertility			
5. Heart Disease				23. Art (IVF Or FET)			
6. Hypertension				24. History of Abnormal Pap			
7. Cancer				25. History of STI			
8. Hematologic Disorders				26. Psychiatric Illness			
9. Anemia				27. Depression/Postpartum Depression			
10. Gastrointestinal Disorders				28. Trauma/Violence			Prepreg / Preg / # Years Use
11. Hepatitis/Liver Disease				29. Tobacco (Smoked, Chewed, ENDS, Vaped) (AMT/Day)			
12. Kidney Disease/UTI				30. Alcohol (AMT/Wk)			
13. Deep Vein Thrombosis				31. Drug Use (Including Opioids) (Uses/Wk)			
14. Diabetes (Type 1 Or Type 2)							
15. Gestational Diabetes				32. Polycystic Ovary Syndrome			
16. Autoimmune Disorders				33. Other			

*P= Personal F= Family

COMMENTS: _____

Version 8. Copyright 2016 The American College of Obstetricians and Gynecologists   (AA128)   12345/09876

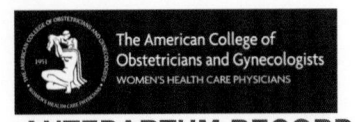

| Patient Name: | Birth Date: - - | ID No.: | Date: - - |

Genetic Screening*

Condition	Patient	Partner	Other	Relationship
Congenital Heart Defect				
Neural Tube Defect				
Hemoglobinopathy Or Carrier				
Cystic Fibrosis				
Chromosome Abnormality				
Tay–Sachs				
Hemophilia				
Intellectual Disability/Autism				
Recurrent Pregnancy Loss/Stillbirth				
Other Structural Birth Defect				
Other Genetic Disease (eg, PKU, Metabolic Disease, Muscular Dystrophy)				

Teratogen Exposures Since LMP/Conception

	Yes	No	Details/Date
Prescription Medications			
Over The Counter Medications			
Alcohol			
Illicit Drugs			
Maternal Diabetes			HGB A1C
Other			
Uterine Anomaly/DES			

*If a patient has been screened for a genetic disorder previously, the results should be documented but the test should not be repeated.

COMMENTS/COUNSELING: _____

Infection History	Yes	No		Yes	No
1. Live with Someone with TB or Exposed to TB			6. HIV Infection		
2. Patient or Partner has History of Genital Herpes			7. History Of Hepatitis		
3. Rash or Viral Illness Since Last Menstrual Period			8. Recent Travel History Outside Of Country		
4. Prior GBS-Infected Child			9. Other (See Comments)		
5. History of STIs: (Check All That Apply) ☐ Gonorrhea ☐ Chlamydia ☐ HPV ☐ Syphilis ☐ PID					

COMMENTS: _____

INTERVIEWER'S SIGNATURE: _____

Immunizations	Yes (Month/Year) ___/___	No	If No, Vaccine Indicated?*	Immunizations	Yes (Month/Year) ___/___	No	If No, Vaccine Indicated?*
TDAP (Each pregnancy; between 27–36 weeks)				Hepatitis A (When Indicated)			
Influenza† (Each pregnancy as soon as vaccine is available)				Hepatitis B (When Indicated)			
Varicella†				Meningococcal (When Indicated)			
MMR (Rubella-containing vaccine)†				Pneumococcal (When Indicated)			
HPV							

*Yes/No & date to be administered

†All live vaccines are contraindicated in pregnancy, including the live intranasal influenza, MMR, and varicella vaccines. All women who will be pregnant during influenza season (October through May) should receive inactivated influenza vaccine at any point in gestation. Administer the HPV, MMR, and varicella vaccines postpartum if needed. The Tdap vaccine can be given postpartum if the woman has never received it as an adult and did not get it during pregnancy.

Initial Physical Examination

Date: ___/___/___ BP/Prepregnancy Weight: _____ Height: _____ BMI: _____

1. Heent	Normal	Abnormal	11. Vulva	Normal	Condyloma	Lesions
2. Teeth	Normal	Abnormal	12. Vagina	Normal	Inflammation	Discharge
3. Thyroid	Normal	Abnormal	13. Cervix	Normal	Inflammation	Lesions
4. Breasts	Normal	Abnormal	14. Uterus Size	Weeks		Fibroids
5. Lungs	Normal	Abnormal	15. Adnexa	Normal	Mass	
6. Heart	Normal	Abnormal	16. Rectum	Normal	Abnormal	
7. Abdomen	Normal	Abnormal	17. Clinical Pelvimetry	Concerns	No Concerns	
8. Extremities	Normal	Abnormal				
9. Skin	Normal	Abnormal				
10. Lymph Nodes	Normal	Abnormal				

COMMENTS (Number and explain abnormals): _____

EXAM BY: _____

Version 8. Copyright 2016 The American College of Obstetricians and Gynecologists (AA128) 12345/09876

Patient Addressograph

| Patient Name: | | Birth Date: — — | ID No.: | Date: — — |

Drug Allergy: _____ Latex Allergy ☐ Yes ☐ No Postpartum Contraception Method: _____
Counseled About LARC? ☐ Yes ☐ No

Is Blood Transfusion Acceptable? ☐ Yes ☐ No   Antepartum Anesthesia Consult Planned ☐ Yes ☐ No

Problems	Plans	Resolved?
1.		
2.		
3.		
4.		
5.		

Medication List (Including Opioids)	Start Date	Stop Date
1.	— —	— —
2.	— —	— —
3.	— —	— —
4.	— —	— —
5.	— —	— —

EDD Confirmation								Pregnancy Weight Gain	
Lmp:	— —	=		= EDD	— —			Prepregnancy Weight	
Initial Exam:	— —	=	Wks	= EDD	— —			Height	
Ultrasonography:	— —	=	Wks	= EDD	— —			BMI	
Final Edd:	— —		IVF Transfer:		— —			Estimated Weight Gain	
Initialed By:								Recommended Weight Gain	

Prepregnancy Weight _____

BMI _____

Date	Weeks Gest. (Best Est.)	Weight	Blood Pressure	Urine (Albumin/Glucose)	Pain Scale* (0–10)	Fetal Movement	Preterm Labor Signs/Symptoms: +=Present ○=Absent	FHR	Fundal Height (CM)/EFW	Presentation	Edema	Cervix Examination (DIL./EFF. STA.) Length On Ultrasonography	Next Appointment	Provider (Initials)	Comments:
— —															
— —															
— —															
— —															
— —															
— —															
— —															
— —															
— —															
— —															
— —															
— —															

*Describe the intensity of discomfort ranging from 0 (no pain) to 10 (worst possible pain).

Version 8. Copyright 2016 The American College of Obstetricians and Gynecologists   (AA128)   12345/09876

Patient Addressograph

Patient Name:		Birth Date: - -	ID No.:	Date: - -

Laboratory and Screening Tests

Comments/Additional Labs

Initial Labs	Date	Result	Reviewed
Blood Type	- -	A B AB O	
D (Rh) Type	- -		
Antibody Screen	- -		
Complete Blood Count	- -	HCT/HGB: _____ % _____ g/dL MCV:_____ PLT:_____	
VDRL/RPR (Syphilis)	- -		
Urine Culture/Screen	- -		
HBsAg	- -		
HIV Testing	- -	Pos. Neg. Declined	
Chlamydia (When Indicated)	- -		
Gonorrhea (When Indicated)	- -		
Rubella Immunity	- -		
Other:			

Supplemental Labs	Date	Result	
Hemoglobin Electrophoresis	- -	AA AS SS AC	
PPD/Quanta (When Indicated)	- -		
Pap Test (When Indicated)	- -		
HPV (When Indicated)	- -		
Early Diabetes Screen (When Indicated)	- -	Pos. Neg. Declined	
Varicella Immunity (When Indicated)	- -		
Cystic Fibrosis	- -	Pos. Neg. Declined	
Spinal Muscular Atrophy	- -	Pos. Neg. Declined	
Fragile X	- -	Pos. Neg. Declined	
Tay–Sachs	- -	Pos. Neg. Declined	
Canavan Disease	- -	Pos. Neg. Declined	
Familial Dysautonomia	- -	Pos. Neg. Declined	
Genetic Screening Tests (See Form B)	- -	Pos. Neg. Declined	
Other:			

8–20-Week Aneuploidy Screening	Date Test Performed	Result	
Aneuploidy Screening Offered	- -	Accepted Declined GA Too Advanced	
1st Trimester Aneuploidy Screening	- -	Pos Neg	
2nd Trimester Serum Screening	- -	Pos Neg	
Integrated Screening	- -	Pos Neg	
Cell-Free DNA	- -	Pos Neg	
CVS	- -	Karyotype: 46,XX Or 46,XY/Other_____ Array	
Amniocentesis	- -	Karyotype: 46,XX Or 46,XY/Other_____ Array	
Amniotic Fluid (AFP)	- -	Normal Abnormal	
Other:			

(continued)

PROVIDER SIGNATURE (AS REQUIRED): _____

Version 8. Copyright 2016 The American College of Obstetricians and Gynecologists

Patient Name:	Birth Date: - -	ID No.:	Date: - -

Laboratory and Screening Tests *(continued)*

Late Pregnancy Labs and Screening	Date	Result	Reviewed
Tdap Vaccination (Every Pregnancy; 27–36 Weeks)	- -		
Complete Blood Count	- -	HCT/HGB:_____ % _____ g/dL MCV:_____ PLT:_____	
Diabetes Screen (24–28 Weeks)	- -		
GTT (If Screen Abnormal)	- -	_____Fbs _____1 Hour _____2 Hours _____3 Hours	
D (Rh) Antibody Screen (When Indicated)	- -		
Anti-D Immune Globulin (RhIg) Given (28 Wks Or Greater) (When Indicated)	- -	_____ Signature	
Complete Blood Count	- -	Hct/Hgb:_____ % _____ g/dL MCV:_____ PLT:_____	
Ultrasonography (18–24 Weeks) (When Indicated)	- -		
HIV (When Indicated)*	- -		
VDRL/RPR (Syphilis) (When Indicated)	- -		
Gonorrhea (When Indicated)	- -		
Chlamydia (When Indicated)	- -		
Group B Strep (35–37 Weeks)	- -		
Resistance Testing If Penicillin Allergic	- -		
Other:			

Comments/Additional Labs

*Check state requirements before recording results.

Comments

_____
_____
_____
_____
_____
_____
_____
_____
_____

PROVIDER SIGNATURE (AS REQUIRED): _____

Version 8. Copyright 2016 The American College of Obstetricians and Gynecologists

| Patient Name: | Birth Date: - - | ID No.: | Date: - - |

Plans/Education
By Trimester. Initial And Date When Discussed.

	NA	Date	Follow-Up Needed	Referral	Comments
First Trimester					
Psychosocial Screening					
Desire For Pregnancy		- -			
Depression / Anxiety (Should Be Performed At Least Once During Perinatal Period)		- -			
Alcohol		- -			
Tobacco (Smoked, Chewed, ENDS, Vaped) Cessation Counseling (Ask, Advise, Assess, Assist, And Arrange)		- -			
Illicit/Recreational Drugs/Substance Use (Parents, Partner, Past, Present)*		- -			
Intimate Partner Violence		- -			
Barriers To Care		- -			
Unstable Housing		- -			
Communication Barriers		- -			
Nutrition		- -			
Wic Referral		- -			
Environmental/Work Hazards		- -			
Anticipatory Guidance					
Anticipated Course Of Prenatal Care		- -			
Nutrition Counseling; Special Diet; Dietary Precautions (Mercury, Listeriosis)		- -			
Weight Gain Counseling		- -			
Toxoplasmosis Precautions (Cats/Raw Meat)		- -			
Use Of Any Medications (Including Supplements, Vitamins, Herbs, Or Otc Drugs)		- -			
Sexual Activity		- -			
Exercise		- -			
Dental Care/Refer to Dentist		- -			
Avoidance Of Saunas Or Hot Tubs		- -			
Seat Belt Use		- -			
Childbirth Classes/Hospital Facilities		- -			
Breastfeeding		- -			
Fetal Testing					
Indications For Ultrasonography		- -			
Screening For Aneuploidy		- -			
Second Trimester					
Anticipatory Guidance					
Signs And Symptoms Of Preterm Labor		- -			
Selecting A Newborn Care Provider		- -			
Reproductive Life Planning & Contraception		- -			
Postpartum Care Planning		- -			
Psychosocial Screening					
Tobacco (Smoked, Chewed, ENDS, Vaped) Cessation Counseling (Ask, Advise, Assess, Assist, And Arrange)		- -			
Depression / Anxiety (Should Be Performed At Least Once During Perinatal Period)		- -			
Intimate Partner Violence		- -			

(continued)

*Data from Ewing H. A practical guide to intervention in health and social services with pregnant and postpartum addicts and alcoholics: theoretical framework, brief screening tool, key interview questions, and strategies for referral to recovery resources. Martinez (CA): The Born Free Project, Contra Costa County Department of Health Services; 1990.

Patient Name:		Birth Date: – –	ID No.:	Date: – –

Plans/Education (continued)
By Trimester. Initial And Date When Discussed.

	NA	Date	Follow-Up Needed	Referral	Comments
Third Trimester					
Birth Preferences					
Pain Management Plans		– –			
Trial Of Labor After Cesarean Counseling		– –			☐ TOLAC ☐ Elective RCS
Labor Support Person(S)		– –			
Immediate Postpartum Larc		– –			☐ Implant ☐ LNG-IUS ☐ Copper IUD
Circumcision Preference		– –			☐ Yes ☐ No
Infant Feeding Intention		– –			☐ Exclusive ☐ Mixed ☐ Formula
Anticipatory Guidance					
Fetal Movement Monitoring		– –			
Signs And Symptoms Of Preeclampsia		– –			
Labor Signs		– –			
Cervical Ripening/Labor Induction Counseling		– –			
Postterm Counseling		– –			
Infant Feeding		– –			
Newborn Education (Newborn Screening, Immunizations, Jaundice, SIDS/Safe Sleeping Position, Car Seat)		– –			
Family Medical Leave Or Disability Forms		– –			
Postpartum Depression		– –			
Psychosocial Screening					
Tobacco (Smoked, Chewed, ENDS, Vaped) Cessation Counseling (Ask, Advise, Assess, Assist, And Arrange)		– –			
Depression / Anxiety (Should Be Performed At Least Once During Perinatal Period)		– –			
Intimate Partner Violence		– –			
Postpartum					
Screening					
Depression / Anxiety (Should Be Performed At Least Once During Perinatal Period)		– –			
Infant Feeding Problems		– –			
Birth Experience		– –			
Glucose Screen (If Gdm)		– –			
Anticipatory Guidance					
Infant Feeding		– –			
Pelvic Muscle Exercise/Kegel		– –			
Return To Work / Milk Expression		– –			
Weight Retention		– –			
Optimal Birth Spacing		– –			
Postpartum Sexuality		– –			
Exercise		– –			
Nutrition		– –			
Cardiometabolic Risk (If Gdm / Ghtn)		– –			
Transition Of Care					
Referral Made To Primary Care Provider		– –			
Pregnancy Complications Documented In Medical Record		– –			
Written Recommendations For Follow-Up Communicated To Patient And To Pcp		– –			

Patient Addressograph

| Patient Name: | Birth Date: - - | ID No.: • | Date: - - |

Plans/Education *(continued)*
By Trimester. Initial And Date When Discussed.

Requests

	Date	Initials	
Tubal Sterilization Consent Signed (If Desired).	- -		
History And Physical Have Been Sent To Hospital, If Applicable.	- -		
Update With Group B Streptococcus Results Sent.	- -		

Comments

Patient Addressograph

| Patient Name: | Birth Date: - - | ID No.: | Date: - - |

Plans/Education Notes

Patient Addressograph

Name: _____
        LAST   FIRST   MIDDLE

ID#: _____ EDD: _____

Prenatal Visits

Prepregnancy Weight _____

BMI _____

Date	Weeks Gest. (Best Est.)	Weight	Blood Pressure	Urine (Albumin/Glucose)	Pain Scale* (0–10)	Fetal Movement	Preterm Labor Signs/Symptoms: +=Present O=Absent	FHR	Fundal Height (CM)/EFW	Presentation	Edema	Cervix Examination (DIL/EFF, STA.) Length On Ultrasonography	Next Appointment	Provider (Initials)	Comments:

*Describe the intensity of discomfort ranging from 0 (no pain) to 10 (worst possible pain).

Progress Notes

_____
_____
_____
_____
_____
_____
_____

PROVIDER SIGNATURE (AS REQUIRED): _____

Version 8. Copyright 2016 The American College of Obstetricians and Gynecologists   (AA128)   12345/09876

Patient Addressograph

Name: _____
         LAST   FIRST   MIDDLE
ID#: _____ EDD: _____

Prenatal Visits

Prepregnancy Weight _____

BMI _____

Date	Weeks Gest. (Best Est.)	Weight	Blood Pressure	Urine (Albumin/Glucose)	Pain Scale* (0-10)	Fetal Movement	Preterm Labor Signs/Symptoms: +=Present O=Absent	FHR	Fundal Height (CM)/EFW	Presentation	Edema	Cervix Examination (DIL./EFF; STA.) Length On Ultrasonography	Next Appointment	Provider (Initials)	Comments:
- -															
- -															
- -															
- -															
- -															
- -															
- -															
- -															
- -															
- -															
- -															
- -															
- -															
- -															

*Describe the intensity of discomfort ranging from 0 (no pain) to 10 (worst possible pain).

Progress Notes

_____
_____
_____
_____
_____
_____
_____
_____

PROVIDER SIGNATURE (AS REQUIRED): _____

Version 8. Copyright 2016 The American College of Obstetricians and Gynecologists   (AA128) 12345/09876

Patient Addressograph

| Patient Name: | Birth Date: - - | ID No.: | Date: - - |

Progress Notes

PROVIDER SIGNATURE (AS REQUIRED): _____

Version 8. Copyright 2016 The American College of Obstetricians and Gynecologists

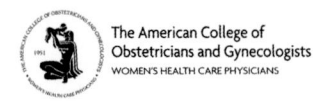

The American College of Obstetricians and Gynecologists
WOMEN'S HEALTH CARE PHYSICIANS

Patient Addressograph

POSTPARTUM CARE PLAN

To be developed prenatally by the patient and her maternity provider and revised as needed after delivery.

Name: _____
        LAST   FIRST   MIDDLE

Care Team

Primary Maternal Provider/Group:	Care Coordinator:
	Home Visitor:
PCP:	MFM:
Infant Medical Provider:	Consultant:
Lactation Support:	Consultant:

Postpartum Visits

Early Visit (Indication) _____ /_____ /_____ At: _____

☐ Hypertension   ☐ Depression/Anxiety   ☐ Wound Check   ☐ Lactation Difficulties   ☐ Medication Titration   ☐ Other: _____

Comprehensive Visit _____ /_____ /_____ At: _____

Reproductive Life Plan

Number Of Children Desired:	Timing Of Next Pregnancy:

Contraceptive Plan

☐ BTL   ☐ Implant   ☐ LNG-IUS   ☐ Copper IUD   ☐ Depot Medroxyprogesterone Acetate (DMPA)   ☐ Combined Ocp   ☐ Progesterone Only Pill

☐ Vasectomy   ☐ Condoms   ☐ Diaphragm   ☐ Lactational Amenorrhea   ☐ Natural Family Planning   ☐ Other

Immediate Postpartum LARC?

☐ Desires   ☐ Declines   ☐ Unsure

Infant Feeding Plan

☐ Exclusive Breastfeeding For _____ Months   ☐ Mixed Feeding   ☐ Formula

Community Resources

☐ WIC Peer Counselor   ☐ Mothers' Groups   ☐ Lactation Warmline   ☐ Return To Work Resources

Pregnancy Complications

Complication _____	Follow-Up Scheduled	Result
☐ GDM	Glucose Screen: _____ /_____ /_____	_____ MG/DL (Fasting) _____ MG/DL (Post 75 G Load)
☐ Preeclampsia ☐ GHTN	BP Check _____ /_____ /_____	_____ /_____ MM HG
☐ Other:		

Mental Health

Risk For Postpartum Depression/Anxiety	Screening (Should Be Performed At Least Once During Perinatal Period)
☐ High ☐ Medium ☐ Low	Date: _____ /_____ /_____ Result:

Postpartum Problems

☐ Perineal/C-Section Wound Pain   ☐ Urinary Incontinence   ☐ Fecal Incontinence   ☐ Dyspareunia/Reduced Sexual Desire   ☐ Fatigue/Sleep Issues

Referrals/Interventions:

Chronic Health Conditions

Problem	Plan
1.	
2.	
3.	
4.	

Version 8. Copyright 2016 The American College of Obstetricians and Gynecologists   (AA197)   12345/54321

Patient Addressograph

POSTPARTUM FORM

Name: _____
        LAST   FIRST   MIDDLE

ID#: _____ EDD: _____

Discharge Date: ____ - ____ - ____

Delivery Information

Delivery At _____ weeks

- ☐ Vaginal
  - ☐ Svd
  - ☐ Vacuum
  - ☐ Forceps
  - ☐ Episiotomy
  - ☐ Lacerations
  - ☐ Tolac
- ☐ Cesarean
  - ☐ Primary (For: _____)
  - ☐ Repeat (For: _____)
  - ☐ Uterine Incision
  - ☐ Low Transverse
  - ☐ Low Vertical
  - ☐ Classical

Labor
- ☐ None
- ☐ Spontaneous
- ☐ Induced
- ☐ Augmented

Anesthesia
- ☐ None
- ☐ Local/Pudendal
- ☐ Epidural
- ☐ Spinal
- ☐ General
- ☐ Other: _____

Postpartum Contraception

	Yes	No
BTL	☐	☐
Implant	☐	☐
LNG-IUS	☐	☐
Copper IUD	☐	☐
Depot Medroxyprogesterone Acetate (DMPA)	☐	☐
Combined OCP	☐	☐
Progesterone-Only Pill	☐	☐
Vasectomy	☐	☐
Condoms	☐	☐
Diaphragm	☐	☐
Lactational Amenorrhea	☐	☐
Natural Family Planning	☐	☐

Other: _____

Delivered By: _____

Postpartum Information

Complications
- ☐ None
- ☐ Hemorrhage
- ☐ Infection
- ☐ Hypertension
- ☐ Diabetes
- ☐ Other: _____

Discharge Information

Neonatal Information

Name Of Baby: _____

Sex
- ☐ Female
- ☐ Male
  - Circumcision ☐ Yes ☐ No

Birth Weight: _____ g

Disposition
- ☐ Home With Mother
- ☐ In Hospital
- ☐ Transfer
- ☐ Neonatal Death
- ☐ Stillbirth
- ☐ Other: _____

Complications/Anomalies:
_____

Newborn Care Provider:
_____

Seen By Newborn Care Provider Before Discharge
- ☐ Yes ☐ No

Received Hepatitis B Birth Dose Prior to Hospital Discharge ☐ Yes ☐ No

Maternal Information

Maternal Age: _____ Gravity And Parity: _____

Regarding Smoking, Chewing, Using A Nicotine Delivery System (ENDS), and Vaping
- ☐ Does Not Use
- ☐ Quit During Pregnancy
- ☐ Current User

HGB/HCT Level: _____

Medications: _____
_____

HIV Status* Known ☐ Yes ☐ No
  - ☐ POS
  - ☐ NEG

Feeding Method ☐ Breast ☐ Bottle

Diagnostic Studies Pending:
_____

Secondary Diagnosis/Preexisting Conditions
- ☐ Asthma
- ☐ Hypertension
- ☐ Diabetes
- ☐ Other: _____

Immunizations Given
- ☐ Anti-D Immune Globulin
- ☐ Tdap Or TD
- ☐ HPV (When Indicated)
  - ☐ No, Received During Pregnancy
  - ☐ No, Received Before Pregnancy
  - ☐ Patient Declined
- ☐ Influenza
- ☐ Varicella
  - ☐ No, Received During Pregnancy
  - ☐ Other: _____
  - ☐ Patient Declined
- ☐ MMR (When Indicated)

Infant Status: _____

☐ If Neonatal Death, Bereavement Counseling

Follow-Up Appt: _____

Date: ____ / ____ / ____

Location: _____

Other: _____

*Check state requirements before recording results.

Interim Contacts or Hospitalizations

Date	Comment

PROVIDER SIGNATURE (AS REQUIRED): _____

Version 8. Copyright 2016 The American College of Obstetricians and Gynecologists   (AA197) 12345/54321

Postpartum Visit

Date: ___ — ___ — ___

Feeding Method:

Contraception Method
- Tubal Sterilization — ☐ Yes ☐ No
- Intrauterine Device (IUD) — ☐ Yes ☐ No
- Depot Medroxyprogesterone Acetate (DMPA) — ☐ Yes ☐ No
- Implant — ☐ Yes ☐ No
- Oral Contraceptives — ☐ Yes ☐ No
- Other: _____

Postpartum Depression Screening:

Intimate Partner Violence Screening:

Discuss Tobacco (Smoked, Chewed, ENDS, Vaped) Relapse Prevention Techniques:

Infant Health:

Interim History:

Follow-Up Lab Studies Ordered
- ☐ Yes ☐ No — Postpartum HCB/HCT: _____
- ☐ Yes ☐ No — Postpartum Glucose Screening If Patient Had Gestational Diabetes: _____
- ☐ Yes ☐ No — Other Studies Requested: _____

Physical Examination

BP: _____ WT: _____ BMI: _____

	Normal	Abnormal
Breasts	☐	☐ _____
Abdomen	☐	☐ _____
External Genitalia	☐	☐ _____
Vagina	☐	☐ _____
Cervix	☐	☐ _____
Uterus	☐	☐ _____
Adnexa	☐	☐ _____
Rectal–Vaginal	☐	☐ _____

Pap Test ☐ Yes ☐ No If No, Due: _____

Allergies:

Immunization Update:

Medications/Contraception:

☐ Dispensed

Interval Care Recommendations

For General Health Promotion:

Plans For Future Pregnancies:

For Reproductive Health Promotion:

Repeat Glucose Screening Needed? ☐ Yes ☐ No
If Yes, Has Patient Been Counseled? ☐ Yes ☐ No
Date Of Repeat Testing:

Return Visit:

Referrals:

Examined By:

Comments

_____
_____
_____
_____
_____
_____
_____
_____

PROVIDER SIGNATURE (AS REQUIRED): _____

Version 8. Copyright 2016 The American College of Obstetricians and Gynecologists (AA197)

Appendix C
Edinburgh Postnatal Depression Scale[1] (EPDS)

Name: _____   Address: _____

Your Date of Birth: _____   _____

Baby's Date of Birth: _____   Phone: _____

As you are pregnant or have recently had a baby, we would like to know how you are feeling. Please check the answer that comes closest to how you have felt **IN THE PAST 7 DAYS**, not just how you feel today.

Here is an example, already completed.

I have felt happy:
- ☐ Yes, all the time
- ☒ Yes, most of the time
- ☐ No, not very often
- ☐ No, not at all

This would mean: "I have felt happy most of the time" during the past week.
Please complete the other questions in the same way.

In the past 7 days:

1. I have been able to laugh and see the funny side of things
   - ☐ As much as I always could
   - ☐ Not quite so much now
   - ☐ Definitely not so much now
   - ☐ Not at all

2. I have looked forward with enjoyment to things
   - ☐ As much as I ever did
   - ☐ Rather less than I used to
   - ☐ Definitely less than I used to
   - ☐ Hardly at all

*3. I have blamed myself unnecessarily when things went wrong
   - ☐ Yes, most of the time
   - ☐ Yes, some of the time
   - ☐ Not very often
   - ☐ No, never

4. I have been anxious or worried for no good reason
   - ☐ No, not at all
   - ☐ Hardly ever
   - ☐ Yes, sometimes
   - ☐ Yes, very often

*5 I have felt scared or panicky for no very good reason
   - ☐ Yes, quite a lot
   - ☐ Yes, sometimes
   - ☐ No, not much
   - ☐ No, not at all

*6. Things have been getting on top of me
   - ☐ Yes, most of the time I haven't been able to cope at all
   - ☐ Yes, sometimes I haven't been coping as well as usual
   - ☐ No, most of the time I have coped quite well
   - ☐ No, I have been coping as well as ever

*7 I have been so unhappy that I have had difficulty sleeping
   - ☐ Yes, most of the time
   - ☐ Yes, sometimes
   - ☐ Not very often
   - ☐ No, not at all

*8 I have felt sad or miserable
   - ☐ Yes, most of the time
   - ☐ Yes, quite often
   - ☐ Not very often
   - ☐ No, not at all

*9 I have been so unhappy that I have been crying
   - ☐ Yes, most of the time
   - ☐ Yes, quite often
   - ☐ Only occasionally
   - ☐ No, never

*10 The thought of harming myself has occurred to me
   - ☐ Yes, quite often
   - ☐ Sometimes
   - ☐ Hardly ever
   - ☐ Never

Administered/Reviewed by _____   Date _____

[1]*Source*: Cox JL, Holden JM, and Sagovsky R. Detection of postnatal depression: Development of the 10-item Edinburgh Postnatal Depression Scale. *Br J Psychiatry.* 1987;150:782–786.

Users may reproduce the scale without further permission providing they respect copyright by quoting the names of the authors, the title, and the source of the paper in all reproduced copies.

Edinburgh Postnatal Depression Scale[1] (EPDS)

Postpartum depression is the most common complication of childbearing.[2] The 10-question Edinburgh Postnatal Depression Scale (EPDS) is a valuable and efficient way of identifying patients at risk for "perinatal" depression. The EPDS is easy to administer and has proven to be an effective screening tool.

Mothers who score above 13 are likely to be suffering from a depressive illness of varying severity. The EPDS score should not override clinical judgment. A careful clinical assessment should be carried out to confirm the diagnosis. The scale indicates how the mother has felt *during the previous week*. In doubtful cases it may be useful to repeat the tool after 2 weeks. The scale will not detect mothers with anxiety neuroses, phobias, or personality disorders.

Women with postpartum depression need not feel alone. They may find useful information on the websites of the National Women's Health Information Center <www.4women.gov> and from groups such as Postpartum Support International <www.chss.iup.edu/postpartum> and Depression after Delivery <www.depressionafterdelivery.com>.

SCORING

QUESTIONS 1, 2, and 4 (without an *)
Are scored 0, 1, 2, or 3 with top box scored as 0 and the bottom box scored as 3.

QUESTIONS 3, 5–10 (marked with an *)
Are reverse scored, with the top box scored as 3 and the bottom box scored as 0.

- Maximum score: 30
- Possible depression: 10 or greater
- Always look at item 10 (suicidal thoughts)

Users may reproduce the scale without further permission, providing they respect copyright by quoting the names of the authors, the title, and the source of the paper in all reproduced copies.

Instructions for Using the Edinburgh Postnatal Depression Scale:

1. The mother is asked to check the response that comes closest to how she has been feeling in the previous 7 days.
2. All the items must be completed.
3. Care should be taken to avoid the possibility of the mother discussing her answers with others. (Answers come from the mother or pregnant woman.)
4. The mother should complete the scale herself, unless she has limited English or has difficulty with reading.

[2]Source: Wisner KL, Parry BL, Piontek CM. Postpartum Depression *N Engl J Med.* 2002 Jul 18;347(3):194–199.

Index

Note: Page numbers followed by "*f*," "*t*," and "*b*" refer to figures, tables, and boxes, respectively.

Abdominal examination, 87
Abdominal pain, 155, 167, 174
Abdominal pregnancy, 172–173
Abdominal wall, 121
Ablative methods, 396–397
Abnormal labor patterns, 100, 101*t. See also*
      Normal labor
  first-stage disorders, 101
    augmentation, 101–102
    continuous labor support, 102
  second-stage disorders, 102
Abnormal uterine bleeding (AUB), 332, 334
  diagnosis of, 335–336
  luteal phase defect, 335
  midcycle spotting, 335
  treatment, 336
ABO hemolytic disease, 208
Abortion. *See* Miscarriage
Abused woman, identifying, 318*b*
Acanthosis nigricans, 341
Acanthotic pattern, 382
Accelerated starvation, 50
Accelerations, of fetal heart rate, 107–109, 108*t*
Acetaminophen, 219
Achondroplasia, 78
Acidemia, 117
Acidosis, 117
Acquaintance rape, 312
Acquired immune deficiency syndrome (AIDS),
      213–214, 260
  management, 214
  pathophysiology, 213
  screening and testing, 213–214
Actinomycin D, 377
Active phase of labor, 87
Acute cystitis, 188
Acute fatty liver of pregnancy, 186–188
Acute reactions, 373
Acyclovir, 211, 257
Add-back therapy, 278
Additive, 371
Adenoacanthoma, 411
Adenocarcinoma, 391, 411
Adenomyosis, 279, 280
Adenosis, 291
Adenosquamous carcinoma, 411
Adjuvant (systemic) therapy, 293
Adnexa, bimanual examination of, 12
Adnexal masses, in pregnancy, 168, 189–190
Adnexal space, 415
Adrenal androgen excess disorders, 342
  adrenal neoplasms, 343
  congenital adrenal hyperplasia (CAH), 342–343
  Cushing syndrome, 343
  treatment, 343
Adrenal crisis, 199
Adrenal function, 50
Adrenal neoplasms, 343
Adrenal steroidogenesis, 339*f*
Adrenarche, 347
Adrenocorticotropic hormone (ACTH), 338
Adult respiratory distress syndrome, 188
Aerobic exercise, contraindications to, 65*t*
Aggravated criminal sexual assault, 313
Aggressive suctioning, 166
Airway management in newborn resuscitation, 117*f*
Alcohol, 69–70
Alkylating agents, 68*t*, 370
Alkylating cancer chemotherapy, 350

Alkylating-like agents, 370
Alleles, 77
Allergic contact dermatitis, 382
Alloimmunization, 203–208
  assessment, 206–207
  diagnosis, 205
  isoimmunization management, to red cell antigens,
      207–208
  natural history, 204
  prevention, 207
α-fetoprotein (AFP) levels, 81
Ambulation, 122
  and position in labor and at delivery, 90–91
Amenorrhea, 167, 233, 332, 356
  causes, 332–333
  treatment, 333
American College of Obstetricians and Gynecologists
  antepartum record, 433–444
  postpartum care plan, 445–447
  well-woman recommendations for annual assessment
    ages 13–18, 428*t*
    ages 19–39, 429*t*
    ages 40–64, 430*t*
    ages 65 years and older, 431*t*
Amine ("whiff") test, 245
Amlodipine, 197*t*
Amniocentesis, 83, 149, 205
Amnioinfusion, 110
Amniotic fluid, 159
  ferning pattern from, 160
  assessment of, 206
  embolism, 132
  volume of, 63, 165
Amniotic fluid index (AFI), 64
Amniotic membranes, 96
Amniotomy, 101
Ampicillin, 188
Ampulla, 39
Anagen (growth) phase, 51
Analgesia, 122
Anamnestic response, 205
Anaphase, 73
Anaphase I, 74
Anaphase II, 74
Anatomy, 33
  bony pelvis, 33–36
  ovaries, 40
  uterine tubes, 39
  uterus and pelvic support, 37–39
  vagina, 36–37
  vulva and perineum, 36
Ancillary tests, 110
  fetal blood pH/lactate, determination of, 111
  fetal stimulation, 110–111
  pulse oximetry, 111
Androblastoma. *See* Sertoli-Leydig cell tumors
Androgen production and androgen action, 337–340
Androgens, 68*t*
Android pelvis, 36
Androstenedione, 337
Anemia, 201–203, 204
Anencephaly, 164*t*
Aneuploidy, 74
Angiotensin-converting enzyme (ACE) inhibitors, 67*t*,
      195, 199
Anogenital cancer, 15
Anovulation, 356
Anovulatory uterine bleeding, 335
Antagonistic, 371

Anteflexed position, 12
Antenatal management, 137–138
Antenatal visits, subsequent, 59
  blood pressure and urinalysis, 59
  physical findings, 59
    fetal heart rate, 60
    fetal presentation, 60–61
    fundal height measurement, 59–60
    uterine palpation, 60
  weight, 59
Antepartum, 57, 164
Antepartum patient education, 64
  breastfeeding, 66
  employment, 64
  exercise, 64
  nutrition and weight gain, 65
  sexual activity, 66
  teratogens, 66–67
    alcohol, 69–70
    herbal remedies, 67
    ionizing radiation, 67
    medications, 67
    methyl mercury, 67
    substance abuse, 70
    tobacco use, 70
  travel, 66
Anteverted position, 12
Anthropoid type, 36
Antibiotic prophylaxis, 314
Antibody response, 204
Anticipation, 77
Anti-D immunoglobulin, 207
Antihypertensive medication, 195
Anti-I antibody, 205
Anti-immunoglobulin D, 122
Anti-Lewis antibody, 205
Antimetabolites, 370
Antineoplastic drugs, 370, 371
Antiphospholipid antibodies, 174
Antiphospholipid antibody syndrome, 173
Antitumor antibiotics, 370
Antiviral drugs, 257
Anxiety disorders, 223
Apert syndrome, 78
Apgar scoring system, 112–114
Aplasia cutis, 182
Appendicitis, 189, 415
Apt test, 156
Arias-Stella reaction, 170
Aromatase inhibitors (AIs), 293, 371
Arrest disorders, 100
Arrhenoblastoma, 424. *See also* Sertoli-Leydig cell tumors
Arterial blood gas assessment during pregnancy, 46
Artificial ROM, 93
Asherman syndrome, 131, 333, 334*f*
Aspirin and acetaminophen, 68*t*
Assisted reproductive technologies (ARTs), 134, 168,
      360–362
Asthma severity and control, classification of, 199
Asthma therapy, 199
Asymptomatic bacteriuria, 188
Asynclitism, 99
Atelectasis, 303
Atopic dermatitis, 382
Atresia, 322
Atrophic urethritis, 348
Atrophic vaginitis, 249, 348
Atypia, 406
Atypical, favor neoplastic AIS, 391

451

Atypical glandular cells (AGCs), 391
Atypical squamous cells (ASCs), 391
Atypical squamous cells of undetermined significance
	(ASC-US), 391, 394f, 395f
Augmentation, 101–102
Autoimmune disorders
	and menopause, 350
Autosomal dominant, 77
Autosomal recessive, 77
Autosomes, 73
Azoospermia, 359

B19 infection, 217
Back pain, 71
Bacterial vaginosis (BV), 245, 246–247
Balanced reciprocal translocations, 76
Balanced translocation, 76
Ballard scoring system, 112, 113t
Balloon, 333
Barrier contraceptives, 234
	condoms, 235
	diaphragm, 235–236
	spermicides, 236
	sponge, 235
Bartholin glands, 36
Basal body temperature, 355
Baseline, 108t
Baseline variability, 108t
Bell's palsy, 221
Beneficence, 22
Benign cystic teratoma, 418
Benign ovarian neoplasms, 417
	benign epithelial cell neoplasms, 417–418
	benign germ cell neoplasms, 418–420
	benign stromal cell neoplasms, 420
Benign vaginal masses, 387
Benzodiazepines, 69t
β-adrenergic receptor agonists, 150t
β-blockers, 68t
β-hCG discriminatory value, 169
Betamethasone, 154
Bethesda System (2014), 392
Bicornuate uterus, 40, 40f
Bilateral salpingo-oophorectomy, 301
Bilirubin release, 204
Bimanual examination, 11–12
	of adnexa, 12
	of uterus, 12
Bimanual pelvic examination, 152
Biochemical hyperthyroidism, 18
Biophysical profile (BPP), 62, 63–64, 165
Bipolar disorders, 223
Birth asphyxia, 105, 112
Bladder, 37
	function, 123
Bleeding, 153
	third-trimester. See Third-trimester bleeding
Bleomycin, 372t
Blood component therapy, 129t
Blood pressure
	assessment, 44
	categories, 6t
	and urinalysis, 59
Blood urea nitrogen (BUN), serum levels of, 48
Bloody show, 86
Body (corpus), 37
Body mass index (BMI), 21t, 59
Bohr effect, 46
Bone demineralization, 348
Bone mineral density (BMD), 19
Bony pelvis, 33–36, 35f
Borderline malignancies, 421
Borderline ovarian tumors, 421
Bowel and bladder function, 123
Brachial plexus injury, 164
Brachytherapy, 373
Bradycardia, 107
Braxton Hicks contractions, 86
BRCA1 gene, 84, 292
BRCA2 gene, 84, 292
Breakthrough bleeding, 232
Breast, 51

abscess, 122
anatomy, 285, 286f
clinical anatomy and associated examination
	schema of, 7f
engorgement, 122
examination, 6–7, 8f
Tanner staging of breast and pubic hair
	development, 328f
Breast, diseases of, 285
	benign breast disease, 289
		benign breast masses, 290–291
		breast masses, 290
		mastalgia, 289
		nipple discharge, 289–290
	breast cancer, 16–17, 122, 291
		Gail model, 292
		histologic types of, 292
		and ovarian cancer, 84
		risk factors, 291–292
		staging, 292–293
		treatment, 293–294
	evaluation of, 287f
		diagnosis algorithm, 289
		diagnostic testing, 287–288
		patient history, 287
		physical examination, 287
		risk factors for breast cancer, 287f
	screening guidelines, 294
Breastfeeding, 66, 214. See also Lactation and breastfeeding
	hospital practices to encourage and support, 115b
	practices to promote, 114
Breast imaging, 296–297
Breast/ovarian familial cancer syndrome, 422
Breast self-awareness, 7
Breast self-examination (BSE), 7
Breech extraction, 139
Breech presentation, 104–105
	types of, 104f
Brenner cell tumor, 418
Broad ligament, 33, 37
Brow presentation, 99
Bruising, 152
Bulking agents, 268

Calcium-channel blockers, 68t, 150t
Calcium therapy, 349
Caldwell-Moloy pelvic types, 36f
Cancer metastatic to the ovary, 424
Cancer screening, 16, 84
	breast cancer, 16–17
	cervical cancer, 17
	colorectal carcinoma, 17
Candida species, 247
Candidiasis, 245
C antigen, 204
Capacity, 23
Caput succedaneum, 94
Carbohydrate metabolism, 50
Carboplatin, 372t, 426
Carcinoma of the Bartholin gland, 387
Carcinosarcomas, 424
Cardiac activity, 171
Cardiac arrhythmias, 198
Cardiac disease, 198
Cardiac output, 43
Cardinal ligament, 37
Cardinal movements of labor, 87, 91f
Cardiovascular lipid changes, menopause and, 349–350
Cardiovascular system, 43, 121
	anatomic changes, 43
	diagnostic tests, 44
	functional changes, 43–44
	physical findings, 44
	symptoms, 44
Carnett sign, 282
Carpal tunnel syndrome, 220
Carrier testing, 82
Case-based approach, 24
Catecholamine, 333
Catecholestrogens, 350
Cell cycle and cancer therapy, 369
	chemotherapy, 369–370, 372t

endocrine therapy, 370
	chemotherapy regimens, 371
	combination chemotherapy, 371
	toxicity of chemotherapy, 371
G_0 phase (resting phase), 369
G_1 phase (postmitotic phase), 369
G_2 phase, 369
generation time, 369
M phase (mitosis), 369
novel chemotherapeutic agents, 373
radiation therapy, 371–373
S phase (synthesis phase), 369
Cell cycle (phase) nonspecific chemotherapeutic
	agents, 369
Cell cycle (phase) specific chemotherapeutic agents, 369
Cellular hyperplasia, 141
Cellular hypertrophy, 141
Central nervous system (CNS), sex hormones' role in, 348
Centromere, 76
Cephalexin, 188
Cephalopelvic disproportion, 99
c-erb-B2, 293
Cerebral palsy, 106, 107t
Certificate of merit, 26
Cervical carcinoma, 17, 389, 398
	biopsy, 298
	clinical evaluation, 398–399
	management, 399–400
	prevention, 401
	spread patterns of, 400f
	staging of, 399t
Cervical cerclage, 138, 174
Cervical conization, 300
Cervical insufficiency, 149, 174
Cervical intraepithelial neoplasia (CIN), 17, 389, 391
	classification, 391–392
	etiology, 389–391
	evaluation of abnormal cervical cytology test results,
		392–394
	follow-up, 398
	management guidelines for, 394–396
	risk factors, 391
	treatment, 395–398
Cervical position, 12
Cervical pregnancy, 172
Cervical ripening, 96
Cervical ripening agents, 165
Cervicitis, 4, 250, 252
	diseases characterized by, 253t
Cervix, 37, 165
	anatomy of, 390f
	and vagina, 121
Cesarean delivery, 96, 104, 137, 145, 154, 180
	decision making, 96
		maternal mortality, risk of, 97
		maternal request, cesarean by, 97
		trial of labor after, 97
Chadwick sign, 58
Chain of evidence, 314
Chancroid, 260
Chaperone, 6
Chief complaint (CC), 4
Child sexual assault, 316–317
Chlamydia, 215–216
Chlamydia infection, 18, 167
Chlamydia trachomatis, 18, 215, 252–254
Chloasma (melasma), 51
Choanal atresia, 182
Cholecystitis, 189
Cholelithiasis, 189
Chorioamnionitis, 160
Choriocarcinomas, 377
Chorionicity, 134
	in twin pregnancies, 135f
Chorionic villus sampling (CVS), 73, 83, 142
Chromatin, 73
Chromopertubation, 358
Chromosomal abnormalities
	commonly diagnosed, 75t
	previous pregnancy affected by, 78
Chromosome number, abnormalities in, 74
Chromosome replication and cell division, 73
	meiosis, 73–74

mitosis, 73
Chromosomes, 72, 73
Chromosome structure, abnormalities in, 76, 76t
　deletions, 76
　insertions, 76
　inversions, 76
　translocations, 76
Chronic pelvic pain, 279, 281
　assessment, 281–282
　conditions that increase the risk of, 282–283
　therapy, 283
　　follow-up, 284
　　medical therapy, 283–284
　　surgical therapies, 284
Circulating cell-free fetal DNA, 81
Circumcision, 118
Cisplatin, 372t, 426
Class II human leukocyte antigens, 380
Clear cell carcinoma, 411
Climacteric, 345
Clinical breast examination, 16
Clinical decision making, principle-based ethical approach to, 23t
Clinical management, ethical steps for, 23–25
Clinical pelvimetry, 99
Clitoris, 36
Cloaca, 33
Cloacal membrane, 33
Clomiphene, 360
Clomiphene citrate, 334, 360
Coagulation defects, 132
Coagulopathy, in pregnancy, 156
Codons, 72
Coelomic metaplasia, 271
Cognitive dysfunction, 316
Colonoscopy, 17
Colorectal cancer, 17
　screening for, 17
Colorectal carcinoma, 17
Colostrum, 51, 125
Colposcopy, 298, 379, 393
　with directed biopsy, 393
Combination chemotherapy, 371
Combined oral contraceptives, 281
Comparative genomic hybridization (CGH), 83
Competence, 23
Complete abortion, 174
Complete abruption, 155
Complete blood count (CBC), 203
Complete moles, 374
　features of, 375t
Complete placenta previa, 153
Complex hyperplasia, 406
Compound presentations, 99
Computed [axial] tomography (CAT/CT), 275, 296
Concealed hemorrhage, 155
Concurrent blockade, 371
Condoms, 235
Condyloma acuminata, 214
Condyloma lata, 215
Condylomata acuminata, 384
Confidentiality, 25
Conflicts of interest, 25
Congenital adrenal hyperplasia (CAH), 29, 329, 342–343
Congenital anomalies, 178
Congenital malformations, 200
Congenital syphilis, 215
Congenital varicella, 217
Conization, 300
Conjoined twins, 134
Conservative management, 174
Conservative surgery, 278
Constipation, 49, 71
Constitutional hirsutism, 343
Continuity of care, 13
Continuous labor support, 102
Contraception, 123, 225
　barrier contraceptives, 234
　　condoms, 235
　　diaphragm, 235–236
　　spermicides, 236
　　sponge, 235

emergency contraception, 237
factors affecting the choice of, 226–227
fertility awareness methods, 236
　basal body temperature method, 237
　calendar methods, 237
　cervical mucus methods, 237
　lactational amenorrhea, 237
　symptothermal method, 237
hormonal contraceptives, 232
　effects of, 233
　mechanisms of action, 232–233
　patient evaluation for, 233–234
　ring and patch, 234
ineffective methods, 238
injectable hormonal contraceptives, 231–232
long-acting reversible contraception (LARC), 227
　implantable hormonal contraceptives, 227–229
　intrauterine contraception, 229–231
postpartum contraception, 238
postpartum sterilization, 123–124
types of, 228t
Contraceptive history, 4
Contraceptive sponge, 235
Contraceptive vaginal ring, 234
Contraction stress test (CST), 62, 63
Controlled ovarian hyperstimulation (COH), 360
Cordocentesis, 83
Cornu, 37
Cornual pregnancy, 172
Corpus albicans, 324
Corpus hemorrhagicum, 417
Corpus luteum, 322
Corpus luteum cysts, 416–417
Cortical cords, 30
Corticosteroids, 151
Couvelaire uterus, 156
Cramping, 174
Craniopharyngioma, 331
Creatinine, serum levels of, 48
Critical titer, 206
Crossing over, in meiosis, 73
Cryotherapy, 298, 396–397
Culdocentesis, 170
Cushing syndrome, 343
Cyclic mastalgia, 289
Cyclophosphamide, 372t, 377
Cystitis, 188
Cystocele, 262
Cyst of the canal of Nuck, 383
Cystourethroscopy, 267
Cytokinesis, 73
Cytological atypia, 406
Cytomegalovirus (CMV), 216
Cytoreductive surgery, 426
Cytosine–adenine–guanine (CAG), 73

Dactinomycin/actinomycin D, 372t
Daily fetal movement counting, 165
Danazol, 68t, 366, 343–344, 404
D antigen, 204
Date of onset of the last normal menses, 59
Date rape, 312
Death of one fetus, 137
Decelerations, FHR, 109
Decision makers, Identifying, 23
Defendant(s), 26
Dehiscence, 123
Dehydroepiandrosterone (DHEA), 337
Delayed capillary refill, 128
Deletions, replication errors, 73
Delivery maneuvers, 139
Delivery of anterior and posterior shoulders, 96
Delivery room assessment of the newborn, 112
　Apgar scoring system, 112–114, 114t
　Ballard scoring system, 112
Deoxyribonucleic acid (DNA), 72
Depot medroxyprogesterone acetate (DMPA), 231–232, 275
Depression
　and anxiety, 221–222
　and sexual dysfunction, 307

Depth of myometrial invasion, 412
Dermatitis, 382
Dermoid cyst, 418, 419f
Descent, 87
Desquamative inflammatory vaginitis, 249
Detrusor muscle, 266
Diabetes mellitus, 19–20, 177–178
　classification of diabetes in pregnancy, 177–178
　fetal morbidity and mortality, 178
　　congenital anomalies, 178
　　macrosomia, 178–179
　　polyhydramnios, 179
　　spontaneous abortion and stillbirth, 178
　gestational diabetes, 180–181
　　infection, 181
　　labor and delivery of patients with diabetes, 181
　　laboratory screening, 180
　　management, 180–181
　physiology of glucose metabolism, in pregnancy, 178
　progestational diabetes, 179–180
　　antepartum fetal monitoring, 179
　　management, 179–180
　　maternal complications, 179
　screening and diagnostic criteria for, 20t
　Type I, 173, 177
　Type II, 177
Diabetic ketoacidosis (DKA), 177
Diabetic nephropathy, 179
Diagonal conjugate, 36
Diamnionic/dichorionic twins, 134
Diamnionic/monochorionic twins, 134
Diaphragm, 235–236
Diastasis recti, 121
Diastolic blood pressure, 195
Dichorionic gestation, 137
Dietary cravings, 49
Digital examination, 160
Dihydrotes-tosterone (DHT), 337
Dilation and curettage (D&C), 299, 407
Dilation and evacuation, 299
Dimethyl sulfoxide, 284
Dinoprostone, 130
Diploid, 73
Direct carrier testing, 82
Direct visualization, 170
Discordant growth, 138
Disjunction, 74
Distended neck veins, 44
Diuretics, 68t
Dizygotic twins, 134
Dizziness, 44
Docusate, 71
Domestic violence, 312, 317
　counseling, 318
　definition, 317–318
　indicators of physical abuse in, 317t
　RADAR model of the physician's approach to, 318b
　risk factors, 318
Dominant gene, 77
Dopamine, 306
Doppler ultrasound, 64, 206
Doppler velocimetry, 143f
Dorsal lithotomy position, 90
Down syndrome, 61, 78, 80t, 81, 82
Doxycycline, 216
Drospirenone, 232
Ductal carcinoma in situ (DCIS), 291
Ductal ectasia, 289
Ducts of Skene (paraurethral) glands, 36
Due date, 163
Dyschezia, 273
Dysgerminomas, 423, 423f
Dysmaturity syndrome, 163, 164
Dysmenorrhea, 279
　combined oral contraceptives, 281
　diagnosis, 279–281
　etiology, 279
　therapy, 281
Dyspareunia, 272, 280
Dysplasia, 391
Dyspnea of pregnancy, 45
Dystocia, 98, 100, 100f

Eantigen, 204
Early deceleration, 108t
Early FHR decelerations, 109
Early-onset infection, 209
Early pregnancy loss, history of, 78
Eccrine sweating, 51
Eclampsia, 195, 196–199
Eclamptic seizure, 196–197
Ectopic pregnancy, 61, 167
  contraindications to medical therapy for, 171
  incidence of types of, 168
  non-fallopian tube, 171–173
    abdominal pregnancy, 172–173
    cervical pregnancy, 172
    heterotopic pregnancy, 172
    interstitial pregnancy, 172
    ovarian pregnancy, 171–172
  surgical management of, 172
  tubal, 167
    clinical findings, 168
    diagnostic procedures, 169–170
    differential diagnosis, 168–169
    management, 170–171
    pathophysiology and risk factors, 167
    symptoms, 167–168
Ectropion, 153
Eczema, 382
Edema, 46, 70, 186
Edinburgh Postnatal Depression Scale (EPDS), 449–450
Effacement, 87
  and dilation, 88f
Eisenmenger syndrome, 198
Electrocautery, 241f
  -based methods, 240–241
Electronic fetal monitoring (EFM), 106
EMACO, 377
Embryology, 29
  external genitalia, development of, 33
  genital ducts, development of, 32–33
  ovary, development of, 30–31
Embryonal cell carcinomas, 424
Emergency contraception (EC), 237, 314
Empathic communication, 3
Employment, 64
Endocervical AIS, 391
Endocrine disorders, 177–183
  diabetes mellitus, 177–178
    classification of diabetes in pregnancy, 177–178
    gestational diabetes, 180–181
    progestational diabetes, 179–180
  thyroid disease, 182
    laboratory screening, 182
    management of, diagnosed during and after pregnancy, 183
    management of existing thyroid disease in pregnancy, 182–183
    pathophysiology, 182
Endocrine system, 49
  adrenal function, 50
  thyroid function, 49–50
Endodermal sinus tumors, 424
Endometrial ablation, 299, 336
Endometrial biopsy (EMB), 298, 407
Endometrial cancer, 410
  diagnosis, 411
  hormone therapy after treatment for, 413
  pathogenesis and risk factors, 411
  prognostic factors, 411–412
  recurrent endometrial carcinoma, 413
  treatment, 412–413
Endometrial carcinomas, 406, 413
  histologic types of, 411t
Endometrial curettage, 170
Endometrial hyperplasia, 406
  atypical hyperplasia and endometrioid intraepithelial neoplasia, 406
  evaluation, 407
    endometrial evaluation, 407–408
    ultrasound, 408–409
  hyperplasia without atypia, 406
  management, 409
    beyond medical therapy, 409

medical therapy, 409
  pathophysiology and risk factors, 406–407
  patient history, 407
  risk factors for, 408t
  World Health Organization's classification of, 407t
Endometrial implants, 274f
  locations of, 272f
Endometrial polyps, 409–410
Endometrial response, 355
Endometrial stromal sarcoma, 413
Endometrial tumors, types of, 410f
Endometrioid tumor, 418, 423
Endometriosis, 271, 279
  diagnosis, 273
    classification, 275, 276–277f
    imaging studies, 275
  differential diagnosis, 273
  pathogenesis, 271
  pathology, 272
  signs and symptoms, 272–273, 274f
    dysmenorrhea and dyspareunia, 272–273
    infertility, 273
  sites of, 273t
  treatment for, 275
    expectant management, 275
    medical therapy, 275–278
    surgical therapy, 278
Endometritis, 160
Endometrium, 37
Engagement, 87
Enhanced breast self-awareness, 7
Enhancer sequences, 72
Enterocele, 262
Entrainment, 364
Enzyme-linked immunosorbent assay (ELISA), 18, 213
Epidural block, 92
Epilepsy, 220
Episiotomy, 94, 94f
Epithelial cell ovarian carcinoma, 421–423
Epithelial cell tumors, 417
Epithelial hyperplasia, 291
Erb-Duchenne palsy, 164
Estimated date of delivery (EDD), 59, 163
Estrogen, 178, 233, 285, 308, 322, 349
Estrogen administration, puberty and, 330
Estrogen and progestin therapy, combined, 350–351
Estrogen deficiency, 269
"Estrogen dependent" endometrial carcinoma, 411
"Estrogen-independent" endometrial carcinoma, 411
Estrogen production, two-cell theory of, 323f
Estrogen receptors (ERs), 349
Estrogen therapy, 413
  for menopause, 350
Estrone, 346
Ethical decision making, contemporary approaches to, 23t
Ethics, 22
  principle-based ethics, 22–23
  steps for ethical clinical management, 23–25
Ethinyl estradiol, 232
Ethnicity, 79
Etoposide, 372t, 377
Euthyroid state, 49
Excessive weight gain, 180
Excisional methods, 398
Exercise, 64
Exfoliative cytology, 17
Expedited partner therapy, 252
Expert witnesses, 26
Expulsion, 87
Extension, 87
External cephalic version (ECV), 61, 104, 139
External female genitalia, 36
External genitalia, 29
  development of, 33
  examination of, 9
  inspection and examination of, 9
  male and female external genitalia, development of, 34f
External os, 37, 389
External rotation, 87
Extirpative surgery, 278
Extragonadal estrogen, 346
Extramammary pain, 289

Extrauterine gestational sac, ectopic pregnancy with, 169f
Extrauterine pregnancy, 164t

Face presentation, 99
Fallopian tube cancers, management of, 426
Fallopian tube disease, 424
  benign disease of fallopian tube and mesosalpinx, 424
  carcinoma of fallopian tube, 424–425
Fallopian (uterine) tubes (oviducts), 39
Falope ring, 241
False-negative nitrazine test, 159
False-positive nitrazine test, 159
Famciclovir, 257
Family history, 5
Fatigue, 71
Fecal immunochemical testing (FIT), 17
Fecal occult blood testing (FOBT), 17
Fecundability, 353
Fecundity, 353, 354
Female infertility, procedures used in the evaluation of, 357b
Female orgasmic disorder, 307t
Female reproductive system, anomalies of, 40–41
Female sexual interest/ arousal disorder, 307t
Female sexual response, physiology of, 305–306
Feminist ethics approach, 24
Fern test, 159
Ferriman-Gallwey scale, modified, 338f
Fertility awareness methods, 236
  basal body temperature method, 237
  calendar methods, 237
  cervical mucus methods, 237
  lactational amenorrhea, 237
  symptothermal method, 237
Fetal activity, 62
Fetal adrenal hypoplasia, 164t
Fetal alcohol syndrome (FAS), 70
Fetal and placental physiology, 51
  fetal circulation, 51–54
  gonads, 55
  hemoglobin and oxygenation, 54
  kidney, 54
  liver, 54
  placenta, 51
  thyroid gland, 54
Fetal asphyxia, 117
Fetal assessment, specific techniques of, 62
  fetal growth, assessment of, 62
  fetal maturity, assessment of, 64
  fetal well-being, assessment of, 62
    biophysical profile, 63–64
    contraction stress test, 62–63
    Doppler ultrasound of umbilical artery, 64
    nonstress test, 62
Fetal biometry measurements, 142
Fetal blood pH/lactate, determination of, 111
Fetal breathing, 161
Fetal circulation, 51–54, 52–53f
Fetal diagnostic procedures, 82
  amniocentesis, 83
  chorionic villus sampling, 83
  comparative genomic hybridization (CGH), 83
  FISH, 83
  karyotype, 83
  percutaneous umbilical blood sampling, 83
Fetal factors, 98–99
Fetal fibronectin, 138
Fetal glucose level, 181
Fetal growth, assessment of, 62
Fetal growth abnormalities, 140
  intrauterine growth restriction, 140–144
  macrosomia, 144–145
  risk factors associated with, 141t
Fetal head, 89
  station and engagement of, 89f
Fetal head crowns, 94
Fetal heart activity, detection of (fetal heart tones), 58
Fetal heart rate (FHR), 60, 92, 101, 106
  accelerations, 107
  decelerations, 109–110
  patterns, 107
  periodic FHR changes, 107
  variability, 107

Fetal heart tones, 189
Fetal macrosomia, 144
Fetal malformations, 196
Fetal–maternal bleeding, 190, 204
Fetal maturity
  assessment of, 64
  transitional time of, 160
Fetal presentation, 60–61
Fetal skin sampling, 83
Fetal stimulation, 110–111
Fetal surveillance, 143
Fetal testing, nonreassuring, 164
Fetal tissue (muscle and liver) biopsy, 83
Fetal well-being
  assessment of, 62
    biophysical profile, 63–64
    contraction stress test, 62–63
    Doppler ultrasound of umbilical artery, 64
    nonstress test, 62
  evaluation of, 92
Fetomaternal bleeding, 153
Fetoscopy, 83
Fever, 302
Fibrocystic changes of the breast, 291
Fibroids, 402
Fibromas, 383, 424
Fibrosarcoma, 424
Filshie clip, 241
Fine-needle aspiration biopsy, 288
First- and second-trimester screening, combined, 61
First division (meiosis I), 73
First stage of labor, 87
First-trimester pregnancy loss, 174
First-trimester screening, 61, 80
  circulating cell-free fetal DNA, 81
  serum screening, 80
  ultrasound screening, 80–81
Flexion, 87
Fluid management and oral intake, 91–92
Fluid passing, 159
Fluorescence in situ hybridization (FISH), 76, 83
Fluoroquinolones, 215
5-Fluorouracil, 214
Folate deficiency, 202
Folic acid, 82, 202
Follicle-stimulating hormone (FSH), 321, 345
Follicular cyst, 416
Follicular maturation, 345
Forceps, 103
Fourth stage of labor, 87
Fracture risk assessment tool (FRAX), 19
Fragile X syndrome, 78, 350
Free T_4, 182
Frenulum, 36
Friedman curve, 87, 100
Functional ovarian cysts, 416
  corpus luteum cysts, 416–417
  follicular cyst, 416
  theca lutein cyst, 417
Functioning tumors, 424
Fundal height, 142
  measurement, 59–60, 60
Fundus, 37

Gail model, 292
Galactocele, 122
Galactorrhea, 4, 334
Gallstones, 189
Gartner cysts, 40, 41f
Gartner duct cysts, 387
Gastroesophageal reflux, 49
Gastrointestinal disorders, 184–186
  nausea and vomiting of pregnancy (NVP), 184–186
    diagnosis, 185–186
    symptoms, 184–185
    treatment, 186
Gastrointestinal system, 48
  anatomic changes, 48
  diagnostic tests, 49
  functional changes, 48–49
  physical findings, 49
  symptoms, 49

Gemcitabine hydrochloride, 372t
General anesthesia, 92
Genes, definition and function, 72–73
Gene therapy, 373
Genetic code, 72
Genetic disorders, prenatal diagnosis of, 82
  carrier testing, 82
  fetal diagnostic procedures, 82
    amniocentesis, 83
    chorionic villus sampling, 83
    comparative genomic hybridization (CGH), 83
    FISH, 83
    karyotype, 83
    percutaneous umbilical blood sampling, 83
  genetic counseling, 83–84
Genetic disorders, risk factors for, 78
Genetic predisposition, 5
Genetics, basic concepts in, 72
  chromosome number, abnormalities in, 74
  chromosome replication and cell division, 73
    meiosis, 73–74
    mitosis, 73
  chromosome structure, abnormalities in, 76
    deletions, 76
    insertions, 76
    inversions, 76
    translocations, 76
  patterns of inheritance, 77
    autosomal dominant, 77
    autosomal recessive, 77
    mitochondrial inheritance, 78
    multifactorial inheritance, 78
    X-linked inheritance, 77–78
Genetics in gynecology, 84
  breast and ovarian cancer, 84
Genetic testing, 359
Genital ducts, 29
  development of, 32–33
Genital herpes, 256–257
Genital ridges, 30
Genital tract biopsy, 297
  cervical biopsy, 298
  endometrial biopsy (EMB), 298
  vaginal biopsy, 298
  vulvar biopsy, 297–298
Genital tubercle, 33
Genital ulcers, diseases characterized by, 251t
Genital warts, 15, 389
Genitopelvic pain/penetration disorder, 307t
Genotype testing, 205
Germ cells, 73
Germ cell tumors, 417, 418, 423–424
Gestational age, 160, 165
  initial assessment of, 59
Gestational diabetes, 177, 180
  infection, 181
  labor and delivery of patients with diabetes, 181
  laboratory screening, 180
  management, 180
    diet and glucose monitoring, 180
    medical therapy, 180–181
Gestational diabetes mellitus (GDM), 177
Gestational hypertension, 59, 191–192
Gestational trophoblastic neoplasia (GTN), 374
  classification of, 376b
  epidemiology, 374
  hydatidiform mole, 374
    clinical presentation, 374–376
    postevacuation management, 376
    treatment, 376
  malignant GTN, 377
    placental site tumors, 378
    treatment, 377
Gingival disease, 49
Glomerular filtration rate, 121
Glucose, 50
Glucose challenge test, 62
Glucose intolerance, 180
Glucose-rich urine, 181
Glucose tolerance test, 62, 181
Glucosuria of pregnancy, 178
Glycosylated hemoglobin levels (HgbA$_{1c}$), 178
GnRH-dependent sex hormone production, 328

GnRH-independent sex hormone production, 328
GnRH secretion, 322
Gonadal/genital ridges, 30
Gonadal stromal cell tumors, 424
Gonadotropin-releasing hormone (GnRH), 366
Gonadotropin-releasing hormone agonists, 283, 404
Gonads, 29, 55
  development of, 31f
Gonococcal ophthalmia, 215
Gonorrhea, 18, 215
Granuloma inguinale, 260
Granulosa cells, 322
Granulosa cell tumor, 424
Granulosa theca cell tumors, 420
Graves' disease, 182
Graves speculum, 10
Gravida, 5b
Gravidity, 4
Greater pelvis (false pelvis), 33
Group B streptococcus (GBS), 62, 209
  GBS prophylaxis, 160
Growth fraction, 369
Gubernaculum, 30
Gynecoid pelvis, 36
Gynecologic cancers, female risk of developing, 16t
Gynecologic history, 4–5
Gynecologic procedures, 295, 297
  cervical conization, 300
  colposcopy, 298
  cryotherapy, 298
  dilation and curettage (D&C), 299
  endometrial ablation, 299
  genital tract biopsy, 297
    cervical biopsy, 298
    endometrial biopsy (EMB), 298
    vaginal biopsy, 298
    vulvar biopsy, 297–298
  hysterectomy, 301–302
  hysteroscopy, 299
  imaging studies, 295
    breast imaging, 296–297
    computed axial tomography (CAT/CT), 296
    hysterosalpingography (HSG), 297
    magnetic resonance imaging (MRI), 296
    ultrasonography, 295–296
  intraoperative considerations, 302
  laser vaporization, 298–299
  minimally invasive and robotic surgery, 300–301
  postoperative considerations, 302–303
  pregnancy termination, 299–300
  preoperative considerations, 302
  urogynecology procedure, 302
Gynecology, 1

HAIR-AN syndrome, 341
Hand-off, 26
Handwashing, 26
Haploid, 73
Hb Barts disease, 202
Head, molding of, 94f
Headaches, 70, 219–221
Health evaluation, of women, 3
  medical history, 3
    chief complaint (CC), 4
    family history, 5
    gynecologic history, 4–5
    history of present illness (HPI), 4
    review of systems (ROS), 6
  pelvic examination, 9
    bimanual examination, 11–12
    inspection and examination of external genitalia, 9
    position of the patient and examiner, 9
    rectovaginal examination, 12–13
    speculum examination, 9–11
  physical examination, 6
    breast examination, 6–7, 8f
    vital signs, 6
Heartburn, 70–71
Heart disease, classification of
  in pregnancy, 198
Hegar sign, 58
HELLP syndrome, 188, 192, 197–198

Hematocrit (Hct), 201
Hematologic disease, 201–203
　anemia, 201–203
　　folate deficiency, 202
　　hemoglobinopathies, 202
　　hereditary hemolytic anemias, 202
　　iron-deficiency, 201–202
Hematologic system, 46
　diagnostic tests, 46
　symptoms and physical findings, 46
Hematoma, 123, 132
Hematometra, 176
Hematopoietic system, 121
Hematosalpinx, 170
Hemizygous, 77
Hemoglobin (Hb), 201
　oxygenation, 54
　hemoglobin A (HgbA), 54
　hemoglobin F (HgbF), 54
Hemoglobinopathies, 202, 203
Hemolysis, 204
Hemolytic disease, 204
Hemoperitoneum, 170
Hemorrhoids, 49, 71, 123
Heparin and low-molecular weight heparins, 68t
Hepatic disorders unique to pregnancy, 186
　acute fatty liver of pregnancy, 186–188
　intrahepatic cholestasis of pregnancy, 186
　preeclampsia and HELPP syndrome, 188
Hepatitis, 211–213
Hepatitis A virus (HAV), 212
Hepatitis B e antigen (HBeAg), 212
Hepatitis B immunoglobulin (HBIg), 212
Hepatitis B surface antigen (HBsAg), 212
Hepatitis C virus (HCV), 212–213
Hepatitis D virus (HDV), 213
Hepatitis E virus (HEV), 213
Herbal remedies, 67
Hereditary disease, 5
Hereditary epithelial ovarian cancer, 422
　endometrioid tumors, 423
　epithelial cell ovarian carcinomas, 423
Hereditary hemolytic anemias, 202
Hereditary nonpolyposis colorectal cancer type A (HNPCC type A), 84
Her2/neu, 293
Herpes simplex virus (HSV), 210–211
Heteroploidy, 74
Heterotopic pregnancy, 172
Heterozygous, 77
Hidradenitis suppurativa, 383
Hidradenoma, 384
High-density lipoprotein, 20
High-grade squamous intraepithelial lesions (HSILs), 391, 395
High-grade squamous intraepithelial lesions of the vulva (vulvar HSIL), 384–385
Hirsutism, 337
　evaluation of, 339f
Histologic grade, 412
History of present illness (HPI), 4
HNPCC type B, 84
Homozygous, 77
Hormonal contraceptives, 232
　mechanisms of action, 232–233
　patient evaluation for, 233–234
　ring and patch, 234
Hormone therapy (HT), 346, 351
　alternatives to, 351–352
　cautions in, 351
Horn, 40
Hospital stay, 121
Hot flushes and vasomotor instability, 347–350
Hulka clip, 241
Human chorionic gonadotropin (hCG), 58, 80, 374
Human immunodeficiency virus (HIV), 18, 213, 260
Human papillomavirus (HPV), 213, 214, 252, 257–258
　DNA testing, 394
　high-risk HPV types, 389
　immunization, 15
　vaccine, 214, 401b
Human placental lactogen (hPL), 178
Huntington disease, 73

Huntington gene, 73
Hydatidiform mole, 374
　clinical presentation, 374–376
　postevacuation management, 376
　treatment of, 376
Hydralazine, 197t
Hydramnios, 136
Hydrocele, 383
Hydrochlorothiazide, 197t
Hydronephrosis, 403
Hydropic placental villi, 374
Hydrops fetalis, 202, 205
Hydrotubae profluens, 425
Hydroureter, 403
21-Hydroxylase deficiency, 329, 342
11β-Hydroxylase deficiency, 343
5-Hydroxytryptamine (5-HT) 1A and 2C, 306
Hymen, 37
Hyperandrogenism, 340
Hyperarousal, 316
Hyperbilirubinemia, 115
Hypercoagulable state, 46
Hyperemesis gravidarum, 49, 70, 183, 184
Hypergonadotropic hypogonadism, 330
Hyperkeratosis, 381
Hyperpigmentation, 51
Hypertension, 20, 186
　chronic, 191
　　management of, 195
　　treatment of, 197
Hypertensive disorders, 191
　classification, 191–192
　　chronic hypertension, 191
　　eclampsia, 192
　　gestational hypertension, 191–192
　　HELLP syndrome, 192
　　preeclampsia, 192
　evaluation, 194–195
　management, 195
　　chronic hypertension, 195
　　preeclampsia, 195–196
　pathophysiology, 193
　　effects on organ systems and fetus, 193–194
　　potential causes of maternal vasopasm, 193–194
　in pregnancy, 192
Hyperthecosis, 341
Hyperthyroidism, 182
Hyperviscosity syndrome, 143
Hypogonadotropic hypogonadism, 330–331
Hypomenorrhea, 332
Hypothalamic–pituitary dysfunction, 332–333
Hypothalamic–pituitary–gonadal axis, 321
　GnRH secretion, 322
　ovarian steroid hormone secretion, 322
　pituitary gonadotropin secretion, 322
Hypothalamic thermoregulation center, 326
Hypothyroidism, 20, 183
Hypoxic-ischemic encephalopathy (HIE), 106
Hysterectomy, 172, 284, 301–302, 404, 407, 412
　and menopause, 350
Hysterosalpingography (HSG), 242, 297, 356–357, 358f
Hysteroscopy, 242, 243f, 299, 357–358, 404

Iatrogenic androgen excess, 343
　danazol, 343–344
　oral contraceptives, 344
Ifosfamide, 372t
IgG antibodies, 205
IgM isoform, 204
Ill newborn, initial care of, 115
　male circumcision, 118–119
　neonatal resuscitation, 115–117, 116f
　newborn screening, 119
　umbilical cord blood banking, 117–118
　umbilical cord blood gases, 117
Immature teratomas, 423
Immunization history, of patient, 4
Immunizations, 14–15, 122–123
Imperforate anus, 115
Imperforate hymen, 331
Implantable hormonal contraceptives, 227–229
Implantation bleeding, 173

Inaccurate/unknown dates, 163, 164t
Inclusion cysts, 383, 387
Incomplete abortion, 174
Increased second heart sound split with inspiration, 44
Independent assortment, 74
Indirect carrier testing, 82
Indirect Coombs test, 207
Induced abortion, 175–176
　complications, 175–176
Induction chemotherapy, 371
Infectious diseases, 209
　acquired immune deficiency syndrome (AIDS), 213–214
　chlamydia, 215–216
　cytomegalovirus, 216
　gonorrhea, 215
　Group B streptococcus (GBS), 209
　hepatitis, 211–213
　herpes simplex virus (HSV), 210–211
　human papillomavirus, 214
　parvovirus, 217–218
　rubella, 211
　syphilis, 215
　toxoplasmosis, 216–217
　varicella, 217
　Zika virus, 218
Infertility, 4, 353
　counseling, 362
　endometriosis and, 273
　etiology of, 353
　evaluation of, 353–358
　　uterine abnormalities, 356f
　male infertility, 358–359
　psychological stress associated with infertility, 353
　treatment, 360
　　assisted reproductive technologies, 361–362
　　intrauterine insemination, 360–361
　　ovarian stimulation, 360
　unexplained infertility, 359
Inflammatory bowel disease, 415
Influenza virus A, 199
Influenza virus B, 199
Informed consent, 25
Infundibulopelvic ligament, 37
Infundibulum, 39
Inheritance, patterns of, 77b
Injectable hormonal contraceptives, 231–232
Insertions, replication errors, 73
Inspection, 4
Insulin, 180
Insulinase, 178
Integrated screening, 82
Interferon, 214
Intermenstrual bleeding, 4
Intermittent auscultation, 106
Internal female reproductive organs, 38f
Internal iliac, 37
Internal os, 389
Internal reproductive organs, development of, 33f
Internal rotation, 87
Interphase, 73
Interspinous diameter, 36
Interstitial cystitis, 283
Interstitial deletion, 76
Interstitial implants, 373
Interstitial portion, 39
Interstitial pregnancy, 172
Intimate partner violence, 317
Intracavitary devices, 373
Intracavitary fluid collection, 169
Intracytoplasmic sperm injection (ICSI), 359
Intrahepatic cholestasis of pregnancy, 186
Intramural leiomyoma, 402
Intraoperative therapy, 373
Intrapartum, 164
Intrapartum care, 86
　labor, evaluation for, 86
　　abdominal examination, 87
　　fetal station, 88–89
　　vaginal examination, 87–88
　labor, mechanism of, 90
　labor, stages of, 89–90
　labor induction, 96

cervical ripening, 96
    membrane manipulation, 96
    oxytocin administration, 96
maternal changes before onset of labor, 86
normal labor and delivery, 90
    general management, 90–92
    management of labor, 92–96
    pain control, 92
    trial of labor after cesarean delivery, 97
Intrapartum fetal surveillance, 105
  ancillary tests, 110
    determination of fetal blood pH or lactate, 111
    fetal stimulation, 110–111
    pulse oximetry, 111
  pathophysiology, 106
    cerebral palsy, 106
    neonatal encephalopathy, 106
  persistently nonreassuring fetal heart rate pattern, 111
Intrapartum management, 138
  complications, 139
  delivery maneuvers, 139
Intrauterine contraception, 229–231
Intrauterine devices (IUDs), 225, 333
Intrauterine growth restriction, 140
  diagnosis, 142–143
  etiology of, 141–142
  neonatal management, 143–144
  pathophysiology, 141
  significance, 140–141
Intrauterine infection, 160
Intrauterine insemination (IUI), 359, 360–361
Intrauterine pressure catheters (IUPCs), 98
Intrauterine synechiae (Asherman syndrome), 173, 174
Invasive mole, 377
Invasive squamous carcinoma, 391
In vitro fertilization (IVF), 359, 361
Ionizing radiation, 67, 371
Iron-deficiency anemia, 201–202, 403
Irregular bleeding, 4
Irregular ovulation, 164t
Irritable bowel syndrome (IBS), 282–283
Irritant contact dermatitis, 382
Isotretinoin, 69t
Isthmus, 39

Jarisch-Herxheimer reaction, 215
Jaundice, 115
Justice, 22

Kallmann syndrome, 330
Karyotype, 73, 83
Karyotyping, 174
Kegel exercises, 121, 267
Kell antigen, 208
Kernicterus, 205
Kick counts, 62
Kidney, 54
Kleihauer-Betke test, 153, 190, 207
Klumpke paralysis, 164
Krukenberg tumor, 424

Labetalol, 197t
Labia majora, 36
Labia minora, 36
Labioscrotal swellings, 33
Labor, 98
  cardinal movements of, 91f
  mechanism of, 90
  median duration of the various phases and stages of, 89–90, 90t
Labor, evaluation for, 86
  fetal station, 88–89
  initial evaluation, 86
    abdominal examination, 87
    vaginal examination, 87–88
Laboratory values in each trimester of pregnancy, 47t
Labor induction, 96
  cervical ripening, 96
  membrane manipulation, 96
  oxytocin administration, 96

Lacerations of lower genital tract, 130–131
Lactational amenorrhea, 125
Lactation and breastfeeding, 125
  contraindications, 125
  lactational amenorrhea, 125
  nipple care, 125
  prolactin release, 125
Laminaria, 96, 96f
Lanugo, 111
Laparoscopic-assisted vaginal hysterectomy (LAVH), 301–302
Laparoscopy, 170, 300, 301f, 357–358
Large for gestational age (LGA), 144
Laryngoscopy, 166
Laser coagulation, 179
Laser vaporization, 298–299
Last menstrual period (LMP), 4, 163
Late deceleration, 108t
Late FHR decelerations, 109
Latency period, 160
Latent phase of labor, 87, 100
Late-onset infection, 209
Leg cramps, 71
Leiomyomata, 279, 402
  common types of, 403f
  in pregnancy, 405
Leiomyosarcoma, 402, 413
Leopold maneuvers, 60, 87, 104f, 145
Lesser pelvis (true pelvis), 33
Leukocytosis, 121
  of pregnancy, 189
Leukorrhea of pregnancy, 51
Levothyroxine, 183
Lichen planus, 381
Lichen sclerosus, 379–381
Lichen simplex chronicus, 381
Lie, 87
Lightening, 86
Light-headedness, 44
Light vaginal bleeding, 4
Linea alba, 51
Linea nigra, 51
Linear salpingostomy, 171
Lipid disorders, 20
Lipid metabolism, 50
Lipomas, 383
Liposomal doxorubicin, 372t
Lispro, 180
Lithium, 69t
Lithotomy position, 9, 9f
Liver, 54
Lobular carcinoma in situ (LCIS), 291
Local block, 92
Localized vulvodynia, 382–383
Lochia, 120, 120–121
Lochia alba, 120
Lochia rubra, 120
Lochia serosa, 120
Long-acting reversible contraception (LARC), 227
  implantable hormonal contraceptives, 227–229
  intrauterine contraception, 229–231
Low-density lipoprotein, 20
Lower genital tract, lacerations of, 130–131
Lower UTIs, 269
Low-grade squamous intraepithelial lesion (LSIL), 391, 395f, 396f
Low-grade squamous intraepithelial lesion of the vulva (vulvar LSIL), 384
Low-grade systolic ejection murmurs, 44
Low-lying placenta, 153
Low operative vaginal delivery, 103
Lumbar lordosis, 50
Lumpectomy (breast conservation therapy), 293
Luteal phase, 321
Luteal-phase cyst, 417
Luteal phase defect, 335
Luteal phase endometrial biopsy, 355
Luteinization, 324
Luteinizing hormone (LH) surge, 321
Lymphogranuloma venereum (LGV), 260
Lynch I syndrome, 84
Lynch II syndrome, 84
Lynch syndrome, 423

Macrosomia, 144–145, 163, 164, 178–179
  diagnosis, 145
  etiology, 144–145
  management, 145
Magnesium sulfate, 150t
Magnesium toxicity, 196
Magnetic resonance imaging (MRI), 17, 275, 288, 296
  -guided focused ultrasound surgery, 405
Maintenance chemotherapy, 371
Major congenital malformation, 173
Male circumcision, 118–119
Male infertility, 358
  causes of, 359
  semen analysis, 358–359
Malignant epithelial cell tumors, 421
Malignant epithelial serous tumors, 421
Malignant germ cell tumors, 421
Malignant mesodermal sarcomas, 424
Malignant mucinous epithelial tumor, 421
Malignant ovarian neoplasms, 420
  borderline ovarian tumors, 421
  cancer metastatic to the ovary, 424
  epithelial cell ovarian carcinoma, 421–422
  germ cell tumors, 423–424
  gonadal stromal cell tumors, 424
  hereditary epithelial ovarian cancer, 422–423
  histologic classification and staging, 421
  ovarian cancers, 424
  pathogenesis and diagnosis, 420–421
  rare germ cell tumors, 424
  risk factors and early symptoms, 420
Malignant potential, 417
Malignant stromal cell tumors, 421
Malignant thecoma, 424
Maloccurrence and malpractice, differentiating between, 26
Mammography, 287–288, 296–297
Marfan syndrome, 78, 198
Marginal abruption, 155
Marginal previa, 153
Marital rape, 312
Mask of pregnancy, 51
Massive hemorrhage, 172
Mastalgia, 289
Mastectomy, 293
Mastitis, 122
Mastodynia, 363
Maternal age, advanced, 78
Maternal and fetal complications, 180
Maternal cardiac arrhythmias, 199
Maternal changes before onset of labor, 86
Maternal factors, 99–100, 141–142, 144
Maternal glucose level, 181
Maternal hypoxia, 200
Maternal-infant bonding, 122
Maternal infection, 200
Maternal mortality, risk of, 97
Maternal physiology, 43
  cardiovascular system, 43–44
  hematologic system, 46
  respiratory system, 44–45
Maternal request, cesarean by, 97
Maternal stabilization, 190
Maternal systems, 50
  breasts, 51
  musculoskeletal, 50
  ophthalmic, 51
  reproductive tract, 51
  skin, 50–51
Maternal vasospasm, potential causes of, 193
Mayer-Rokitansky-Küster-Hauser syndrome, 331
McCune–Albright syndrome, 329
McRoberts maneuver, 105
Meconium, 111
  passage of, 164, 166
Meconium aspiration syndrome (MAS), 111, 163, 164
Medical abortion, 175
Medical history, 3
  chief complaint (CC), 4
  history of present illness (HPI), 4
  past history, 4
    family history, 5

Medical history (*Cont.*)
  gynecologic history, 4–5
  review of systems (ROS), 6
Medical liability, 25
  action, 25–26
  confidentiality, 25
  conflicts of interest, 25
  informed consent, 25
Medical maloccurrence, 26
Medical malpractice, 26
Medical management, 171
Medical records, 26
Meigs syndrome, 420
Meiosis, 73, 73–74
  stages of, 74*f*
Melanocyte-stimulating hormone, 51
Melanoma, 387
Membrane manipulation, 96
Memory changes, menopause and, 348
Menarche, 4, 327
Menopause, 2, 4, 345
  alternatives to hormone therapy, 351–352
  cautions in hormone therapy, 351
  effects of, 347*f*
  and female life expectancy, 346*f*
  hot flushes and vasomotor instability, 347
  management of, 350
    combined estrogen and progestin therapy, 350–351
    estrogen therapy, 350
  menstruation and, 345–346
  primary ovarian insufficiency, 350
    alkylating cancer chemotherapy, 350
    autoimmune disorders, 350
    genetic factors, 350
    hysterectomy, 350
    smoking, 350
  symptoms and signs of
    cardiovascular lipid changes, 349–350
    menstrual cycle alterations, 346–347
    mood changes and memory changes, 348
    osteoporosis, 348–349
    skin, hair, and nail changes, 348
    sleep disturbances, 347–348
    vaginal dryness and genital tract atrophy, 348
Menorrhagia, 402
Menstrual cycle alterations, menopause and, 346–347
Menstrual history, 4
Mentum anterior face presentation, 99
Mesonephric (wolffian) duct, 32
Mesovarium, 40
Messenger RNA (mRNA), 72
Menstrual diary, 364
Metabolic and cardiovascular disorders, 19
  diabetes mellitus, 19–20
  hypertension, 20
  lipid disorders, 20
  obesity, 20–21
  osteoporosis, 19
  thyroid disease, 20
Metabolic syndrome, 340–341
Metabolism, 50
Metaphase, 73
Methimazole, 182
Method or perfect use failure rate, 226
Methotrexate, 68*t*, 171, 172, 175, 372*t*, 377
Methyldopa, 197*t*
  and hydralazine, 68*t*
Methylergonovine maleate, 130
Methyl mercury, 67
15-Methyl prostaglandin, 130
Metronidazole, 68*t*, 248
Microhematuria, 188
Microsurgical epididymal sperm aspiration, 359
Midcycle spotting, 335
Midpelvis operative vaginal delivery, 103
Midposition position, 12
Midtrimester preterm premature rupture of membranes, 161
Mifepristone, 175
Migraine headaches, 219
Migrating gonads, route of
  in a female fetus, 32*f*
Minilaparotomy, 241–242

Minimally invasive and robotic surgery, 300–301
Miscarriage, 173–175
  etiology, 173
  spontaneous abortions, 173–174
    recurrent pregnancy loss, 174
    types of, 173–174
  treatment, 174–175
Misoprostol, 130, 175
Missed abortion, 174
Missense mutations, 72
Mitochondrial inheritance, 78
Mitosis, 73
  stages of, 73*f*
Mitotic inhibitors, 370
Mittelschmerz, 324, 354
Mixed endometrial stromal and smooth muscle tumors, 413
Modified biophysical profile, 165
Modified Ritgen maneuver, 94
Molar pregnancy, preoperative evaluation of, 376*b*
Molding, 93
Molimina, 363
Molluscum contagiosum, 261
Monoamnionic/monochorionic twins, 134
Monoamniotic twins, 137
Monochorionic-diamnotic pregnancies, 136
Monochorionic-monoamniotic twins, 139
Monozygotic twins, 134
Montevideo unit (MVU), 98
Mood changes, menopause and, 348
Morning sickness, 49, 70, 184
Motivational interviewing, 3
Mucinous cystadenocarcinoma, 421
Mucinous cystadenoma, 418, 419*f*
Müllerian agenesis, 40, 331
Müllerian (paramesonephric) abnormalities, 40
Multichannel urodynamic testing, 267
Multifactorial inheritance, 78
Multifetal gestation, 134
  antenatal management, 137–138
  diagnosis, 137
  intrapartum management, 138
    complications, 139
    delivery maneuvers, 139
  morbidity and mortality in, 136*t*
  natural history, 134–135
  risks of, 135
    death of one fetus, 137
    monoamniotic twins, 137
    twin-twin transfusion syndrome, 136–137
  ultrasonography, 138
Multifetal pregnancy reduction, 137
Multigravida, 5*b*
Multipara, 5*b*
Multiple birth rate, 134
Multiple sclerosis (MS), 220
Musculoskeletal, 50
Mutation, 72
Myolysis, 404
Myomas, 402
Myomectomy, 405
Myometrium, 37

Nabothian cysts, 391
Naegele rule, 59
Narcotic antagonists, 117
Nausea and vomiting of pregnancy (NVP), 49, 70, 184–186
  dietary and lifestyles measures for managing symptoms of, 186
  pharmacologic management of, 187
  selected differential diagnosis of, 185
Neisseria gonorrhoeae (Gonorrhea), 254–256
Neoadjuvant chemotherapy, 371
Neonatal encephalopathy, 106
Neonatal resuscitation, 115–117
  algorithm for, 116*f*
Neonatal thyroid dysfunction, 182
Nephrolithiasis, 188
Neural tube defects (NTDs), 202
  screening for, 81–82
Neurofibromatosis, 77, 78

Neurologic disorders, 192, 219
  Bell's palsy, 221
  carpal tunnel syndrome, 220
  epilepsy, 220
  headaches, 219–221
  multiple sclerosis (MS), 220
Neutral protamine hagedorn (NPH), 180
Nevi, 384
Newborn, immediate care of, 112
  initial care of the ill newborn, 115
    male circumcision, 118–119
    neonatal resuscitation, 115–117, 116*f*
    newborn screening, 119
    umbilical cord blood banking, 117–118
    umbilical cord blood gases, 117
  initial care of the well newborn, 112
    delivery room assessment of the newborn, 112–114
    jaundice, 115
    routine care, 114–115
Newborn resuscitation, airway management in, 117*f*
Newborn screening, 119
New York heart Association Functional Classification of Heart Disease, 198
Nifedipine, 197*t*
Night sweats, 347
Nipple care, 125
Nitrazine test, 159
Nitrofurantoin, 68*t*, 188
Nocturia, 266
Noncyclic mastalgia, 289
Non–fallopian tube ectopic pregnancy, 171–173
Nonfunctional ovarian neoplasms, 417
Noninflammatory vulvar pathology, 379
Nonmaleficence, 22
Nonreassuring fetal status, 105
Non-sense mutations, 72
Nonsteroidal anti-inflammatory drugs (NSAIDs), 69*t*, 150*t*, 219, 281, 366
Nonstress test (NST), 62, 63*f*, 165
Nontreponemal screening tests, 215
Norepinephrine, 305
Normal labor and delivery, 90, 98. See also Abnormal labor patterns
  fetal factors, 98–99
  general management, 90
    ambulation and position in labor and at delivery, 90–91
    fetal well-being, evaluation of, 92
    fluid management and oral intake, 91–92
  management of labor, 92
    first stage, 92–93
    second stage, 93–94
    third stage, 94–95
    fourth stage, 95–96
  maternal factors, 99–100
  pain control, 92
  uterine contractions, 98
19-Nortestosterones, 232
Nuchal region, 61
Nuchal translucency (NT), 61, 80
Nulligravida, 5*b*
Nullipara, 5*b*
Nutrition and weight gain, 65

Obesity, 20–21, 340
Obstetric conjugate, 33
Obstetric lacerations, classification of, 96*t*
Occipitoposterior position, 99
Occlusion of the fallopian tubes, 240
Ofloxacin, 216
Oligohydramnios, 160, 163, 164, 196
Oligomenorrhea, 332
Oligo-ovulation, 340, 356
Oocyte, 30
Oogonia, 30
Open glottis pushing, 93
Operative delivery, 102
  classification, 103
  forceps, 103
  indications and contraindications, 103
  vacuum extraction, 103–104
Ophthalmic manifestations, 51

Oral contraceptives (OCs), 275, 336, 344
Organ systems and fetus, effects on, 193–194
Osteopenia, 19
Osteoporosis, 19
  menopause and, 348–349
  nonhormonal regimens for, 349t
Outlet operative vaginal delivery, 103
Ovarian/adnexal masses, 189
Ovarian and adnexal disease, 415
  benign ovarian neoplasms, 417
    benign epithelial cell neoplasms, 417–418
    benign germ cell neoplasms, 418–420
    benign stromal cell neoplasms, 420
  differential diagnosis, 415
  evaluation of, 415–416
  fallopian tube disease, 424
    benign disease, 424
    carcinoma, 424–425
  functional ovarian cysts, 416
    corpus luteum cysts, 416–417
    follicular cyst, 416
    theca lutein cyst, 417
  malignant ovarian neoplasms, 420
    borderline ovarian tumors, 421
    cancer metastatic to the ovary, 424
    epithelial cell ovarian carcinoma, 421–422
    germ cell tumors, 423–424
    gonadal stromal cell tumors, 424
    hereditary epithelial ovarian cancer, 422–423
    histologic classification and staging, 421
    ovarian cancers, 424
    pathogenesis and diagnosis, 420–421
    rare germ cell tumors, 424
    risk factors and early symptoms, 420
  management of ovarian and fallopian tube cancers, 426
Ovarian cancer, 84, 420, 424
  diagnosis of, 421
  early warning signs of, 421b
  symptoms of, 420
Ovarian dysgenesis, 40
Ovarian failure, causes of, 333f
Ovarian fibroma, 420
Ovarian follicle development during the reproductive cycle, 323f
Ovarian function, return of, 121
Ovarian hyperstimulation syndrome, 360
Ovarian neoplasms, 341
  Sertoli-Leydig cell tumors, 342
  uncommon virilizing ovarian tumors, 342
Ovarian pregnancy, 171–172
Ovarian steroid hormone secretion, 322
Ovary, 40
  development of, 30–31
  serous cystadenoma of, 418f
Overflow incontinence, 267
Ovulation, 321
  long-term suppression of, 420
  induction, 360
Ovulation tests, 355
Oxygen consumption, 44
Oxytocin, 96, 160, 306

Paclitaxel, 372t, 426
Paget disease, 385–386
Painful bleeding, 152
Painless bleeding, 152, 153
Palmar erythema, 50
PALM-COEIN, 335
Palpation, 4
  of the pregnant uterus, 60
Papillary serous adenocarcinoma, 411
Papillomas, 291
Pap test, 17, 214, 387
  collection, 11f
Paracentric inversion, 76
Parallel veins, 37
Paramesonephric (Müllerian) duct, 32, 33f
Parametrium, 37
Paraovarian cysts, 424
Partial abruption, 155
Partial moles, 374
  features of, 375t
  hydropic villi of, 376f
Partial rupture, 156
Parvovirus, 217–218
Passive immunity, 55
Past history, 4
  family history, 5
  gynecologic history, 4–5
Paternal age, advanced, 78
Paternal antigen status, significance of, 205
Patient autonomy, 22
Patient capacity and patient competency, 24
Patient education, 124
Patient–physician partnership, 2–3, 3t
Patient safety, 26
Patient self-screening, 16
Patterns of inheritance, 77
  autosomal dominant, 77
  autosomal recessive, 77
  mitochondrial inheritance, 78
  multifactorial inheritance, 78
  X-linked inheritance, 77–78
Peak velocity, 206
Pederson speculum, 10
Pediculosis pubis (pubic lice), 261
Pedunculated leiomyoma, 402
Pelvic adhesions, 357
Pelvic diameters and estimating the obstetric conjugate, 35f
Pelvic examination, 9
  bimanual examination, 11–12
  external genitalia, inspection and examination of, 9
  lithotomy position during, 9f
  rectovaginal examination, 12–13
  speculum examination, 9–11
Pelvic inflammatory disease (PID), 4, 255, 279, 282
Pelvic inlet, 87
Pelvic muscle training, 267
Pelvic organ prolapse, 262
Pelvic Organ Prolapse Quantification (POP-Q), 263
Pelvic outlet, 87
Pelvic pressure, 403
Pelvic relaxation classified by stage, 265f
Pelvic support defects, 262–264, 263f
  differential diagnosis, 264
  evaluation of, 264
  treatment of, 264–266
Pelvic surgery, 39
Pelvimetry, 33
Pelvis, 33
  positions of the uterus within, 39f
  size of, 33
Penetrance, 77
Pentosan polysulfate sodium, 284
Percutaneous epididymal sperm aspiration, 359
Percutaneous umbilical blood sampling (PUBS), 82, 83, 142, 206
Pericentric inversion, 76
Perihepatitis (Fitz-Hugh-Curtis syndrome), 255
Perimenopause, 4, 345
Perinatal depression, 125–126
  risk factors for, 126b, 221
  validated screening tools for, 221t
Perinatal morbidity, 153
Perinatal mortality, 153
Perineum, 36
  care of, 123
Peripartum cardiomyopathy, 198–199
Persistent GTN, 377
Persistently nonreassuring fetal heart rate pattern, 111
Persistent/malignant disease, 374
Pertinent negatives, 4
Pessaries, 264–265, 266f
  placement of, 138
Petechiae, 152
Pfannenstiel, 301
"Phasic" formulations, 232
Phenytoin, 68t
Physical abuse, 317
Physical examination, 6
  breast examination, 6–7, 8f
  vital signs, 6
Physiology
  endocrine system, 49
  adrenal function, 50
  thyroid function, 49–50
  gastrointestinal system, 48
    anatomic changes, 48
    diagnostic tests, 49
    functional changes, 48–49
    physical findings, 49
    symptoms, 49
  maternal systems, 50
    breasts, 51
    musculoskeletal, 50
    ophthalmic, 51
    reproductive tract, 51
    skin, 50–51
  metabolism, 50
    carbohydrate metabolism, 50
    lipid metabolism, 50
    protein metabolism, 50
  renal system
    anatomic changes, 48
    diagnostic tests, 48
    functional changes, 48
    physical findings, 48
    symptoms, 48
Pica, 49, 65
Pituitary gonadotropin secretion, 322
Placenta, 51, 141
Placenta accreta, 131, 154, 155
Placenta increta, 131, 154, 155
Placental abruption, 152, 155–156
  characteristics of, 155t
  complete abruption, 155
  complications, 156
  diagnosis and management, 155–156
  low-lying placenta, 153
  marginal abruption, 155
  partial abruption, 155
  risk factors, 155
Placental site tumors, 378
Placental sulfatase deficiency, 164t
Placenta percreta, 131, 154, 155
Placenta previa, 152, 153–155
  characteristics of, 155t
  complete, 153
  complications, 154–155
  diagnosis, etiology, and risk factors, 153–154
  management, 154
  partial, 153
  and placental abruption, characteristics of, 155
  transvaginal sonogram of, 154
Plaintiff(s), 26
Plasma iodide levels, 182
Platypelloid pelvis, 36
Podophyllin, 214
Polycystic ovary syndrome (PCOS), 334, 340, 356
  HAIR-AN syndrome, 341
  hyperthecosis, 341
  metabolic syndrome, 340–341
  obesity, 340
  treatment, 341
Polyhydramnios, 179
Polymastia, 285
Polymerase chain reaction (PCR) testing, 210
Polythelia, 285
Pomeroy tubal ligation, 241, 242f
Position of patient and examiner, 9
Postabortal syndrome, 175–176
Postcoital bleeding, 4
Postdates, 163
Posterior pelvic cul-de-sac, 37
Postmenopausal bleeding, 411
  causes of, 412t
Postpartum blues, 222
Postpartum care, 120
  immediate postpartum period, management of, 121
    ambulation, 122
    analgesia, 122
    bowel and bladder function, 123
    breast care, 122, 123t
    care of the perineum, 123
    contraception, 123–124
    hospital stay, 121
    immunizations, 122–123

Postpartum care (*Cont.*)
　　lactation and breastfeeding, 125
　　maternal–infant bonding, 122
　　patient education, 124
　　postpartum complications, 122
　　sexual activity, 124
　　weight loss, 124
　perinatal depression, 125–126
　puerperium, physiology of, 120
　　abdominal wall, 121
　　cardiovascular system, 121
　　cervix and vagina, 121
　　hematopoietic system, 121
　　involution of the uterus, 120
　　lochia, 120–121
　　renal system, 121
　　return of ovarian function, 121
Postpartum complications, 122
Postpartum contraception, 238
Postpartum depression (PPD), 222–223
Postpartum hemorrhage (PPH), 127
　amniotic fluid embolism, 132
　coagulation defects, 132
　general management of patients, 128–129
　hematomas, 132
　lower genital tract, lacerations of, 130–131
　management of the patient with, 128*b*
　precautionary measures to prevent/minimize, 130*b*
　prevention, 133
　recognition and early detection, 127–128
　retained placenta, 131
　　abnormal placental separation, 131–132
　risk factors for, 127*b*
　uterine atony, 129
　　surgical management, 130
　　uterotonic agents, 130
　uterine inversion, 132
　uterine rupture, 132–133
Postpartum mood disorders, categories of, 222*t*
Postpartum psychosis, 223
Postpartum sterilization, 123–124
Postpartum thyroiditis, 182, 183
Post-term gestations, 163
Post-term pregnancy, 163–166
　diagnosis, 165
　effects, 163–164
　　dysmaturity syndrome, 164
　　macrosomia, 164
　　meconium aspiration syndrome (MAS), 164
　　oligohydramnios, 164
　factors associated with, 164*t*
　management, 165–166
　　fetal assessment, 165
　　labor induction, 165–166
Posttraumatic stress disorder, 316
Postvoid residual (PVR) volume, 267
Precocious sexual development, causes of, 329*b*
Preconception and antepartum care, 56
　antepartum patient education, 64
　　breastfeeding, 66
　　common symptoms, 70–71
　　employment, 64
　　exercise, 64–65
　　nutrition and weight gain, 65
　　sexual activity, 66
　　teratogens, 66–70
　　travel, 66
　initial prenatal visit, 58
　　gestational age, initial assessment of, 59
　　risk assessment, 58
　preconception counseling and care, 56–57
　pregnancy, diagnosis of, 57–58
　screening tests, 61–62
　subsequent antenatal visits, 59
　　blood pressure and urinalysis, 59
　　physical findings, 59–61
　　weight, 59
　ultrasound, 61
Preeclampsia, 179, 188, 192
　management of, 195
　risk factors for, 192
　with severe features, 196
Preexisting renal disease, 189
Pregestational diabetes mellitus, 177
Pregnancy

　and amenorrhea, 332
　-associated urinary stasis, 188
　causes of bleeding in second half of, 153*b*
　diagnosis of, 57–58
　fern test, 159
　immunology of, 55
　termination, 299–300
　test, 58
Pregnancy-associated plasma protein A (PAPP-A), 80
Prehypertension, 20
Premature rupture of membranes (PROM), 158–162
　clinical impact, 158
　diagnosis, 159–160
　　fern test, 159
　　nitrazine test, 159
　　ultrasonography, 159
　etiology and risk factors, 158–159
　evaluation and management, 160–162
Prematurity and multifetal gestations, 136*t*
Premenarchal age group, 415
Premenstrual dysphoric disorder (PMDD)
　daily record of severity of problems, 367*f*
　definition of, 363
　diagnostic criteria, 364, 365
　etiology, 363–364
　incidence, 363
　nonpharmacologic treatment, 365–366
　oophorectomy, 367
　pharmacologic treatment
　symptoms, 363
Premenstrual symptoms, 4
Premenstrual syndrome (PMS)
　daily record of severity of problems, 367*f*
　definition of, 363
　diagnostic criteria, 364
　differential diagnosis of, 366
　etiology, 363–364
　incidence, 363
　oophorectomy, 367
　pharmacologic treatment
　symptoms, 363
Prenatal screening, 79
　first-trimester screening, 80
　　circulating cell-free fetal DNA, 81
　　serum screening, 80
　　ultrasound screening, 80–81
　integrated screening, 82
　second-trimester screening, 81
　　neural tube defects (NTDs), screening for, 81–82
　　triple and quadruple screening tests, 81
　　ultrasound screening, 81
Prenatal visit, initial, 58
　gestational age, initial assessment of, 59
　risk assessment, 58
Presacral neurectomy, 281
Presence/absence of meconium, 93
Preterm birth, 147, 153
Preterm labor, 147, 148*f*
　causes, 147
　factors associated with, 148*b*
　factors improving outcomes, 147–148
　management of, 150
　　corticosteroids, 151
　　tocolytics, 150–151
　prediction of, 148
　　cervical changes, 149
　prevention, 149
　suspected preterm labor, 149
Preterm premature rupture of membranes (PPROM), 160
　midtrimester preterm premature rupture of membranes, 161–162
　24 weeks to 31 completed weeks, 161
　32 weeks to 33 completed weeks, 161
Preventive care, 14. *See also* Screening and preventive care
Primary amenorrhea, 332
Primary dysmenorrhea, 279
　pain and associated systemic symptoms in, 280*t*
Primary fallopian tube carcinoma, 424
Primary oocytes, 30
Primary ovarian insufficiency, 350
Primary postpartum hemorrhage, 122
Primary prevention, 14
Primary pulmonary hypertension, 198
Primary sex cords, 30
Primary syphilis, 259
Primigravida, 5*b*

Primipara, 5*b*
Primordial follicles, 30
Primordial germ cells, 30
Principle-based approach, 24
Principle-based ethics, 22–23
Prior pregnancy, abruption in, 155
Procidentia, 263
Progestational agents, 371
Progestational diabetes, 179–180
　antepartum fetal monitoring, 179
　management, 179
　maternal complications, 179
Progesterone, 138, 178, 285, 322, 354
Progesterone challenge test, 334
Progesterone therapy, 275
Progestin-only oral contraceptives, 232–233
Progestins, puberty and, 330
Progestin supplementation, 404
Progestin therapy, 350–351
Prolactin release, 125
Proliferative and secretory phases, 322
Prolonged deceleration, 108*t*
Prolonged latent phase, 101
Prometaphase, 73
Promoter sequences, 72
Prophase, 73
Prophylactic administration of tocolytics, 138
Prophylactic antibiotics, 302
Prostaglandin $F_{2\alpha}$ ($PGF_{2\alpha}$), 279
Prostaglandins, 323
Protein metabolism, 50
Proteinuria, 179, 186
Protraction disorders, 100
Pruritus, 49
Psammoma bodies, 421
Pseudoephedrine, 69*t*
Pseudogestational sac, 169, 170
Pseudomyxomatous peritonei, 422
Psoriasis, 381–382
Psychiatric disorders, 221
　anxiety disorders, 223
　bipolar disorders, 223
　depression and anxiety, 221–222
　postpartum depression, 222–223
　postpartum psychosis, 223
　schizophrenia, 223
Psyllium hydrophilic mucilloid, 71
Ptotic kidney, 415
Ptyalism, 49
Pubarche, 327
Puberty, 327
　abnormalities of pubertal development, 327
　　delayed puberty, 329–331
　　precocious puberty, 328–329
　ethnicity and onset of, 328*t*
Pudendal block, 92, 93*f*
Puerperium, physiology of, 120
　abdominal wall, 121
　cardiovascular system, 121
　cervix and vagina, 121
　hematopoietic system, 121
　lochia, 120–121
　ovarian function, return of, 121
　renal system, 121
　uterus, involution of, 120
Pulsatile GnRH, 330
Pulse oximetry, 111
Punch biopsies, 379
Pushing, 93
Pyelonephritis, 181, 188

Q-tip test, 264
Quadruple screen, 81
Quickening, 58
Quinolones, 68*t*

Radial scar, 291
Radiation absorbed dose (rad), 373
Radiation-induced breast cancer, 292
Radiation therapy, 426
Raloxifen, 289
Rape trauma syndrome, 316
Rapid HIV testing, 214

Rare germ cell tumors, 424
Recommended daily allowances (RDAs), 65
Rectosigmoid carcinoma, 415
Rectovaginal examination, 12–13, 13f
Rectovaginal fistula, 267
Rectum, 37
Recurrent pregnancy loss, 174
Recurrent second-trimester abortions, 173
Redistribution in the cell cycle, 373
Reduction division, 73
Renal and ureteral calculi, 415
Renal system, 121
　anatomic changes, 48
　diagnostic tests, 48
　functional changes, 48
　physical findings, 48
　symptoms, 48
Reoxygenation, 371, 373
Replication error, 72–73
Repopulation, 371
Reproductive-age group, 353, 415
Reproductive and sexual coercion, 317
Reproductive cycles, 321
　clinical manifestations of hormonal changes, 324
　　breasts, 326
　　endocervix, 325
　　endometrium, 324
　　hypothalamic thermoregulation center, 326
　　vagina, 326
　hypothalamic–pituitary–gonadal axis, 321
　　GnRH secretion, 322
　　ovarian steroid hormone secretion, 322
　　pituitary gonadotropin secretion, 322
　luteal phase, 324
　menstruation and the follicular phase, 321, 323
　ovarian follicle development during, 323f
　ovulation, 324
Reproductive tract, 51
Respiratory/cardiac illness, 45
Respiratory disorders, 199
　asthma, 199
　influenza, 200
Respiratory distress syndrome (RDS), 64
Respiratory system, 44
　anatomic changes, 44
　diagnostic tests, 46
　functional changes, 44–45
　physical findings, 45
　symptoms, 45
Restriction fragment length polymorphisms, 82
Resuscitation, 115
Retained placenta, 131
　abnormal placental separation, 131–132
Retroflexed position, 12
Retrograde menstruation, 271
Retropubic colposuspension and sling procedures, 268
Retroverted position, 12
Review of systems (ROS), 6
Rh (CDE) system, 204
Rh D-negative, 204
Rh D-positive, 204
Rheumatic heart disease, 198
Rh immunoglobulin, 171
Ribonucleic acid (RNA), 72
Ring chromosome, 76
Ritgen maneuver, modified
　vaginal delivery assisted by, 95f
Robertsonian translocation, 76
Rome III criteria, 282
Round ligament pain, 71
Rubella, 122, 211
Rugation, 338
Rupture of membranes (ROM), 86

Sacrospinous ligament, 37
Sacrum, 33
Safe medication practices, 26
Salpingectomy, 171
Salpingitis, 167
Salpingitis isthmica nodosa, 167
Sarcoma botryoides, 388
Sarcomas, 406
Schizophrenia, 223
Sclerosing adenosis, 291

Screening and preventive care, 14
　immunizations, 14–15
　metabolic and cardiovascular disorders, 19
　　diabetes mellitus, 19–20
　　hypertension, 20
　　lipid disorders, 20
　　obesity, 20–21
　　osteoporosis, 19
　　thyroid disease, 20
　secondary prevention, 15
　　breast cancer, 16–17
　　cervical cancer, 17
　　characteristics of screening tests, 16
　　colorectal carcinoma, 17
　sexually transmitted diseases, 18
　　chlamydia infection, 18
　　gonorrhea infection, 18
　　human immunodeficiency virus, 18
　　syphilis, 18–19
Screening mammography, 16
Screening tests, 14, 61–62, 79
　characteristics of, 16
　criteria for, 16t
Sebaceous cysts, 383
Seborrheic dermatitis, 382
Sebum production, 51
Secondary dysmenorrhea, 279, 403
　causes of, 280b
Secondary postpartum hemorrhage, 122
Secondary prevention, 14
Secondary syphilis, 259
Second meiotic division (meiosis II), 74
Second-stage arrest, 102
Second-stage disorders, 102
Second stage of labor, 87
Second-trimester pregnancy loss, 174
Second-trimester screening, 61, 81
　neural tube defects (NTDs), screening for, 81–82
　triple and quadruple screening tests, 81
　ultrasound screening, 81
Segmental resection, 171
Selective estrogen receptor modulators (SERMs), 289, 349, 371
Selective serotonin reuptake inhibitors (SSRIs), 68t, 222, 366
Semen analysis, 358–359
Seminiferous (or testis) cords, 30
Septic abortion, 175
Septic shock, 188
Sequential blockade, 371
Serosa, 37
Serotonin, 306
Serotoninergic dysregulation
　and premenstrual dysphoric disorder, 364
Serous cystadenoma, 417
Sertoli-Leydig cell tumors, 342, 420, 424
Serum creatinine, 189
Serum human chorionic gonadotropin levels, 169
Serum pregnancy tests, 58
Serum progesterone, 169, 355
Serum screening, 80
Settlement, 26
Sex chromosome abnormalities, 74
Sex hormone–binding globulin (SHBG), 338
Sexual abuse, 317
Sexual activity, 66, 124
Sexual assault, 312
　child sexual assault, 316–317
　definitions and types of, 312–313
　and domestic violence. See Domestic violence
　emotional issues, 316
　management, 313–316
　physician's role in evaluation of, 313b
　posttraumatic stress disorder, 316
　posttreatment evaluation, 314
Sexual disorders
　biologic and psychological risk factors for, 309b
　medical risk factors for, 309b
Sexual dysfunction, 307
　categories of, 307t
　depression and, 307
　screening for, 308–309

　factors affecting, 307
　　depression, 307
　　medical conditions, 307–308
　　medications, 307, 308b
　　psychological factors, 308
　human sexual response, 304
　　intimacy-based model, 305
　　physiology of female sexual response, 305–306
　　traditional model, 304–305
　management, 308
　　additional history, 309
　　establishing a diagnosis, 310
　　risk factors, 309–310
　　screening for sexual dysfunction, 308–309
　negative and positive feedback loops of sexual function, 305f
　sexual dysfunction, 307
　sexual identity, 304
　treatment, 310–311
Sexually transmitted diseases (STDs), 18
　chlamydia infection, 18
　gonorrhea infection, 18
　human immunodeficiency virus, 18
　risk factors for, 18t
　screening recommendations for, 210t
　syphilis, 18–19
Sexually transmitted infections (STIs), 250, 260–261
　Chlamydia trachomatis (Chlamydia), 252–254
　general diagnostic principles, 250
　genital herpes, 256–257
　HIV and AIDS, 260–261
　human papillomavirus (HPV), 257–258
　Neisseria gonorrhoeae (Gonorrhea), 254–256
　prevention, 252
　screening, 250–252
　syphilis, 258–260
Shoulder dystocia, 103, 105, 106f, 163, 164, 180
Shoulders, delivery of anterior and posterior shoulders, 96f
Sickle cell anemia, 203
Sickle cell disorders, 202, 203
Sickle cell trait, 203
Sigmoid diverticular disease, 415
Signet-ring cell type, 424
Simple fibroadenomas, 291
Simple hyperplasia, 406
Single-channel urodynamic testing, 267
Single-gene (Mendelian) disorders, 77
Sinusoidal pattern, 108t
Skin, 50–51
Skin nevi, 51
Sleep disturbances, menopause and, 347–348
Small for gestational age (SGA), 140
Smoking, and menopause, 350
Sniffing position, 117
Sojourn time interval, 16
Somatic cells, 73
Spastic quadriplegia, 106
Spectral karyotyping (SKY), 83
Speculum examination, 9–11
Speculum insertion, 10, 11f
Spermatogenesis, 359
Spermicides, 236
Spider angiomata, 50
Spinal anesthesia, 92
Spironolactone derivative, 232
Spongiotic pattern, 382
Spontaneous abortion, 173
　recurrent pregnancy loss, 174
　　first-trimester pregnancy loss, 174
　　second-trimester pregnancy loss, 174
　and stillbirth, 178
　types of, 173–174
Squamocolumnar junction (SCJ), 37, 389
Squamous cell cancer (SCC) of the vulva, 381
SRY (sex-determining region on Y), 29
Step-care therapeutic approach, 200
Sterilization, 239
　decision for, 244
　of men, 239–240
　as a method of contraception, 239
　reversal of tubal ligation, 243–244
　of women, 240
　　hysteroscopy, 242
　　laparoscopy, 240–241
　　minilaparotomy, 241–242

Sterilization (*Cont.*)
    noncontraceptive benefits, 243
    side effects and complications, 242–243
Stress urinary incontinence, 48, 266–267
Striae gravidarum, 50, 121
Stromal cell tumors, 417, 420
Sublethal injury, repair of, 371
Submucous leiomyoma, 402, 403
Subserosal leiomyoma, 402
Substance abuse, 70
Subtotal hysterectomy, 301
Succenturiate, 131
Successful conception, steps in, 354*f*
Sulfonamides, 68*t*
Supine exercises, 64
Supine hypotensive syndrome, 90
Suppressive therapy, 257
Supracervical hysterectomy, 301
Surgical conditions, 189–190
    adnexal masses in pregnancy, 189–190
    appendicitis in pregnancy, 189
    cholelithiasis in pregnancy, 189
    pregnant patients, considerations for, 189
Surgical errors, reducing the likelihood of, 26
Surgical management, 171
Surrogate decision maker, 24
Survival, 158
Sweeping the membranes, 165
Symphysis–fundal height, measurement of, 145
Symphysis pubis, 33
Syncope, 44
Synergistic, 371
Synthetic progesterones, 409
Syphilis, 18–19, 215, 258–260
Systemic corticosteroids, 200
Systolic blood pressure, 195

Tachycardia, 107, 128
Tachypnea, 128
"Talk before you touch," 8
Tamoxifen, 289, 409
Teletherapy, 373
Telogen (resting) phase, 51
Telophase, 73
Tension headaches, 219
Teratogenicity, 68*t*
    fear of, 186
Teratogens, 66
    alcohol, 69–70
    herbal remedies, 67–69
    ionizing radiation, 67
    medications, 67
    methyl mercury, 67
    substance abuse, 70
    tobacco use, 70
Terminal deletion, 76
Term premature rupture of membranes, 158, 160
Testis-determining factor, 29
Test of cure, 254
Testosterone, 337
    and anabolic steroids, 68*t*
Testosterone receptors, 338
Tetanus–diphtheria–acellular pertussis vaccine, 122
Tetracyclines, 68*t*, 215
Thalassemias, 202, 203
Theca lutein cysts, 375, 376, 417
Thecomas, 424
Thelarche, 327
Third spacing, 193
Third stage of labor, 87
Third-trimester bleeding, 152
    history and physical examination, 152–153
    placental abruption, 155
        complications, 156
        diagnosis and management, 155–156
        risk factors, 155
    placenta previa, 153
        complications, 154–155
        diagnosis, etiology, and risk factors, 153–154
        management, 154
    uterine rupture, 156

vasa previa, 156
    tests, 156
Third-trimester screening, 62
Thorax, maternal, 44
Threatened abortion, 173
Thromboembolism, 46
Thrombophilias, 173
Thyroid-binding globulin (TBG), 182
Thyroid disease, 20, 182
    laboratory screening, 182
    management of existing thyroid disease in pregnancy, 182–183
    management of thyroid disease diagnosed during and after pregnancy, 183
        biochemical hyperthyroidism, 183
        postpartum thyroiditis, 183
    pathophysiology, 182
Thyroid disorders, 380
Thyroid function, 49–50
Thyroid gland, 54
Thyroid-stimulating hormone (TSH), 182
Thyroid storm, 182
    symptoms of, 183*b*
Thyrotoxicosis, 182
Tobacco use, 70
Tocodynamometer, 98, 99*f*, 149
Tocolytics, 148, 150
    contraindications, 151
Tocometry, 190
Topoisomerase inhibitors, 370
Topotecan, 372*t*
Total hysterectomy, 301
Total thyroxine (T4), 182
Toxoplasmosis, 216–217
Transabdominal ultrasonography, 33
Transcription, 72
Transdermal contraceptive patch, 234
Transformation zone (TZ), 37, 391
Transitional care, 114–115
Translation, 72
Transvaginal sonogram, 154
Transvaginal ultrasound, 59, 149, 153–154, 169, 408
    for cervical length screening, 138
Transverse diameter, 36
Trauma, in pregnancy, 190
    fetal–maternal hemorrhage, 190
    management, 190
Travel, 66
Treponemal-specific tests, 215
Treponema pallidum, 215, 259
Tretinoin, 69*t*
Trials of labor after cesarean (TOLAC), 97
Trichomoniasis, 245, 248
Triglycerides, 20
Triple and quadruple screening tests, 81
Triple screen, 81
Trisomy 13, 61
Trisomy 16, 74
Trisomy 18 (Edward syndrome), 61, 74
Trisomy 21 (Down syndrome), 74
Trisomy 13 (Patau syndrome), 74
True labor, 86
T-score, 19
Tubal abortion, 167
Tubal ectopic pregnancy, 167
    clinical findings, 168
    diagnostic procedures, 169
        culdocentesis, 170
        endometrial curettage, 170
        laparoscopy, 170
        serum human chorionic gonadotropin levels, 169
        serum progesterone level, 169–170
        transvaginal ultrasonography, 169
    differential diagnosis, 168–169
    management, 170–171
    pathophysiology and risk factors, 167
    symptoms, 167–168
Tubal ligation, 167
Tubal rupture, 167
Tubal sterilization, 167
Tubo-ovarian abscesses (TOAs), 255
Tumor debulking, 426

Tumors of low malignant potential, 421
Tumor vaccines, 373
Tunica albuginea, 30
Turner syndrome, 61
Turtle sign, 105
Twin pregnancy, 137
    chorionicity in, 135*f*
    delivery of second twin, 139*f*
Twin–twin transfusion syndrome (TTTS), 136–138
Typical use failure rate, 226

Ultrasonography, 61, 138, 159, 275, 288, 295–296
    dating, 165
    of umbilical artery blood flow velocity, 62
Ultrasound, 59, 61, 80–81, 149, 155, 206
Umbilical artery blood gases, 117
Umbilical artery Doppler velocimetry, 144*f*
Umbilical cord blood banking, 117–118
Umbilical cord blood gases, 117
Umbilical cord care, 114
Umbilical cord compression, 164
Unbalanced translocation, 76
Uncomplicated urinary tract infection, 188
Uncorrected tetralogy of Fallot, 198
Undifferentiated endometrial sarcoma, 413
Upper urinary tract infection, 269
Ureter and uterine artery, relative locations of, 39*f*
Ureterovaginal fistula, 267
Urethritis, 250, 254
    diseases characterized by, 253*t*
Urethrocele, 262
Urethrovaginal fistula, 267
Urinary calculi, 188
Urinary frequency, 48
Urinary incontinence, 264, 266
    characteristics of, 266*t*
    evaluation, 267
    treatment, 267–269
    types, 266–267
Urinary tract disorders, 188–189
    asymptomatic bacteriuria and uncomplicated urinary tract infection, 188
    nephrolithiasis and urinary calculi, 188
    preexisting renal disease, 189
    pyelonephritis, 188
        treatment, 188
Urinary tract infections (UTIs), 48, 188, 269, 415
    clinical history, 269
    laboratory evaluation, 269–270
    risk factors for, 269*t*
    treatment, 270
Urine culture, 188
Urine LH kits, 355
Urodynamic testing, 267
Urogenital diaphragm, 36, 37*f*
Urogenital folds, 33
Urogenital ridges, 29
Urogenital system, early development of, 30*f*
Urogynecology procedure, 302
Urorectal septum, 33
Uterine and vaginal anomalies, 40*f*
Uterine artery, 37
Uterine atony, 128, 129
    management of, 129–130
Uterine contractions, 86, 98
Uterine corpus, cancer of, 406
    endometrial cancer, 410
        diagnosis, 411
        hormone therapy after treatment for endometrial carcinoma, 413
        pathogenesis and risk factors, 411
        prognostic factors, 411–412
        recurrent endometrial carcinoma, 413
        treatment, 412–413
    endometrial hyperplasia, 406
        atypical hyperplasia and endometrioid intraepithelial neoplasia, 406
        evaluation, 407–409
        hyperplasia without atypia, 406
        management, 409
        pathophysiology and risk factors, 406–407

patient history, 407
risk factors for, 408t
World Health Organization's classification of, 407t
endometrial polyps, 409–410
uterine sarcoma, 413–414, 413f
Uterine dehiscence, 132, 156
Uterine inversion, 132
Uterine leiomyoma and neoplasia, 173, 402
diagnosis, 403–404
effect of leiomyomata in pregnancy, 405
symptoms, 402–403
treatment, 404
Uterine malignancy, 402
Uterine palpation, 60
Uterine rupture, 132–133, 156
Uterine sarcoma, 413–414, 413f
Uterine surgery, 154
Uterine tubes, 39
Uteroplacental insufficiency, 106, 141, 164
Uteroplacental unit, 106
Uterosacral ligament, 37
Uterus, 37
bimanual examination of, 12
involution of, 120
and pelvic support, 37–39
positions of, within the pelvis, 39f
Uterus and adnexa, bimanual examination of, 12f
Uterus didelphys, 40

Vaccinations for women, 15t
Vacuum extraction, 103–104
Vacuum extractor, 104f
Vagina, 36–37
Vaginal artery, 37
Vaginal biopsy, 298
Vaginal birth, 33
Vaginal birth after cesarean (VBAC), 97
Vaginal bleeding, 152, 155, 167
Vaginal breech delivery, 104–105
Vaginal cancer, 388
Vaginal delivery, 111, 164
assisted by modified Ritgen maneuver, 95f
low operative, 103
midpelvis operative, 103
outlet operative, 103
Vaginal discharge, 71
Vaginal dryness and genital tract atrophy, menopause and, 348
Vaginal examination, 87–88
Vaginal hemorrhage, 153
Vaginal hysterectomy, 301

Vaginal intraepithelial neoplasia (VAIN), 387–388
Vaginal plate, 32
Vaginal speculum, 10f
Vaginitis, 4
Valacyclovir, 257
Valproic acid and carbamazepine, 68t
Valsalva maneuver, 93
Vanishing twin syndrome, 137
Variable deceleration, 108t
Variable expressivity, 77
Variable FHR decelerations, 109
Varicella, 217
Varicose veins and hemorrhoids, 71
Vasa previa, 156
Vascular and lymphatic dissemination, 271
Vascular spiders, 50
Vasectomy, 240f
Vaso-occlusive crisis, 202, 203
Velamentous insertion, 156
Vertex presentation, various positions in, 88f
Vesicouterine, 267
Vesicovaginal fistula, 267, 267f
Vibroacoustic stimulation, 109
Vincristine, 372t, 377
Virilization, 337
Virtue-based approach, 24
Vital signs, 6
Vitamin A, 69t
Vitamin K, 54
Vitamin K1 oxide, 115
Von Willebrand disease, 152
Vulva, 36
biopsy, 297–298
and perineum, 36
Vulvar and vaginal disease and neoplasia, 379
benign vulvar disease, 379
dermatitis, 382
lichen planus, 381
lichen sclerosus, 379–381
lichen simplex chronicus, 381
localized vulvodynia, 382–383
psoriasis, 381–382
vulvar lesions, 383–384
Paget disease, 385–386
vaginal disease, 387
benign vaginal masses, 387
vaginal cancer, 388
vaginal intraepithelial neoplasia (VAIN), 387–388
vulvar cancer, 386–387
vulvar intraepithelial neoplasia (VIN), 384
high-grade squamous intraepithelial lesions of the vulva (vul-var HSIL), 384–385

low-grade squamous intraepithelial lesion of the vulva (vulvar LSIL), 384
Vulvar dermatitis, 382
Vulvar dermatoses, clinical characteristics of, 383t
Vulvar intraepithelial lesions, grading systems for, 384t
Vulvovaginal ecosystem, normal, 245–246
Vulvovaginitis, 245
atrophic vaginitis, 249
bacterial vaginosis (BV), 246–247
clue cells, 247f
diagnosis and treatment, 246t
trichomonal vulvovaginitis, 248–249
vulvovaginal candidiasis, 247–248

Waning fertility, 5
Warfarin, 68t
Warming, 114
Weak D antigen, 204
Weight, maternal, 59
Weight loss, 124
Well newborn, initial care of, 112
delivery room assessment of the newborn, 112
Apgar scoring system, 112–114, 114t
Ballard scoring system, 112
jaundice, 115
routine care, 114
practices to promote breastfeeding, 114
transitional care, 114–115
umbilical cord care, 114
vital signs, 114
warming, 114
Western blot test, 213
White's classification of diabetes, in pregnancy, 178
WHO Surgical Safety Checklist, 27f
Withdrawal bleed, 234
WNT4 gene, 29

X-linked inheritance, 77–78

Yuzpe method, 237

Zavanelli maneuver, 105
Zero station, 86
Zidovudine, 213
Zika virus, 218
Zona basalis, 131
Zona spongiosa, 131
Z-score, 19